R00007 26729

ANNALS OF THE NEW YORK ACADEMY OF SCIENCES

Volume 266

PATHOBIOLOGY OF INVERTEBRATE VECTORS OF DISEASE

Edited by Lee A. Bulla, Jr. and Thomas C. Cheng

D0095699

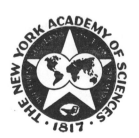

The New York Academy of Sciences
New York, New York
1975

Copyright, 1975, by The New York Academy of Sciences. All rights reserved. Except for brief quotations by reviewers, reproduction of this publication in whole or in part by any means whatever is strictly prohibited without written permission from the publisher.

Library of Congress Cataloging in Publication Data

Conference on Pathobiology of Invertebrate Vectors of Disease, New York, 1975.
Pathobiology of invertebrate vectors of disease.

(Annals of the New York Academy of Sciences; v. 266)
Sponsored by The New York Academy of Sciences.

1. Invertebrates as carriers of diseases—Congresses. 2. Invertebrates—Diseases—Congresses. I. Bulla, Lee A. II. Cheng, Thomas Clement. III. New York Academy of Sciences. IV. Title. V. Series: New York Academy of Sciences. Annals; v. 266. Q11.N5 vol. 266 [QL362] 592'.02

ISBN 0-89072-020-7   75-43621

PCP
Printed in the United States of America
ISBN 0-89072-020-7

ANNALS OF THE NEW YORK ACADEMY OF SCIENCES

VOLUME 266

November 28, 1975

PATHOBIOLOGY OF INVERTEBRATE VECTORS OF DISEASE *

Editors and Conference Chairmen
LEE A. BULLA, JR. AND THOMAS C. CHENG

Advisory Committee
GRANT ST. JULIAN, ANDREW SPIELMAN, J. WILLIAM
VINSON, AND JOHN A. WISE

CONTENTS

* This series of papers is the result of a conference entitled Pathobiology of
Invertebrate Vectors of Disease, held by The New York Academy of Sciences on
March 17, 18, and 19, 1975.

303369

Part V. Pathobiology of Noninsect Invertebrates

Part VI. Mollusk-Parasite Interactions

Financial support was received from:

- HOFFMANN-LA ROCHE INC.
- SANDOZ, INC.

INTRODUCTORY REMARKS

Lee A. Bulla, Jr.

Agricultural Research Service
U.S. Grain Marketing Research Center
Manhattan, Kansas 66502

Thomas C. Cheng

Institute for Pathobiology
Center for Health Sciences
Lehigh University
Bethlehem, Pennsylvania 18015

Pathobiology is the study of diseased organisms. It encompasses not only the study of pathologic conditions but also the biology of causative agents and response reactions. The Conference on Pathobiology of Invertebrate Vectors of Disease was organized to provide an interdisciplinary and comparative analysis of such factors as they concern invertebrates. Because of the diversity of problems related to invertebrate disease vectors, we tried to provide broad coverage that includes certain aspects of microbiology, parasitology, and invertebrate physiology, biochemistry, immunology, and development. At the same time, we felt an obligation to relate fundamental principles to practical problems. Consequently, we organized this Conference to cut across the boundaries of biomedicine, agriculture, and environmental sciences, and we selected participants according to this goal.

The collection of papers presented in this monograph is by no means definitive, but, hopefully, it does provide a broader view of the variety of research problems in invertebrate pathobiology and will stimulate new ideas for researchers who are working with invertebrates and for those investigators who are concerned with the implications of invertebrate vectors and causative agents in vertebrate diseases.

We are deeply appreciative of the following people who helped organize this Conference and this monograph: B. J. Bogitsh, G. St. Julian, A. Spielman, J. W. Vinson, R. F. Whitcomb, and J. A. Wise.

PATHOGENIC RICKETTSIAE AND THEIR ARTHROPODS: AN INTRODUCTION

J. William Vinson

Department of Microbiology
Harvard University School of Public Health
Boston, Massachusetts 02115

Rickettsiae or rickettsia-like microorganisms are found associated with a wide variety of arthropods. Only a few of them produce disease when introduced into human tissues. The rickettsiae pathogenic for man are divided into five groups on the basis of their biologic behavior and differences in the antigens that they synthesize. Recent studies [1, 2] on the molar percentages of guanine plus cytosine of the DNA of several species of rickettsiae tend to confirm the validity of this separation. Two members of the typhus group are pathogenic for man: *Rickettsia prowazeki,* transmitted by the human body louse, causes epidemic typhus; *R. mooseri (typhi),* transmitted by the oriental rat flea, causes murine or endemic typhus. A recent addition to this group is *R. canada,*[3] isolated from a tick and not yet clearly incriminated as an agent of human disease. Members of the spotted fever group, exemplified by *R. rickettsi,* are symbionts of several genera of ticks. The single exception is *R. akari,* which is carried by a mouse mite. Also in the genus *Rickettsia* is *R. tsutsugamushi,* the agent of scrub typhus. It is carried in several species of mites and is marked by antigenic diversity among strains.

Clearly separated from these three groups are *Rochalimaea quintana,* the agent of trench fever carried by the human body louse, and *Coxiella burneti,* the agent of Q fever, which, though found in ticks, is generally wafted to man as an aerosol from products of infected livestock.

The papers that follow consider various aspects of the intimate and frequently complex relationships between some rickettsial species and the arthropods that transmit them to man.

Wisseman *et al.* begin with an important aspect of what might be called the microepidemiology of epidemic typhus. They have demonstrated that antibody ingested by the body louse in a blood meal from a typhus-immune host is degraded into small fragments, presumably by proteolytic enzymes in the louse gut. The fragments were identified by immunologic techniques. Also destroyed was that portion of the antibody responsible for opsonization of typhus rickettsiae. Opsonization of rickettsiae renders them vulnerable to engulfment and destruction by professional phagocytes and constitutes the major immunologic defense against rickettsiae. This finding suggests that *R. prowazeki* in the feces of lice feeding on a person with specific antibodies would be capable of infecting the next person in the man-louse-man chain of infection.

Also concerned with epidemic typhus, Murray and Torrey demonstrate that *Pediculus humanus capitus,* the human head louse, can in the laboratory be readily infected with the agent of epidemic typhus and that infection is as fatal for them as it is for body or clothes lice. It consequently appears to be a mystery why head lice are not responsible for transmitting epidemic typhus under natural conditions. Head and body lice are closely related to each other. It appears likely that during the course of the evolutionary relationships of man and lice that head lice adapted themselves first to a parasitic existence on man and then later modified their behavior to live on clothes when *Homo sapiens* began to cover himself with skins and fibers. It is possible to "domesticate" wild head lice to laboratory conditions so that they deposit eggs on cloth and become accustomed to one meal a day. They can mate with body lice. *P.h. capitus* is easily transmitted from person to person, especially among children, as the current epidemics of head louse infestation demonstrate. The fact remains, however, that so far, head lice have not been implicated in the transmission of *R. prowazeki*. In Mexico, for example, epidemic typhus is confined to the cool regions of the altiplano, where both head and body lice are found, and is not reported from the tierra caliente, the hot country along the coasts of both the Pacific Ocean and the Gulf of Mexico, where only head lice exist.

Ito *et al.* report observations on the ultrastructure of *R. mooseri* and the oriental rat flea. Because very little information is available on the ultrastructure of *X. cheopis*, or of any other flea, we describe the fine structure of the gut in the first part of the report. In contrast to the pathogenesis of *R. prowazeki* infection in body lice, which procedes inexorably until the gut epithelium is destroyed, *R. mooseri* infection in the rat flea appears to cause only minimal damage to the gut epithelium. Nidi of undifferentiated cells are in any case available for replacement of gut epithelial cells. *R. mooseri* that proliferated in the flea epithelium were larger than those that grew in either cell culture or in the yolk sac of chick embryos, which suggests that this site may furnish the most favorable environment for their propagation.

R. prowazeki, *R. quintana*, and *R. mooseri* are not transmitted transovarially in their insect vectors. By contrast, spotted fever and scrub typhus rickettsiae can be transmitted vertically from one generation of arthropod to the next. Many questions about vertical transmission of these microorganisms have remained unsolved. The last four papers in this session attempt to clarify some of the mechanisms involved in transovarial transmission.

Burgdorfer and Brinton report the results of a quantitative study on transovarial transmission of *R. rickettsi* in three important tick vectors of Rocky Mountain spotted fever. They found that naturally infected females transmitted rickettsiae via eggs to 100% of their progeny. The invasion of germinal cells by rickettsiae began during feeding of nymphal females, and efficiency of transovarial transmission appeared to depend upon the extent of rickettsial reproduction. In some cases, massive infection of engorged females proved fatal or adversely affected oviposition and egg development.

Three papers are devoted to elucidation of problems connected with vertical transmission of *R. tsutsugamushi* in their chigger vectors. Manipulations with this diminutive and active arthropod require great meticulousness and must surely be among the most laborious procedures used during experiments with rickettsial agents. Roberts *et al.* discuss identification of scrub typhus rickettsiae in the life stages of *Leptotrombidium fletcheri*. By means of immunofluorescent techniques, they demonstrated the presence of *R. tsutsugamushi* in all stages of development and in all organs at some time during development. The ovary was the most frequently infected organ in adult females, whereas in unfed larvae, the principal infected sites were the salivary gland and midgut. These studies substantiate the existence of transstadial transmission of *R. tsutsugamushi* in the mite vector.

Both Walker *et al.* and Traub *et al.* report on a problem central to the ecology of scrub typhus: Are mites the reservoir of *R. tsutsugamushi,* maintaining the microorganisms in nature without replenishment by means of a chigger-infected small mammal-chigger cycle? Both groups approached the problem by determining if uninfected chiggers could acquire scrub typhus infection by feeding on rickettsemic mice and if females so infected could transmit the rickettsiae to their progeny. Although the main goals of the two groups were the same, their experimental approaches diverged. Walker *et al.* used relatively small numbers of mites and tested them individually. Traub *et al.* used pools of large numbers of mites and tested them as pools. Both showed that chiggers could acquire infection by feeding on an infected rodent. Walker *et al.* found no evidence for transovarial transmission of infected females, whereas Traub *et al.,* by use of mass methods, found that transovarial transmission of acquired infection occurred in only one of 23 *L. deliense* pools tested. These findings suggest the importance of naturally infected chiggers as the reservoir of scrub typhus. Traub *et al.,* however, list 11 reasons to suggest that small mammals "may also serve as a wellspring for maintenance of the rickettsial cycle in nature." These speculations should provide an impetus for years of study.

REFERENCES

1. TRERYAR, F. J., JR., E. WEISS, D. B. MILLAR, F. M. BOZEMAN & R. A. ORMSBEE. 1973. DNA base composition of rickettsiae. Science **180:** 415–417.
2. SCHRAMEK, S. 1968. Isolation and characterization of deoxyribonucleic acid from *Coxiella burneti.* Acta Virol. **12:** 18–22.
3. McKIEL, J. A., E. J. BELL & D. B. LACKMAN. 1967. *Rickettsia canada:* a new member of the typhus group of rickettsiae isolated from *Haemaphysalis leporispalustris* ticks in Canada. Can. J. Microbiol. **13:** 503–510.

MODIFICATION OF ANTITYPHUS ANTIBODIES ON PASSAGE THROUGH THE GUT OF THE HUMAN BODY LOUSE WITH DISCUSSION OF SOME EPIDEMIOLOGIC AND EVOLUTIONARY IMPLICATIONS *

C. L. Wisseman, Jr., J. L. Boese,† A. D. Waddell,
and D. J. Silverman

Department of Microbiology
University of Maryland
School of Medicine
Baltimore, Maryland 21201

INTRODUCTION

Arthropod-borne diseases pose some fascinating and complex biologic questions, especially when the arthropod vector is also an obligate parasite that depends for nutrition and survival upon the blood or tissue juices of the vertebrate host of the microbial agent. In such instances, the vertebrate is a dual host to two parasites, the vector and the microbial agent. The vertebrate host is not neutral in this relationship but reacts to both vector and microbe in a variety of ways, which range from behavioral, for example, tail swishing, twitching of the platysma muscles, and submersion in water or mud holes, to inflammatory and immunologic. The immunologic responses of the vertebrate host to the arthropod vector have received some attention.[1-3] The responses of the vertebrate host, especially the human host, to the microbial agent have received far more attention, although even here the information is far from complete. However, only scant attention has been paid to the effect of factors from the vertebrate host upon the interactions between agent and vector and between agent and subsequent vertebrate hosts in the transmission cycle, especially in those instances in which the microbe is limited to the gut of the vector.

The man-louse (*Pediculus humanus humanus L.*) -rickettsia (*Rickettsia prowazeki*) system of epidemic or louse-borne typhus fever is an excellent, relatively simple example of the biologic system just described.[4, 5] Man is the dual vertebrate host and responds to both vector and rickettsia in a variety of ways, for example, behavioral, cultural, physiologic (inflammatory, immunologic). The body louse is an obligate ectoparasite; it depends entirely upon the blood of the human host for nutrition.[6] The rickettsia is an obligate intracellular microbial parasite that can survive and grow in the cells of both the vertebrate host and the midgut of the vector.[7-11] The rickettsia regularly kills the louse vector.[4, 6, 10, 11]

One of the responses of the human host to *R. prowazeki* infection is the

* Supported in part by Contract DADA-17-71-C-1007 with the U.S. Army Research and Development Command, Office of the Surgeon General, Department of the Army, and NIAID Training Grant, Public Health Service, AI 00016. Dr. Boese was a Postdoctoral Trainee supported by the training grant.

† Present address: Food & Drug Administration, Public Health Service, Baltimore, Md. 21201.

6

production of antibodies specific for rickettsial antigens, which appear in the blood after the first few days of disease. Both antibodies and rickettsiae coexist in the blood for a few days, during which time the typhus fever patient remains infective for body lice that feed upon him. This situation persists until defervescence, when the rickettsiae disappear from the blood but not from all tissues, whereas the antibodies persist in the blood for many years.[4, 5, 10]

We have studied certain facets of the interaction between antibodies in typhus convalescent serum and *R. prowazeki*. Thus, although these antibodies are not rickettsiacidal, they do opsonize the rickettsiae and prepare them for destruction within professional phagocytes of the host defense system without, however, interfering with the capacity of antibody-coated rickettsiae to infect cells that are not professional phagocytes.[12-17, 47, 48]

In a previous paper,[10] we called attention to the influence of some factors in the blood of the human host on the interaction between *R. prowazeki* and its vector, the body louse. In that study, we demonstrated that antibodies present with rickettsiae in the blood meal of the louse did not prevent the latter from infecting and growing in the louse midgut cells. Moreover, rickettsiae, excreted in the feces of infected lice that had fed upon a typhus-immune host, have on their surface substances that react with immunofluorescent reagents specific for the IgG species of human immunoglobulins. In a subsequent paper,[11] we demonstrated by electron microscopy that the rickettsiae embedded in such dried louse feces retain their typical morphologic features without evidence of a shift to "dormant" forms.

It is well known that the feces of *R. prowazeki*-infected body lice from typhus-immune subjects are highly infectious for nonimmune people and that they retain their infectivity for a relatively long time (reviewed in References 10 and 11), despite the fact that the rickettsiae are coated with antibodies. These facts pose some interesting problems when we consider the possible interactions between these rickettsiae and the defense mechanisms of the next human host in the transmission cycle. They suggest the possibility that the antibodies in the feces and on the fecal rickettsiae may have been altered by the digestive enzymes of the louse gut in such a way that they retain the capacity to combine with antigenic determinants on the rickettsia but have lost their capacity to express their usual biologic functions, which operate as defense mechanisms for the human host.

A milestone in the understanding of immunoglobulin structure and function was the introduction by Porter [18] of proteolytic enzymes as tools to cleave the antibody molecule into discrete fragments that could be separated and studied independently. These studies, along with the subsquent studies of many others, have helped to define the structure of immunoglobulins and have identified specific regions of the molecule that are responsible for specific combination with antigen (the variable region of the Fab fragment) and subsequent biologic function, such as activation of the complement cascade and attachment to receptor sites on the plasma membrane of various types of cells [the Fc fragment and perhaps some portion of the $F(ab')_2$ fragment].[19-35]

In this paper, we present evidence that human IgG molecules that pass through the louse gut undergo various degrees of partial, perhaps selective, degradation. Although some surviving fragments retain the capacity to bind with rickettsial antigens, these fragments have lost much or all of the original biologic functions of IgG molecules. The lowly louse, thus, seems to have anticipated Porter's classic experiments by a time factor measurable only on an evolutionary scale. We suggest that this phenomenon may be of importance in the epidemiology of typhus, that it may have been a selective influence in the choice of microorganism that could occupy this unique ecologic niche, and that similar phenomena may be operational on some other microbial agents transmitted to vertebrates by hematophagous arthropods.

MATERIALS AND METHODS

Louse Feces

In the course of other studies,[10] the feces of uninfected (LF) and *Rickettsia prowazeki*-infected [LF(i)] human body lice fed upon a typhus-immune human subject were collected in a special apparatus under conditions of controlled humidity. Individual batches of louse feces were stored separately in plastic tubes in a desiccator held in a —20° C freezer. Feces stored for more than 12 months yielded satisfactory results.

Louse Feces Extracts

Weighed quantities of louse feces were suspended in measured quantities of either phosphate-bufferd saline (PBS), pH 7.5, or Veronal®-buffered saline (VBS), pH 8.6, and were thoroughly ground in a motor-driven Porter-Elvejem-type tissue homogenizer equipped with a Teflon® pestle (Virtis Co., Gardner, N.Y.), keeping the specimen cold in an ice-water bath. For the feces from uninfected lice to be used to study the presence and state of antibodies present, the homogenate was cleared of particulate matter by high-speed centrifugation (av. 28,620g for 30 min). In such cases, the sediment was discarded, and the supernatant fluid was used for study. On the other hand, for feces from *R. prowazeki*-infected lice, the sediment was saved for further processing and study of the rickettsiae present in the louse feces; the supernatant fluid was also used for studies on the antibodies.

Usually, the supernatant from the high-speed centrifugation was employed without further treatment in antibody studies. In some instances, however, such as the sucrose gradient centrifugation studies, where the density of the crude extract was at times too great to permit layering on top of the gradient without uncontrolled mixing, or when infected louse feces were homogenized in a relatively large volume of buffer, the fluid was first dialyzed overnight in a viscose tube against buffer (usually PBS) and was concentrated to the desired volume by placing the small dialysis tube in a beaker of solid Carbowax® (polyethylene glycol). Because of the limited supply of louse feces, the volume of extracts that contained concentrations of the substances studied adequate to measure by methods available was generally very small. Some characteristics of the serum and louse feces extracts used in the studies reported here are listed in TABLE 1.

Immunologic Reagents

Serum from the typhus-immune host who served as louse feeder was drawn during the period of louse feeding and feces collection. Normal human serum and serum as a source of human complement was obtained from a healthy young adult human female, who had no detectable typhus antibodies or history of exposure or immunization against typhus. After clotting and retraction for 3 hr at 37° C, the serum was removed, clarified by centrifugation, quick-frozen in small aliquots in glass-sealed ampoules in a dry ice-alcohol mixture, and stored at —70° C. Precipitating antisera against human antibodies and their components, in addition to other serum components, used in agar diffusion and immunoelectrophoresis studies were obtained from a variety of commercial sources. The following antisera were obtained from Hyland Laboratories (Los Angeles, Calif.): antihuman serum for immunoelectrophoresis precipitin test (goat), antihuman IgG (goat), antihuman IgA, antihuman IgM, antihuman γGκ, antihuman γGλ. The following antisera were obtained from the Research

TABLE 1

SERUM AND LOUSE FECES EXTRACTS USED IN THIS STUDY

Material	Designation	Diluent	Louse Feces (mg/ml)	Diameter of Precipitation Ring (mm)	Apparent * IgG Concentration (mg/ml)
Human serum (ca. 1:10) (V-19504)	S	PBS, pH 7.5	—	7.9	0.55
Louse feces (uninfected)	LF-2	VBS, pH 8.6	58	6.9	(0.31)
Louse feces † (uninfected)	LF-3	PBS, pH 7.5	160	8.8	(0.92)
Louse feces † (infected)	LF(i)	PBS, pH 7.5		6.6	(0.27)

* Determined by radial immunodiffusion on Meloy low-level IgG plates. (Values for louse feces extracts may not be accurate because of presence of IgG degradation products.)

† Dialyzed and reconcentrated prior to use.

Products Division of Miles Laboratories, Inc. (Kankakee, Ill.): antihuman IgG (Pentex), antihuman Fab fragment of IgG (Miles-Yeda, Ltd.), antihuman Fc fragment of IgG (Miles-Yeda, Ltd.), antihuman albumin (rabbit) (Pentex).

Conjugated antisera specific for various human antibodies and their components and for complement components were also obtained from commercial sources: fluorescein-conjugated antihuman globulin (horse origin) (Progressive Laboratories, Inc., Baltimore, Md., distributed by Roboz Surgical Instrument Co., Washington, D.C.), fluorescein-conjugated IgG fraction of rabbit antihuman IgG (heavy chain) (Cappel Laboratories, Inc., Downingtown, Pa.), ferritin-conjugated IgG fraction of rabbit antihuman IgG (heavy chain) (Cappel), antihuman C′3 (Meloy Laboratories, Inc., Springfield, Va.), and antihuman C′4 (Meloy).

Immunologic Methods

Immunodiffusion (Ouchterlony type) was performed either in 1% agarose (Sea Kem, Marine Colloids Inc., distributed by Bausch and Lomb Co., Rochester, N.Y.) gels in Veronal buffer (pH 8.6) in the LKB (LKB Instruments, Inc., Rockville, Md.) slide system, with custom-built cutters or in precut rehydratable agarose films for micro-Ouchterlony technique (Marine Colloids Inc., Rockland, Maine). Immunoelectrophoresis, by the slide microtechnique of Scheidegger,[36] was performed in 1% agarose gels in Veronal buffer (pH 8.6) in the LKB apparatus, usually at 250 V and 10 mA per tray of six slides for 40–60 min. Precipitin bands were photographed either without staining, by dark-field illumination, or after staining with Amido-Schwartz 10 B stain.[36]

Fluorescent antibody studies for the detection of antibodies and complement were performed with the general principles outlined by Goldwasser and Shepard.[37, 38] Methods for the detection of antibody or antibody fragments that react with typhus rickettsiae made use of antigen slides prepared from *R. prowazeki*-infected chick embryo cells in which the rickettsiae were in the early log phase of growth.[49] When necessary, 0.1–0.5% Evans blue and yolk sac homogenate were included in the reaction mixtures to suppress nonspecific fluorescence. Preparations were examined under an American Optical Co. Microstar microscope equipped with a vertical uv illuminator.

Sucrose Density Centrifugation

Antibody fragments were separated according to size by the sedimentation rate method on 4.8-ml 5–20% sucrose (w/v) gradients [39] in a SW-65 rotor in an L-4 Spinco ultracentrifuge at speeds of 42,000–47,000 rpm at 3–5° C for 18–20 hr. Six-drop fractions, which yielded 47–50 fractions per gradient, were collected from each gradient. Peaks and distribution of substances that reacted with antihuman IgG antiserum were determined by radial immunodiffusion [40, 41] in Meloy low-range IgG plates. Diameters of the precipitin zones only were plotted for the gradient fractions, because the standard curve determined with intact IgG molecules would not necessarily be applicable to the various degradation products detected. The distribution of Fab- and Fc-reacting fragments on the gradients was determined by simple immunodiffusion of individual fractions against precipitating antisera specific for the Fab or Fc components of the IgG molecule.

Miscellaneous

Opsonization was measured with human polymorphonuclear leukocytes by methods previously described,[16] with a highly purified preparation of formalin-killed *R. prowazeki*. Agglutination tests were performed by the micro-agglutination technique of Fiset *et al*.[42]

The sediments from the centrifuged extracts described above were used to detect IgG or IgG fragments on the surface of rickettsiae in infected louse feces. The sediments, after washing by centrifugation in PBS (pH 7.5), were resuspended in a very small volume of PBS. Aliquots were treated in suspension with either fluorescein-labeled anti-Ig or ferritin-conjugated anti-IgG. In the fluorescein technique, the reaction was allowed to proceed for 60 min at ambient temperature, after which time the suspension was diluted with PBS, centrifuged (av. 28,620g for 30 min), and washed with PBS by centrifugation. The well-drained pellet was finally resuspended in a very small quantity of buffered glycerine and examined, as a wet mount under a coverslip, under the fluorescence microscope. For the ferritin-conjugated anti-IgG, the reaction was permitted to continue overnight at 4° C, after which time the rickettsia-containing material was sedimented and washed as described above. The pellet was resuspended in a small quantity of PBS, followed by the addition of cold 1% glutaraldehyde in 0.2 M cacodylate buffer (pH 7.4). After overnight fixation at 4° C, the rickettsiae were washed three times by centrifugation in cacodylate buffer, fixed in 1% osmium tetroxide for 1 hr, and embedded in Epon® 812 as described previously.[11] Ultrathin sections (60–80 nm) were cut on a Porter-Blum MT-2 ultramicrotome with a DuPont diamond knife. The sections were picked up on 300-mesh Formvar®-carbon-coated copper grids and were double stained, first with an aqueous solution of uranyl acetate (0.5%) and then with Reynolds lead citrate. The sections were examined in a Siemens Elmiskop IA electron microscope that operates at 80 kV that was equipped with a 400-μm condenser and a 50-μm objective aperture.

Results

Confirmation of Antiimmunoglobulin-Reactive Substances on the Surface of Rickettsiae from Infected Louse Feces

Because the drying and fixation in cold acetone of LF(i) homogenates for detection of immunoglobulin on rickettsiae in the previous study[10] may have denatured some antibody molecules, some fluorescent antibody studies were repeated by reacting the unfixed, but washed, rickettsiae directly with the fluorescein-labeled anti-Ig in suspension, washing and examining as a wet mount. Brilliant fluorescence was observed for objects the size and shape of rickettsiae, with little or no background staining of the debris present in such homogenates. Electron microscopic examination of ultrathin sections of similar preparations reacted with ferritin-conjugated anti-IgG revealed objects with ultrastructural features compatible with those of *R. prowazeki* in louse feces,[11] surrounded by a halo of ferritin molecules (Figure 1). Additionally, structures compatible with rickettsiae in various stages of autolysis, probably the result of prolonged incubation in PBS prior to fixation, were seen with ferritin on their surface. Thus, the presence of substances that react with anti-IgG antisera on the surface of rickettsiae in the feces of infected lice fed upon an immune host is confirmed.

Interestingly, in contrast to our unpublished ultrastructural study of *R. prowazeki* within host cells or liberated from them by gentle methods,[50] little evidence for the presence of a microcapsule was seen in these electron micrographs, because the ferritin was most often closely associated with the outer bilayer with no significant intervening electron-lucent space. It is unknown if this finding indicates the lack of a microcapsule on the rickettsiae as they occur in the louse feces or if much of it has been removed by the harsh grinding and washing, as was noted earlier by Anacker *et al.*[43] The latter alternative, together with the possible autolytic processes, may also account for the fact that many structures of presumed rickettsial origin did not appear to have ferritin specifically associated with them.

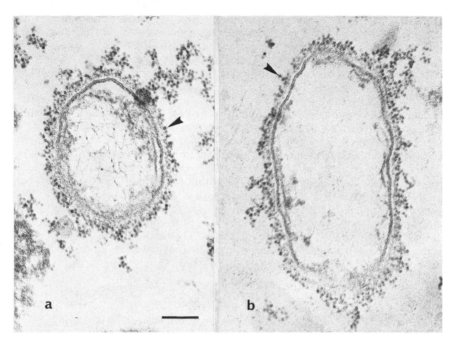

FIGURE 1. Reaction of ferritin-conjugated rabbit antihuman IgG with surface of *Rickettsia prowazeki* from feces of infected *Pediculus h. humanus* L. fed upon typhus immune human subject. Electron micrographs of ultrathin sections. Marked auto-lytic changes of cytoplasm, more marked in b, are the result of prolonged incubation in buffer that contained the conjugate prior to fixation. Arrows point to ferritin conjugate halo external to bilayer of cell wall. Bar in a = 100 nm.

Demonstration of Altered Immunoglobulins and Other Selected Serum Proteins in Louse Feces Extracts by Immunodiffusion

Ouchterlony-type double-diffusion tests with diluted whole serum and louse feces extracts failed to detect IgM in the extracts. Extremely faint staining of diffuse areas in tests with anti-IgA serum suggested the possible presence of minute amounts of IgA, but these results were no more conclusive for the presence of this immunoglobulin than were the fluorescent antibody studies of the previous report.[10]

In contrast, strong precipitin bands were regularly formed with anti-IgG antibodies (FIGURE 2). One anti-IgG serum (Pentex) gave a single band with serum but multiple bands (up to three or more) with louse feces extracts (FIGURE 2a and d). One of these bands fused with the single serum band in a reaction of identity, whereas the others crossed or spurred, which suggested IgG-reactive components that had undergone mild to marked alterations. Another anti-IgG serum (Hyland) gave only one clear band in the louse feces extract, which was not identical with that of the serum (FIGURE 2e). On occasion, another faint diffuse band could be detected with this serum. These results suggest that louse feces extracts contain, in addition to a small quantity of relatively unaltered IgG, as measured by fusion of a precipitin band with that of serum, large amounts of several markedly altered anti-IgG-reactive substances, possibly IgG degradation products.

Similar tests with antisera against the Fab and Fc fragments of IgG showed that louse feces extracts contain substances that precipitate with both reagents. However, whereas the extracts gave a single strong precipitin line with anti-Fab antiserum that appeared to fuse with the corresponding band in serum (FIGURE 2b), these same extracts yielded at least three bands with anti-Fc antiserum, none of which seemed to fuse with the single band in serum (FIGURE 2c and f). These results suggest the possibility of greater alteration of the Fc portion of the IgG molecule than of the surviving Fab portion by passage through the louse gut.

Anti-β1c/1a antiserum gave a single precipitin band with both serum and LF extracts that appeared to fuse (FIGURE 2g). However, antialbumin antiserum produced a very heavy precipitation reaction with both serum and LF

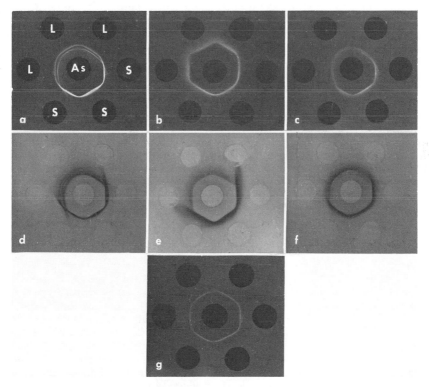

FIGURE 2. Alteration of IgG in louse feces extracts demonstrated by Ouchterlony-type double immunodiffusion against various antisera. L, louse feces extract; S, 1:10 dilution of host serum; As, antiserum. Antiserum (As): a and d, anti-IgG (Pentex); e, anti-IgG (Hyland); b, anti-Fabγ; c and f, anti-Fcγ; g, anti-β1c/1a. Louse feces extract (L): a–c and g, LF-3; d–f, LF-2.

extracts (not shown). There was spur formation between the serum and LF extract albumin bands, which again suggested alteration of this molecule in the LF extract.

Demonstration of IgG Fragments in Louse Feces Extracts by Immunoelectrophoresis

The presence of multiple altered IgG components in LF extracts, which differed markedly in their migration in an electric field, was clearly demonstrated by immunoelectrophoresis (FIGURE 3). Although the precipitin patterns of diluted serum and LF extracts produced by antiserum against whole human serum appear superficially similar (FIGURE 3a), which would indicate multiple precipitable serum components in LF extracts, closer examination reveals substantial differences. The differences with respect to IgG are better illustrated by the use of precipitating antisera against IgG and its Fab and Fc components. Thus, the Pentex anti-IgG antiserum revealed at least three, and perhaps four, components in the LF extract as opposed to the single band in the dilute serum (FIGURE 3b). The Hyland anti–IgG antiserum appeared to detect two of the three components (FIGURE 3c); it failed to react with the fast-migrating component detected by the Pentex serum. The anti-Fab antiserum, which yielded only a single band in the LF extract, fusing with that of the serum, has in immunodiffusion detected two of the three or four LF extract anti-IgG-reactive bands (FIGURE 3d). On the other hand, the anti-Fc antiserum detected a fast-moving and a slow-moving band that seemed to correspond to two of the three or four bands detected by the Pentex anti-IgG antiserum and perhaps to one of the bands detected by anti-Fab serum (FIGURE 3e). Thus, immunoelectrophoresis has revealed at least three separate forms or fragments of the IgG molecule in LF extracts. Their patterns and reaction with specific subcomponent antisera suggest that one component may be derived primarily from the Fc portion of the IgG molecule, a second one primarily from the Fab portion, and a third one that contains components of both portions.

Demonstration of Heterogeneity of Molecular Size of IgG Fragments in Louse Feces Extracts by Sucrose Density Gradient Centrifugation

Centrifugation of serum and LF extracts through a sucrose density gradient revealed the expected single compact band of IgG for the dilute serum, whereas in the louse feces extracts, anti-IgG-, as well as anti-Fab- and anti-Fc-, reactive components were distributed throughout the gradient, from about the level of the intact marker IgG (7S) to about the level expected of dissociated Fab and Fc fragments (about 3.5S) (FIGURE 4). In addition, a second component, detectable as a faint second ring on the radial immunodiffusion plates, appeared near the top of the gradient, above the 3.5S level. Although it reacted with the anti-IgG serum in the immunodiffusion plates, it was not detected with antisera specific for the Fab or Fc fragments. This region may consist of various small fragments of the IgG molecule only detectable by a potent serum broadly reactive against all components of the molecule.

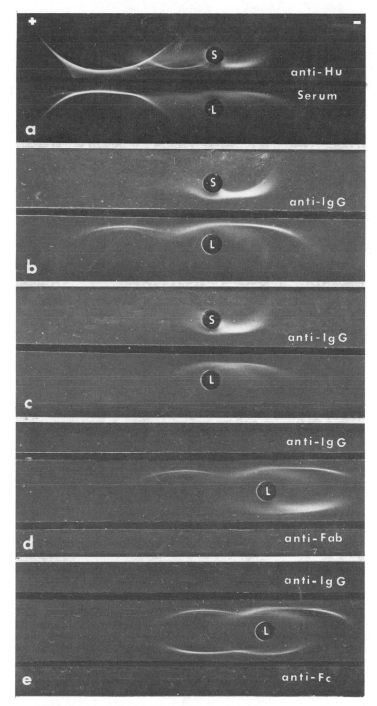

FIGURE 3. Comparison by immunoelectrophoresis of IgG in louse feces extract with that in diluted host serum. S, 1:10 dilution of host serum; L, louse feces extract (LF-3).

Biologic Activities of Immunoglobulins in Louse Feces Extracts

The crude louse feces extracts theoretically should contain immunoglobulins othe¢ than IgG and its degradation products. However, only IgG was present in detectable quantities, and, therefore, the reactions of crude LF extracts should

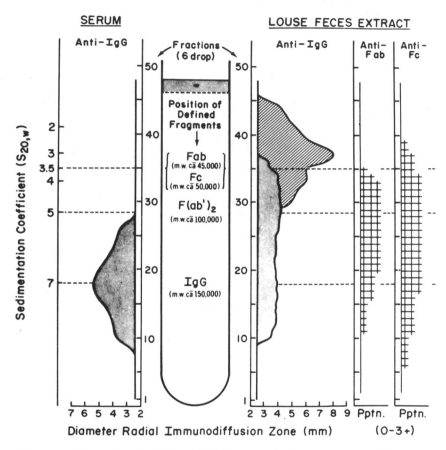

FIGURE 4. Separation of IgG and IgG fragments in human serum and louse feces extract according to sedimentation rate by ultracentrifugation in a 5–20% sucrose gradient. Louse feces extract was dialyzed LF-3; serum was 1:10 dilution of host serum. Position of IgG and IgG fragments was determined by radial immunodiffusion measurements of gradient fractions in plates that contained anti-IgG antiserum; that of Fab-reactive and Fc-reactive fractions was determined by simple double immunodiffusion. Cross-hatched area represents the second ring that formed around the wells of the radial immunodiffusion plates with fractions near top of gradient (low-sedimentation-rate substances). Centrifuged at 46,468 rpm for 18.6 hr at 3° C in an SW-65 rotor.

reflect almost entirely those of IgG and its fragments. Louse feces extracts were tested for the following antibody functions.

1. When applied to *R. prowazeki* antigens by the indirect fluorescent antibody technique, components detectable by fluorescent anti-IgG were found to

bind to the rickettsiae, which suggests that the extracts contain some Fab or $F(ab')_2$ or larger components with the variable region intact.

2. Although the capacity of crude LF extracts to agglutinate *R. prowazeki* varied from preparation to preparation [LF-3, 1:8; LF(i), <2] and, when present, was low compared with diluted serum (≥ 32), the fact that some agglutination did occur suggests that fragments that contain intact $F(ab')_2$ portions are present at times in low amounts.

Fractions of sucrose density gradients of diluted serum and louse feces extract (LF-2) were tested for *R. prowazeki* agglutinating activity by adding agglutinating antigen to each fraction that had been collected in microtiter plates (FIGURE 5). The gradient was used in such a manner to detect primarily immunoglobulins with a sedimentation coefficient of 7S or less so as to be able to identify degradation products of IgG. As a result, the intact IgG molecules were driven near the region of the IgM molecules, the sedimentation of which was being restricted by the bottom of the centrifuge tube. Thus, agglutinating activity in the serum gradient extended from the bottom of the tube to a level above the sensitivity of the immunodiffusion assay method for IgG. On the other hand, no rapidly sedimenting agglutinating activity was detected in the LF extract, a finding consistent with the failure to detect IgM immunoglobulins by precipitin formation in double-diffusion tests with anti-IgM antiserum. Agglutinating activity was detected in the LF extract from the level of the upper portion of the serum IgG peak to the lower portion of the peak that one would expect with intact $F(ab')_2$ fragments. In view of other findings below and the gradient above, these findings suggest that the agglutinins in this LF extract consisted primarily of large IgG molecular fragments that retained intact $F(ab')_2$ portions associated with substantial, but partially degraded, Fc portions.

3. By the fluorescent antibody technique for detection of complement fixation,[37, 38] it was easy to demonstrate that antibodies from serum that had combined with the *R. prowazeki* antigen would fix human C'3. LF extracts, on the other hand, failed to fix human C'3 under the same conditions. This finding suggests that the bulk of the IgG fragments that combine with the rickettsial antigen either have a defective C_H2 portion of the Fc component or have lost it entirely.[23, 24, 28-33]

4. Convalescent typhus serum contains antibodies that opsonize rickettsiae for enhanced phagocytosis by professional phagocytes.[12, 13, 16, 17] The initial stage of immune opsonization is thought to be an attachment of the Fc portion of the antibody molecule to receptor sites on the phagocyte plasma membrane.[19-24, 34, 35] By use of methods that we developed earlier to study phagocytosis and opsonization by typhus immune serum,[16] we found that, whereas the diluted serum caused massive phagocytosis of *R. prowazeki* by human polymorphonuclear leukocytes (74% PMN phagocytizing with 5.72 RLB per PMN), the most concentrated LF extract prepared (LF-3) failed to stimulate phagocytosis to any appreciable degree (15% PMN phagocytizing with 0.38 RLB per PMN), which is about the level of phagocytosis to which the system was adjusted for normal serum. Thus, the altered IgG in LF extracts also lacks the capacity to initiate this important biologic function of some antibody species.

DISCUSSION

The experimental data presented in this report indicate that human immunoglobulins in a blood meal, upon passage through the gut of the human body

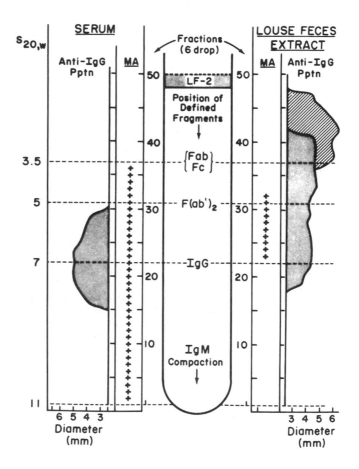

FIGURE 5. Distribution of *R. prowazeki*-agglutinating antibody and antibody fragments in serum and louse feces extract according to sedimentation rate on 5–20% sucrose gradient. Louse feces extract was LF-2; serum was 1:10 dilution of host serum. Position of substances reactive with anti-IgG antiserum was determined by radial immunodiffusion. The broad band of agglutinins from bottom of tube up through IgG band with serum results from restriction of free sedimentation of IgM and its accumulation toward bottom of tube in this gradient. Centrifuged at 42,000 rpm for 18.4 hr at 5° C in an SW-65 rotor.

louse, are greatly modified, altered, or destroyed, presumably by enzymes of the louse midgut. Potent precipitating antisera specific for the heavy chains of IgG, IgM, and IgA were used to detect, in extracts of louse feces, surviving immunoglobulin fragments of sufficient size and antigenicity to yield precipitates visible by immunodiffusion and immunoelectrophoretic techniques. No material reactive with anti-IgM serum, and only traces of material reactive with anti-IgA serum, were found in the louse feces extracts. In contrast, strong precipitin reactions were obtained with anti-IgG sera. However, information gained from immunodiffusion, immunoelectrophoresis, and sucrose density rate sedimentation studies indicated that very little, if any, intact IgG was present. Indeed, these methods gave evidence to indicate that the material that precipitated with anti-IgG serum was, in fact, a complex mixture of molecular fragments that ranged in size from nearly as large as the intact IgG molecule to smaller than intact Fab or Fc fragments. Some of these fragments reacted with anti-Fc serum only, some with anti-Fab serum only, and some with both sera.

Although the Fc component determines some of the biologic functions of the antibody molecule, such as initiation of the classic complement cascade and attachment to receptor sites on the plasma membrane of professional phagocytes,[19-35] Fc fragments that are not also combined with functional Fab portions, the variable regions of which determine antibody specificity and, indeed, actually combine with antigenic determinents, are essentially biologically useless in defense against microbial agents. Therefore, tests for surviving antibody function by the immunoglobulin fragments in louse feces extracts relied upon reactions that were dependent first upon a functional variable portion of Fab fragment. Some of the tests required, in addition, functional integrity of the Fc and other portions of the molecule.

That extracts of the feces of lice fed upon a typhus-immune subject contained IgG fragments with intact variable regions of the Fab fragment was demonstrated by the fact that these extracts contained substances, detectable by fluorescein-conjugated anti-Ig and anti-IgG, that would regularly bind specifically to *R. prowazeki* surface antigens. The irregular presence in louse feces extracts of agglutinins for *R. prowazeki* indicated that at times, at least $F(ab')_2$ fragments were present, but the single sucrose density gradient, the fractions of which were tested for agglutinating activity, indicated that, in this particular preparation, the agglutinating fragments were larger than the definitive $F(ab')_2$ fragment but smaller than the intact IgG molecule; that is, they probably retained portions of the Fc fragment.

Two tests were performed for retention of biologic activity of fragments bearing intact variable regions of the Fab fragment, namely, capacity to fix complement and capacity to opsonize rickettsiae for enhanced phagocytosis by human polymorphonuclear leukocytes. In neither instance were the tests positive. This finding suggests that, even though some fairly large fragments of the IgG molecule, which retain the capacity to bind specifically to *R. prowazeki* antigens, are present in the feces of lice, the digestive enzymes of the louse have altered them sufficiently, so that any portion of the Fc region that still remains on the molecule no longer has the capacity to initiate these biologic functions of the intact IgG molecule. However, evidence has been published to indicate that the component of an IgG molecule required to activate the alternate complement pathway resides in the $F(ab')_2$ portion of the molecule.[31, 33] It is not possible to determine from our data if the failure to detect C′3 fixation by the alternate pathway in agglutinating preparations represents an inadequacy of the method or if it, indeed, indicates some subtle changes in the surviving $F(ab')_2$ fragments.

Very little is known about the digestive enzymes of the midgut of the human body louse. Because blood is the midgut's sole source of nutrients, it is reasonable to assume that at least some blood proteins or portions of proteins are digested completely to amino acids or lower peptides by proteolytic enzymes. No information is available on the possible presence of enzymes that would digest carbohydrate portions of the IgG molecule. It is not known if the antibody fragments that survive in louse feces simply represent incomplete digestion of blood proteins or if they represent end-products of proteolytic enzymes and/or carbohydrases with specific, limited types of action on IgG molecules. Nor is it known if some changes in function are due solely to the action of proteolytic enzymes or if specific digestion of carbohydrate groups may also have contributed. No quantitative measurements have been made to determine what proportion of the ingested IgG molecules survives in the feces as identifiable antibody fragments. Operationally, however, regardless of mechanism, some IgG fragments with some identifiable antibody activities, namely, the capacity to bind with rickettsial antigens, do survive.

The single measurement of the louse midgut pH that we have found in the literature,[44] which is near neutrality, suggests that any extracellular proteolytic enzymes that might be present would probably have an optimal activity in this pH range and, possibly, would be expected to have an action more similar to those of trypsin, chymotrypsin, and certain peptidases than to that of pepsin, the action of which on IgG molecules has also been studied. (The amount of proteolysis due to endocytosis of blood proteins with intracellular digestion, a process known to occur in some arthropods,[45] has been, to our knowledge, totally unexplored for the human body louse.) The reported action of trypsin and chymotrypsin on IgG molecules appears to be complex; they act on both Fc and Fab ends of the molecule.[25-27] Thus, fragments may be present that are detectable by immunodiffusion techniques with potent antisera but that would not be detected by tests that depend upon function residing in either Fab or Fc regions. However, as suggested above, from a biologic viewpoint, such fragments are operationally unimportant, because they no longer have the capacity to bind with specific antigens.

Thus, concentrating on those surviving IgG fragments that retain the capacity to combine with rickettsial antigens, it is clear that the louse gut enzymes have performed a molecular dissection on the Fc fragment which has destroyed its capacity to initiate the biologic functions that are commonly associated with defense mechanisms, that is, the capacity to fix complement in the classic system and the capacity to opsonize the rickettsiae. We have already demonstrated that typhus rickettsiae are resistant to the lethal action of antibody-mediated complement action [51] but are sensitized by antibodies that prepare them for destruction within macrophages,[13] even though similarly sensitized *R. prowazeki* still retain the capacity to infect cells that are not professional phagocytes, including those of the louse gut.[10, 14] The alteration of the Fc fragment by louse gut enzymes to render the molecule incapable of opsonizing rickettsiae, by destroying its capacity to bind the receptor sites on the phagocyte cell membrane, therefore assumes great biologic and epidemiologic significance. Thus, although the rickettsiae excreted in the feces of a louse feeding upon an immune person are coated with antibody fragments that retain the capacity to combine with rickettsial antigens, as demonstrated in the previous publication [10] and confirmed more rigorously here, the louse gut proteolytic enzymes have selectively destroyed the portion of the antibody molecule that could initiate the only known function of antibody in resistance to infection, namely, opsonization followed by intracellular destruction by a professional phagocyte. It is not surprising, therefore, that the feces from such lice are highly infectious for man.

These circumstances suggest an extraordinary adaptation, or selection, of *R. prowazeki* to an unique ecologic niche that is especially conducive to survival in the man-louse-man transmission cycle, in which man has the capacity to respond with specific antirickettsial factors that do not operate in the vector and the vector has the capacity to destroy the capacity of these factors to operate in the next human link in the transmission chain.

An interesting extension, not specifically tested in this study, rests on the fact that *R. prowazeki* infection of the louse midgut progressively destroys the lining cells that simultaneously serve as host cells for the rickettsiae and producers of the proteolytic enzymes.[4, 6, 10, 11] Because these cells are not regenerated, it can be assumed that as the rickettsial infection progresses, the alteration of antibodies by louse gut enzymes should decrease toward the peak of rickettsial infection and rickettsiae excreted by a maximally infected louse feeding upon an immune host may actually be coated with some minimally altered, or unaltered, antibody molecules that might retain a significant component of biologic function. If such rickettsiae, upon transmission to another host, first encounter a professional phagocyte, instead of some other kind of cell, their "infectivity" might actually be reduced. Although typhus, in epidemic form, is a formidable disease, it is conceivable that this phenomenon of decreasing alteration of antibody molecules may actually serve as a restraining force or negative feedback mechanism, in transmission, because a single heavily infected louse may contain over 10^8 rickettsiae,[10] which is a sufficient amount to infect millions of people if optimally disseminated.

A further speculative point is a correlation between the fact that the vectors of rickettsial agents of human disease are blood-sucking arthropods and the metabolism of the rickettsiae. The major constituent of the vector food is protein, which is digested to varying degrees. The fact that the rickettsiae that have been studied do *not* derive their energy from oxidation or glycolysis of carbohydrates but, instead, utilize glutamate for energy metabolism [7-9] may also represent an adaptive mechanism to the peculiar ecologic niche that they inhabit. Thus, although the different groups of organisms that cause the "rickettsial diseases" of man differ in many important ways from one another and probably represent organisms of diverse origin, as suggested by examination of the various phenotypic properties and DNA base composition,[7-9, 46] convergent evolutionary processes may have selected certain common features as essential for survival as an intracellular parasite in the blood-sucking arthropod-vertebrate host cycle in which they exist, for example, energy derived from oxidation of products of proteolytic digestion, resistance to lysozyme and to killing by antibody and complement, and infectivity of antibody-coated rickettsiae for cells that are not professional phagocytes. At the same time, certain divergent evolutionary processes within groups have led to diversification in other properties, such as surface antigens, which leads to the development of strains that are currently recognized taxonomically as species or serotypes within a group.

We believe that some of the principles elucidated by the example of louse-borne epidemic typhus may have more general application to varying degrees to certain other systems in which an infectious agent is transmitted by blood-sucking arthropods to vertebrate hosts, especially when the microorganism is confined to the gut of the arthropod vector.

SUMMARY

Evidence is presented to indicate that proteolytic and perhaps other enzymes of the louse midgut, essential to the nutrition of the louse, perform molecular dissection on the antirickettsial antibodies present in the blood of a typhus-immune host that selectively destroys, along with other functions, the portion of the antibody that determines the only known function by which antirickettsial antibodies may operate in host defense mechanisms, namely, opsonization of rickettsiae for enhanced ingestion by professional phagocytes and subsequent destruction.

The epidemiologic significance of these findings is discussed in relation to the progressive destruction of cells that produce digestive enzymes of the louse midgut that occurs with progressive rickettsial infection, and the possibility of a negative feedback mechanism in transmission is introduced.

Speculations that involve evolutionary concepts of both convergent and divergent varieties with respect to rickettsiae, potentially operational in a system that consists of an obligate blood-sucking arthropod vector and a vertebrate host capable of adaptive responses to both vector and rickettsial agent, are presented.

REFERENCES

1. FEINGOLD, B. F., E. BENJAMINI & D. MICHAELI. 1968. The allergic responses to insect bites. Annu. Rev. Entomol. **13:** 137–158.
2. BENJAMINI, E. & B. F. FEINGOLD. 1970. Immunity to arthropods. *In* Immunity to Parasitic Animals. G. J. Jackson, R. Herman & I. Singer, Eds. Vol. 2: 1061–1134. Appleton-Century-Crofts. New York, N.Y.
3. BOESE, J. L. 1974. Rabbit immunity to the rabbit tick *Haemaphysalis leporispalustris* (ACARI:IXODIDAE). I. Development of resistance. J. Med. Entomol. **11:** 503–512.
4. SNYDER, J. C. 1965. Typhus fever rickettsiae. *In* Viral and Rickettsial Infections of Man. F. L. Horsfall, Jr. & I. Tamm, Eds. 4th edit. Chap. 49: 1059–1094. J. B. Lippincott Co. Philadelphia, Pa.
5. WISSEMAN, C. L., JR. 1972. Concepts of louse-borne typhus control in developing countries: the use of the living attenuated E strain typhus vaccine in epidemic and endemic situations. *In* Immunity in Viral and Rickettsial Diseases. A. Kohn & M. A. Klingberg, Eds. : 97–130. Plenum Publishing Corporation. New York, N.Y.
6. BUXTON, P. A. 1946. The Louse. An Account of the Lice Which Infect Man, Their Medical Importance and Control. 2nd edit. : 164. The Williams & Wilkins Co. Baltimore, Md.
7. WISSEMAN, C. L., JR. 1968. Some biological properties of rickettsiae pathogenic for man. Zentr. Bakteriol. Parasitenk. Abt. I Orig. **206:** 299–313.
8. ORMSBEE, R. A. 1969. Rickettsiae (as organisms). Annu. Rev. Microbiol. **23:** 275–295.
9. WEISS, E. 1973. Growth and physiology of rickettsiae. Bacteriol. Rev. **37:** 259–283.
10. BOESE, J. L., C. L. WISSEMAN, JR., W. T. WALSH & P. FISET. 1973. Antibody and antibiotic action on *Rickettsia prowazeki* in body lice across the host-

vector interface, with observations on strain virulence and retrieval mechanisms. Amer. J. Epidemiol. **98**: 262–282.

11. SILVERMAN, D. J., J. L. BOESE & C. L. WISSEMAN, JR. 1974. Ultrastructural studies of *Rickettsia prowazeki* from louse midgut cells to feces: search for "dormant forms." Infect. Immunity **10**: 257–263.

12. GAMBRILL, M. R. & C. L. WISSEMAN, JR. 1973. Mechanisms of immunity in typhus infections. II. Multiplication of typhus rickettsiae in human macrophage cell cultures in the non-immune system: influence of rickettsial strains and of chloramphenicol. Infect. Immunity **8**: 519–527.

13. GAMBRILL, M. R. & C. L. WISSEMAN, JR. 1973. Mechanisms of immunity in typhus infections. III. Influence of human immune serum and complement on the fate of *Rickettsia mooseri* within human macrophages. Infect. Immunity **8**: 631–640.

14. WISSEMAN, C. L., JR., A. D. WADDELL & W. T. WALSH. 1974. Mechanisms of immunity in typhus infections. IV. Failure of chicken embryo cells in culture to restrict growth of antibody-sensitized *Rickettsia prowazeki*. Infect. Immunity **9**: 571–575.

15. ANDRESE, A. P. & C. L. WISSEMAN, JR. 1971. In vitro interactions between human peripheral macrophages and *Rickettsia mooseri*. *In* Proceedings of the 29th Annual Meeting of the Electron Microscopy Society of America. C. J. Arceneaux, Ed. : 39, 40. Claitor's Publishing Division. Baton Rouge, La.

16. WISSEMAN, C. L., JR., J. R. GAULD & J. G. WOOD. 1963. Interaction of rickettsiae and phagocytic host cells. III. Opsonizing antibodies in human subjects infected with virulent or attenuated *Rickettsia prowazeki* or inoculated with killed epidemic typhus vaccine. J. Immunol. **90**: 127–131.

17. WISSEMAN, C. L., JR. & H. TABOR. 1964. Interaction of rickettsiae and phagocytic host cells. V. Early cellular response of man to typhus rickettsiae as revealed by the skin window technique, with observations on *in vivo* phagocytosis. J. Immunol. **93**: 816–825.

18. PORTER, R. R. 1959. The hydrolysis of rabbit gamma globulin and antibodies with crystalline papain. Biochem. J. **73**: 119–127.

19. COHEN, S. & R. R. PORTER. 1964. Structure and biologic activity of immunoglobulins. Advan. Immunol. **4**: 287–349.

20. COHEN, S. & C. MILSTEIN. 1967. Structure and biological properties of immunoglobulins. Advan. Immunol. **7**: 1–89.

21. EDELMAN, G. M. & W. E. GALL. 1969. The antibody problem. Annu. Rev. Biochem. **38**: 415–466.

22. DORRINGTON, K. J. & C. TANFORD. 1970. Molecular size and conformation of immunoglobulins. Advan. Immunol. **12**: 333–381.

23. NATVIG, J. B. & H. G. KUNKEL. 1973. Human immunoglobulins: classes, subclasses, genetic variants and idiotypes. Advan. Immunol. **16**: 1–59.

24. SPIEGELBERG, H. L. 1974. Biologic activities of immunoglobulins of different classes and subclasses. Advan. Immunol. **19**: 259–294.

25. NATVIG, J. B. & M. W. TURNER. 1971. Localization of Gm markers to different molecular regions of the Fc fragment. Clin. Exp. Immunol. **8**: 685–700.

26. TURNER, M. W., H. H. BENNICH & J. B. NATVIG. 1970. Pepsin digestion of human G-myeloma proteins of different subclasses. I. The characteristic features of pepsin cleavage as a function of time. Clin. Exp. Immunol. **7**: 603–625.

27. TURNER, M. W., A. KOMVOPOULOS, H. BENNICH & J. B. NATVIG. 1972. Antigenic and immunological characteristics of tryptic and chymotryptic subfragments from the Cγ3 homology region of human immunoglobulin G. Scand. J. Immunol. **1**: 53–62.

28. KEHOE, J. M. & M. FOUGEREAU. 1969. Immunoglobulin peptide with complement fixing activity. Nature (London) **224**: 1212, 1213.

29. AUGENER, W., H. M. GREY, N. R. COOPER & H. J. MÜLLER-EBERHARD. 1971.

The reaction of monomeric and aggregated immunoglobulins with C1. Immunochemistry **8:** 1011–1020.

30. ELLERSON, J. R., D. YASMEEN, R. A. PAINTER & K. J. DORRINGTON. 1972. A fragment corresponding to the C_H2 region of immunoglobulin G (IgG) with complement fixing activity. FEBS Lett. **24:** 318–322.

31. OSLER, A. G. & A. L. SANDBERG. 1973. Alternate complement pathways. Progr. Allergy **17:** 51–92.

32. TARANTA, A. & E. C. FRANKLIN. 1961. Complement fixation by antibody fragments. Science **134:** 1981, 1982.

33. SCHEER, P. H. & E. L. BECKER. 1965. Pepsin digestion of rabbit and sheep antibodies. The effect on complement fixation. J. Exp. Med. **118:** 891–904.

34. BERKEN, A. & B. BENACERRAF. 1966. Properties of antibodies cytophilic for macrophages. J. Exp. Med. **123:** 119–144.

35. INCHLEY, C., H. M. GREY & J. W. UHR. 1970. The cytophilic activity of human immunoglobulins. J. Immunol. **105:** 362–369.

36. CROWLE, A. J. 1961. Immunodiffusion. : 1–333. Academic Press, Inc. New York, N.Y.

37. GOLDWASSER, R. A. & C. C. SHEPARD. 1959. Fluorescent antibody methods in the differentiation of murine and epidemic typhus sera; specificity changes resulting from previous immunization. J. Immunol. **82:** 373–380.

38. GOLDWASSER, R. A. & C. C. SHEPARD. 1958. Staining of complement and modifications of fluorescent antibody procedures. J. Immunol. **80:** 122–131.

39. TRAUTMAN, R. & K. M. COWAN. 1968. Preparative and analytical ultracentrifugation. *In* Methods in Immunology and Immunochemistry. Volume II. Physical and Chemical Methods. C. A. Williams & M. W. Chase, Eds. Chap. 7: 81–118. Academic Press, Inc. New York, N.Y.

40. MANCINI, G., A. O. CARBONARA & J. F. HEREMANS. 1965. Immunochemical quantitation of antigens by single radial immunodiffusion. Immunochemistry **2:** 235–254.

41. FAHEY, J. L. & E. M. McKELVEY. 1965. Quantitative determination of serum immunoglobulins in antibody-agar plates. J. Immunol. **94:** 84–90.

42. FISET, P., R. A. ORMSBEE, R. SILBERMAN, M. G. PEACOCK & S. H. SPIELMAN. 1969. A microagglutination technique for detection and measurement of rickettsial antibodies. Acta Virol. **13:** 60–66.

43. ANACKER, R. L., E. G. PICKENS & D. B. LACKMAN. 1967. Details of the ultrastructure of *Rickettsia prowazeki* grown in the chick yolk sac. J. Bacteriol. **94:** 260–262.

44. POPOW, P. P. & R. D. GOLZOWA. 1933. Zur Kenntnis der Wasserstoffionenkonzentration im Darm einiger blutsaugender Arthropoden. Arch. Schiffs-Trop. Hyg. **37:** 465, 466.

45. ROCKSTEIN, M. 1964. The Physiology of Insecta. Academic Press, Inc. New York, N.Y.

46. TYERYAR, F. J., JR., E. WEISS, D. B. MILLAR, F. M. BOZEMAN & R. A. ORMSBEE. 1973. DNA base composition of rickettsiae. Science **180:** 415–417.

47. WISSEMAN, C. L., JR. To be published.

48. DALTON, D. D. & C. L. WISSEMAN, JR. To be published.

49. WADDELL, A. D. et al. In preparation.

50. BROWN, D. T. et al. In preparation.

51. WISSEMAN, C. L., JR. et al. To be published.

VIRULENCE OF *RICKETTSIA PROWAZEKI* FOR HEAD LICE *

E. S. Murray and S. B. Torrey

Department of Microbiology
Harvard School of Public Health
Harvard University
Boston, Massachusetts 02115

INTRODUCTION

Lice that infest man colonize in three separate areas: the clothes, the hair of the head, and the hair in the pubic area. The separateness of these colonizations is sufficiently distinct for human lice to be categorized as body (or clothes) lice, head lice, and crab (or pubic) lice.

The crab louse (*Pediculis pubis*) is markedly different anatomically and physiologically from both head and body lice; we will address ourselves to the subject of virulence of *R. prowazeki* for the crab louse in a subsequent paper. Head and body lice are considered by some entomologists to belong to two distinct species: *Pediculis humanus corporis* and *capitis*. However, the majority opinion seems to be that head and body lice are at opposite ends of a single species.[1] Regardless of taxonomic differences, it is clear that, geographically on man, colonies of head lice rarely migrate to the clothes and colonies of body (clothes) lice rarely migrate to the hair on the head; furthermore, almost without exception, eggs of head lice are laid on hair and eggs of body (clothes) lice are laid on clothes.

During this century, a further distinction between body and head lice has become clear-cut in the developed nations. Since 1900, infestation with body lice has markedly decreased in the United States, Western Europe, and in other nations with high standards of living. There remains, however, a wide prevalence of head lice, particularly on school children, in many of these countries. Sporadically, head lice reach epidemic proportions, such as in England in 1972, when more than 150,000 school children were reported infested. In Boston during the winter of 1973–74, an epidemic of head lice plagued the schools. Two school nurses who provided us with combed-out head lice informed us that they had examined the clothes and heads of hundreds of children with head lice. They insisted that they had not found any lice living in the clothes.

This greater prevalence of head lice over body lice is now also becoming noticeable in traditional endemic typhus areas of Eastern and Southeastern Europe, such as Bosnia, Yugoslavia.[2] Head lice are therefore still prevalent in the world and are becoming more available to be the sole transmitters of typhus, if they do transmit it.

Transmission of typhus from man to man by the human body louse (*P.*

* Supported mainly by contract DADA 17-70-C-0054 with the Research and Development command through the office of the Surgeon General, Department of the Army, Washington, D.C. and partly by the training program in Rickettsiology and Virology 5T1-AI0014-15 of the NIAID.

humanus corporis) was demonstrated by Nicolle *et al.* in 1909. Since 1909, Nicolle's discovery has been confirmed many times, and no other vector (except, possibly, the flea in certain atypical instances) has been implicated in the typhus transmission cycle.

However, there is little accurate information on the significance of head lice in the transmission of typhus. In 1912, Goldberger and Anderson [3] conducted inconclusive studies on the infectability of the head louse. Weyer's experiments [4] were also suggestive but not conclusive.

The present study was performed to determine whether head lice could be infected with *R. prowazeki,* and, if so, would the infection be fatal to the louse and would the rickettsiae be shed in the feces and therefore be available, as with infected body lice, to transmit and disseminate the disease.

MATERIALS AND METHODS

Source of Lice

Body lice used in this experiment were obtained from a normal colony of *P. humanus corporis* that had been adapted to feeding on a rabbit. This colony was supplied by the United States Department of Agriculture in 1964 and has been maintained with daily feedings on a succession of rabbits in our laboratory for more than 10 years. Lice are maintained by placing them on a shaved rabbit's belly and allowing them to feed for approximately 30 min daily. Between feedings, the lice are kept in a desiccator in a 29°C incubator with humidity maintained at about 60%. At intervals of 1–2 years, lice from this colony are removed, sacrificed, dissected, smeared on slides, and stained by Giemsa, Giménez, or immunofluorescence for the presence of rickettsiae. No rickettsiae have ever been demonstrated in smears of lice from this colony.

All head lice used in this experiment were obtained from Boston school children with obvious head louse infestations. A special fine-toothed comb was used to comb out the adult and instar lice into plastic bags. In the laboratory, lice were retrieved from the plastic bags and placed in a special metal louse feeding capsule.†

Physiologic Characteristics of Head Lice

There were no characteristic marks of head lice. However, head lice appeared to be more active than body lice. Furthermore, they preferred to move around on hairs rather than on felt cloth, which body lice preferred. The most obvious characteristic was that head lice consumed very little food, even when starved. Frequently, it was necessary to inspect a head louse under a dissecting microscope to determine if it had imbibed blood. A body louse usually fed itself to repletion, with a large, maximally distended abdomen. In addition, head lice would not, or could not, effectively feed through the bolting silk that covered one face of the metal feeding box. In contrast, all stages of body lice, from nymph to adult, readily fed through the bolting silk.

---

† These special feeding boxes were designed and donated by Dr. Anka Sitar of the Institute of Health Protection of Serbia, Belgrade, Yugoslavia.

Strain of Infecting Rickettsia

The Ankara strain of *R. prowazeki* was used to infect both body and head lice in this experiment. The Ankara strain was obtained from a case of classic louse-borne typhus in Ankara, Turkey by Dr. John C. Snyder in 1943. The pool of rickettsiae used was the 16th yolk sac passage in embryonated eggs of the original Ankara strain. Ankara pool 66H1397–50% yolk sac in PGS [5] was thawed, diluted to 10%, and spun at 1000 rpm for 10 min. The middle layer was removed and refrozen at −80°C to be used later (see below).

Manner of Infecting Lice

Rabbit Inoculation

We chose to infect lice by intravenous inoculation of a rabbit in the manner described by Snyder and Wheeler.[6] The lice were subsequently fed on the shaved belly of the infected rabbit. On the Day 0 of infection, 5.25 ml of 10% Ankara strain yolk sac material (see above) was thawed. This material was inoculated into the ear vein of a recently weaned 800-g rabbit.

Head Lice

The prepared colony of 39 wild head lice was immediately (11:30 AM) put on the cleanly shaved belly of the rabbit in a metal corral and was allowed to feed for 30 min, after which time the head lice ran about; they showed no interest in feeding. All 39 lice were examined under a dissecting microscope. No red blood could be seen in the gut of seven of the lice; these lice were discarded. The remaining 32 lice were put in a 29°C incubator. Four hours later, 16 (or 50% of those that fed initially) were placed on the same infected rabbit for a second feeding in the same manner. Most of these 16 lice fed for 15–30 min before detaching and starting to run around aimlessly. They were put back into the metal box in the 29°C incubator, rejoining the remaining 16 head lice that had fed only once. Thereafter, these head lice were fed and handled as described later.

Body Lice

Sixty body lice (50 adults and 10 newly hatched nymphs) were placed on the shaved rabbit's belly in a metal corral at 3:30 PM (4 hr after the inoculation, see above). They were allowed to feed for approximately 30 min, at which time almost all had fed to repletion, with distended abdomens. The 55 fed lice were put in a metal feeding box and placed in the 29°C incubator. Thereafter, they were fed and manipulated as described in the next section.

Method of Feeding Lice After They Were Infected with R. prowazeki

Body lice were fed on the forearm of one of us (E.S.M.) once daily at approximately 9 AM. The body lice were kept continually in a metal feeding box, one face of which was covered with bolting silk, which had holes large enough for the lice to feed through but not large enough for even the nymphs to escape. It was found that the body lice would feed to repletion once a day through the bolting silk with the metal box strapped tightly to the forearm. This was happily convenient by allowing the author (E.S.M.) to strap the body louse metal feeding box on the right forearm and take the head lice out of their metal box and put them on the skin of the left forearm. Thus, the right hand was free to manipulate the head lice. After the 9-AM feeding, the body lice were kept in the 29°C incubator until 5 PM and then were put in a pocket close to the body and kept there from 5 PM to approximately 9 AM the next day.

Head lice were fed loose on the forearm of the author (E.S.M.) three times a day, usually at 9 AM, 5 PM, and 11 PM. Head lice were allowed to feed as long as they desired. However, they rarely fed to repletion, almost always only partially. Between feedings, they were kept in a metal feeding box. Between 9:30 AM and 5 PM, they were maintained in a 29°C incubator (see *Body Lice*). Between 5 PM and 9 AM the next day, they were kept in a pocket close to the body. Head lice did not feed well through the bolting silk in the metal box feeder. They were always removed from the box and allowed to feed while free on the skin.

Immunofluorescent Testing of the Lice and Feces

Collecting Dead Lice

The metal feeding box that contained the infected body lice was opened only once every 24 hr, namely, when they were fed, at about 9 AM. Any dead lice were removed at this time and placed in a separate small vial at ±4°C until processed. The infected head lice were examined three times daily at approximately 9 AM, 5 PM, and 11 PM. Dead lice were removed and placed at ±4°C in separate vials until processed.

Smearing Lice

The technique for smearing lice was developed by Dr. Jacob A. Gaon of the Department of Epidemiology in the Sarajevo Medical School, Sarajevo, Yugoslavia. A small drop of water was placed slightly away from the center of a microscope slide. The louse to be smeared was placed in the drop and under a dissecting microscope. With a cataract knife, a cut was made at the junction of the thorax and abdomen. Then, under ordinary vision, the abdomen was pulled away from the thorax and dragged into the dry central area of the slide, where, as it was dragged, the gut tissues dried out, were pulled apart, and then were stretched into thin layers suitable for staining.

Feces of lice were emulsified in very small drops of sterile water and dried on the slide.

Immunofluorescent (IF) Staining of Louse Smears

A simple standard three-layer indirect IF test was performed. The louse (or feces) smears represented the *R. prowazeki* antigen to be tested for its presence or absence. A high titered (1:5120) human serum from a Brill Zinsser disease patient was used at 1:80 (or 64 units) as the known positive *R. prowazeki* serum or second layer. Antihuman γ-globulin conjugated with fluorescein isothiocyanate was used as the third layer.

RESULTS

Developing a Stable Colony of Normal Wild Head Lice

One of the major impediments to performing the experiment became evident immediately atfer obtaining our first dozen wild head lice. The lice died quickly when we fed them once a day, which was our usual procedure. When we changed to two feedings per day, they still died. We noticed that they ate very little at each feeding. They appeared much more sensitive to variations in humidity and temperature. They were also more active and seemed to exhaust their blood meal rapidly. Moreover, they could not feed regularly through bolting silk in a feeding box, in contrast to the ability of our departmental colony of rabbit-fed body lice to do so.

We finally developed a feeding method by which we could keep head lice alive for a reasonable period of time (20–30 days) for experimentation. We did not attempt to develop a scheme for maintaining an optimal egg-laying colony for several generations. Our method consisted of feeding lice obtained in the wild outside a feeding box on the clean skin of the forearm, putting them on and picking them off after they ceased feeding. Three feedings were given at approximately 8-hr intervals at 9 AM, 5 PM, and 11 PM.

Precautions and Procedures with Lice After Infection with R. prowazeki

The lice were tightly taped inside a metal feeding box and were then sealed in a petri dish before being placed inside a pocket and kept close to the skin from 5 PM to 9 AM. Between 9 AM and 5 PM, the metal feeding box was kept in a desiccator jar inside a 29°C incubator at about 60% humidity. After the lice were infected with virulent *R. prowazeki,* they had to be handled by the author alone in special isolated areas.

The author had contracted louse-borne typhus in a laboratory in Cairo, Egypt in 1944 and had a serum antibody titer of 1:320 against *R. prowazeki* at the time of the experiment. A previous experiment with *R. prowazeki* strain E had demonstrated that blood meals that contained *R. prowazeki* antibodies did not alter the infection in the louse. Wisseman *et al.*[7] have also shown that typhus antibodies are not inhibitory in the louse gut.

Difficulties in Maintaining Wild Head Lice

TABLE 1 summarizes some of the difficulties involved in preparing a group of wild head lice for experimentation. On Day 0, two groups of lice were obtained in plastic bags. Lice had been combed into the bags from children's infested heads. On Day 1, 28 of 42 adults and 26 of 40 instars fed on the author's arm. By Day 2, all 28 adults who had fed survived, whereas only 14 instars remained of the original 40.

By Day 7, the daily mortality rate had markedly decreased, but there were only 20 survivors of 42 original adults and 8 survivors of 40 instars. Instars exhibited a high mortality rate at first but after adaptation appeared sturdier and lived longer than adults.

With only 28 seasoned head lice available on the day of the experiment, we added a group of 11 new wild head lice, mixed adults and instars, which had been sent to us the night before. Therefore, we had 39 head lice for the infection experiment, although we expected a high mortality from the unseasoned 11 mixed lice.

Louse Infection Data

On 6/19/74, we selected 50 adults and 10 newly hatched instars from our normal rabbit-fed colony of body lice. On the same day, we had 39 head lice

TABLE 1

PREPARING A NORMAL HEAD LOUSE COLONY FOR EXPERIMENTAL INFECTION

Beginning Date 6/12/74	Louse Feedings			
	Adults		Instars	
	Fed		Fed	
Day	Total	Dead *	Total	Dead *
0	42	—	40	—
1	28/42	—	26/40	—
2	28/28	14	14/26	14
3	21/28	0	10/14	12
4	20/21	7	8/10	4
7	20/20	1	8/8	2
Total	20/42	22	8/40	32

* Found dead in the morning before feeding.

(see above). The 39 head and 60 body lice were infected as described in the MATERIALS AND METHODS. TABLES 2 and 3 record the results after infection of the lice. The first three lines of TABLE 2 summarize the deaths from Days 0 to 4. The body lice fed well, 55 of 60 in one feeding. Of the 39 head lice, 32 fed poorly to fairly well in one or two feedings (see MATERIALS AND METHODS). By the fourth postinfection day, only 33 of 55 body lice and 16 of 32 head lice had survived. These 49 lice, which were manipulated in detail, represent the main part of the experiment.

TABLE 3 records the deaths from Day 5 onward as they occurred each day and the results of IF tests on the dead lice smeared and of tests on batches of feces removed from the feeding boxes on various days and tested by IF. As can be seen, all head lice dead from Days 5 to 9 were positive; of the 16 lice alive on Day 5, only three survived until Day 9, and these three, when sacrificed and tested, were also found to be infected with R. prowazeki. Of the 28 body lice alive on Day 5, five survived until Day 15. Of the 23 that died, 18 were positive;

TABLE 2

HEAD AND BODY LICE INFECTED BY FEEDING ON RABBIT
INOCULATED INTRAVENOUSLY WITH *R. prowazeki*
[TEST FOR INFECTION: IMMUNOFLUORESCENCE (IF)]

Day After Infection	Data	Body Lice	Head Lice
0	total lice put on infected rabbit	60	39
0	total successfully fed	55 *	32 †
0–4	total dead	22	16
0–4	no. lice infected / total tested	0/3	2/6 ‡
5–9	no. lice infected / total tested	—	16/16
6–15	no. lice infected / total tested	22/28	—

* One 30-min feeding only: it began 4 hr after rabbit infected intravenously.

† Two 30-min feedings: one immediately after infecting the rabbit intravenously (all 32) and another 4 hr later for ½ colony (16).

‡ One positive on Day 0, another positive on Day 2.

TABLE 3

HEAD AND BODY LICE INFECTED BY FEEDING ON RABBIT
INOCULATED INTRAVENOUSLY WITH *R. prowazeki*
[TEST FOR INFECTION: IMMUNOFLUORESCENCE (IF)]

Day After Infection	Body Lice No. Lice Infected / Total Examined	Feces	Head Lice No. Lice Infected / Total Examined	Feces
0–4	see TABLE 2		see TABLE 2	
5	0/5 *		1/1 *	+, ++ †
6	4/4	±, ± †	5/5	++++, +++
7	3/4	±, ++	—	+++, +++
8	1/1	+, ++	3/3	+++, +++, ++++
9	3/3	++	7/7	
10	0/1	+++	3 L=live	
11	1/1	+++	3 M=moribund	
12	4/5		1 D=dead	
13	0/1	++, +++		
14	—			
15	6/8 5 L, 3 D			
Control lice	0/4	(—)	0/4	(—)

* Numerator, number of lice positive for *R. prowazeki;* denominator, total number tested by IF.

† ±, Suspicious; +, few definitely with rickettsiae; ++, +++, ++++. moderate to massive rickettsial infection.

four of the five living and sacrificed on Day 15 were positive for *R. prowazeki.*
Feces from head lice were moderately positive for *R. prowazeki* on Day 5
and were heavily positive by Day 8. Feces from body lice were only suspicious
on Day 6, definitely positive on Day 7, and quite strongly positive on Day 10
and later.

Smears of four normal head lice and four normal body lice and the feces
they passed were negative for *R. prowazeki.*

Referring again to TABLE 2, of the many lice of both kinds that died through
the fourth experimental day, three body lice and six head lice were tested.
None of the body lice were positive by IF, but two of the six head lice had a
few distinct rickettsiae by IF.

From Days 5 to 9, all 16 dead and sacrificed head lice were positive for
R. prowazeki. From Day 6, when the first body louse was demonstrated to
be positive, through the 15th day of experimental infection, 22 of the 28 body
lice were positive by IF.

In a previous pilot study that employed various staining methods, IF was
superior to either Giemsa or Giménez. In this pilot experiment, seven of eight
head lice infected with the Ankara strain of *R. prowazeki* were positive for
rickettsiae by the IF test. Because of the superior results with IF in testing
smears of lice and feces in the pilot test, we used this test exclusively in the
main experiment.

DISCUSSION

This experimental work clearly demonstrates that the head louse (*P.
humanus capitis*) is highly susceptible to virulent *R. prowazeki.* From the fifth
day of infection onward, all 16 head lice tested, the 13 that died and three that
were sacrificed alive on the ninth postinfection day, displayed massive infection
of gut tissues.

As mentioned previously, in a pilot experiment prior to the main experiment,
seven of eight head lice infected with the Ankara strain of *R. prowazeki* were
demonstrated by IF to be infected with typhus rickettsiae. Furthermore, in both
the pilot and the main experiment, all pooled feces of infected head lice from
the sixth day onward were demonstrated by IF to be heavily contaminated with
R. prowazeki rickettsiae. Head lice, therefore, appear to be potential transmitters of *R. prowazeki* under optimal epidemiologic circumstances.

It was surprising that the body lice that fed on the same infected rabbit in
the main experiment exhibited a slightly lower infection rate (78%) and a
longer time lag for the infection to develop (maximum 15 days). There are
several possible explanations.

The head lice fed for 30 min on the rabbit *immediately* after it had been
infected intravenously with *R. prowazeki.* Because of an accident, we were not
able to feed the body lice on the same rabbit until 4 hr after it had been intravenously infected. Snyder and Wheeler fed groups of body lice on a rabbit at
various intervals after intravenous infection of *R. prowazeki.* Their results
make an interesting comparison with ours.

Of 49 body lice fed on an infected rabbit immediately after it had been
infected with *R. prowazeki* intravenously, 48 (98%) were positive for rickettsiae
on smear testing. Of a second group of 19 body lice that were placed on the

same rabbit for the first time 8½ hr after the intravenous infection, only 13 (68%) were ultimately demonstrated to be infected. Thus, the body lice fed later had both a lower infection rate and a longer survival time as a group than those fed immediately. This result may be a partial or complete explanation for our differences between infections in the body and head lice.

However, there were other differences in experimental details that might be significant. For example, the body lice were only examined once daily, at which time dead lice were removed to the refrigerator. Head lice, conversely, were examined three times daily; therefore, head lice were removed more promptly after death, so that head louse smears and test samples were, in general, in better condition than those from body lice. Furthermore, the three small feedings per day of the head lice might produce quite different infection conditions in the gut when compared to the single daily gut-distending blood meal that the body louse had to digest. Finally, a domesticated colony of body lice fed over several decades on rabbit blood may possibly have developed some natural immunity to typhus.

One may question why we fed half (16) of the head louse colony a second time 4 hr after the first meal. In fact, we were distressed by the small amount of blood ingested by most head lice at the first meal. For almost half of the lice, we had to use a dissecting scope to determine the presence of red blood in the gut. We were not certain that the head lice had imbibed sufficient blood to become infected. However, when we fed the head lice a second time on the rabbit, we were more concerned that the rabbit blood might be toxic to the lice.[8] Therefore, we "scatter-basketted our eggs" and only gave half of the head louse colony infected rabbit blood on the second occasion; we hoped for at least some infectious meals and some survivors. Unfortunately, our data are not sufficiently precise to state the exact toxicity of the rabbit blood or to make a firm conclusion as to whether mortality of lice that fed twice on the rabbit was higher than that for those that fed only once.

SUMMARY

Wild head lice were obtained by combing out adult and instar lice from the uncut hair of school children. Normal body lice were selected from a colony of rabbit-adapted body lice obtained from the United States Department of Agriculture and maintained in the Department of Microbiology for more than 10 yr. Thirty-nine head lice and 60 body lice were fed on a rabbit that had been injected intravenously with a 10% suspension of a yolk sac pool from eggs heavily infected with the Ankara strain of virulent *R. prowazeki*. Five days after infection, 33 body lice and 16 head lice had survived and were feeding on a volunteer. Between Days 5 and 9, 13 head lice were dead or moribund and all of them were positive by IF for *R. prowazeki*. The three surviving head lice were also positive. Tests on the 33 body lice showed that 22 were positive for *R. prowazeki*, including four of the five body lice that survived until Day 15. In summary, head lice can be readily infected with *R. prowazeki* and disseminate virulent *R. prowazeki* organisms in their feces. Thus, theoretically, head lice appear to be highly potential as transmitters of *R. prowazeki* under optimal epidemiologic circumstances.

ACKNOWLEDGMENTS

We thank Drs. John C. Snyder, Andrew Spielman, and J. William Vinson for their invaluable advice and help in designing the experiment and in working out technical details of handling the lice. We also thank Mrs. Barbara Walsh and Mrs. Rita Cunningham for their imaginative and expert technical assistance in providing live entomologic specimens. Mrs. Judith Spielman provided indispensable assistance in growing and processing infectious inocula and in infecting the rabbit.

REFERENCES

1. BUXTON, P. A. 1939. The Louse. Edward Arnold & Co. London, England.
2. GAON, J. A. 1973. Louse eradication programs in Yugoslavia. *In* Proceedings of the International Symposium on the Control of Lice and Louse-Borne Diseases. Pan American Health Organization Scientific Publication No. 263. Washington, D.C.
3. GOLDBERGER, J. & J. F. ANDERSON. 1912. The transmission of typhus fever with especial reference to transmission by the head louse (*Pediculus capitis*). Public Health Rep. (US) **27:** 297–307.
4. WEYER, F. 19xx. Personal communication.
5. BOVARNICK, M. R., J. C. MILLER & J. C. SNYDER. 1950. The influence of certain salts, amino acids, sugars and proteins on the stability of rickettsiae. J. Bacteriol. **59:** 509–522.
6. SNYDER, J. C. & C. M. WHEELER. 1945. The experimental infection of the human body louse *Pediculus humanus corporis* with murine and epidemic louse-borne typhus strains. J. Exp. Med. **32:** 1–20.
7. WISSEMAN, C. L., JR., J. L. BOESE, A. D. WADDELL & D. J. SILVERMAN. This monograph.
8. VINSON, J. W. 1962. Personal experience with lice and rabbit blood in Mexico.

MURINE TYPHUS RICKETTSIAE IN THE ORIENTAL RAT FLEA *

S. Ito, J. W. Vinson, and T. J. McGuire, Jr.

Department of Anatomy
Harvard Medical School
and Department of Microbiology
Harvard University School of Public Health
Boston, Massachusetts 02115

INTRODUCTION

Rickettsia mooseri, the etiologic agent of murine typhus, is transmitted from its natural rodent host to man by the oriental rat flea, *Xenopsylla cheopis*.[1] When these rickettsiae are imbibed in an infectious blood meal, they propagate in the midgut epithelium of the flea and are excreted in the feces, which thus becomes the actual vehicle of infection.[2-4] A similar sequence of events occurs in the transmission of epidemic typhus rickettsiae by the infected human body louse. Adult rat fleas may under normal circumstances live for many months. Infection of the flea with *R. mooseri* can occur only during the parasitic adult stage, and the life-span of the flea is not shortened by the infection.[5]

Although electron microscopic features of the infection of the body louse by *Rickettsiae prowazeki* have been examined in several studies,[5-12] no comparable investigations have been made of rickettsial infection in oriental rat fleas. Indeed, ultrastructural studies on the flea midgut epithelium have so far been limited to a short report by Reinhardt *et al.*[13] on the midgut of the oriental rat flea and two other species and to an earlier description by Richards and Richards[14] of a novel beaded layer that forms the basement lamina that underlies the midgut epithelium of the flea, *Ctenophthalmus*.

Herein, we intend to provide further information on normal midgut epithelium of *X. cheopis* and to elucidate some of the ultrastructural features of the infection of this species by murine typhus rickettsiae.

MATERIALS AND METHODS

The Wilmington strain[15] of *R. mooseri* used in the present study represents the eighth passage in the yolk sacs of developing chick embryos since it was received in this laboratory in 1946. The stock pool of this strain was a 50% suspension of infected yolk sac in sucrose-PG,[13] aliquots of which were stored at −70° C.

Our colony of *Xenopsylla cheopis*, originally obtained from the United States Department of Agriculture, Entomology Research Division, Gainesville, Florida, has been maintained in our laboratory. Rearing procedures followed those recommended by Cole.[16] Fasted adult fleas of unknown age were used

* Supported in part by grant AI 11508 from the National Institute of Allergy and Infectious Diseases.

in some trials, but in most of the experiments, recently metamorphosed, unfed adults were employed.

Fleas were infected with *R. mooseri* by feeding them on infected mice. Adult albino mice that weighed 20–30 g were inoculated intraperitoneally with 0.5 ml of a 1% suspension of the stock pool of *R. mooseri*, a concentration that caused death of mice in from 3 to 5 days. A mouse infected 3 days previously was placed in a small wire mesh cage that contained food pellets and a piece of potato. The cage was then suspended in the jar that contained approximately 100 fleas in a bed of fine sterilized sand and kept at about 25° C. The mouse was restricted in the jar until it died from the infection. A second, and sometimes a third, infected mouse was sequentially caged with the fleas to ensure a high percentage of infected fleas. Mice were autopsied, and infection with rickettsiae was verified by examination of Giménez-stained smears of peritoneal exudate, spleen, and liver cells.

To provide comparative information on the ultrastructure of *R. mooseri*, Vero cells infected with this rickettsia were examined electron microscopically. Cells were propagated in 25-ml plastic tissue culture flasks in medium 199 with 10% fetal calf serum. No antibiotics were used in the medium. Forty-eight to 72 hr after culturing the cells, when a monolayer was formed, the medium was withdrawn and 1 ml of a 20% suspension of the stock pool of *R. mooseri* in sucrose-PG was layered over the cells. After incubation for 30 min at 37° C, the inoculum was aspirated, and the cell monolayer was rinsed twice with fresh medium and cultured in 5 ml of the same medium at 37° C. Progress of infection in the cells was checked by daily examination of Giménez-stained smears.[15]

Fleas in various nutritional states were anesthetized by chilling them in a container on crushed ice. The midgut was dissected from the flea on a wax plate in a drop of fixative. After several trials with various fixatives and combinations, the most reproducible fixation for the midgut tissue was found to be a mixture of 3% paraformaldehyde, 4% glutaraldehyde, and 0.05% trinitrocresol in 0.05 N phosphate buffer. To make this fixative, 0.5 ml of a 50% glutaraldehyde solution was mixed with 0.05 ml of a 50% solution of hydrogen peroxide according to the method of Peracchia et al.[17] This mixture was then added to the formaldehyde and trinitrocresol fixative, which was made up in phosphate buffer.[18] The midguts were fixed for 1 hr at 4° C, washed with the same buffer solution, and postosmicated with 1% OsO_4 in phosphate buffer. The tissue was then treated with 1% uranyl acetate in a maleate buffer at pH 5.2, rapidly dehydrated through graded ethanol solutions, and embedded in a mixture of diepoxyoctane and dodecenyl succinic anhydride according to Luft.[19] The infectious yolk sac inoculum, samples of infected mouse spleen, liver and peritoneal scrapings, and infected cell cultures were fixed and embedded in a similar manner. Thin sections of all tissues were stained with uranyl acetate and lead citrate and were examined by transmission electron microscopy.

For freeze-fractured replicas of tissues and rickettsiae, flea midguts and infected tissue culture cells were fixed for 30 min at 4° C in a mixture of 2% paraformaldehyde, 2.5% glutaraldehyde in cacodylate buffer at pH 7.4 that contained 2 mg/ml $CaCl_2$. The tissue was washed in cacodylate buffer, infiltrated for 2 hr with 20% buffered glycerol at room temperature, mounted on disks, frozen in liquid Freon® 22 (chlorodifluoromethane), and stored in liquid nitrogen. Specimens were fractured in a Balzers apparatus (Balzers High Vacuum Corp.), and the platinum-carbon replicas were cleaned in a 4–6% sodium hypochlorite solution and collected on grids after several distilled water washes.

OBSERVATIONS

Ultrastructure of the Flea Midgut Epithelium

The midgut of the flea forms a significant part of the digestive tract and is the major site for storage, digestion, and absorption of the blood meals. Simple cuboidal to pseudostratified columnar cells form the midgut epithelium, which varies in thickness, depending on the degree of distention by its contents. The lumenal surface of these cells bears numerous microvilli arranged in a typical striated border. There is no cuticular border over the midgut epithelium, and, unlike the majority of insects, a peritrophic membrane is absent.

An electron micrograph of a portion of an epithelial cell (FIGURE 1) illustrates some of the features of the flea midgut. Only one type of epithelial cell, which is low cuboidal in shape in greatly distended midguts and tall columnar in empty collapsed midguts, seems to be present. These cells contain a nucleus often located in the apical part of the cell, and elaborate nucleoli (FIGURES 1 & 2) are consistent features of the nuclei. Mitochondria are moderately numerous, particularly in the apical cytoplasm, immediately beneath the microvilli. Some cells contain concentrated lamellar arrays of granular endoplasmic reticulum, but this cell component is usually scattered throughout the cytoplasm (FIGURES 1, 3 & 4). Occasional dense lysosome-like bodies and multivesicular bodies are present, and some cells contain numerous clear vacuoles. Smooth endoplasmic reticulum and Golgi complexes are inconspicuous components and are only rarely encountered.

The apical surface is covered with a uniform array of microvilli about 100 nm in diameter and 1–2 μm long. Their outer aspect is coated with a filamentous surface coat, which is not visible when the lumen is filled with blood. The core of the microvilli contains fine filaments that extend a short distance into the apical cytoplasm.

The lateral cell borders at the apical end of the cell have extensive areas of continuous junctions or zonula continua, which are characteristic of arthropod epithelia in place of the better known tight junction. In low-power micrographs (FIGURES 2, 3, 5 & 6), this junction appears as a continuous dense line that forms as much as one third of the lateral cell border. At higher magnifications, the trilaminar plasma membranes are seen to be about 5 nm thick, and the intercellular space of the continuous junction is about 15 nm wide. The extracellular space contains a substance of high density, and no distinct striations or structural specializations are visible. In freeze-fractured replicas, the continuous junction is represented by a series of single or multiple ridges on the A face and grooves on the B face (FIGURE 7). Typical septate junctions, areas of gap junctions (with particles on the B face, that is, gap junction B; FIGURE 8), scattered segments of tight junctions, and occasional desmosomes are also present along the lateral cell border.

The basal cell membrane is very irregular and forms numerous infoldings on the basal labyrinth described by Reinhardt *et al.*[10] Some of these infoldings are continuous with the lateral cell membrane (FIGURE 1). Immediately underlying the cell is an unusual beaded layer (FIGURES 1, 9 & 15). This structure was described in detail for a different genus of flea, *Ctenophthalmus*, by Richards and Richards[14] and resembles the structure in *Xenopsylla*.[13] The beaded layer and its underlying basement lamina-like structure form a smooth contoured base that only rarely extends into the basal folds of the epithelium.

Between the base of the epithelial cell, with its beaded layer, and the hemo-

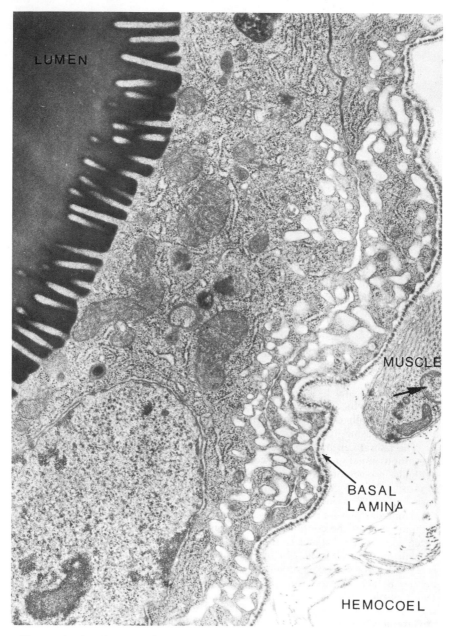

FIGURE 1. An electron micrograph of parts of two midgut epithelial cells from a control *Xenopsylla cheopis*. The blood-filled lumen is very dense. Mitochondria, rough-surfaced endoplasmic reticulum, and some dark lysosome-like inclusions fill much of the apical cytoplasm. A prominent basal labyrinth with much clear extracellular space is present. Along the base of the cell, the basal lamina with its beaded layer underlies the epithelium. Part of a striated muscle cell lies in the space between the basal lamina and the boundary layer that borders the hemocoel. In the muscle cell (arrow), an indigenous rickettsia-like oragnism is present. ×19,000.

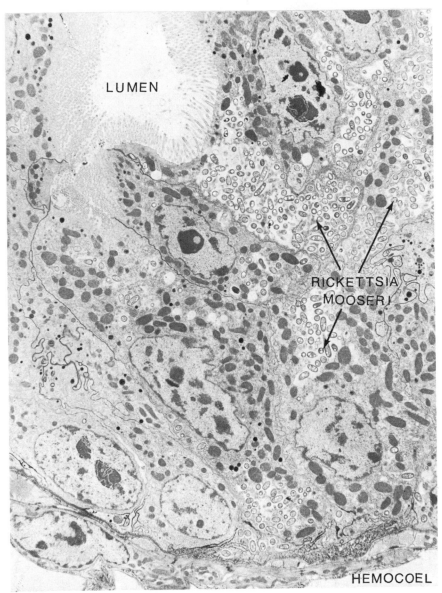

FIGURE 2. A low-power view of infected flea midgut cells in a region interpreted to be a cell nest. Most of the fully differentiated cells contain moderate numbers of infectious microorganisms. Near the lower left, there are two cells with basal nuclei, and these cells may be undifferentiated precursor cells. They are not infected with rickettsiae. ×2500.

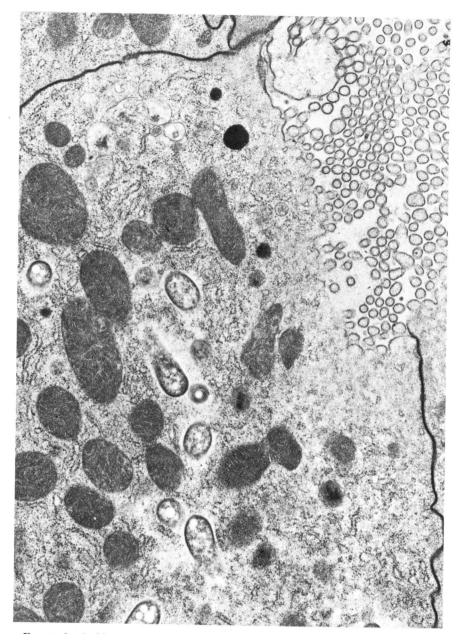

FIGURE 3. A thin section through the apical cytoplasm of a flea midgut cell that is lightly infected with *R. mooseri*. The microorganisms are scattered among the numerous mitochondria. A zone of low density surrounds the rickettsiae. The dense lateral cell borders are the usual appearance of the zonula continua at low magnification. ×27,000.

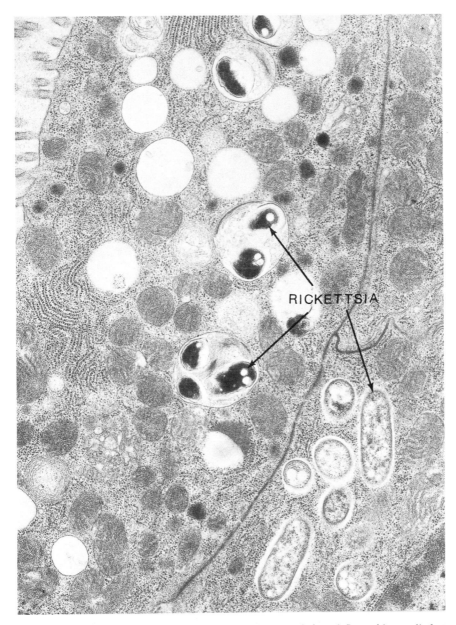

FIGURE 4. An electron micrograph of an *R. mooseri* infected flea midgut cell that has sequestered all of the rickettsiae in lysosomal vacuoles. These microorganisms appear to be homogeneous and dense, but the clear vacuolar spaces still remain. In contrast, rickettsiae in the cell at the lower right are not enclosed in a vacuole and appear to be normal. ×20,000.

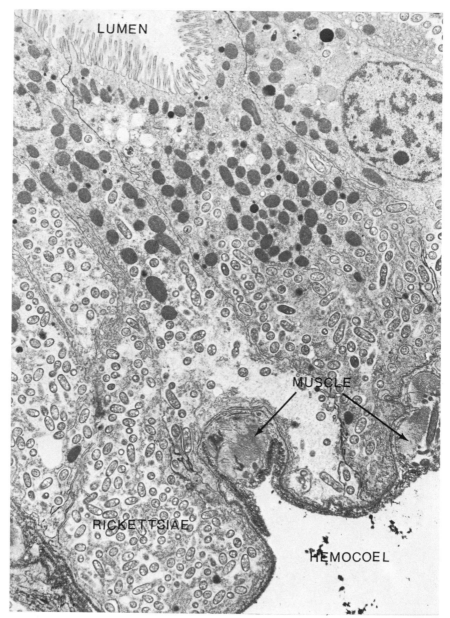

FIGURE 5. A low-power electron micrograph of midgut epithelium from a fasting flea. The cells are moderately infected with *R. mooseri*. Most of the rickettsiae are localized in the basal cytoplasm, where the basal labyrinth is no longer prominent. The midgut muscle fibers lie in furrows of epithelial cells. The hemocoel is separated from the base of the epithelium by the midgut investment, which is attenuated in this specimen. Several dividing rickettsiae are present. ×6100.

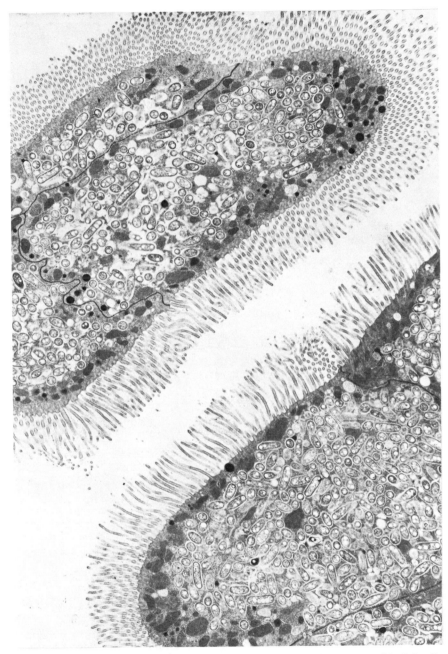

FIGURE 6. A tangential section of the apical parts of several midgut epithelial cells crowded with *R. mooseri*. In these cells, where proliferation of rickettsiae has resulted in a mass of tightly packed microorganisms, dividing forms are infrequently encountered. Note that the rim of apical cytoplasm, which is packed with mitochondria, is not penetrated by rickettsiae. ×5200.

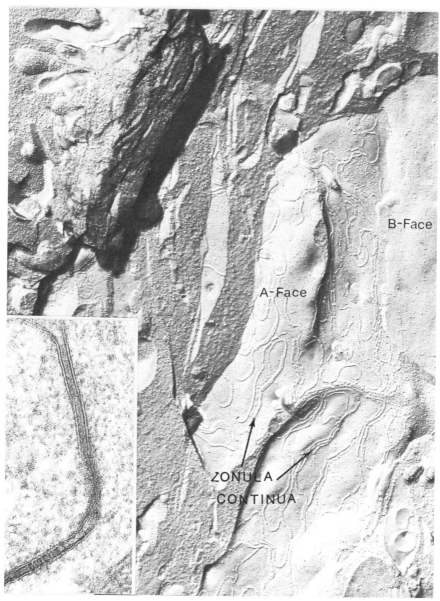

FIGURE 7. A freeze-fractured replica of apical portions of the flea midgut epithelium. A large part of the field includes the A face of the lateral plasma membrane with an extensive array of the zonula continua or continuous junction. On the A face, this junction appears as a series of single or multiple ridges and on the B face as fine grooves. The inset is a high-magnification thin section at the lumenal border. The trilaminar plasma membranes of the zonula continua are separated by a space filled with dense material. Near the lower left, faint striations of this junction are visible in this space. ×41,000; inset, ×120,000.

coel is a layer of variable thickness, the midgut investment, that contains striated muscle cells arranged circumferentially and longitudinally, a moderate amount of connective tissue filaments and collagen fibers, and a few connective tissue cells and tracheoles (FIGURES 1, 2, 5 & 15). An acellular, amorphous layer, the bounding layer, delineates the basal complex from the hemocoel. This complex

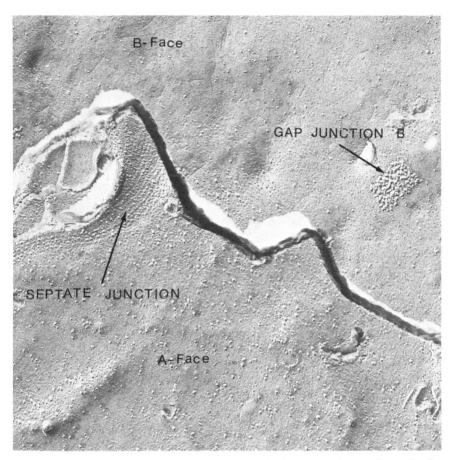

FIGURE 8. Freeze-fracture replica of the lateral plasma membranes from the flea midgut epithelium. The A-face fracture includes a linear array of beaded particles of a septate junction. A gap junction B with particle clusters on the B face of the membrane is also present. ×68,000.

is so varied in its width that in some areas, the beaded layer basal lamina is adjacent to the bounding layer of the hemocoel (FIGURE 5).

In widely scattered sites, there are small nidi or cell nests where undifferentiated basal cells rest on the beaded layer. Most of these cells apparently do not extend to the lumen. They contain a less well-organized or differentiated cytoplasm and are presumed to divide and differentiate into new epithelial cells (FIGURE 2).

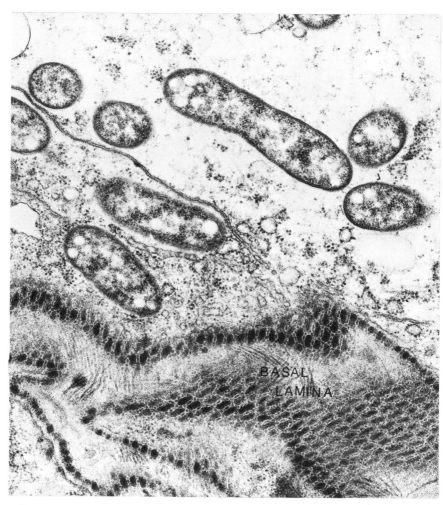

FIGURE 9. Part of the basal cytoplasm of infected flea midgut cells and its obliquely sectioned basal lamina. The upper epithelial cell has a cytoplasm of very low density, in contrast to the lower cell. Both contain rickettsiae that have numerous vacuole-like clear areas, particularly near their poles. Note the relative absence of a capsule-like halo around the microorganism in this preparation. The portion of the basal lamina that is sectioned tangentially illustrates the unique appearance of the beaded layer. ×33,000.

Ultrastructure of the Infected Midgut Epithelium

The number of rickettsiae found in the infected flea midgut epithelial cells varies from a very few scattered microorganisms (FIGURES 2, 3 & 5) to many hundreds of densely packed rickettsiae (FIGURES 6 & 12). The mode of entry of the infectious rickettsiae into the cytoplasmic matrix of the host cell is not known. Once in the cytoplasm, they are not segregated from other cytoplasmic organelles and lie directly in the cytoplasm. In many cells, the microorganisms are separated from the host cell cytoplasm by a thin rim or halo of low density (FIGURES 6, 13 & 14). However, examples of rickettsiae without such a clear space around them are also present (FIGURE 9). There is some reason to suspect that this halo may be exaggerated during specimen preparation. When concentrations of rickettsiae are arrayed in focal areas of the cytoplasm, those areas are very often marked by a lowered density, rarified matrix of host cell cytoplasm, as is evident in FIGURES 2, 3 & 5. These areas still contain rough surfaced endoplasmic reticulum and mitochondria and do not exhibit obvious disruptive or degenerative changes.

The concentration and close packing of *R. mooseri* in the flea midgut cell may be so high that they are a dense mass (FIGURES 6 & 12). In these states, dividing binary forms are still present but less common than in the earlier stages of infection, when fewer rickettsiae are present. Binary forms in various stages of fission are quite common (FIGURE 5). Less frequently encountered are bead chains of three or four rickettsiae (FIGURES 5 & 13).

In lightly infected cells, the rickettsiae are often localized in focal areas of a few organisms or other clusters of larger numbers. These areas may be in the basal cytoplasm, paranuclear zone, or in the apical cytoplasm. A narrow zone that is usually not invaded by rickettsiae, even in very heavily infected cells, is the rim of apical cytoplasm immediately beneath the microvillous border (FIGURES 6 & 12). This band of cytoplasm usually contains numerous mitochondria, in contrast to the basal region of the midgut cell, which has numerous infoldings and relatively few mitochondria.

The process of epithelial cell lysis or extrusion was infrequently encountered, so that the process of cell renewal has not been observed. However, some examples of rickettsia-filled cells in the process of being disrupted were seen (FIGURE 12). In this particular case, the apical cytoplasm bulges into the gut lumen, the plasma membrane is ruptured in numerous sites, and the microvilli are disorganized. These changes are presumed to represent the process for release of rickettsiae into the gut lumen. In the present study, only limited numbers of *R. mooseri* were observed free in the gut lumen. This was true whether midguts were examined soon after feeding on an infectious blood meal or in later stages when numerous infected cells were conspicuous.

Most of the rickettsiae found in the epithelial cells of the flea midgut are not found in vacuoles, but there are occasional organisms found in lysosomal vacuoles. These enclosed rickettsiae may be in various stages of condensation and disruption. In some cells, all or most of the microorganisms are sequestered in vacuoles (FIGURE 4).

Indigenous rickettsia-like microorganisms were never observed in uninfected control flea midgut epithelial cells, and several fleas fed on infected mice also revealed no rickettsiae in the epithelial cells. However, rickettsia-like microorganisms were found in some control flea muscle cells around the midgut epithelial cells (FIGURES 1 & 15). These microorganisms are directly embedded in the muscle cell cytoplasm and coexist with mitochondria. Some are enclosed in a tight-fitting membrane, presumed to be infolded plasma membrane. They seem to cause no drastic disruption of the muscle cell ultrastructure, but myofilaments are displaced and, in some cells, focally disorganized. In some animals, occasional microorganisms were found free in the connective tissue space among the collagenous fibers. The number of these extraepithelial cell rickettsiae was never very high, and their presence was variable. Fewer than half of the fleas examined regularly contained rickettsiae in the midgut striated muscle cells. In fleas exposed to *R. mooseri,* the presence of microorganisms in the muscle cells was also variable. In other words, even the heavy infection of the epithelium did not seem to influence the presence or absence or increase the number of rickettsiae in the muscle cells and extracellular space.

The morphology of these extraepithelial cell rickettsiae is very similar to *R. mooseri* in the epithelial cell, but they tend to be slightly thinner in diameter and commonly more than 2 μm in length, whereas only exceptional *R. mooseri* measure more than 2.5 μm in length. They also contain clear vacuolar areas, but their size and number are never as high as in the *R. mooseri* that proliferate in the epithelium.

Ultrastructure of R. mooseri

In structure, *R. mooseri* generally resembles other rickettsiae. Its morphology is not greatly changed whether examined in preparations of the original chick yolk sac inoculum (FIGURES 11 & 14, *right*), in infected tissue culture cells (FIGURE 16), in infected mouse cells (FIGURE 10), or in the flea midgut epithelial cells. There are, however, some differences in the size and internal characteristics of rickettsiae grown in different host cells. *R. mooseri* examined in the infected chick yolk sac inoculum are 0.2–0.3 μm in width and rarely more than 1 μm in length, even when they are undergoing binary fission (FIGURE 14, *right*). These dimensions are similar to those of rickettsiae found in mouse polymorphonuclear leukocytes infected with the yolk sac inoculum (FIGURE 10). In contrast, rickettsiae that proliferate in tissue culture cells (FIGURE 16), or in the flea midgut epithelium are larger and measure 0.30–0.45 μm in width or diameter and up to 2.5 μm in length. The great majority of longitudinal profiles, however, are no more than 1–1.5 μm long. The limiting investment of rickettsiae is the cell wall and the underlying plasma membrane. These two components and the intervening zone are about 25 nm thick (FIGURES 13, 14 & 17). The trilaminar cell wall is about 10 nm thick and is composed of a thin outer leaflet about 2 nm thick, a clear space about 3 nm thick, and an inner dense component about 5 nm thick. The inner dense line of the cell wall may also appear to have a narrow clear zone in its center. The trilaminar plasma membrane, which is about 5 nm thick, is often difficult to distinguish

FIGURE 10 (*top*). A polymorphonuclear leukocyte from mouse peritoneal exudate after infection with *R. mooseri.* Several rickettsiae, some of which contain small clear vacuole-like areas, are visible in the cytoplasm. ×27,000.

FIGURE 11 (*bottom*). *R. mooseri* in the yolk sac inoculum used to infect mice on which fleas were infected. A binary form undergoing fission and a rod-shaped organism are shown. The rickettsiae are similar in size and appearance to those found in the infected mouse cell. ×55,000.

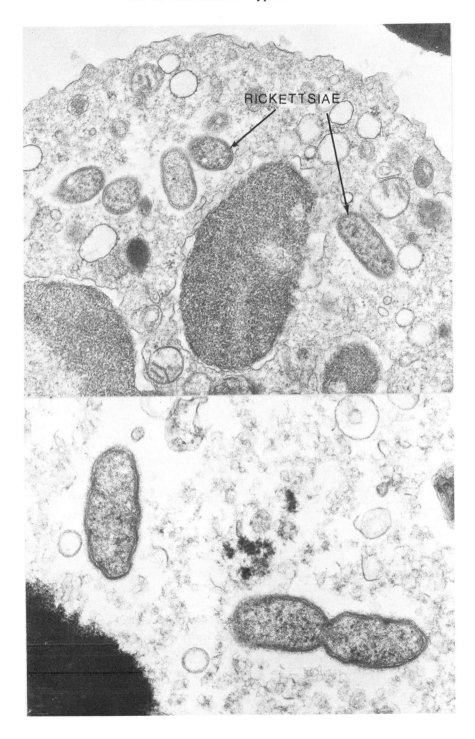

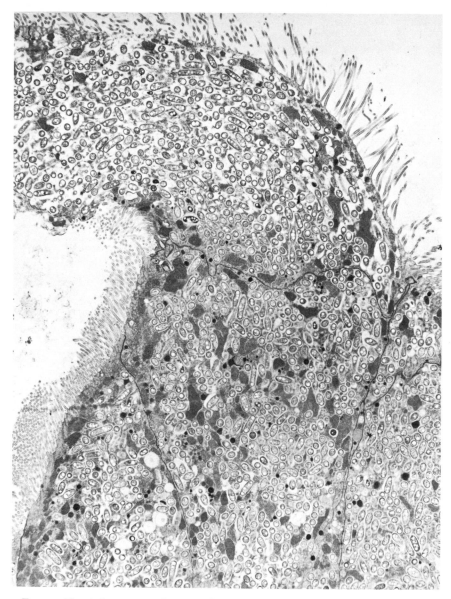

FIGURE 12. A low-power electron micrograph of an extruding epithelial cell and parts of several other flea midgut epithelial cells heavily packed with *R. mooseri*. The uppermost cell is in the process of disruption. Its striated border is disorganized, discontinuities of the plasmalemma are apparent, and very little cytoplasmic matrix remains. In contrast, the intact cells also contain a very high concentration of rickettsiae but retain their organization. ×3300.

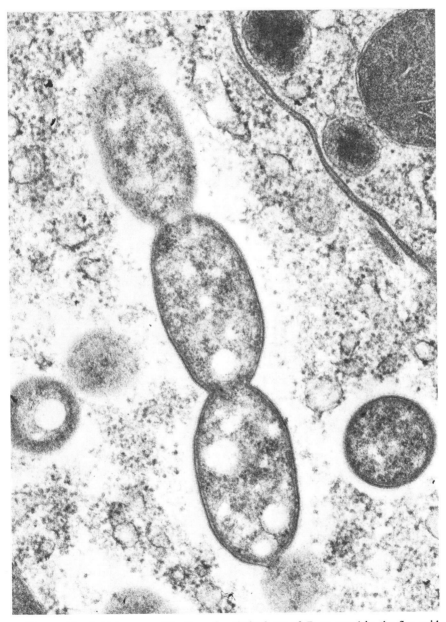

FIGURE 13. A higher magnification of a chain form of *R. mooseri* in the flea midgut. The division furrows have begun to separate the microorganisms into four units. At the upper right, areas of gap junctions and possible focal tight junctions are visible. ×62,000.

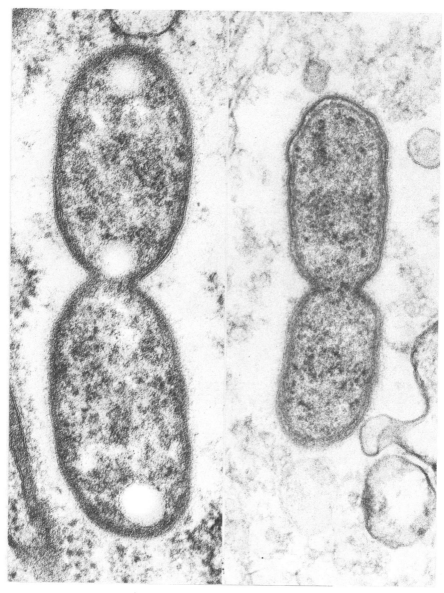

FIGURE 14. *Left: R. mooseri* in the flea midgut epithelial cell undergoing binary fission. The cytoplasm contains several clear vacuole-like areas in addition to its usual contents. ×88,000. *Right: R. mooseri* in the chick yolk sac inoculum used for these studies. Note that the rickettsiae in the yolk sac are markedly smaller than are the corresponding dividing forms in the louse gut cell. The actual magnification of this Figure is slightly higher than that of FIGURE 14, *left.* ×90,000.

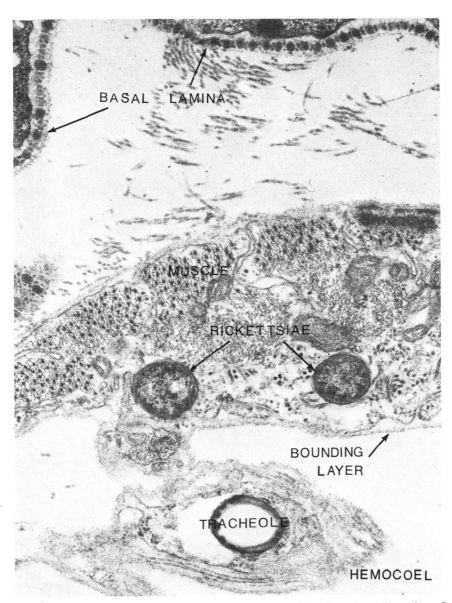

FIGURE 15. A micrograph of the midgut investment of the flea. A small portion of the epithelial cell with its basal lamina is present. The hemocoel with the bounding layer is near the bottom of the illustration. The striated muscle cell sectioned transversely includes myofilaments, mitochondria, and corss-sectioned profiles of two indigenous rickettsia-like microorganisms. Note that the myofilaments in their vicinity are disorganized and partially disrupted. ×63,000.

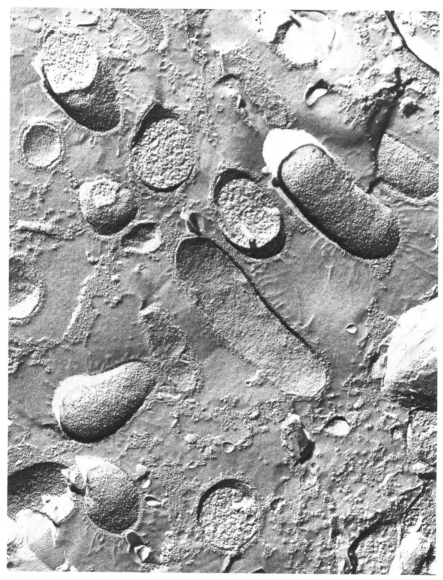

FIGURE 16. A freeze-fractured replica of *R. mooseri* propagated in the cytoplasm of a tissue culture cell. The membrane fractures are, in large part, through the plasma membrane and not through the cell wall. The A face (convex) contains numerous paticles, whereas the B face (concave) is relatively free of particles. On the outer surface of the cell wall, there are radiating structures that may be due to the surface coat on the rickettsiae. ×37,000.

and is separated from the cell wall by a 10-nm space filled with material of intermediate density.

On the free surface of the cell wall, there may be a layer of fine filamentous material that radiates outward (FIGURES 14 & 17). This component and its surrounding clear halo appear to form a capsule-like investment around the rickettsiae. Its presence, however, is not consistent, and it may be thicker in some preparations and nearly absent in others.

The cytoplasm of *R. mooseri* contains a moderate number of particles, identified in other rickettsiae as ribosomes, and a meshwork of fine filaments that represents the DNA component of the cytoplasm. In addition, clear vacuolar areas, without a limiting membrane, that measure up to 150 nm in diameter are particularly abundant in *R. mooseri* that proliferate in the flea midgut cells (FIGURES 2, 3, 5, 6, 9, 12–14 & 17). Sections of rickettsiae may include profiles of eight or more of these clear areas. Some may be partially or completely filled with a homogeneous substance of low density, whereas others appear to be void of any structured inclusion. They are readily perforated in thin sections and appear as holes in the specimen (FIGURE 17). These vacuolar areas are present but much less prominent in murine typhus rickettsiae found in the yolk sac inoculum, infected mouse cells, or in cell cultures.

DISCUSSION

The present report is an attempt to elucidate the ultrastructural features of the oriental rat flea midgut and to describe the distribution and proliferation of *R. mooseri* in these fleas. Previous studies on the fine structure of flea midguts have been limited to the short paper by Reinhardt *et al.*,[13] who described the salient features in three different species: *Xenopsylla cheopis*, *Echidnophaga gallacea*, and *Junga penetrans*. The flea intestinal epithelia is not exceptionally different from other insects that have been studied in greater detail, such as the mosquito.[20-22]

A common feature of arthropod epithelial cell junctions is the presence of the poorly understood type of cell junction, the zonula continua or continuous junction. It was first described in insect intestinal epithelium by Noirot and Noirot[23] and subsequently in several other studies.[24-27] Though very different in its structure from the well-known tight and septate junctions, it apparently performs some similar functions. Histochemical studies indicate the presence of a glycoprotein component in the junctional structure,[24] and studies on lanthanum penetration into the junction reveal penetration between the continuous bars.[27] The continuous junction has some of the morphologic features of tight junctions and septate junctions; it seems to be a combination of these two forms. Its role in the flea gut is obscure. The distribution and significance of the septate desmosomes, gap junctions B, segments of tight junctions, and desmosomes in the flea midgut remain to be studied in greater detail.

An unusual and apparently rather unique structural specialization of the basement membrane of the flea midgut is the beaded layer described by Richards and Richards[14] and Reinhardt *et al.*[13] for several different genera of fleas. The present observations are in general accord with the earlier reports. A feature that has not been emphasized in previous reports is the thin amorphous layer associated with the outer surface of the beaded layer. Electron micrographs of our preparations suggest that this layer is similar to the typical basal lamina of

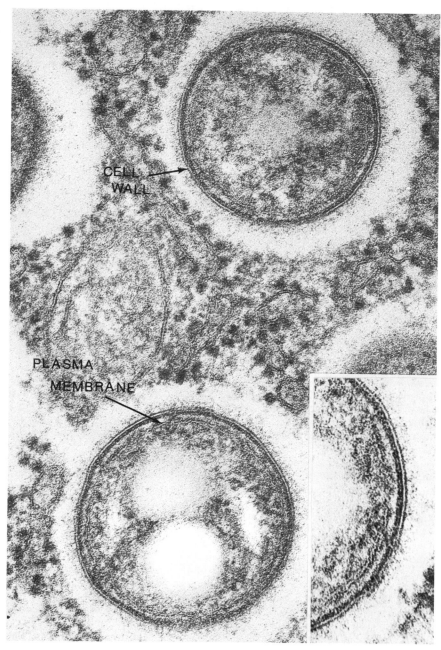

FIGURE 17. Higher-magnification electron micrographs of *R. mooseri* in the flea gut epithelial cell. The cell wall is a trilaminar structure, the inner leaflet of which has a dense layer attached to its surface. This dense layer may also appear to be layered in favorable views (see inset). The plasma membrane is separated from the cell wall by a space of about 10 nm. The clear vacuole-like spaces have a content of moderate density. The lowermost space has an actual perforation in the specimen and appears as a clear hole. ×160,000; inset, ×235,000.

other epithelia and that it is also quite like the bounding layer of the midgut investment adjacent to the hemocoel.

Although infectious rickettsiae somehow penetrate the midgut epithelial cell, presumably by endocytosis, the actual process has not been observed. A search for features of this process in static, fixed cells may be difficult, because the process may be rapid. Nevertheless, once in the cytoplasm, the rickettsiae seem to undergo proliferation without apparently causing profound deleterious effects on the host cell. Ultrastructurally, none of the normal cytoplasmic organelles of the flea midgut cells seem to be disrupted.

The presence of the halo or microcapsule described by Silverman *et al.*[12] was confirmed in some of our preparations. Some of these structures may well represent some type of capsular material that is not preserved in the thin-sectioned specimens. In some of the clear spaces, fine filamentous elements radiate from the outer surface of the cell wall and resemble structures described for elements of the glycocalyx or cell surface coats.[28, 29] These features are also found on freeze-fractured specimens of *R. mooseri* (FIGURE 16). However, specimens with little or no capsular space are also present. This finding may indicate that the capsule is a differentiated structural investment of rickettsiae found only in particular developmental states. It should be noted, however, that part of the halo-like capsular space may be due to the preferential shrinkage of the microorganism during specimen preparation. In our earlier attempts to study intracellular proliferation of pathogenic rickettsiae, we found that the choice of fixatives and embedding media may enhance or reduce the prominence of the halo. The precise nature or role of this layer around the cell wall of pathogenic rickettsiae in flea midgut epithelial cells remains to be determined. It seems probable, however, that some type of surface structure must allow the rickettsiae to enter and remain in the host cell cytoplasm, to enjoy all the gracious hospitality therein, and receive sufficient energy and metabolic precursors. Of the various host cells examined, the flea midgut epithelial cell allows the most abundant and concentrated proliferation of *R. mooseri*. This suggests that the conditions here are most favorable for proliferation of this rickettsia.

The present studies do not indicate that the rapid segregation and disruption of intracellular *R. mooseri* is a major process in the elimination of this infection from the epithelial cell. Only occasional vacuole-enclosed rickettsiae undergoing autolytic changes were observed. This finding does not rule out the possibility that this process may be important in the long-term survival of the infected fleas.

The empty vacuolar spaces in the cytoplasm of *R. mooseri*, particularly abundant during propagation in the flea gut, are similar to the spaces previously noted for *R. prowazeki* in the louse gut cells.[12] These vacuolar spaces were prominent and rather characteristic of *R. prowazeki*. The present observation of numerous vacuoles of similar nature in *R. mooseri* suggests that they may be a common feature of many rickettsiae. Silverman *et al.*[12] suggested that in *R. prowazeki,* these vacuoles might possibly be storage granules. Their abundance in *R. mooseri* when they are in a very active phase of proliferation adds further support to their role as storage sites for metabolic or structural precursor substances.

The presence of rickettsia-like organisms in some control fleas is not entirely unexpected, because many arthropods are known to harbor natural bacteria or rickettsia-like microorganisms in many of their tissues. To confirm the identification of the rickettsiae in our inoculum, indirect immunofluorescent tests were performed on the original yolk sac inoculum and on rickettsiae in the peritoneal exudate recovered from mice ill or dead from infection with *R. mooseri*. In both cases, the rickettsiae reacted strongly with typhus antibody. In contrast, negative results were obtained when numerous control flea guts were tested in the same system. These findings suggest that the indigenous rickettsiae probably do not react with typhus antibody.

It is obvious that much further work is needed to understand more fully the precise pathobiology of the flea as a vector for murine typhus. Work is under way to compare the infection produced by *R. mooseri* in the rat flea with that produced by the same rickettsia in the human body louse. Despite some similarities in the mode of transmission of the rickettsial agents by their insect vectors, major differences occur in their host-parasite relationships. The louse is killed by typhus rickettsial infection, thus truncating the period during which it can transmit the disease, whereas the relatively long life of the flea is not abbreviated by a similar infection. This difference has important implications for the epidemiology of the two rickettsial diseases. Starting with the newly hatched first nymphal instar, the normal span of the human body louse is about 40 days.[30] Because all stages of the louse suck blood, infection can occur at any stage. Infection causes death of the louse in 8–12 days. On the other hand, adult rat fleas live for many months. Infection of the flea with *R. mooseri* can occur only during the parasitic adult stage, and the life-span of the flea is not shortened by the infection.[5]

The precise reason for the difference in the response of lice and fleas to the rickettsial infections is not clear, but it seems highly likely that profound differences in the biology of the two insects, rather than relative differences in virulence, are responsible. The flea midgut epithelium is renewed by cells from cell nests, but such renewal is not known to occur in the midgut of the human body louse. Experiments have shown that *R. mooseri* also produces fatal infection of the louse, whereas it does not cause a lethal infection in the oriental rat flea.[31-33]

Continued study of the insect host as a vector in rickettsial diseases should further our understanding of such parameters as infectious process, proliferation, host cell response, longevity of microorganism and host, ultrastructural changes or modulation, species identification at the cellular level, characterization by antibody localization, and other aspects. The present report is an initial step in this direction.

REFERENCES

1. DYER, R. E., A. RUMREICH & L. F. BADGER. 1931. Typhus fever. A virus of the typhus type derived from fleas collected from wild rats. Publ. Health Rep. **36:** 334–338.
2. DYER, R. E., E. T. CEDER, W. G. WORKMAN, A. RUMREICH & L. F. BADGER. 1932. Typhus fever. Transmission of endemic typhus by rubbing either crushed infected fleas or infected flea feces into wounds. Publ. Health Rep. **47:** 131–133.
3. CEDER, E. T., R. E. DYER, A. RUMREICH & L. F. BADGER. 1931. Typhus fever: typhus virus in feces of infected fleas (Xenopsylla cheopis) and duration of infectivity of fleas. Publ. Health Rep. **40:** 1–9.
4. MOHR, W., F. WEYER & E. ASSHAUER. 1972. Murines Fleckfieber. *In* Infectionskrankheiten. O. Gsell, S. Gallen & W. Mohr, Eds. Vol. IV : 57, 58. Springer-Verlag. Berlin, Federal Republic of Germany.

5. BLANC, G. & M. BALTAZAR. Longevite du virus de typhus murin chez la puce (*Xenopsylla cheopis*). Compt. Rend. **202:** 1461–1463.

6. SHKOLNIK, L. Y., B. G. ZATULOVSKY & N. M. SHESTOPALOVA. 1966. An electron microscope study of ultrathin sections from infected louse guts and chick embryo yolk sacs. Acta Virol. **10:** 260–265.

7. ANACKER, R. L., E. G. PICKENS & D. B. LACKMAN. 1967. Details of the ultrastructure of *Rickettsia prowazekii* grown in the chick yolk sac. J. Bacteriol. **94:** 260–262.

8. JADIN, J., J. CREEMERS, J. M. JAIN & P. GIROUD. 1968. Ultrastructure of *Rickettsia prowazeki*. Acta Virol. **12:** 7–11.

9. HIGASHI, N. 1968. Recent advances in electron microscope studies on ultrastructure of rickettsiae. Zentr. Bakteriol. Parasitenk. Abt. I Orig. **206:** 277–283.

10. BULEVSKAYA, S. A. & V. F. IGNATOVICH. 1971. New electron microscopic data on structural formations in the cytoplasm of *Rickettsia prowazeki*. Acta Virol. **15:** 510–514.

11. SHKOLNIK, L. Y. & B. G. ZATULOVSKY. 1971. Electron microscopy of vaccine and Breinl strains of *Rickettsia prowazeki* in louse gut cells. Acta Virol. **15:** 102–106.

12. SILVERMAN, D. J., J. L. BOESE & C. L. WISSEMAN, JR. 1974. Ultrastructural studies of Rickettsia prowazeki from louse midgut cells to feces: search for "dormant" forms. Infect. Immunity **10:** 257–263.

13. REINHARDT, C., V. SCHULZ, H. HECKER & T. A. FREYVOGEL. 1972. Zur ultrastruktur des Mitteldarmepithels bei flohen (Insecta, Siphonaptera). Rev. Suisse Zool. **79:** 1130–1137.

14. RICHARDS, A. G. & P. A. RICHARDS. 1968. Flea Ctenophthalmus: heterogeneous hexagonally organized layer in the midgut. Science **160:** 423–425.

15. MAXCY, K. F. 1929. Endemic typhus fever of the southeastern United States: reaction of the guinea pig. Publ. Health Rep. **44:** 589–600.

16. COLE, M. M. 1971. Technique of rearing Xenopsylla cheopis. United States Department of Agriculture, Agricultural Research Service, Entomology Research Division. Gainesville, Fla.

17. PERACCHIA, C., B. S. MITTLER & S. FRENK. 1970. Improved fixation using hydroxyalkylperoxides. J. Cell Biol. **47:** 156a.

18. ITO, S. & M. J. KARNOVSKY. 1968. Formaldehyde-glutaraldehyde fixatives containing trinitro compounds. J. Cell Biol. **39:** 168a.

19. LUFT, J. H. 1973. Embedding media—old and new. *In* Advanced Techniques in Biological Electron Microscopy. J. K. Kochler, Ed. : 1–34. Springer-Verlag New York Inc. New York, N.Y.

20. HECKER, H., T. A. FREYVOGEL, H. BRIEGEL & R. STEIGER. 1971. The ultrastructure of midgut epithelium in *Aedes aegypti* (L.) (Insecta, Diptera) males. Acta Trop. **28:** 274–285.

21. HECKER, H., T. A. FREYVOGEL, H. BRIEGEL & R. STEIGER. 1971. Ultrastructural differentiation of the midgut epithelium in female *Aedes aegypti* (Insecta, Diptera) imagines. Acta Trop. **28:** 79–104.

22. REINHARDT, C. & H. HECKER. 1973. Structure and function of the basal lamina and of cell junctions in the midgut epithelium (stomach) of female *Aedes aegypti* L. (Insecta, Diptera). Acta Trop. **30:** 213–236.

23. NOIROT, C. & C. T. NOIROT. 1967. Un nouveau type de junction intercellulaire (zonula continua) dans l'intestin moyen des insectes. Compt. Rend. **264:** 2796–2798.

24. DALLAI, R. 1970. Glycoproteins in the zonula continua of the epithelium of the midgut in an insect. J. Microsc. **9:** 277–280.

25. SATIR, P. & N. B. GILULA. 1973. The fine structure of membranes and intercellular communications in insects. Annu. Rev. Entomol. **18:** 2–24.

26. FLOWER, N. E. 1974. Plasma membrane differentiations in the midgut of a lepidopteran larvae, Ephestra kuhniella. *In* Eighth International Congress on Elec-

tron Microscopy. J. V. Sanders & D. J. Goodchild, Eds. Vol. **2:** 224, 225. Australian Academy of Science. Canberra, Australia.

27. NOIROT, T. C. & C. T. NOIROT. 1974. Junctions septees et junctions continues chez les insectes. Etude apres impregnation par le lanthane et par cryofracture. *In* Eighth International Congress on Electron Microscopy. J. V. Sanders & D. J. Goodchild, Eds. Vol. **2:** 228, 229. Australian Academy of Science. Canberra, Australia.

28. ITO, S. 1974. Form and function of the glycocalyx on free cell surfaces. Phil. Trans. Roy. Soc. London Ser. B **268:** 55–66.

29. BENNETT, H. S. 1969. *In* Handbook of Molecular Cytology. A. Lima-de-Faria, Ed. : 1263–1293. North-Holland Publishing Company. Amsterdam, The Netherlands.

30. BUXTON, P. A. 1939. The Louse. Edward Arnold & Co. London, England.

31. MOOSER, H. 1945. Die Beziehungen des murinen Fleckfiebers zum klassichen Fleckfieber. Acta Trop. (Suppl.) **4.**

32. SNYDER, J. C. & C. M. WHEELER. 1945. The experimental infection of the human body louse, *Pediculus humanus corporis,* with murine and epidemic louse-born typhus strains. J. Exp. Med. **82:** 1–20.

33. FULLER, H. S. 1954. Human body lice. IV. Direct serial passage of typhus rickettsiae by oral infection. Proc. Soc. Exp. Biol. Med. **85:** 151–153.

MECHANISMS OF TRANSOVARIAL INFECTION OF SPOTTED FEVER RICKETTSIAE IN TICKS

Willy Burgdorfer and Lyle P. Brinton

Rocky Mountain Laboratory
National Institute of Allergy and Infectious Diseases
Public Health Service
National Institutes of Health
United States Department of Health, Education, and Welfare
Hamilton, Montana 59840

Field investigations by Ricketts [1] in western Montana on Rocky Mountain spotted fever established the principal features responsible for the persistence of *Rickettsia rickettsii* in nature. Unfamiliar with the causative agent, Ricketts proved conclusively that the wood tick, *Dermacentor andersoni,* is the vector. He further demonstrated that the etiologic agent acquired by immature ticks from a variety of small mammals, particularly rodents and lagomorphs, is maintained transstadially and may be transmitted via eggs to the progeny of infected female ticks. [2]

Ricketts' observations on transovarial infection were based on infectivity of larval ticks derived from females that were infected as adults by feeding on guinea pigs sick with spotted fever. Because no more than half of the females transmitted rickettsiae via eggs, he concluded that under natural conditions, this phenomenon does not occur in more than 50% of infected tick females. He also pointed out that the brood of an infected female may include many uninfected larvae.

Although these findings were confirmed by many workers, quantitative data that pertain to transovarial infection did not become available until 1954, when Price [3] reported that transovarial transmission in the field occurs about 30% of the time and that, when it does occur, rickettsiae are not passed to all filial ticks. Unfortunately, experimental data were not given, although the results were based "on a great many studies carried out with several strains of *R. rickettsii* and several lots of *D. andersoni.*" In a similar study with a low-virulence strain of *R. rickettsii* in *D. variabilis,* the same author [4] found that 30–40% of female ticks that had been infected as larvae and as nymphs by feeding on rickettsemic meadow voles passed rickettsiae to their offspring. Filial infection rates, determined by injection of oviposited eggs and engorged larvae into chick embryos, varied. Fifty percent of the transmitting females laid eggs, of which one of every 10 was infected, 15% showed one of every two to four eggs infected, and 35% had one of every 20–40 eggs infected. Similar results were obtained with engorged filial larval ticks.

In contrast to these findings, Burgdorfer [5] reported almost 100% transovarial and filial infection rates for *D. andersoni* infected either experimentally or naturally with virulent strains of *R. rickettsii.* Applying direct immunofluorescence to the examination of eggs, larvae, nymphs, and adults, this author found that rickettsial infections were retained throughout all developmental stages of the first filial generation and were again passed to 100% of eggs and larvae of the second generation. Since publication of these observations, studies were extended to determine whether transmission and filial infection rates of similar magnitude would occur in subsequent generations. Also, experiments were initiated to evaluate transovarial passage of different strains of *R. rickettsii* in naturally infected *D. andersoni, D. variabilis,* and *Haemaphysalis leporispalustris.* Additional investigations were performed with laboratory-reared *D. andersoni, H. leporispalustris,* and *Amblyomma americanum.* The results of these studies are reported here.

MATERIALS AND METHODS

The strains of *R. rickettsii* used included LOST HORSE-1958, SAW-TOOTH ♀-2, WACHSMUTH-1973, 275-F, 7421, ALABAMA ♀-2, TVA ♀-2, ARKANSAS-198, and ARKANSAS-200. Origin and characteristics of these strains and the modes to establish them in ticks follow.

The LOST HORSE-1958 strain was isolated in 1958 from a *D. andersoni* removed from a golden-mantled ground squirrel (*Spermophilus lateralis tescorum*) captured on the west side of the Bitter Root Valley, Montana. It was established in the parental tick generation by feeding laboratory-reared *D. andersoni* larvae on guinea pigs that had been inoculated intraperitoneally with suspensions of ticks previously infected with this strain.

The SAWTOOTH ♀-2 and WACHSMUTH-1973 strains were detected by hemolymph test[7] in individual *D. andersoni* females from the Sawtooth Canyon in the Bitter Root Valley in 1961 and from a spotted fever patient hospitalized in Hamilton, Montana, respectively. Both females were placed for feeding and mating on guinea pigs and subsequently provided the first filial generations.

The 275-F strain was originally isolated in chicken eggs by Dr. E. J. Bell from a pool of *D. andersoni* collected in eastern Montana in 1962. The strain had two initial egg passages and 27 subsequent guinea pig passages before it was established in laboratory-reared *D. andersoni* females through intracelomic injection of rickettsial suspensions.

The 7421 strain came from a pool of *H. leporispalustris* removed in 1961 from a snowshoe hare (*Lepus americanus*) captured in the Bitter Root Valley, Montana. It was established in laboratory-reared *H. leporispalustris* by feeding nymphs on rickettsemic snowshoe hares.

The ALABAMA ♀-2 strain was detected by hemolymph test in a fully engorged *H. leporispalustris* nymphal female removed in 1972 from a cotton-tail rabbit (*Sylvilagus floridanus*) from the Wilson Dam area in northwestern Alabama. Upon development to the adult stage, this tick was placed together with a normal laboratory-reared male on a snowshoe hare for feeding and mating.

The TVA ♀-2 strain and the ARKANSAS-198 and ARKANSAS-200 strains were detected by hemolymph test, respectively, in a *D. variabilis* female from the Land Between the Lakes area of the Tennessee Valley Region in 1970 and in two separate *D. variabilis* females collected by Dr. J. L. Lancaster near Fayetteville, Arkansas in 1972. Filial generations from each of these ticks were established by allowing the parental females to feed and mate on guinea pigs.

The LOST HORSE-1958, SAWTOOTH ♀-2, and WACHSMUTH-1973 strains of *R. rickettsii* are of the virulent type. Male guinea pigs developed fever (39.8–41.7°C) for 5–12 days and severe scrotal reactions. The 275-F strain is less virulent; in male guinea pigs, it produced fever for 3–6 days but no scrotal swelling. The 7421 and ALABAMA ♀-2 strains from *H. leporispalustris,* in addition to the TVA ♀-2, ARKANSAS-198, and ARKANSAS-200 strains from *D. variabilis,* were found to be avirulent for male guinea pigs; that is, they do not evoke fever or scrotal swelling.

The techniques used for rearing and maintaining ticks were essentially those described by Kohls.[6] Guinea pigs served as hosts for *D. andersoni* and *A. americanum;* domestic and cottontail rabbits were the experimental hosts for *D. variabilis* and *H. leporispalustris.* For feeding, larval and nymphal ticks were placed free on animals; adult ticks were confined in feeding capsules.

To establish the first filial generations of naturally and experimentally infected ticks, females found infected by the hemolymph test and laboratory-reared normal males were placed together for feeding and mating on hosts. Upon repletion, the females were held individually in cotton-stoppered glass vials for oviposition. Transovarial and filial infection rates for each tick generation were determined by conventional and fluorescence microscopy. For this purpose, smears prepared from each of 25–50 eggs, larvae, or nymphs from as many as 50 individual females were stained either by Giménez' method [8] or with anti-*R. rickettsii* conjugates.[5] Infection rates for adult ticks were determined by examination of stained tissue smears or by the hemolymph test. Usually, 5–10 infected females were used to obtain subsequent filial generations.

Rickettsial development in the ovarian tissues of infected nymphal and adult female ticks was followed by direct immunofluorescence and electron microscopy. Ticks and their tissues were treated as outlined by Tobie *et al.*[9] and by Brinton and Burgdorfer.[10]

RESULTS

Naturally Infected Ticks

As summarized in TABLE 1, all naturally infected *D. andersoni, D. variabilis,* and *H. leporispalustris* females passed their rickettsiae to 100% of their progeny. The SAWTOOTH ♀-2 strain of *R. rickettsii* has so far been maintained through 12 generations and still produces 100% transovarial and filial infection rates. To evaluate whether such high infection rates are possibly due to reinfection of tick females during each feeding, several lines of ticks were maintained for six generations on immunized animals only. This procedure neither affected infection rates nor altered the biologic characteristics of the SAWTOOTH ♀-2 strain of *R. rickettsii.*

Continuous transovarial infection appeared to have an adverse effect on the biologic development of ticks. Beginning with the fifth filial generation of *D. andersoni* infected with the SAWTOOTH ♀-2 strain, increasing numbers of replete females died within 1–2 weeks after engorgement. The majority of ticks that survived oviposited about one third to one half the number of eggs deposited by normal ticks. Unusually high mortality among engorged females and failure of oviposited eggs to develop were also recorded for *D. variabilis* infected with any of the three strains of *R. rickettsii.*

TABLE 1

FILIAL INFECTION RATES PRODUCED BY TICKS NATURALLY INFECTED WITH *R. rickettsii*

Tick Vectors	Strains of R. rickettsii	Number of Filial Generations Investigated	Filial Infection Rates (%)
D. andersoni	SAWTOOTH ♀-2	12	F_{1-2} :100*
			F_{3-12}:100
		6†	F_{1-6} :100
	WACHSMUTH-1973	1	F_1 :100
D. variabilis	TVA ♀-2	6	F_{1-6} :100
	ARKANSAS-198	3	F_{1-3} :100
	ARKANSAS-200	3	F_{1-3} :100
H. leporispalustris	ALABAMA ♀-2	2	F_{1-2} :100

* Results previously reported.[5]
† Ticks fed on immunized animals only.

Experimentally Infected Ticks

Tick females infected with *R. rickettsii*, either by feeding on rickettsemic animals or by injection of rickettsial suspensions, produced transovarial and filial infection rates similar to those infected naturally (TABLE 2). As previously reported,[5] 40 *D. andersoni* females that were infected with the LOST HORSE-1958 strain of *R. rickettsii* by feeding on infected guinea pigs passed rickettsiae to 100% of their progeny, and four of five F_1 females transmitted to 100% of their offspring. In the progeny from the fifth female, all F_2 larvae and nymphs examined harbored rickettsiae, but only 28 of 30 adults were positive. However, tick lines established from five infected F_2 females

TABLE 2

FILIAL INFECTION RATES PRODUCED BY TICKS EXPERIMENTALLY INFECTED WITH *R. rickettsii*

Tick Vectors	Strains of R. rickettsii	Number of Filial Generations Investigated	Filial Infections Rates (%)
D. andersoni	LOST HORSE-1958	6	F_1 :100*
			F_2 :93–100*
			F_{3-6}:100
	275-F	6	F_1 :10–86
			F_{2-6}:100
H. leporispalustris	7421	4	F_1 :24, 100
			F_{2-4}:100
A. americanum	SAWTOOTH ♀-2	2	F_{1-2}:100

* Results previously reported.[5]

transmitted to 100% of their filial ticks through four additional tick generations (FIGURE 1).

Each of 10 *D. andersoni* females injected intracelomically with the 275-F
strain transmitted ovarially, but filial infection rates varied from 10 to 86%.
However, the progeny of five infected F_1 females were 100% infected and
maintained rickettsiae through four additional generations.

Only four of 64 *H. leporispalustris* females that had fed as nymphs on
rickettsemic snowshoe hares gave a positive hemolymph test. Two of these
fed, mated, and oviposited properly. Both transmitted rickettsiae via eggs, one
to 100% and the other to 24% of filial ticks. Five hemolymph test-positive F_1
females of each line of ticks used to establish subsequent filial generations

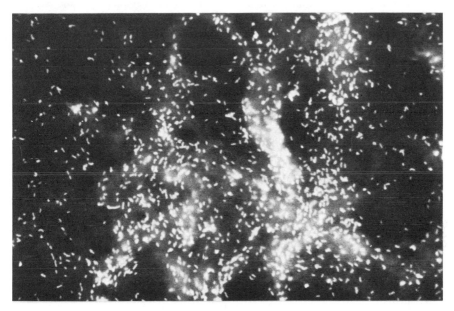

FIGURE 1. Smear of *D. andersoni* egg of the fourth filial generation infected with
R. rickettsii, LOST HORSE-1958 strain (fluorescent antibody staining, ×1050).

transmitted rickettsiae to 100% of their progeny, which maintained infections
through at least two additional generations.

To study transovarial passage of a virulent strain of *R. rickettsii* in laboratory-reared *A. americanum*, larval ticks of this species were fed on guinea
pigs infected with the SAWTOOTH ♀-2 strain. After the ticks had developed
to adults, 310 females were examined for rickettsial infections by the hemolymph test. Twelve (3.8%) were infected and were fed together with normal
males on guinea pigs. Four females eventually produced viable eggs that provided the first filial generations. All eggs, larvae, nymphs, and adults examined
from each of these females were infected, and rickettsiae were again passed
ovarially by each of five F_1 females to 100% of their offspring. When ready
for feeding, 10 F_2 females were used to establish the third filial generation. All

10 females fed and mated properly, but seven of them died within a few days after repletion, and the remaining three oviposited small quantities of eggs that failed to develop. In another attempt to initiate the F_3 generation, additional lots of F_2 females were fed and mated. Although all ticks engorged properly, the majority of females died shortly after dropping, and the remaining ones either failed to oviposit or produced eggs that would not develop. Microscopic examination of smears prepared from freshly deposited eggs revealed masses of rickettsiae in all instances.

Histologic Studies

Microscopic studies that pertained to rickettsial development in the ovarian tissues were limited to the SAWTOOTH ♀-2 strain of *R. rickettsii* in nymphal and adult females of *D. andersoni* and *A. americanum*. In unfed nymphal females, these tissues consist of oogonia and interstitial cells.[11, 12] Ovaries of all nymphal ticks examined were infected with rickettsiae that appeared to be limited to interstitial cells. Rickettsial invasion of germinal cells was found to occur during feeding of nymphs and during their development to adults. Oocytes of freshly molted adults always contained rickettsiae distributed either singly or in groups (FIGURE 2). Interstitial cells at this time were uniformly and heavily infected.

In the ovaries of starved adult females, rickettsiae appeared to be in a latent growth phase, as evidenced by absence of division forms and by the flaccid condition of the rickettsial cytoplasm, which resulted in a pulling away of the plasma membrane from the cell wall. During feeding of adult females, the rickettsiae in developing oocytes and epithelial cells were found to enter a renewed growth phase, as indicated by the turgid cytoplasm of organisms and by the presence of division forms within cells (FIGURE 3). In one instance, a rickettsia undergoing binary fission was also seen in the tunica propria.

Fluorescent antibody-stained sections of ovarian tissues from unfed, partially engorged, and replete *D. andersoni* females revealed massive rickettsial infections in all germinal cells (FIGURE 4) and in the supporting epithelium. Unlike the previously reported study,[5] rickettsial development was noted not only in the cytoplasm but occasionally also in the nuclei of oocytes.

DISCUSSION

It has been speculated that transovarial passage of spotted fever rickettsiae to 100% of filial ticks, as reported previously for *D. andersoni*, may be an exception rather than the rule or may apply to virulent strains of *R. rickettsii* only. Results of the present study show that this phenomenon also occurs in *D. andersoni* experimentally infected and in *D. variabilis* and *H. leporispalustris* naturally infected with less virulent strains.

Efficiency of transovarial infection depends primarily on the degree of rickettsial development in ovarian tissues, as suggested by the results obtained with experimentally infected ticks. Females with generalized massive infections transmitted rickettsiae to 100% of their progeny; those with mild rickettsial infections or those in which rickettsial development was still in an initial phase at the beginning of oviposition produced considerably lower per-

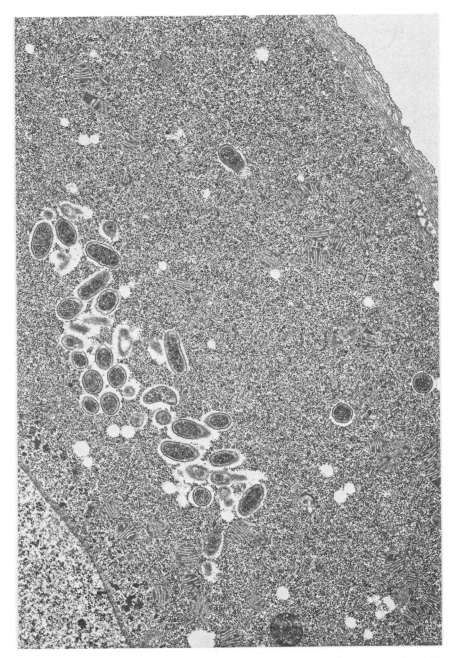

FIGURE 2. *R. rickettsii* in perinuclear ooplasm of developing oocyte from *D. andersoni* ($\times$ 10,000).

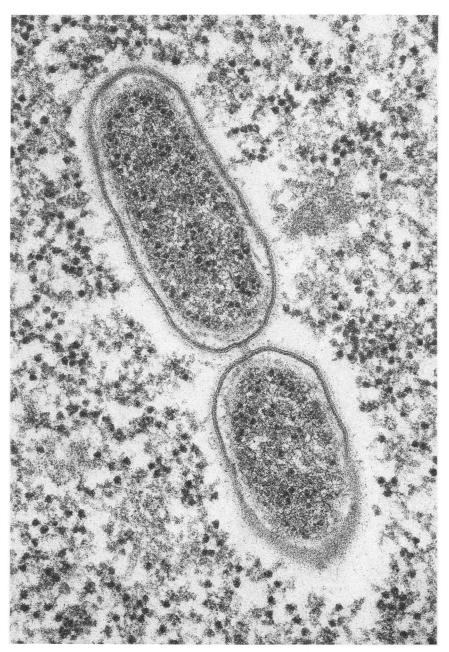

FIGURE 3. Division form of *R. rickettsii* in ooplasm of developing oocyte from *D. andersoni*. Note binary fission nearly completed (×81,000).

centages of infected filial ticks. Thus, of the two *H. leporispalustris* females, one transmitted rickettsiae to 100%, the other to only 24% of progeny. Similarly, intracelomic injection of the 275-F strain of *R. rickettsii* into *D. andersoni* resulted in filial infection rates that varied from 10 to 86%. These findings, to some extent, are comparable with those reported by Ricketts,[2] who infected *D. andersoni* females by allowing them to feed on guinea pigs sick with spotted fever. Infections established under such experimental conditions apparently do not develop sufficiently to include all germinal cells. In particular, eggs deposited during early phases of oviposition may not be infected, because formation of the chitinious vitelline membrane, which is initiated as early as 5–6 days after the tick begins to feed, prevents penetration of rickettsiae into

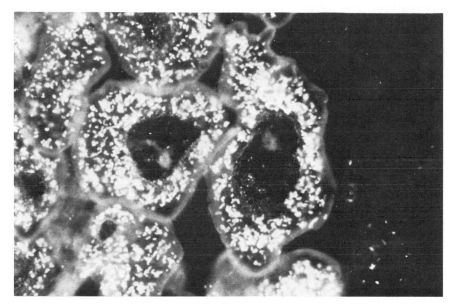

FIGURE 4. Section through ovary of completely engorged *D. andersoni* infected with *R. rickettsii*. Note rickettsiae in each oocyte (fluorescent antibody staining, ×1050).

oocytes. However, because the vitelline membrane is not formed in a uniform and simultaneous manner due to asynchronous oocyte development, rickettsiae are found only in the eggs that are laid during later phases of oviposition. Once rickettsial infections become generalized, as must have occurred in the naturally infected parental females, and in all infected F_1 females examined, rickettsiae are passed to 100% of filial ticks. Electron microscopic observations suggested that rickettsial infections in oocytes are due to both intracellular multiplication and penetration of extracellular organisms, from the hemocele, via the tunica propria.

All strains of *R. rickettsii* studied produced in ovarially infected ticks massive infections that did not decrease in intensity as a result of continuous transovarial passage. The feeding of ovarially infected *D. andersoni* on immunized animals for six generations also had no effect on degree of infections. This finding, to some extent, is in agreement with previously reported results [13] of experiments in which two additional strains of virulent *R. rickettsii* were maintained ovarially through six generations of ticks fed on immunized guinea pigs only. One of these strains, like the SAWTOOTH ♀-2, produced 100% filial infection rates throughout the entire study. However, the other strain behaved differently from the third generation on, when several lines of ticks revealed the presence of atypical rickettsial antigen no longer infectious for guinea pigs. The progeny of females infected with such atypical rickettsiae were uniformly negative. Because degradation in virulence and subsequent disappearance of rickettsiae in ticks have so far been recorded for only one strain of *R. rickettsii,* it appears premature to speculate that continuous ingestion of antibody-containing blood was responsible for these phenomena.

There was strong evidence that continuous transovarial passage of rickettsiae may lead to massive rickettsial development, responsible for the unusually high mortality among certain engorged tick females, and for the quantitatively poor oviposition and frequent failure of egg development.

With regard to the high mortality recorded for *A. americanum* infected experimentally with the SAWTOOTH ♀-2 strain, it should be noted that several previous attempts failed to infect this tick with virulent strains of *R. rickettsii* isolated from *D. andersoni.*[14] In one instance, rickettsial infections could be maintained for three generations. However, the F_3 females, as in the present study, either died prior to oviposition or produced eggs that did not develop.

It has been argued that transovarial transmission is such an efficient means by which *R. rickettsii* is maintained and distributed in nature that it should lead to higher infection rates than the <1–13.5% reported in the literature. This argument, however, as logical as it may sound, does not hold true, because infection of ticks with *R. rickettsii* depends primarily on the initial concentration of rickettsiae ingested. It has been shown in rather limited studies [15] that the minimal dosages required to infect 50% of larval *D. andersoni* with virulent *R. rickettsii* range between 10 and 100 guinea pig infectious doses per 0.5 ml of blood. Rickettsial concentrations of this magnitude and even higher ones have been demonstrated in a variety of experimentally infected tick hosts, but only for very short periods of time. Ticks that fed during peak rickettsemias invariably showed high infection rates, whereas those that fed during initial or final stages of rickettsemias ingested insufficient quantities of rickettsiae to become permanently infected. Indeed, little is known about duration and concentrations of rickettsemias experienced by rodents and other small mammals in nature, but in view of the low infection rates in field-collected adult ticks, it appears that such rickettsemias may be even milder and shorter than those observed under laboratory conditions.[15] Thus, transovarial infection may represent a far more important mechanism for maintaining *R. rickettsii* in nature than infection of ticks by feeding on rickettsemic hosts.

There are many biologic and ecologic factors, such as unfavorable climatic conditions, failure to find a suitable host, and lack of mating, that limit the number of ticks in nature. It is therefore safe to assume that relatively few larval ticks infected ovarially or by feeding on rickettsemic hosts reach the adult stage and pass rickettsiae to their offspring.

It is not known whether under natural conditions, transovarial infection initiates rickettsial development to the same degree as recorded in the laboratory. Studies of *R. montana* in *D. andersoni* revealed that rickettsial infections decreased in intensity as a result of continuous transovarial passage.[14] Although such decreases, or the previously reported [13] degradation in virulence, were not evident in the present study, it is conceivable that such phenomena may occur more readily in ticks in nature.

Finally, one may also speculate that even under natural conditions, certain strains of *R. rickettsii* develop in their tick vectors to such an extent that biologic functions, such as egg maturation, oviposition, and embryogenesis, are adversely affected.

SUMMARY

In a quantitative study of transovarial infection of various tick vectors by the spotted fever agent, *R. rickettsii*, it was found that naturally infected *D. andersoni*, *D. variabilis*, and *H. leporispalustris* females transmitted rickettsiae via eggs to 100% of their progeny. In one instance, infection was maintained through 11 generations and was again passed to 100% of ticks of the 12th generation.

Electron microscopic examination of ovarially infected ticks suggested that rickettsial invasion of germinal cells begins during feeding of nymphal females. Direct immunofluorescent staining of ovarian tissues of unfed, partially engorged, and replete females revealed massive rickettsial infections in the cytoplasm of every oocyte; occasionally, rickettsiae were found also in the nuclei.

Efficiency of transovarial infection appears to depend on the extent of rickettsial reproduction in ovarian tissues. *D. andersoni*, *H. leporispalustris*, and *A. americanum* infected either by feeding on rickettsemic animals or by intracelomic injection of rickettsial suspensions transmitted ovarially, but filial infection rates varied from 10 to 100%. However, practically all infected F_1 females passed rickettsiae to 100% of their progeny.

All strains of *R. rickettsii* studied produced generalized massive tick infections, which, in some instances, proved fatal for engorged females or adversely affected oviposition and subsequent egg development.

REFERENCES

1. RICKETTS, H. T. 1909. Some aspects of Rocky Mountain spotted fever as shown by recent investigations. Med. Rec. **76:** 843–855.
2. RICKETTS, H. T. 1907. Further experiments with the wood tick in relation to Rocky Mountain spotted fever. J. Amer. Med. Ass. **49**(15): 1278–1281.
3. PRICE, W. H. 1954. Variation in virulence of *"Rickettsia rickettsii"* under natural and experimental conditions. *In* The Dynamics of Virus and Rickettsial Infections. F. W. Hartman, F. L. Horsfall, Jr. & J. G. Kidd, Eds. : 164–183. McGraw-Hill Book Company. New York, N.Y.
4. PRICE, W. H. 1954. The epidemiology of Rocky Mountain spotted fever. II. Studies on the biological survival mechanism of *Rickettsia rickettsii*. Amer. J. Hyg. **60:** 292–319.
5. BURGDORFER, W. 1963. Investigation on "transovarial transmission" of *Rickett-*

sia rickettsii in the wood tick, *Dermacentor andersoni.* Exp. Parasitol. **14**(2): 152–159.

6. KOHLS, G. M. 1937. Tick rearing methods with special reference to the Rocky Mountain wood tick, *Dermacentor andersoni* Stiles. *In* Culture Methods for Invertebrate Animals. P. S. Galtsoff, F. E. Lutz, P. S. Welch & J. G. Needham, Eds. : 246–256. Comstock Publishing Associates. Ithaca, N.Y.

7. BURGDORFER, W. 1970. Hemolymph test. A technique for detection of rickettsiae in ticks. Amer. J. Trop. Med. Hyg. **19**(6): 1010–1014.

8. GIMÉNEZ, D. F. 1964. Staining rickettsiae in yolk-sac cultures. Stain Technol. **39**(3): 135–140.

9. TOBIE, J. E., W. BURGDORFER & C. L. LARSON. 1961. Frozen sections of arthropods for histological studies and fluorescent antibody investigations. Exp. Parasitol. **11**(1): 50–55.

10. BRINTON, L. P. & W. BURGDORFER. 1971. Fine structure of *Rickettsia canada* in tissues of *Dermacentor andersoni* Stiles. J. Bacteriol. **105**(3): 1149–1159.

11. BRINTON, L. P. & J. H. OLIVER, JR. 1971. Gross anatomical, histological, and cytological aspects of ovarian development in *Dermacentor andersoni* Stiles (Acari: Ixodidae). J. Parasitol. **57**(4): 708–719.

12. BRINTON, L. P. & J. H. OLIVER, JR. 1971. Fine structure of oogonial and oocyte development in *Dermacentor andersoni* Stiles (Acari: Ixodidae). J. Parasitol. **57**(4): 720–747.

13. BURGDORFER, W. & M. G. R. VARMA. 1967. Trans-stadial and transovarial development of disease agents in arthropods. Annu. Rev. Entomol. **12**: 347–376.

14. BURGDORFER, W. Unpublished results.

15. BURGDORFER, W., K. T. FRIEDHOFF & J. L. LANCASTER, JR. 1966. Natural history of tick-borne spotted fever in the USA. Susceptibility of small mammals to virulent *Rickettsia rickettsii.* Bull. World Health Org. **35**(2): 149–153.

IDENTIFICATION OF *RICKETTSIA TSUTSUGAMUSHI* IN THE LIFE STAGES OF *LEPTOTROMBIDIUM FLETCHERI* WITH ISOLATION AND IMMUNOFLUORESCENCE TECHNIQUES *

L. W. Roberts, E. Gan, G. Rapmund,[†] C. T. Chan,
S. M. Ramasamy, and J. S. Walker [‡]

*United States Army Medical Research Unit
Institute for Medical Research
Kuala Lumpur, Malaysia*

B. L. Elisberg [§]

*Walter Reed Army Institute of Research
Washington, D.C. 20012*

INTRODUCTION

The infection of *Leptotrombidium* mites, *L. deliense*-group, with *Rickettsia tsutsugamushi* was one of the earliest findings in epidemiologic and laboratory investigations of chigger-borne rickettsiosis, that is, scrub typhus.[1-6] However, the dynamics of infection in the mites has remained relatively obscure, and the information available has been very fragmentary until recently. In the late 1960s, Rapmund *et al.*[7] published the results of experiments in which larvae from successive generations were fed individually on mice and demonstrated the occurrence of very high transovarial transmission and filial infection in an infected colony of *L. fletcheri* maintained in the laboratory. However, many questions still remained, because the small amount of data available on isolations from the various developmental stages did not support high transstadial transmission rates, which had to exist to have $\geq 90\%$ transovarian transmission rate in positive mites. The above findings led some investigators [8] to postulate that the rickettsiae were reactivated during the feeding stage of the larvae after being in an eclipse or occult phase during the other developmental stages. Traub and Wisseman pointed out in their recent review [9] that isolation from certain developmental stages, that is, unfed larval, nymph, and adult mites from field collections, were usually very low or negative, whereas isolation rates from engorged larvae were higher. Russian workers during the 1960s reported on the presence of rickettsiae in various life stages.[10-12] However, few details are available, and the results are difficult to evaluate.

* In conducting the research described in this report, the investigators adhered to the *Guide for Laboratory Animal Facilities and Care,* as promulgated by the Committee on the Guide for Laboratory Animal Facilities and Care of the Institute of Laboratory Animal Resources, National Academy of Sciences, National Research Council.

† Present address: Walter Reed Army Institute of Research, Washington, D.C. 20012.

‡ Present address: United States Army Medical Research Institute of Infectious Diseases, Fort Detrick, Frederick, Md. 21701.

§ Present address: Food & Drug Administration, Bureau of Biologics, Bethesda, Md. 20014.

We conducted several experiments over a 6-year period to examine trans-stadial transmission and to determine in what organs the rickettsiae were distributed in each developmental stage. Mites from a colony of *L. fletcheri* described by Rapmund *et al.*[7] were used.

Experimental Methods for Isolation

The methods used to isolate rickettsiae from the various developmental stages of the mites have already been described in detail.[13] In brief, a single larva from a known positive adult was fed on one mouse, that is, a ratio of one larva to the ear of one mouse. Each mouse was then tested for infection with *R. tsutsugamushi*. Larvae were maintained separately after feeding, and when they had attained the selected stage of development, they were ground in 0.25 ml of Snyder's diluent in the well of a small hemagglutination plate. One-tenth milliliter of the mite tissue suspension was then injected intraperitoneally into each of two mice. A liver and spleen suspension from the two mice was injected

TABLE 1

Isolation of Rickettsiae from Different Developmental Stages of Mites from an Infected *L. (L.) fletcheri* Colony

	Deutova	Engorged Larvae	Nympho-phanes	Nymphs	Teleio-phanes	Adults
No.	13	20	18	19	20	21
Larvae transmitting rickettsiae to mice (%)	—	100	100	100	100	100
No. infected mites	1	19	17	9	12	4
Percent	8	95	94	47	60	19

intraperitoneally at 14 days into five second-passage mice. If any of the second-passage mice died, a third passage was made with a liver and spleen suspension from the second-passage mice. All surviving second- and third-passage mice treated with antibiotics were challenged with lethal doses, that is, 10^{3-4} mouse intraperitoneal lethal doses ($MIPLD_{50}$), of the Karp strain of *R. tsutsugamushi*. Survival of challenged mice is evidence of rickettsial infection transmitted to the mouse during larval feeding.

Isolation Results

Table 1 presents the results obtained from our isolation attempts. Except for deutova, isolations were attempted from approximately 20 mites at each stage of metamorphosis, with 10 offspring from each of two different positive female adults. All individuals transmitted *R. tsutsugamushi* during feeding as larvae, but rickettsiae were isolated from only some of the individuals at each postlarval stage. The bottom line of Table 1 gives the percentage of individuals that were positive at each stage. It can be observed that high rates of isolation were obtained from both the engorged larvae and the nymphophane stages, whereas lower rates were obtained at the nymph, teleiophane, and adult stages. In earlier experiments that utilized the same colony,[7] unengorged larvae of six different females were examined, and rickettsiae were isolated from 51 of 59 individuals for an 86% isolation rate. Although these data proved that rickettsiae could be isolated from all developmental stages, they did not identify the organs of the mites that were infected.

Fluorescent Antibody Methods

The next series of experiments to be presented were designed to investigate the distribution of rickettsiae in organs. We used the fluorescent antibody and microdissection techniques developed and perfected by Burgdorfer and Lackman in their detailed studies of *R. rickettsiae* in ticks.[14, 15] The fluorescent conjugates used in this study were monospecific for the Kato and Karp strains. We established that the rickettsiae in the *L. fletcheri* colony [7] are antigenically closely related to the Kato strain and to a lesser extent also to the Karp strain.[16] The direct staining technique with rhodamine as a counterstain was employed. Extreme care was taken at all times to avoid contamination of the internal organs by the exoskeleton during microdissection, because it autofluoresced with a brilliant green color. Three tissue smears were made from each organ; one was stained with normal rabbit γ-globulin conjugated with fluorescein isothiocyanate, one with the Kato conjugate, and the third with the Karp conjugate. Organs from mites from a known negative colony of *L. fletcheri* were also included as controls on an intermittent basis. Specimens were considered positive if specific fluorescence and typical rickettsial morphologic features were observed.

Fluorescent Antibody Results

Infection rates in various internal organs are shown in TABLE 2. Interestingly, many rickettsiae were detected in the salivary gland and midgut of unfed larvae. This, of course, constitutes an optimum situation for transmission to a mammalian host during feeding. We attempted to microdissect engorged larvae but found it was impossible because of the extreme friability of the mite tissues in the engorged stage. Significantly ($p < 0.001$) fewer organs were positive in the nymphophane than in the unfed larvae (TABLE 2). The salivary glands of the nymphophane did not contain rickettsia, whereas 80% of those of unfed larvae contained organisms. Eighty percent of the adult ovaries were positive by the fluorescent antibody test. Thus, it appears that the location of rickettsia within mites may shift from one organ to another during the various development stages, but all stages are infected. This apparent organ difference between the various stages may, however, be due to tissue reorganization during metamorphosis.

FIGURE 1 depicts fluorescent rickettsiae in the salivary gland of an unfed larva and in an egg from a positive adult female.

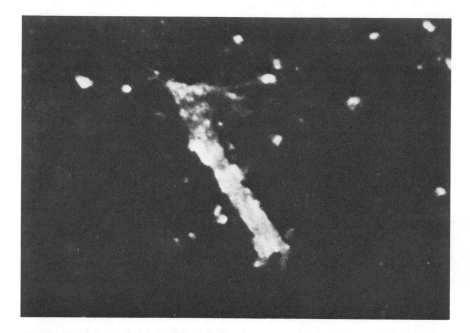

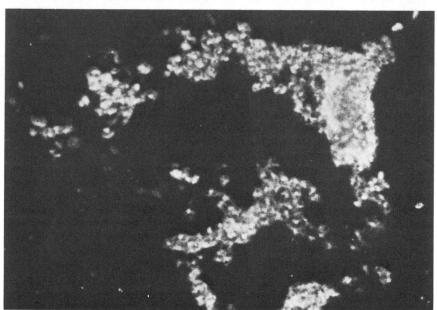

FIGURE 1. Fluorescent rickettsiae in salivary gland of unfed larvae (*top*) and in egg from positive adult female (*bottom*).

TABLE 2

IMMUNOFLUORESCENT IDENTIFICATION OF *R. tsutsugamushi* IN ORGANS
OF INFECTED, LABORATORY-REARED *L.* (*L.*) *fletcheri* *

| | Organ | | | | | | Organ Totals | |
| | Salivary Glands | Mid-gut | Excretory Tubule | Epidermal | Ovary | Hemolymph | No. | % |
Stage								
Unfed larvae	8/10	9/10	— †	—	—	7/10	24/30	80
Nymphophanes	0/10	2/10	0/10	0/10	—	5/10	7/50 ‡	14
Nymphs	5/10	4/10	2/10	5/10	8/10	4/10	28/60	47
Teleiophanes	7/10	5/10	6/10	4/10	2/10	5/10	29/60	48
Adults	5/10	4/10	3/10	4/10	8/10	4/10	28/60	47
Total No.	25/50	24/50	11/40	13/40	18/30	25/50		
%	50	48	28	33	60	50		

* After Roberts *et al.*[17]
† Organ either not present in stage or too small for adequate examination.
‡ p <0.001, Chi square with Yate's correction factor.

DISCUSSION

TABLE 3 summarizes our results on detection of transstadial transmission by mouse isolation and microdissection combined with the fluorescent antibody technique. The difference between the ability of the two techniques to determine the presence of rickettsiae was most pronounced with the eggs. The fluorescent antibody test demonstrated that 92% of the eggs contained rickettsiae, whereas we were unsuccessful in 132 attempts to isolate rickettsiae from individual mite

TABLE 3

COMPARISON OF TRANSSTADIAL TRANSMISSION AS DETERMINED BY ISOLATION
AND IMMUNOFLUORESCENCE TECHNIQUES

| | Isolation | | Immunofluorescence * | |
Developmental Stage	No.	% Positive	No.	% Positive
Eggs	132	0	12	92
Deutova	13	8	—	—
Larvae				
Unfed	59	86	12	92
Engorged	20	95	—	—
Nymphophanes	18	94	13	54
Nymphs	19	47	15	87
Teleiophanes	20	60	14	86
Adults	21	19	15	100

* After Roberts *et al.*[17]

eggs by mouse inoculation. Isolation failure may have been due to mechanical factors. The egg was so small that it was almost impossible to assure complete disruption and suspension of contents in diluent, even though the procedure was performed under a dissecting microscope. Alternately, isolation failure could have been due to small numbers of rickettsiae in the egg, that is, less than one minimal infectious dose for a mouse. The other significant disparity between the two techniques occurred in the adult mites, where rickettsiae were found in all 15 examined by the fluorescent antibody test, whereas mouse isolation identified only four of 21 individuals as positive (19%). Again, mechanical factors or number of rickettsiae present could be responsible for the observed discrepancy. The fluorescent antibody results demonstrated that the ovary was the most frequently involved organ in the adult. If the hemolymph had been similarly involved, the isolation rate from adult mites might have been much higher. The data for the other stages either are in close agreement, for example, unfed larvae, or the differences were smaller than in eggs and adults.

CONCLUSIONS

In conclusion, we feel, first, that these data have demonstrated that rickettsiae are not completely masked nor in an occult phase in the mite, because the organisms can be both isolated and visualized by fluorescent antibody techniques in all life stages. Second, all organs are positive at some time during the life cycle of the arthropod, but the presence of rickettsiae in a particular organ appears to vary with the developmental stage of the mite. For example, the principal organs infected were the salivary gland and midgut in unfed larvae and the ovary in adult females. These data, however, do not allow precise determination of the complete dynamics of the rickettsial infection in the various life cycle stages of the mites. Finally, and most importantly, the distribution of rickettsia in the various developmental stages of the mite is consistent with the known life cycle of the infection in nature.

REFERENCES

1. FLETCHER, W. & J. W. FIELD. 1927. The tsutsugamushi disease in the Federated Malay States. Bull. Inst. Med. Res. F.M.S. 1: 1–26.
2. FLETCHER, W., J. E. LESSLAR & R. LEWTHWAITE. 1928. The aetiology of the tsutsugamushi disease and tropical typhus in the Federated Malay States. A preliminary note. Part I. Trans. Roy. Soc. Trop. Med. Hyg. 22: 161–174.
3. FLETCHER, W., J. E. LESSLAR & R. LEWTHWAITE. 1929. The aetiology of the tsutsugamushi disease and tropical typhus in the Federated Malay States. Part II. Trans. Roy. Soc. Trop. Med. Hyg. 23: 57–70.
4. LEWTHWAITE, R. 1930. Clinical and epidemiological observations on tropical typhus in the Federated Malay States. Bull. Inst. Med. Res. F.M.S. 1: 1–42.
5. LEWTHWAITE, R. & S. R. SAVOOR. 1940. Rickettsia diseases of Malaya. Identity of tsutsugamushi and rural typhus. II. Morbid anatomy and histology. Lancet 1: 305–311.
6. FULLER, H. S. 1947. Infestation of man in Burma with trombiculid mites, with special reference to Trombicula deliensis. Amer. J. Hyg. 45: 363–371.
7. RAPMUND, G., R. W. UPHAM, JR., W. D. KUNDIN, C. MANIKUMARAN & C. T. CHAN. 1969. Transovarian development of scrub typhus rickettsiae in a colony of vector mites. Trans. Roy. Soc. Trop. Med. Hyg. 63: 251–258.

8. TRAUB, R. & L. P. FRICK. 1950. Chloramphenicol (Chloromycetin) in the chemoprophylaxis of scrub typhus (tsutsugamushi disease). V. Relation of number of vector mites in hyperendemic areas to infection rates in exposed volunteers. Amer. J. Hyg. **51**: 242–247.

9. TRAUB, R. & C. L. WISSEMAN, JR. 1974. The ecology of chigger-borne rickettsiosis (scrub typhus). J. Med. Entomol. **11**: 237–303.

10. MIROLYUBOVA, L. V., N. I. KUDRYASHOVA & I. V. TARASEVICH. 1966. Use of the serologico-fluorescent method of determining the natural infection of red mites by *Rickettsia tsutsugamushi*. Zh. Mikrobiol. Epidemiol. Immunobiol. **43**(7): 36–38.

11. KUDRYASHOVA, N. I., I. V. TARASEVICH & L. F. PLOTNIKOVA. 1967. On the methods of studying natural infection of chiggers with *Rickettsia tsutsugamushi*. Parazitologya **1**: 339–341 (in Russian).

12. KULAGIN, S. M., I. V. TARASEVICH, N. I. KUDRYASHOVA & I. M. COPACHENKO. 1967. On the natural focus of scrub typhus in the south of the Primorye areas of the USSR. Acta Med. Biol. **15**(Suppl.): 49–52.

13. WALKER, J. S., C. T. CHAN, C. MANIKUMARAN & B. L. ELISBERG. This monograph.

14. BURGDORFER, W. 1961. Evaluation of the fluorescent antibody techniques for the detection of Rocky Mountain spotted fever rickettsiae in various tissues. Pathol. Microbiol. **24**(Suppl.): 27–39.

15. BURGDORFER, W. & D. LACKMAN. 1960. Identification of *Rickettsia rickettsii* in the wood tick, *Dermacentor andersoni*, by means of fluorescent antibody. J. Infect. Diseases **107**: 241–244.

16. WALKER, J. S., E. GAN, F. M. BOZEMAN & B. L. ELISBERG. 1972. Unpublished data.

17. ROBERTS, L. W., D. M. ROBINSON, G. RAPMUND, J. S. WALKER, E. GAN & S. RAM. 1975. Distribution of *Rickettsia tsutsugamushi* in organs of *Leptotrombidium* (*Leptotrombidium*) *fletcheri* (Prostigmata: Trombiculidae). J. Med. Entomol. **12**: 345–348.

ATTEMPTS TO INFECT AND DEMONSTRATE TRANSOVARIAL TRANSMISSION OF R. TSUTSUGAMUSHI IN THREE SPECIES OF LEPTOTROMBIDIUM MITES *

J. S. Walker,† C. T. Chan, and C. Manikumaran

*United States Army Medical Research Unit
Institute for Medical Research
Kuala Lumpur, Malaysia*

B. L. Elisberg ‡

*Walter Reed Army Institute of Research
Washington, D.C. 20012*

INTRODUCTION

It has been generally assumed that the genus *Rattus* was the natural reservoir of *Rickettsia tsutsugamushi*.[1-4] However, in recent years, this assumption has been questioned, most recently in the excellent review article by Traub and Wisseman.[5] If a mammalian host is to be infected with *R. tsutsugamushi*, transovarial transmission is necessary, because the only morphologic development stage of the mite that feeds on a mammalian host is the larval stage. In addition, except under rare instances, the larval stage normally only feeds once on a mammalian host. Traub and Wisseman [5] stated that an understanding of the ecology of the disease depended upon the definition of three important parameters or questions: the possible role of the chiggers themselves as the principal natural reservoir of *R. tsutsugamushi*, the ability of chiggers to acquire rickettsiae during the feeding process, and the zoogeography of the vectors and mammalian hosts of chigger-borne rickettsiosis.

The experiments presented here were designed to answer two questions: can chiggers during the process of feeding on infected rodents acquire rickettsiae and develop an infection that is passed transtadially, and if infection of the mite occurs at the time the larvae feed, can the subsequent adult females pass it transovarially? Corollary questions that were considered were: are there differences among rickettsial strains that affect the ability of the larvae to acquire the infection from the rodent and the subsequent maintenance of the infection, do wild rodents that are hosts in nature differ from laboratory mice in their ability to transmit rickettsiae to larvae that are feeding on them, and do different

---

* In conducting the research described in this report, the investigators adhered to the *Guide for Laboratory Animal Facilities and Care,* as promulgated by the Committee on the Guide for Laboratory Animal Facilities and Care of the Institute of Laboratory Animal Resources, National Academy of Sciences, National Research Council.

† Present address: United States Army Medical Research Institute of Infectious Diseases, Fort Detrick, Frederick, Md. 21701.

‡ Present address: Food & Drug Administration, Bureau of Biologics, Bethesda, Md. 20014.

members of *Leptotrombidium deliense*-group vary in their ability to acquire rickettsiae and transmit them?

INFECTION IN MICE

We based the design of our experiments on the work reported by Burgdorfer *et al.* over the years concerning their *Rickettsia rickettsii* studies with ticks.[6-8] Burgdorfer has demonstrated that one of the most important factors involved in an arthropod's ability to acquire rickettsiae from an infected rodent is the duration and level of rickettsemia. Thus, the first series of experiments was designed to determine the relationship between the dose used to infect mice and the resultant rickettsemia. The presence and numbers of rickettsiae in the skin of the infected mouse were also determined, because larvae feed on cell

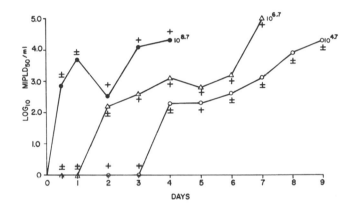

FIGURE 1. Effect of dose of Karp strain *R. tsutsugamushi* on rickettsemia and skin positivity of mice. Infecting doses: ● = $10^{8.7}$ MIPLD$_{50}$; △ = $10^{6.7}$ MIPLD$_{50}$; ○ = $10^{4.7}$ MIPLD$_{50}$. Skin subinoculation: + = 4/4 positive; ± = 1/4 to 3/4 positive.

debris and on the lymph in the skin rather than on blood from vessels in the subdermal layers of the skin, as ticks do.

FIGURE 1 illustrates the effect of rickettsial dose on rickettsemia in mice and on the time at which the skin became infected. The highest intraperitoneal dose, $10^{8.7}$ mouse intraperitoneal lethal doses (MIPLD$_{50}$), was followed by high rickettsemia; we demonstrated that the skin contained rickettsiae by the mouse isolation technique. However, the disease in these mice was of short duration, and the mice died before the larvae could have fully engorged. The second level, $10^{6.7}$ MIPLD$_{50}$, was the one selected for further study, because with $10^{4.7}$ MIPLD$_{50}$, the number of rickettsiae isolated from blood was lower and isolation from skin was not uniform after infection.

FIGURE 2 illustrates the results of a more detailed study, in which mice infected with $10^{6.9}$ MIPLD$_{50}$ of the Karp strain were sacrificed every 12 hr for 4½ days and rickettsemia and skin levels were determined. We took great care to remove, under a dissecting microscope, all subcutaneous tissue and

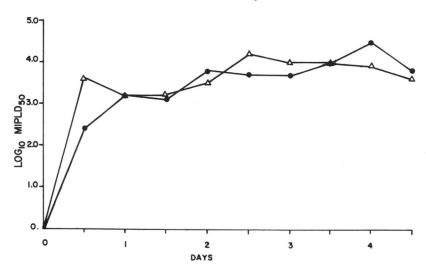

FIGURE 2. Mean level of rickettsiae in blood and skin of mice inoculated ip with 6.9 $\log_{10}$ MIPLD$_{50}$ Karp strain of *R. tsutsugamushi;* ●/ml blood, △/100 mg skin.

blood vessels before the skin was minced and ground for inoculation into mice; however, we realized that not all vessels, particularly those embedded in the dermis itself, could be removed. The level of rickettsiae in the skin from 2 to 4 days is approximately 10^4 MIPLD$_{50}$. In subsequent experiments, we usually employed an infecting dose of 10^6–10^7 MIPLD$_{50}$ for the mouse; the chiggers were placed on the mice at 48 hr postinoculation. The larvae usually had fully engorged and dropped off the mouse 48–60 hr later.

EXPERIMENTAL DESIGN

FIGURE 3 details the techniques used in the subsequent series of experiments. All mice utilized in these studies were sensitized to mites before infecting them. The rationale for prior sensitization was that Dr. Traub and others felt that sensitization to the salivary secretions of the chiggers might play a role in subsequent acquisition of rickettsia by the larvae. Our sensitization method involved the feeding of 90 uninfected *L. fletcheri* larvae in both ears and on the backs of normal mice; if they were not available, the *Blankaartia* larvae were used to maintain the sensitization schedule, because they were available in large numbers. This feeding was performed every 2 weeks for 4 months prior to infecting the mice with rickettsia. By this procedure, the mice were exposed to chiggers feeding on nine separate occasions for a total of 810 larvae in the specific sites where the larvae would be placed in subsequent infection experiments. An infected mouse that had been sensitized to chiggers and infected 48 hr earlier was exposed to mites by placing 20 larvae in each ear and also on its back for a total of 60 larvae per mouse. The pan under the cage was divided, as illustrated, so that the chiggers that dropped off the ears fell in the front of the pan, and those from the back fell into the rear of the pan.

After the larvae from known negative colonies had engorged on the infected mouse and dropped off into the water, they were removed, transferred to clay pots in groups of approximately 10, and held for further study. At each stage of metamorphosis, two mites were removed, and isolation of rickettsiae was attempted. The first isolation period was at 24 hr, which will be subsequently referred to as postlarval (PL) stage. The nymphophane (Np) stage was sampled at approximately 7 days, the nymph (N) stage at 13 days, teleiophane (T) stage at 31 days, and the adult (A) stage at approximately 45 days. The individual mites at various stages were ground in the wells of hemagglutination plates with the aid of a dissecting microscope in 0.25 ml of Snyder's diluent, and the suspension was inoculated intraperitoneally into each of two mice. At 14 days, these mice were killed, and a pooled suspension of their liver and spleens was inoculated into five more mice. If no deaths occurred in these five mice, they were challenged at 28 days with a lethal dose (10^3–10^4 MIPLD$_{50}$) of the Karp strain. If deaths or severe illness occurred, a liver and spleen suspension of the five mice was inoculated again into still another five mice that were treated with chloramphenicol and subsequently challenged as above.[9] When the mites reached the adult stage, each female was held separately and mated with a male from a proven negative colony. Five or more larvae from each adult were individually fed on one mouse, that is, one larva to one mouse. The engorged larvae were collected after feeding and held separately pending isolation of rickettsiae from the mouse on which it had fed. This isolation was accomplished by killing the mouse at 14 days and preparing suspensions of its liver and spleen, which were inoculated into five more mice. If there were no deaths, these mice were challenged at 28 days; if the challenged mice died, we considered the larvae negative. If the challenged mice survived, which would indicate the presence of specific immunity, they were positive. If deaths occurred, the scheme that we have outlined was followed. All observations were

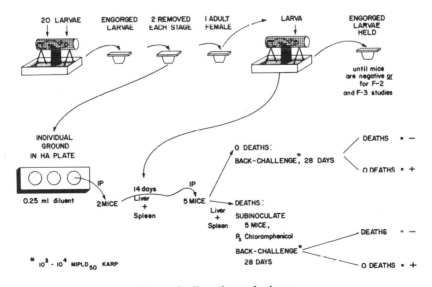

FIGURE 3. Experimental scheme.

based on individual larvae feeding separately one per mouse, and complete records were kept on each mite.

RESULTS

TABLE 1 illustrates our first attempt to infect two species of *Leptotrombidium* mites. There were no obvious differences between the larvae fed on the back and those in the ears; therefore, the data have been consolidated for purposes of presentation. In the first experiment with *L. deliense,* only one of 14 mites tested during the postfeeding developmental stage acquired rickettsiae from an infected mouse. The positive mite was found in the nymphophane stage. The second and third experiments were entirely negative, and in the fourth one, two of 16 mites acquired rickettsiae detected at the nymphophane stage. We tested a total of 19 F_1 generation larvae from the first experiment, none of which harbored rickettsiae. To test host adaptation, a phenomenon that is known to be necessary for some viruses, we carried some of these mites through F_2 and F_3 generations, without evidence for transovarial transmission being obtained. In four experiments with *L. fletcheri* mites, no evidence of rickettsial acquisition or transovarial passage was obtained.

TABLE 2 presents the results of a similar series of experiments in which the infecting strain in the mouse was a mixture of the Karp and Gilliam strains. Again, *L. deliense* acquired rickettsiae from feeding on an infected mouse. Postlarval and nymphophane stages were positive. *L. fletcheri* again failed to pick up rickettsiae; no transovarial transmission was detected in either species.

The experiment described in TABLE 3 took into consideration rickettsial strain adaptation. It could be possible that rickettsiae either have to be adapted to a host or are host specific. Therefore, to infect the mice, we used an isolate from an infected *L. fletcheri* colony [10] at the 11th generation that had only undergone two mouse passages. How long this rickettsial strain has been carried in chiggers and transovarially transmitted is not known, but it is not unreason-

TABLE 1

ATTEMPT TO INFECT TWO SPECIES OF *Leptotrombidium* MITES
WITH *R. tsutsugamushi* (KARP) *

Mouse	Species	No. Mites Positive/ Total	Positive Stage	No. Adults Laying Eggs	No. Offspring Positive/Total		
					F_1 Individuals	F_2 (Pools)	F_3 (Pools)
1	*deliense*	1/14	Np	4	0/19	0/1	—
2		0/16		8	0/42	0/17	0/2
3		0/16		7	0/50	0/11	0/1
4		2/16	Np	6	0/50	—	—
5	*fletcheri*	0/14		2	0/8		
6		0/16		0	—		
7		0/16		0	—		
8		0/16		2	0/19		

* Log_{10} infecting dose: 6.7 MIPLD$_{50}$.

TABLE 2

ATTEMPT TO INFECT TWO SPECIES OF MITES WITH
R. tsutsugamushi (KARP + GILLIAM) *

Mouse	Species	No. Mites Positive/ Total	Positive Stage	No. Adults Laying Eggs	No. Offspring Positive/Total F_1
1	*deliense*	4/8	PL+Np	1	0/5
2		0/6		2	0/10
3		2/6	PL+Np	0	—
4		0/6		3	0/16
5		0/6		4	0/20
6	*fletcheri*	0/10		7	0/35
7		0/10		8	0/37
8		0/8		6	0/29
9		0/4		0	—
10		0/10		5	0/23

* Log_{10} infecting doses: Karp, 7.1 $MIPLD_{50}$; Gilliam, 6.5 $MIPID_{50}$.

able to speculate that it may involve hundreds of years. In unpublished studies, we have identified the infecting strain to be predominantly related antigenically to the Kato strain.[11] Thus, the rickettsiae referred to as Kato in TABLE 3 were isolated from the infected *L. fletcheri* colony. We substituted strain TA 686 for Karp, because it is a recent isolate from Thailand.[12] Strain TA 686 was isolated from a rodent in Thailand in 1962 and had undergone only 36 egg passages at the time we used it in this study. Thus, it had been carried in the laboratory only 10 years compared to Karp, which was isolated in 1943 and had undergone 50 egg passages. In addition, by this time, we had established an uninfected *L. arenicola* colony and were able to include this species in the study. Again, the mites feeding on the infected mice were able to acquire rickettsiae during feeding and passed them transstadially to nymphs, teleiophanes, and adults. However, the adults that laid eggs did not transmit rickettsiae transovarially.

TABLE 4 presents data on the question of whether wild rodents might be better able to transmit rickettsiae to larvae than laboratory white mice. We were able to establish a colony of *Rattus annandalei* at the Institute for Medical Research, Kuala Lumpur. This species is found infected with *R. tsutsugamushi* in nature and becomes infected with low doses of the Karp strain.[4] Transmission experiments were performed on F_1 and F_2 generation rats raised in a laboratory colony that were negative serologically for *R. tsutsugamushi*. Again, three strains of rickettsiae were used, including a Gilliam-like strain, TC 586.[12] This strain was isolated from a pool of chiggers collected in 1962 in Thailand and was used at the 35th egg passage. It can be seen that the *L. deliense* larvae acquired rickettsiae by feeding on the wild rats and that three stages were positive: postlarval, nymphs, and adults. *L. arenicola* larvae did not acquire rickettsiae. No transovarial transmission could be demonstrated in either species.

TABLE 5 summarizes acquisition of rickettsiae from infected rodents and its subsequent transstadial transmission. We were able to identify rickettsiae

TABLE 3

ATTEMPT TO INFECT THREE SPECIES OF MITES WITH *R. tsutsugamushi* (GILLIAM, TA 686, KATO) *

No. of Mice	Mite Species	Rickettsial Strain	No. Mites Positive/Total	Positive Stage	No. Adults Laying Eggs	No. Offspring Positive/Total F_1
2	*deliense*	Kato †	0/20	—	9	0/48
5		Gilliam+TA 686	5/44	PL A	23	0/131
2	*fletcheri*	Kato	1/20	N	1	0/7
4		Gilliam+TA 686	1/40	Np	16	0/74
1	*arenicola*	Kato	2/8	T	1	0/6
1		Gilliam+TA 686	2/10	T	2	0/23

* Log_{10} infecting doses: Kato, 4.0 $MIPID_{50}$; Gilliam, 3.8 $MIPID_{50}$; TA 686, 4.4 $MIPLD_{50}$.
† The colony isolate denoted Kato has been identified as being antigenically predominantly related to the Kato strain.[16]

TABLE 4

ATTEMPT TO INFECT TWO SPECIES OF MITES BY FEEDING ON WILD RATS (*R. annandalei*) INFECTED WITH COMBINATIONS OF *R. tsutsugamushi* STRAINS *

No. of Rats	Mite Species	Rickettsial Strain	No. Mites Positive/Total	Positive Stage	No. Adults Laying Eggs	No. Offspring Positive/Total F_1
3	*deliense*	Karp+TC 586	2/46	Np	9	0/81
2		TC 586+Kato	2/34	PL A	3	0/29
1	*arenicola*	Karp+TC 586	0/20	—	5	0/37
2		TC 586+Kato	0/39	—	14	0/104

* Log_{10} infecting doses: Karp, 6.8 $MIPLD_{50}$; TC 586, 5.5 $MIPID_{50}$; Kato (colony isolate), 3.6 $MIPID_{50}$.

TABLE 5

EVIDENCE FOR TRANSSTADIAL TRANSMISSION IN MITES OF RICKETTSIAE
ACQUIRED FROM INFECTED RODENTS

Species	No. Positive/Total					
	Postlarval (1) *	Nymphophanes (7)	Nymphs (13)	Teleiophanes (31)	Adults (45)	Grand Totals †
deliense	7/58	8/58	0/54	0/36	3/32	18/238
fletcheri	0/38	1/37	1/34	0/28	0/27	2/164
arenicola	0/15	0/16	0/16	4/16	0/14	4/77
Total	7/111	9/111	1/104	4/80	3/73	24/479 (5%)

* Approximate day after feeding as larvae that isolation was attempted.
† Differences among mite species, significant at $p < 0.02$; variance test for homogeneity of the binomial distribution.[13]

in three of the five stages of *L. deliense*, including adults. At some stage of development, all three species of mites were positive. The grand totals listed on the right-hand side of TABLE 5 present the ratio of the number positive for all stages to the total tested. Analysis of the acquisition data by the variance test for homogeneity of the binomial distribution [13] revealed that there were significant differences ($p < 0.02$) between the rates at which the three species of mites acquired rickettsiae from infected rodents. This lack of homogeneity of the acquisition data was the result of the low level observed with *L. fletcheri* (TABLE 5). In the lower right-hand corner is the ratio of the total number of chiggers that were positive to the number of all species tested. A total acquisition rate of at least 5% was noted; that is, our data indicate that 5% of all larvae that feed on infected rodents will acquire rickettsiae from the infected host. If the low rate of isolation from nymph, teleiophane, and adult stages is considered, the actual rate is probably much higher.[11]

TABLE 6 presents the negative results obtained on transovarial transmission. In this series of experiments, 148 adults produced 903 offspring that were tested separately for infection by feeding on an individual mouse; none of them were

TABLE 6

EVIDENCE FOR LACK OF TRANSOVARIAL TRANSMISSION IN
MITES OF RICKETTSIAE ACQUIRED FROM RODENTS

Mite Species	No. of Adults Producing Eggs	No. Offspring Positive/Total		
		Individually Tested F_1	Pools of 4–10 F_2	Pools of 4–10 F_3
deliense	79	0/501	0/29	0/3
fletcheri	47	0/232	—	—
arenicola	22	0/170	—	—
Total	148	0/903	0/29	0/3

positive. In one series of experiments with *L. deliense,* negative results were also obtained through the F_2 and F_3 generations.

DISCUSSION

To determine the probable rate of transovarial transmission of rickettsiae acquired from infected rodents based on our negative data, we made the following assumptions: that the adults that had fed as larvae on infected rodents and subsequently laid eggs acquired rickettsiae at the same rate as the mites tested in the various morphologic stages (TABLE 5); that is, 5% of the 148 adults (TABLE 6) had acquired rickettsiae; and that if these adults were infected, including their ovaries, the transovarial transmission would be 100%, based on the work of Rapmund *et al.*[10] By use of the above assumptions for the 148 adults of all three species that produced 903 F_1 negative offspring (TABLE 6) and by applying the confidence interval estimate of the true proportion P, and with the normal distribution used to approximate the binomial distribution,[14] the transovarial transmission rate of *R. tsutsugamushi* acquired from infected rodents has to be less than 1/10,000. If we use the data for only *L. deliense,* where we had an acquisition rate of 7.5% (18/238), and had 79 adults produce 501 F_1 offspring, all of which were negative (TABLE 6), the transovarial transmission rate has to be less than 1/1,000,000.

We have tested the hypotheses as to whether the species of chiggers influenced acquisition of rickettsia, and the answer is "yes" (TABLE 5), but it did not influence the subsequent transovarial transmission. Utilizing the same type of analysis applied to test differences between species of chiggers,[13] we analyzed the data for rickettsial strains, of which there were five combinations, Karp, Karp-Gilliam, Karp-TC 586, Kato-TC 586, and Gilliam-TC 686, and found no significance between the acquisition proportions of the five combinations at the 5% level. Similarly, there was no significant difference between the ability of wild rodents (*R. annandalei*) and laboratory white mice to transmit rickettsia to larvae of *Leptotrombidium* mites.

We think that we have answered Traub and Wisseman's question [5] about the acquisition of rickettsiae during feeding; the answer is "yes," but they do not appear to become infected in the true sense of the word. Elaborating on this point, we first would like to quote Audy,[15] who reasoned, or speculated, that "It is noteworthy that rickettsiae in their primitive acarine hosts pass through the gut wall and permeate the tissues generally . . ." and that "it is possible that the main factor in ability to transmit rickettsiae among trombiculid mites is permeability of the gut wall." Our data fail to support Audy's thesis. Although we have no direct evidence, the positive acquisition data and negative transovarial transmission data led us to reason that the rickettsiae acquired during feeding on an infected rodent did not permeate the gut wall and infect the hemocytes of the mite hemolymph, which would have led to infection of the ovary. This could be the result of the dose of rickettsiae that the larvae acquire during feeding on rodents. However, mice infected with doses comparable to those used in these studies did run a high rickettsemia, and the skin of the mice was also infected (10^{3-4} MIPLD$_{50}$/100 mg of skin, FIGURE 2). Another possibility is generic susceptibility of the *L. deliense*-group of mites themselves. Although there is no way of determining it at this time, the possibility remains that hundreds or thousands of years ago, mites of the *L. deliense*-group were more susceptible to rickettsial infection than were those in our study and could have acquired their infection from rodents. This possibility would also explain and account for the infected mites that exist at this time and answer the question of how did the infected mites that exist acquire their *R. tsutsugamushi* infections; otherwise, one is left with "the chicken and egg question," for which there is no answer. However, we would like to emphasize, again, that the above explanation is speculation on our part.

We are not concluding that mites under any circumstances cannot acquire and transovarially transmit *R. tsutsugamushi* after feeding on infected rodents, but if this phenomenon does occur, it is such a rare event in nature that it plays little or no role in the epizoology of chigger-borne rickettsiosis. We agree with the suggestion of Traub and Wisseman[5] that the rodent, at this time, only plays a role in the epidemiology of the disease, in that it provides a host for the larvae to feed upon and thus enables the mites to maintain themselves in their various habitats. We think that our data support the conclusion that the mites of the *L. deliense*-group are both the reservoir and the vector of chigger-borne rickettsiosis, or scrub typhus, for all practical purposes.

REFERENCES

1. HARRISON, J. L. & J. R. AUDY. 1951. Hosts of the mite vector of scrub typhus. II. An analysis of the list of recorded hosts. Ann. Trop. Med. Parasitol. **45:** 186–194.
2. TRAUB, R. & C. L. WISSEMAN, JR. 1968. Ecological considerations in scrub typhus. 1. Emerging concepts. Bull. World Health Org. **39:** 209–218.
3. TRAUB, R. & C. L. WISSEMAN, JR. 1968. Ecological considerations in scrub typhus. 2. Vector species. Bull. World Health Org. **39:** 219–230.
4. WALKER, J. S., E. GAN, C. T. CHAN & I. MUUL. 1973. Involvement of small mammals in the transmission of scrub typhus in Malaysia: isolation and serological evidence. Trans. Roy. Soc. Trop. Med. Hyg. **67:** 838–845.
5. TRAUB, R. & C. L. WISSEMAN, JR. 1974. The ecology of chigger-borne rickettsiosis (scrub typhus). J. Med. Entomol. **11:** 237–303.
6. BURGDORFER, W. & M. G. R. VARMA. 1967. Trans-stadial and transovarial development of disease agents in arthropods. Annu. Rev. Entomol. **12:** 347–376.
7. PHILIP, C. B. & W. BURGDORFER. 1961. Arthropod vectors as reservoirs of microbial disease agents. Annu. Rev. Entomol. **6:** 391–412.
8. BURGDORFER, W., K. T. FRIEDHOFF & J. L. LANCASTER, JR. 1966. Natural history of tick-borne spotted fever in the USA. Susceptibility of small mammals to virulent *Rickettsia rickettsii*. Bull. World Health Org. **35:** 149–153.
9. JACKSON, E. M., J. X. DANAUSKAS, J. E. SMADEL, M. COALE & F. M. BOZEMAN. 1957. Occurrence of *Rickettsia tsutsugamushi* in Korean rodents and chiggers. Amer. J. Hyg. **66:** 309–320.
10. RAPMUND, G., R. W. UPHAM, JR., W. D. KUNDIN, C. MANIKUMARAN & C. T. CHAN. 1969. Transovarial development of scrub typhus rickettsiae in a colony of vector mites. Trans. Roy. Soc. Trop. Med. Hyg. **63:** 251–258.
11. ROBERTS, L. W., E. GAN, G. RAPMUND, C. T. CHAN, S. M. RAMASAMY, J. S. WALKER & B. L. ELISBERG. This monograph.
12. ELISBERG, B. L., V. SANGKASUVANA, J. M. CAMPBELL, F. M. BOZEMAN, P. BODHIDATTA & G. RAPMUND. 1967. Physiogeographic distribution of scrub typhus in Thailand. Acta Med. Biol. **15**(Suppl.): 61–67.
13. SNEDECOR, G. W. & W. G. COCHRAN. (Eds.) 1967. Statistical Methods. Chap. 9, Sec. 9.8: 240. The Iowa State University Press. Ames, Iowa.

14. NATRELLA, M. G. (Ed.) 1963. Experimental Statistics. Sec. 7-2. National Bureau of Standards Handbook 91. U.S. Government Printing Office. Washington, D.C.
15. AUDY, J. R. 1961. The ecology of scrub typhus. *In* Studies in Disease Ecology. J. M. May, Ed. : 389–432. Hafner Publishing Co., Inc. New York, N.Y.
16. WALKER, J. S., E. GAN, F. M. BOZEMAN & B. L. ELISBERG. 1972. Unpublished data.

THE ACQUISITION OF *RICKETTSIA TSUTSUGAMUSHI* BY CHIGGERS (TROMBICULID MITES) DURING THE FEEDING PROCESS *

Robert Traub, Charles L. Wisseman, Jr., Marilyn R. Jones, and
James J. O'Keefe

Department of Microbiology
University of Maryland School of Medicine
Baltimore, Maryland 21201

INTRODUCTION

A fundamental concept in the ecology of ectoparasite-borne disease is that of the reservoir, or the wellspring of the infection in nature during interepidemic periods. In the case of chigger-borne rickettsiosis (scrub typhus), it has often been argued that chiggers (larval trombiculid mites) are not only the vectors but also the true reservoirs of the infection and that the small mammals (theraphions) that serve as hosts of the chiggers are of no importance as a source of rickettsiae for the chiggers.[1] This point of view has been based largely upon several factors, namely, the known transovarian transmission of the causative agent, *Rickettsia tsutsugamushi*, from mother to progeny in certain species of chiggers,[2-5] the demonstration of the efficiency of the mechanism of transovarian transmission by Rapmund and his colleagues,[6-8] the difficulty or impossibility to show that chiggers can acquire *R. tsutsugamushi* while feeding on infected hosts in the laboratory,[1, 8-11] the fact that chiggers are unique among vectors in that in their lifetime, they are parasitic only in one stage (i.e., as larvae) and normally attach to, and feed upon, only one vertebrate and therefore could not acquire an infection from one such host and transmit it later directly to a second, and, finally, the widespread belief that chiggers do not imbibe blood but, instead, feed solely on serum exudate when in the parasitic stage and thus are unlikely to come in contact with pathogens that circulate in the blood of the host.[4, 5]

In the present paper, it is shown that, contrary to general belief, chiggers can acquire *R. tsutsugamushi* while feeding on rickettsemic mice and that, when tested by pools of chiggers, this acquisition is relatively frequent. Persistence of acquired rickettsiae for at least 1–2 weeks in the chiggers is demonstrated, and a single case of presumed transovarian transmission to the next generation is reported. The preliminary data presented suggest, somewhat surprisingly, that in nature, under certain conditions, a small but perhaps significant proportion of chiggers may partially feed on one host and then later feed to repletion on a second one, raising the possibility that such "reattached" chiggers may

* Supported by Contract DADA-17-70-C-0047 from the Army Medical Research and Development Command under the auspices of the Commission on Rickettsial Diseases, U.S. Armed Forces Epidemiological Board. Various aspects of the investigations undertaken by the authors and reported herein were also supported by that Contract and its predecessors and by Grant AI-04242 from the National Institutes of Health.

91

transmit acquired rickettsiae. These points, coupled with the observation in our laboratory that chiggers may, indeed, imbibe blood on occasion,[4, 5, 12] indicate that theraphions may perhaps truly be of significance as a source of *R. tsutsugamushi* infection in chiggers in nature, even though the trombiculids themselves apparently constitute the prime reservoir of chigger-borne rickettsiosis.

The approach in this study has primarily been concerned with the acquisition of *R. tsutsugamushi* by chiggers that were presumably free of natural infection; we utilized colonies of six species of chiggers that are known or suspected vectors of chigger-borne rickettsiosis and fed the chiggers on mice that had been inoculated with *R. tsutsugamushi*. The absence of natural infection in the lines of trombiculids was periodically checked by testing aliquots of specimens during the investigations, because the fact that chiggers normally feed only once as parasites precludes preliminary examination of the individual chiggers before they are exposed to rickettsemic mice. We originally planned to compare the course of experimentally induced infection in chiggers with that of naturally infected chiggers. For this purpose, wild-caught specimens of a Malayan species were employed in an attempt to establish colonies based wholly upon demonstrably infected lines of chiggers, but this aspect had to be abandoned before fruition because of lack of funds (which also terminated the entire program). Some of the data are presented for the cultures that contained some naturally infected chiggers because of relevance to the section on the discussion on the reservoirs of chigger-borne rickettsiosis.

DEFINITIONS

Because some terms basic to a discussion of the ecology of ectoparasite-borne infections are used in a variety of senses by different workers or are otherwise ambiguous, it is advisable to discuss terminology at this point. Terms like endemic, intrazootic, theraphion, intramurid, bioendemic, and so on, will be used in the sense of Traub and Wisseman.[5] Others applicable to discussion of such infections are defined as follows:

A reservoir is the regular or permanent source of an infection in nature during the interepidemic period, but it is useful to distinguish between two main types of reservoir: true reservoirs and quasireservoirs. A *true* reservoir is a species, taxon, or group of individuals that shows no clinical signs of illness produced by an etiologic agent that it may routinely harbor, even though the agent may result in serious illness or death if introduced into another host. Examples of true reservoirs are heteromyid and other bioendemic or indigenous desert rodents in endemic areas of sylvatic plague, which readily withstand challenge of millions of lethal doses of *Yersinia pestis* organisms,[5, 13] and various species of *Dermacentor* and other ticks that harbor the rickettsiae of tick typhus.[4, 14, 15] Differences of degree of involvement by true reservoirs may be expressed by the terms primary and secondary. In contrast to the true reservoir, the quasireservoir is one in which the organism is maintained temporarily but which itself may become ill from the infection or become involved in an epizootic, for example, dogs and livestock in leptospirosis. The quasireservoir is often a direct source of infection to man or other mammals by contact, as in rabbits in tularemia or sylvatic plague in prairie dogs (*Cynomys*) or ground squirrels, but transmission by arthropod vectors may also occur, as in both of these examples.

Distinctions between types of host resistance are also useful. A *susceptible* host is an individual with a lack of resistance to an infection, as indicated by clinical signs of disease, or death, for example, urban rats in an epizootic of plague. A *supersensitive* host is one that is extremely susceptible; it dies rapidly after exposure to an etiologic agent, for example, hamsters and experimental leptospirosis. A *tolerant* host, on the other hand, is capable of acquiring and maintaining an infection but does not develop clinical signs, for example, rats with murine typhus infection. A *responsive* host is capable of acquiring an infection, but it is sufficiently resistant, so that not only are there no signs of overt illness but also the infection is of short duration. An *immune* host is one that fails to develop clinical illness or perhaps even a true infection because of the immune response based upon prior contact with the agent. A *refractory* host is a taxon (e.g., genus or species) that is completely resistant to an etiologic agent, not because of the immunity mechanism but presumably because of the processes of evolution and long association. The resistance of desert rodents to plague is in this category. An *intractable* host is an alien one that is utterly unaffected when deliberately exposed to an etiologic agent that it ordinarily never encounters in nature.

The terms are not mutually exclusive, because there, of course, are variations with time: an animal that is susceptible today may become immune later, or vice versa. Also, a host that is *tolerant* may also be an *immune* one, or its lack of clinical response may be due to other reasons.

BACKGROUND

The ecology of chigger-borne rickettsiosis was extensively reviewed by Traub and Wisseman in 1974,[5] in which article may be found more data and references on vectors, possible reservoirs, and so on, than are presented here. Certain points are treated now, briefly, to facilitate discussion and the evaluation and analysis of the approach, methods, and data.

There is no doubt that chiggers are the vectors of chigger-borne rickettsiosis and that the infection is transmitted by the bite of the trombiculid.[4, 5] As indicated by those sources, it is also well established that species of *Leptotrombidium* in the *L.* (*L.*) *deliense* complex are the major vectors, that transovarian transmission of rickettsiae from parental *Leptotrombidium* to progeny occurs, and that such infected F_1 chiggers can transmit *R. tsutsugamushi* while feeding. Transstadial transmission of rickettsiae from larva to nymph and from nymph to adult has also been demonstrated. The studies by Rapmund *et al.*[6-8] amply showed that the mechanism of transovarian transmission is highly effective. Thus, in some tests, virtually all of the infected females passed the infection to some of their offspring, and in such instances, at times 100% of the progeny acquired the infection. Similarly impressive results were obtained by transovarian transmission through all four generations tested, but the duration of such transmission to succeeding generations was not determined. Those investigators also showed that the bite of a single naturally infected chigger was generally sufficient to cause illness and death in a white mouse. Roberts *et al.*[16] provided evidence of the frequent occurrence of *R. tsutsugamushi* in the salivary glands of unfed, naturally infected *L. fletcheri* in Western Malaysia and in the gut or hemolymph of the various stadia.

The evidence for vectorship by *L. deliense* and allies is overwhelming and unquestioned, and the points merely outlined above are in themselves also highly suggestive that the chiggers likewise serve as the reservoirs of the infection in nature, an argument heard even before such recent information became available. It is important to note that, in theory, the trombiculid could be important as a reservoir regardless of whether a particular infection was ultimately derived (i.e., "acquired") from a mammal host, whether it represented a "natural" infection limited to that familial line of mites (perhaps passing into a vertebrate as the chigger feeds but going no further), or was a combination of both. Such distinctions were not generally made in the literature when discussing chiggers as "reservoirs," particularly because it was often assumed that "acquired" infection became "natural" and persisted for at least a few generations.

Philip [3] used epidemiologic information and the phenomenon of transovarian transmission as the basis for flatly claiming that chiggers served as the prime reservoir. Philip and Burgdorfer,[17] while stating that "rodents are undoubted reservoirs" (p. 399), added that "mites must be conceded to play an important role" because of the ability of laboratory reared larval L. deliense to transmit infection upon feeding and because the mites can overwinter as adults. They pointed out that "trombiculids feed not on blood but on lymph and tissues of the hosts' dermis," presumably intimating that as a result, chiggers were not apt to ingest rickettsiae from the host during the feeding process. Among the theoretical grounds for chiggers serving as reservoirs was the point that they normally feed only once on a vertebrate, and under such circumstances, it would be impossible for the chiggers to acquire an infection from one host and later transmit it to another one directly.[4, 5] Only by transovarian transmission could such rickettsiae enter into the ecology of the infection.

Supporting this concept of chiggers as reservoirs, and denigrating the possible role of theraphions as sources of rickettsiae to trombiculids, have been the firm indications in the literature that it is difficult or impossible for chiggers to acquire R. tsutsugamushi by feeding on mice that had been inoculated with virulent strains of the agent. Tamiya,[18] Audy,[1] and Fukuzumi [10] all reported such conclusions, and in Western Malaysia, it was claimed that chiggers failed to acquire rickettsiae, even when feeding on localized sites where special efforts had been undertaken to induce high concentrations of R. tsutsugamushi.[8] Toyokawa,[19] in a complex series of experiments that employed animals inoculated with one serotype and exposed to chiggers under natural conditions where that serotype was absent, concluded that wild chiggers could ingest such rickettsiae. However, there was no evidence to suggest that any growth of rickettsiae occurred in the chigger.[5]

On the other hand, there are many references to the importance of rodents and other small mammals as a source of rickettsiae for perpetuating the cycle in nature, at least as a supplement to the mechanism of transovarian transmission of natural infection.[1, 3, 20-22] There has been a widespread impression that there must be some acquisition of R. tsutsugamushi by chiggers while feeding on rickettsemic hosts, as typified by the following quotation: "The chigger feeds on a host animal infected with rickettsiae and picks up those organisms from it" (p. 5).[23] It had even been stated in 1972 that there is successful transovarian transmission of rickettsiae that results from acquired infection,[24] but this statement was undocumented and is believed to have been made in error, as pointed out in 1974 by Traub and Wisseman.[5]

Perhaps, the main reasons for the common assumption that theraphions must serve as a source of replenishment for the natural cycles of R. tsutsugamushi are that in endemic areas, a large gamut of hosts have been found naturally infected and that as many as 36–50% of the ground-dwelling rodents tested have proven to harbor such rickettsiae.[5, 25] Because such rats, mice, and tupaiads (tree shrews) may each be infested with hundreds or thousands of vector *Leptotrombidium*, it is easy to believe that chiggers can acquire infection while feeding on those hosts. There also have been suggestions that the behavior of chiggers did not necessarily rule out the possibility that they could acquire rickettsiae and perhaps even transmit them to a second host without resorting to the mechanism of transovarian transmission. The evidence that chiggers may at times imbibe blood has recently been reviewed,[4, 5] and in histologic studies undertaken in our laboratory, we have seen a red blood cell within the lumen of the stylostome of a chigger. On the basis of detailed histologic studies, we have suggested that, as a result of the inflammatory response in the host at the site of attachment of the chigger, wandering inflammatory cells that carry intracellular *R. tsutsugamushi* may be brought into the immediate proximity of the chigger's feeding tube.[5] Experimental proof of this hypothesis has not been sought, but it offers a mechanism whereby chiggers could acquire rickettsiae while feeding. Philip[15] claimed that an American pest chigger of the genus *Eutrombicula* could acquire *R. tsutsugamushi* by feeding on rickettsemic mice. Preliminary reports of our findings on the ingestion of such rickettsiae by four species of *Leptotrombidium* and *Gahrliepia ligula* have been made to the Commission on Rickettsial Diseases of the Armed Forces Epidemiological Board.[26-28] As mentioned, the investigations of Toyokawa[19] also indicated that chiggers may acquire rickettsiae orally. During wartime studies in Burma, it was shown that if tissue that contained attached chiggers was sewn into the ear of a white rat, some of the trombiculids would detach and feed on the new host.[29] It therefore seemed possible that under certain circumstances, reattachment might occur in nature, and this hypothesis led to our studies on the subject.[5, 27, 28]

Although a great deal remains to be learned about the antigenic strains of *R. tsutsugamushi*, it is evident that certain strains are extremely widespread, extending across the range of the rickettsiosis, and that there is no apparent correlation between species of vector and antigenic strain of rickettsiae; that is, each serotype may be vectored by several species of chigger. These points have been advanced as support for the belief that theraphions are of consequence in the perpetuation of the rickettsial cycle in nature.[5]

There is some confusion over the important question of how long natural infection persists by transovarian transmission in colonies that are not exposed to rickettsemic hosts. Both Audy[1, 30] and Krishnan *et al.*[31] reported that the infection was lost after their colonies had fed for several generations on uninfected hosts. In contrast, Rapmund *et al.* found that there was remarkably little diminution in the "transovarial infection rate" or the "filial infection rate" in three to five generations of *L. fletcheri*,[7] although the results were not as good when *L. arenicola* was tested.[5, 6] Perhaps, the contradictory findings are due to variations in the virulence of the strains of rickettsiae under study.

MATERIALS AND METHODS

Species of Chiggers

Because the main objective was to evaluate the role of chiggers in acquiring *R. tsutsugamushi* infection from experimentally infected laboratory animals, we decided to use demonstrably or palpably uninfected lines of species known to be efficient vectors of natural infection. For this reason, three established vectors, *Leptotrombidium* (*L.*) *deliense* (Walch), *L.* (*L.*). *fletcheri* (Womersley),† and *L.* (*L.*) *arenicola* Traub, were collected in Kuala Lumpur, Western Malaysia, and transported to Baltimore where mass colonies were established in our laboratory. It was also desirable to assay the potentialities of a species of *Leptotrombidium* suspected as being at least an intrazootic vector in recently discovered areas endemic for chigger-borne rickettsiosis in the mountains of Western Pakistan,[11, 32] namely, *L.* (*L.*) *subintermedium* (Jameson and Toshioka), along with a species of chigger commonly encountered in rodents in those localities and in endemic foci in Assam, Burma, and India and considered a potential vector, namely, *Gahrliepia* (*Schoengastiella*) *ligula* (Radford).[4, 32, 33] Both of these species were collected in large numbers in our studies in Pakistan and taken to Baltimore for colonization. A sixth species, *Ascoschoengastia* (*Laurentella*) *indica* Hirst, a common species on urban, peridomestic, and rural rats in the Asiatic Pacific area, was subsequently collected in Western Malaysia and reared in this program as a model for a species that had not been specifically incriminated as a vector of chigger-borne rickettsiosis,[4, 5] although it had been reported as being naturally infected with *R. mooseri*, the agent of murine typhus, in Indonesia.[34]

Handling of Chiggers

The mass cultures of chiggers were maintained in transparent glass jars of 3-gallon capacity that contained a bottom layer of a hardened mixture of powdered charcoal and plaster of Paris, or charcoal and sterilized loam, inclined at an angle of about 30° and ranging in height from about 1½ to 3 in. After thorough drying to ensure rigidity, this layer was soaked with water, and then it was covered with a bedding layer of 3–4 in. of a mixture of sterile soil (33%) and Vermiculite® (67%). Colonies were started by placing 100–1000 nymphs or adults on the moistened surface of the bedding, and they were free to burrow to depths of appropriate relative humidity. The jars were watered sufficiently frequently to provide surface humidity near the saturation point when the jars were kept at room temperature (about 70° C). Because *L. subintermedium* is a montane species restricted to cool or cold climes, it was generally maintained at 50–60° C at night. The nymphs and adults of *Leptotrombidium* were fed by supplying them with the eggs of the collembolan, *Sinella curviseta*, or by rearing the insects in the same jar as the mites. During the course of the project, it was noted that the postlarval stages of *Gahrliepia* were actively predaceous upon the collembolans,[5] and the insects were therefore regularly supplied to these cultures. When the various cultures developed to the point where 500–1000 larvae were obtainable per mouse host every fortnight, they were regarded as suitable for experiments on the transmission of *R. tsutsugamushi*. At such times, compact clusters of 100–300 chiggers could be observed on the sides of the jar.

---

† This is the species that had formerly been considered as the Malayan representative of *L.* (*L.*) *akamushi* (Brumpt), a taxon that is now regarded as being restricted to Japan.

In addition, smaller, screw-cap culture jars (4 × 2 in.) that contained only a level foundation of plaster of Paris and charcoal were used for rearing. This method was used for three reasons: as a precaution against loss of the mass cultures, to eliminate the possibility that acquired infection might build up in chiggers maintained for successive generations in jars in which infected mice had been placed for short periods to serve as food for the larval mites, and to prevent problems posed by the possibility that some chiggers might acquire some rickettsiae while feeding but detach prematurely, and later attach to a second host ("reattachment") and transmit an infection (see p. 98 and p. 103). These small jars were stocked with appropriate numbers of engorged larvae, and the cultures were maintained until suitable numbers of chiggers of the next generation were available for testing. The jars were then temporarily placed in a special receptacle to permit the chiggers to attach to a laboratory mouse, or the chiggers were collected by hand and placed on the host.

In either case, whether with the mass cultures or the small jars, two to four young adult mice, either normal or infected, depending upon the test, and wearing special collars to keep them from catching and eating the chiggers on their bodies, were placed in jars that contained chiggers about 3–7 days old. (When chiggers that had remained unfed for weeks were used, there was a reduction in the numbers of engorged chiggers recovered.) The mice were exposed to the chiggers for about 2–4 hr, according to the degree of infestation, because it had been noted that in flourishing colonies, a 2-hr exposure was sufficient for attachment of 1000–2000 chiggers, whereas contact for a longer period would result in such a heavy infestation that the mice would die within hours if infected with *R. tsutsugamushi,* or within a day or two if originally healthy. Usually, the mice were exposed in the chigger cultures for only 2 hr. After removal, the mice, still wearing collars, were placed in small restraining cages that prohibited their turning around or scratching effectively. These cages were then inserted in funnels and suspended over water. After engorgement, the chiggers would detach from the hosts and drop into the water, from where they were removed and either used in experiments or saved for colonization. Tropical or subtropical species like *L. deliense, L. fletcheri,* and *L. arenicola* usually engorged within 2–3 days, but the subalpine *L. subintermedium* generally required 4–7 days to engorge. Chiggers were noted as detaching over a 5–7-day period, not only because of individual variations in the time required to engorge but also because some chiggers would wander for hours, or a day or longer, before attaching and commencing to feed.

In tests on the isolation of rickettsiae (see p. 98), pools of engorged larvae or developing postlarvae that contained about 100–200 specimens (mean, 150; range, 70–2000) were inoculated into white mice at varying intervals after detachment from the host. In each case, such cited numbers refer to the actual numbers tested and not to the quantity of chiggers observed or placed upon the host. (Usually, only 40–70% of the chiggers noted on a host were later recovered as engorged larvae.) The mice used to feed chiggers suspected of harboring rickettsiae were also examined to see if they had acquired infection in the process, as mentioned on p. 99.

In our cultures, engorged larvae of *Leptotrombidium* and *G. (S.) ligula* usually entered the quiescent *nymphophane* or prenymph stage about 3–4 days after detachment. The nymphs typically emerged after 7–12 days spent in the nymphophane stage for *L. deliense, L. arenicola,* and *L. fletcheri,* but the quiescent stage lasted about 10–18 days in *L. subintermedium* and, at times, as long as 3 weeks in *G. (S.) ligula*. To facilitate handling and also to reduce the mortality rate due to the formation of mold around quiescent prenymphs, the larvae and developing prenymphs were often retained in water as long as 10–12 days prior to inoculation.

In certain cases, aliquots of the engorged larvae that had fed on rickettsemic mice were retained in special containers for rearing until the next generation (F_1) to test for transovarian transmission of acquired infection with *R. tsutsugamushi*. In such cases, the numbers of F_1 chiggers tested varied from 17 to 2000, with a mean of 140, and the mice were exposed to the mites in special jars.

Reattachment of Chiggers

The following procedures were used to determine whether "reattached" chiggers may acquire rickettsiae from one host during an interrupted feeding and later transmit infection to a second host. Two infected mice per test were exposed to chiggers in the usual way but were killed 6 hr after contact. The carcasses were then suspended over water, and the chiggers were collected from the water within 24 hr. The chiggers that had obviously fed on the mice, that is, those that were about ¼–½ engorged, were retained, and the rest were discarded. The partially engorged larvae were examined again 1 week later, and those that had regressed in size, to the point at which they once again resembled normal unfed larvae, were placed on a new normal mouse at that time. The reattached chiggers that successfully engorged on this second host were tested for *R. tsutsugamushi* infection, as were the mouse hosts themselves.

Conducting valid experiments on reattachment was a laborious and time-consuming procedure. Replication was difficult, because the percentage of larvae prone to reattach would vary tremendously under what seemed to be similar conditions. Large numbers of chiggers were consumed in the experiments, but even so, there seldom were enough engorged reattached chiggers left at the end to start colonies to test their progeny. The entire study had to be terminated before the reattachment phenomenon could be properly investigated.

Isolation of R. tsutsugamushi

Isolations from Chiggers

1. Pools of chiggers, which generally contained 100–200 specimens, were ground in 2 ml of sterile "SPG diluent" of Bovarnick *et al.*,[35] which contained sucrose, phosphate, and glutamate, with a mortar and pestle. 2. The suspension was inoculated intraperitoneally (ip) into four adult white mice at the rate of 0.5 ml per mouse. 3. The mice were observed as long as 14 days for signs of illness, for example, ruffled fur and/or swollen abdomen. 4. The sick mice were autopsied and examined for typical scrub typhus pathologic features, for example, splenomegaly, peritoneal exudate, or ascites. If exudate was present, Giemsa-stained smears of peritoneal scrapings were prepared and examined for rickettsiae. In lines where the presence of *R. tsutsugamushi* had regularly been determined earlier, the results were considered positive if typical rickettsiae were observed in the smears. In other lines, confirmation was made only after

steps 5–8 were followed and positive results obtained. 5. In the absence of illness, abnormal pathologic features, or rickettsiae in smears, or in instances where there had been no confirmed history of scrub typhus infection in the lines, the mice were autopsied 14 days after inoculation (or earlier, if sick). Livers and spleens were removed, and a 20% suspension of these tissues was prepared in SPG and inoculated ip into eight normal mice. 6. These mice were observed and processed as above. However, in the absence of symptoms, three mice were autopsied 14 days after inoculation, and the livers and spleens were frozen at −70° C. 7. At about 30 days after inoculation, the remaining five mice were challenged by ip inoculation with about 1000 LD_{50} of *R. tsutsugamushi*, Karp strain, and then observed for 21 days for resistance to the lethal dose. If the mice succumbed, it was concluded that they had not been immune and therefore could not have been infected with *R. tsutsugamushi* originally. In such instances, the inoculum of chiggers was considered to have been negative for these rickettsiae. 8. If there was significant resistance, for example, 50% survival, the tissues frozen in step 6 were reexamined by additional passage in mice as in steps 1–6 but with liver and spleen tissues substituted for the chigger inoculum. In the meantime, it was tentatively assumed that the mice had become resistant to challenge, because the original chigger inoculum had contained viable *R. tsutsugamushi*. 9. Under special circumstances, the frozen tissues from step 6 were passed blindly for as many as three such passages. 10. The challenge procedure, if positive, was useful in detecting the occasional isolate that may be avirulent or of low virulence, as had been encountered in some of our isolations of *R. tsutsugamushi* in Pakistan.

Isolations from Normal Mice Used to Feed "Infected" Chiggers

In experiments on transovarian transmission of acquired *R. tsutsugamushi* infection, or on transmission of reattached chiggers, it was important to determine whether the mouse hosts had become infected as a result of the chiggers feeding on them. Similar information was needed to check whether natural infection with the agent was present in the colonies of chiggers regarded as "uninfected" and therefore used in tests on acquired transmission of rickettsiae. The procedures were as follows: Approximately 10–14 days after the chiggers had detached, each mouse was sacrificed and a portion of liver and spleen removed. The tissues were suspended in 2 ml of SPG, using a Ten Broeck tissue grinder, and inoculated ip into each of four white mice at the rate of 0.5 ml per mouse. Subsequent procedures were the same as steps 3–9 above.

Miscellaneous Points Regarding R. tsutsugamushi *Infection*

Infective Feedings of Normal Chiggers on Rickettsemic Mice. In this program, the Sialkot (Pakistan) strain of *R. tsutsugamushi*, well studied in our laboratory and known to be of high virulence, was employed throughout in tests aimed to determine whether normal chiggers can acquire *R. tsutsugamushi* infection as a result of feeding on rickettsemic mice. The mice were inoculated ip with 0.5 ml of material of known and standard virulence, empirically calculated so as to kill the mice within 12–14 days.

Various factors were considered in determining the exposure of the chiggers to the infective feeding, and some of these factors were mutually exclusive. On the one hand, there was the need to time the feeding so that high levels of rickettsemia were assured, for example, as late in the disease and as close to the expected date of death as possible. On the other hand, such seriously ill or moribund mice could not withstand the shock of infestation by thousands of chiggers, coupled with the effects of restraint imposed by a large collar on their necks and by imprisonment in tiny cages. Further, some species of chiggers took twice as long to engorge as others, and this required a period of 5–7 days on the host. On the basis of such considerations, for *L. subintermedium,* the mice were exposed to the chiggers for only 4 days after inoculation; for *G. ligula,* exposure was for 6 days, and the remaining *Leptotrombidium* were exposed for 8 days postinoculation. As a rule, the mice were placed in the culture jars for only 2 hr. In the event of death of the mice, either then or when in the restraining cages, the carcasses were retained over water for a minimum of 24 hr, because numbers of engorged chiggers would continue to drop off the hosts.

The chiggers used in the experiments on acquired infection came from cultures labeled "normal," because they had never been exposed to infected mice and showed no signs of harboring natural infection, as noted in the next paragraph. At times, chiggers in other cultures were used in special tests that employed rickettsemic mice exposed for about 2 hr. These colonies were designated "potentially infected," but careful screening likewise failed to disclose any signs of infection in those stock colonies at any time.

Lack of Infection in Chiggers in the "Normal" Colonies. Inasmuch as the main objectives in this series of experiments concerned the acquisition of experimental *R. tsutsugamushi* infection by chiggers, it was imperative that trombiculids used in the investigations were free of such infection prior to testing. It was possible that small numbers of the chiggers in the colonies were naturally infected with the agent and that such infection, although difficult to demonstrate, might persist in certain family lines by the mechanism of transovarian transmission and might account for "false positives" in the study. To foreguard against such a possibility, the stock cultures were regularly tested for signs of infection. Testing was performed by feeding the "normal" chiggers on uninfected mice and then utilizing the standard procedures outlined above to search for *R. tsutsugamushi* infection in adequate samples of engorged chiggers and in the tissues of the host mice. No signs of natural infection have been observed in a minimum of 80 such attempts at isolation of rickettsiae in the various colonies under test. If one adds the negative results from experiments on acquisition of rickettsial infection, more than 200 pools of chiggers or mouse tissues have been examined without an indication of natural infection. Further, at least 50 additional mice used in such experiments have been considered "negative" because of the lack of suggestive pathologic features and the absence of detectable rickettsiae in microscopic examination of smears of tissues.

Natural Infection in L. fletcheri *Chiggers*

Wild-caught, untested *L. fletcheri* chiggers were obtained from the United States Army Medical Research Unit (Malaysia) in an attempt to establish a colony of naturally infected chiggers. After it was shown in our laboratory that *R. tsutsugamushi* was present in samples tested, two procedures were followed to meet the objectives. In each case, only normal mice were used to feed the chiggers. The first method was the definitive approach of establishing cultures ultimately based upon single segregated females whose progeny were shown to include infected individuals, as determined by examination of the tissues of the mice used to feed the F_1 chiggers. (The procedures for isolation of rickettsiae here were the same as those outlined in the second paragraph on pp. 98–99.) In this series of experiments, adults reared from pools of chiggers that contained at least some infected larvae were placed individually in separate vials, and the sex was determined by whether spermatophores or eggs were deposited in the tubes. (The adults were first permitted to remain together in the small rearing jar for a few days to ensure fertilization of the females before segregation.) The F_1 chiggers from such segregated females were fed as a special unit, by themselves, and the tissues of the host mouse were tested for *R. tsutsugamushi*. When reaching adulthood, the F_1 females were segregated in turn, as above, and their progeny (F_2) were handled similarly. (This procedure of using segregated females was not followed beyond the F_2 generation because of the failure to isolate *R. tsutsugamushi* from these particular lines.) The other procedure was aimed at maintenance of mass cultures that contained some naturally infected chiggers. Maintenance was achieved by stock-piling and rearing only the pools of chiggers in which the mice showed evidence of rickettsial infection after the pools had fed. In such cases, the females were not segregated, but, instead, the chiggers were reared as a group. Such cultures, wherein generally only pools with evidence of infection were used for rearing, were maintained for four generations. After that period, there were no isolations of rickettsiae, but the mass culture was tested for an additional period of time sufficient to yield at least four more generations.

RESULTS AND OBSERVATIONS

Acquisition of R. tsutsugamushi *by Uninfected Chiggers After Feeding on Rickettsemic Mice and Not Permitted to Reattach*

Tests with Engorged Larvae and Protonymphs

It is generally believed that after a single meal on a vertebrate host, chiggers continue their development without further parasitism.[5] The results of a series of tests of 138 pools of chiggers regarded as being free of natural infection, and having their sole meal on laboratory mice with *R. tsutsugamushi* rickettsemia, are shown in TABLE 1. (The mean number of chiggers inoculated per pool was about 150.) It can be seen that all five species that had been tested four or more times [namely, four species of *Leptotrombidium* and *Gahrliepia* (*S.*) *ligula*] demonstrated the capacity to acquire *R. tsutsugamushi* during the feeding process. [Because a total of only five pools were tested for *Ascoschoengastia* (*L.*) *indica*, the consistently negative results with that species may represent inadequate sampling, and those data are therefore not considered in the results summarized below.] Of the pools tested on the day when the engorged chiggers had detached from the mice, 60–100% were positive for *R. tsutsugamushi* when examined by standard procedures. For the relatively well-tested *L. arenicola*, 11 of the 12 pools (92%) collected on the first to fourth days after detachment yielded rickettsiae. For all of these species, 10–27% of the

TABLE 1

ISOLATION OF *R. tsutsugamushi* FROM POOLS OF NORMAL CHIGGERS THAT HAD FED ON MICE WITH EXPERIMENTAL RICKETTSEMIA

	Known Major Vector	Results *			
Number of days after detachment of chigger		0	1–4	5–15	21–23
Leptotrombidium (L.) arenicola	yes	3/4 = 75%	11/12=92%	1/4 =25%	
Leptotrombidium (L.) deliense	yes	9/9 =100%	2/3 =67%	4/15=27%	
Leptotrombidium (L.) fletcheri	yes	3/4 = 75%	—	1/5 =20%	
Leptotrombidium (L.) subintermedium	no	20/32= 63%	0/1 = 0%	3/24=13%	
Gahrliepia (S.) ligula	no	3/5 = 60%	3/4 =75%	1/10=10%	0/3=0%
Ascoschoengastia (L.) indica	no	0/2 = 0%	0/1 = 0%	0/2 = 0%	

* Numerators of figures indicate numbers of pools found positive; denominators indicate numbers of pools tested.

pools that had been obtained on the fifth to 15th days after the chiggers had dropped off the hosts were positive. The rate of isolation was significantly lower in the later nymphophane stage than in the newly engorged larvae or recently quiescent chiggers, that is, only 10 positive isolations in 58 attempts (17%) with all five species in the period 5–15 days after detachment, versus 38/54 (70%) and 16/21 (76%) for the early categories. These data suggest that though uninfected chiggers may frequently acquire *R. tsutsugamushi* by feeding on infected mice, those rickettsiae generally *persist* in the mites' tissues rather than appreciably *multiply* therein.

This is the first report of the isolation of *R. tsutsugamushi* from pools of *L. subintermedium* or of *G. (S.) ligula* chiggers for which it can be categorically stated that no other species was represented in the inocula. There was a previous report of an isolation from *G. (S.) ligula* in nature, but the presence of *Leptotrombidium* therein admittedly could not be excluded.[5, 36] The present isolations, of course, presumably were not due to natural infection.

Transovarian Transmission of Rickettsiae After Acquired Infection

If it were indeed correct that in nature, trombiculids feed only once on a vertebrate host in their lifetime, the critical factor as to whether rickettsiae acquired by feeding could ultimately contribute to the infection of a second host, and thus help perpetuate the cycle, is transmission of the acquired infection to the next generation (F_1) of chiggers. The results of experiments on such possible transovarian transmission of acquired infection are summarized in TABLE 2; we used four species of trombiculids and a total of 43 pools of F_1 chiggers reared from parents that had fed as normal larvae on rickettsemic mice. Rickettsiae were isolated only once, namely, from one pool of 28 *L. deliense* of 23 pools tested. On 31 occasions, the tissues of the mice that had been used to feed these F_1 chiggers were also tested for infection, and all results were negative, including the tissues of the mouse that was the host to the above-mentioned positive pool. (As will be mentioned in the DISCUSSION, there are recorded instances of analogous findings in nature, namely, failure to recover *R. tsutsugamushi* in the tissues of rats that had been infested with chiggers which yielded rickettsial strains, and vice versa.[29]

Virulence of Strains

All of the isolations reported on the previous pages were of virulent strains in that they produced pathogenic changes in mice, and so on, and were recovered *without* the repeated serial blind passage undertaken because of limited survival to challenge (as indicated in steps 7–9 in MATERIALS AND METHODS). It must be noted, however, that the sole strain recovered from the F_1 chiggers (from *L. deliense*) *was* a relatively avirulent one and probably would have been overlooked if we had not employed the serial blind passage. This strain was the only one of low pathogenicity isolated during all the studies with acquired infection. (There was one mild strain among the 19 isolated during investigations of the naturally infected cultures of *L. fletcheri*.)

Reattachment of Chiggers and Possible Transfer of Acquired Rickettsiae

The Reattachment Phenomenon

When white mice were exposed to large numbers of chiggers in our laboratory, usually more than 90% of the chiggers attached to the hosts engorged

TABLE 2

POSSIBLE TRANSOVARIAN TRANSMISSION OF ACQUIRED *R. tsutsugamushi* INFECTION IN PROGENY OF UNINFECTED CHIGGERS WHICH HAD FED ON MICE WITH EXPERIMENTAL RICKETTSEMIA. RESULTS OF TESTS INVOLVING INOCULATIONS OF ENGORGED F_1 CHIGGERS AND OF THE TISSUES OF MICE UPON WHICH THEY FED

	L. deliense	*L. arenicola*	*L. fletcheri*	*G. (S.) ligula*
Pools of 17–1000 F_1 chiggers (mean: 140)	1/23 * =4%	0/12	0/3	0/5
Tissues of mouse hosts of these F_1 chiggers	0/19	0/8	0/1	0/3

* Numerator, number of pools found positive; denominator, number of pools inoculated.

fully, whereas the remainder, for unknown reasons, stayed attached for only a short period (6–24 hr instead of about 72–76 hr) and then dropped from the host while only partially fed. Such slightly engorged chiggers usually regressed to normal size within a few days, and about half of them were found to attach to a new host if exposed to one at that time. About half of these "reattached" chiggers engorged and successfully completed their life cycle. Thus, of 1000 unfed chiggers, about 20, as a conservative estimate, were capable of feeding to repletion on a second host after having partially fed on an earlier one. Further, if the original host died or was killed within 6–20 hr after exposure to infestation by chiggers, a significantly greater proportion of the chiggers would detach, namely, 25–50%, whereas 60–75% of the partially fed larvae would later successfully attach to a second host, and nearly all of them developed normally thereafter. Under such conditions, at least 250 chiggers of an original batch of 1000 would feed on two hosts instead of the usual single mouse, even though only a limited degree of engorgement occurred on the first animal.

Transmission of Rickettsiae by Reattached Chiggers

The results of a limited number (seven) of tests with reattached chiggers, which involved *L. arenicola* and *L. deliense,* are shown in TABLE 3, from which it can be seen that *R. tsutsugamushi* was shown to have been present in one pool (of five) of originally uninfected *L. deliense* that had partially fed on a rickettsemic mouse and that, 1 week after the interrupted feeding, later engorged on a second, but normal, mouse. The strain isolated was typical with respect to virulence. This demonstration of rickettsiae, made within 24 hr after engorgement on the uninfected second host, indicates that the aborted meal on the infected host was sufficient for the acquisition and persistence of viable rickettsiae. However, because the tissues of the second host did not yield any rickettsiae upon testing in this case (nor in the five others), there is no evidence at hand to show that the reattached chiggers could actually transmit acquired *R. tsutsugamushi* by biting.

It will be recalled that infected mice were exposed for about 2 hr in the mass cultures of the so-called possibly infected lines of chiggers. If some of the chiggers that acquired rickettsiae by feeding detached prematurely instead of engorging completely, there might have been an opportunity for subsequent

TABLE 3

ATTEMPTS TO ISOLATE *R. tsutsugamushi* FROM REATTACHED CHIGGERS
ORIGINALLY PARTIALLY FED ON INFECTED MICE AND THEN ENGORGING
ON NORMAL MICE ABOUT 1 WEEK LATER

Inocula		Number Positive	Number of Pools	Percent Positive
Pools of 50–141 reattached chiggers	*L. arenicola*	0	2	—
	L. deliense	1	5	20%
Tissues of these mouse hosts	*L. arenicola*	0	1	—
	L. deliense	0	5	—

TABLE 4

ISOLATIONS OF *R. tsutsugamushi* FROM MICE USED TO FEED 86 POOLS OF VARIOUS
GENERATIONS OF *L. fletcheri* CHIGGERS FROM CULTURES
WITH NATURALLY INFECTED CHIGGERS

Generation of Chiggers Tested	Numbers of Chiggers in Pools Feeding on Mice		Numbers of Infected Pools
	Range	Mean	
First filial (F_1)	25–1100	195	2/7
Third filial (F_3)	5–427	73	17/57
Fourth filial (F_4)	21–350	106	0/10
Subsequent $(F_5–F_8)$	25–1100	226	0/11

transmission if such chiggers successfully reattached to a second host 2 weeks later at the time of routine feeding, or if transovarian transmission occurred so as to render the next generation effective. Nevertheless, it is reiterated that careful, repeated, long-term checking of the mass cultures did not disclose any evidence of infection in the test colonies. Apparently, such brief exposure was insufficient to produce infection in reattaching chiggers.

Miscellaneous Observations

Because the studies in this program were ultimately aimed at elucidating the role of certain species of chiggers as vectors of chigger-borne rickettsiosis, incidental data were obtained and are presented here as pertinent to our discussion. It was noted for the first time that *L. intermedium, L. arenicola,* and *G. (S.) ligula* will readily attach to and engorge on man and develop normally thereafter,[5] and this is the first report that *A. (L.) indica* will likewise do so.

It was also observed that detached engorged larvae that fell into water and remained submerged for days or weeks not only continued their development but also could even emerge under water as nymphs and continue to survive there for at least several additional days.[5] Moreover, certain of the pools of nymphophanes that proved positive for *R. tsutsugamushi* in TABLE 1 had been maintained submerged in water for 10 days or more.

Natural Infection in L. fletcheri *Chiggers*

The mice used to feed the first two batches of chiggers reared from the *L. fletcheri* chiggers received from Malaya were positive for natural infection with *R. tsutsugamushi.* Accordingly, both pools of chiggers were saved for rearing stock, and their descendents were divided into subcultures and from the F_3 generations onward were tested for natural infection over a period of several generations. As noted, in most instances, only mites from positive pools were used as breeding stock for the next generation. The results are summarized in TABLE 4, from which it can be seen that in the third generation, 17 of 57 pools (30%) tested (by examining the mouse hosts) were positive for natural infection. In 21 tests of subsequent generations of chiggers by this method, however, there was no evidence of rickettsial infection. In addition, in two pools of F_3 and one of F_4 chiggers *inoculated* into mice, the results were also negative.

Further analysis of the data on the naturally infected cultures of *L. fletcheri* is presented in TABLE 5, which deals with the sizes of the pools of chiggers fed on the mice in tests on isolation of rickettsiae. It is naturally axiomatic that, within limits, the possibility of transmitting *R. tsutsugamushi* increases as the numbers of potentially infected chiggers feeding on the host are increased. It is therefore not surprising that six strains were isolated in 11 attempts (55%) when 100–200 chiggers were placed on the host, whereas only 5% (2/41) of the attempts were positive when small pools (9–49 chiggers) were employed. However, it appears that more than mere numbers of chiggers is involved. Thus, a great many mice were exposed to small pools of fewer than 50 chiggers to augment chances of segregating infected females for individual cultures. A significant number of chiggers (876) were in that category, whereas 1595 and 1173 chiggers were employed in the 50–99 and 100–199 size pools, respectively.

It is noteworthy that when small pools of chiggers were fed on the mice, the total of two strains recovered in the 41 attempts represented an average of 439 chiggers per isolation, whereas for the next two higher groups, the averages per isolation were 228 and 196, respectively. Further analysis of the data is necessary because of the important possibility that there may be a quantitative factor involved in transmission by naturally infected chiggers; that is, it may be more probable that infection resulted when several chiggers that harbored *R. tsutsugamushi* attached to a host than when merely one did so. It is therefore necessary to consider whether the disparity noted above could have been due to a disproportionate number of small pools being tested late in the study, when all the attempts at isolations were negative. Such skewing of the data is ruled out by the fact that only seven pools in the 5–49 chigger category were tested in the F_{4-8} generations and by the figures in TABLE 6, which deals only with the 57 pools tested in the F_3 generation; this group accounts for 17 of the 19 isolations. Thus, the average number of chiggers per isolation was 273 for the small-sized pools, but the average numbers were 149 and 154 for the 50–99 and 100–199 chigger pools, respectively. In other words, the isolation rate for the larger pools was 1.8 times that of the small pools, based on this criterion.

TABLE 5

ISOLATIONS OF *R. tsutsugamushi* FROM MICE USED TO FEED 86 POOLS OF *L. fletcheri* CHIGGERS FROM CULTURES WITH NATURALLY INFECTED CHIGGERS. NUMBERS OF CHIGGERS PER POOL COMPARED WITH NUMBERS OF ISOLATIONS

	Range of Numbers of Chiggers in Pools			
	5–49	50–99	100–199	200–1100
Numbers of pools: positive/total tested	2/41	7/21	6/11	4/13
Total numbers of chiggers in category	876	1595	1173	5625
Average number of chiggers per isolation	439	228	196	1406

TABLE 6

Isolations of *R. tsutsugamushi* from Mice Used to Feed 57 Pools
of Third-Generation (F_3) Chiggers from Naturally Infected Chiggers.
Numbers of Chiggers per Pool Compared with Numbers of Isolations

	Range of Numbers of Chiggers in Pools			
	5–49	50–99	100–199	200–1100
Numbers of pools: positive/total tested	2/29	7/14	6/9	2/5
Total numbers of chiggers in category	545	1016	921	1667
Average number of chiggers per isolation	273	149	154	834

In the experiments aimed at obtaining offspring from individual segregated female *L. fletcheri* reared from pools of chiggers responsible for infecting normal mice by feeding, it was possible to test the progeny of 17 different females. A total of 46 attempts at isolation were made from tissues of mice on which these larvae fed. The numbers of chiggers ranged from five to 250. All results were negative.

All except one of the strains of rickettsiae isolated from the naturally infected *L. fletcheri* were as virulent for the mice as were the strains with which we regularly work. However, one F_3 strain was of low virulence and was nonlethal.

DISCUSSION

It is apparent that the five species of chiggers under study readily acquired *R. tsutsugamushi* when feeding on rickettsemic mice, at least with respect to demonstration by inoculation of pools of trombiculids, because 60–100% of the tests conducted on the day the chiggers detached were positive. Because the results with the three adequately tested species were almost as successful within 4 days after drop-off, it is obvious that there was noteworthy persistence of the rickettsiae for at least that period. It seems doubtful that there was marked proliferation of the rickettsiae within the chiggers, because the isolation rate dropped appreciably (to 10–27%) when protonymphs were tested 5–15 days after detachment.

Once it became clear that chiggers could acquire rickettsiae by feeding, it was rather surprising to learn that even in vector species, there was little or no evidence that true infection resulted. Inasmuch as the infection is acquired by the bite of the vector and is transovarially transmitted in the mite, it was considered axiomatic that the rickettsiae must be widely distributed within the body in the various stages of the trombiculid, for example, at least within the salivary gland of the chigger and within the female genitalia in the adult. (That this is so has just been shown by Roberts *et al.*[16]) On theoretical grounds, it therefore seemed to us likely that once *R. tsutsugamushi* entered the gut of uninfected chiggers feeding on rickettsemic mice, the rickettsiae would rapidly penetrate the walls of the intestine and soon reach other parts of the body. The actual fate of the rickettsiae ingested in our experiments is, of course, unknown, but because the results generally (with one noteworthy exception) indicate persistence rather than reproduction of rickettsiae, it may be that the intestinal walls of the vector chiggers are a fairly effective barrier against *R. tsutsugamushi* within the lumen. (Tarasevich and Rehacek believed that the gut of ticks was impermeable to this agent and that because of this barrier, ticks did not become infected after feeding on such rodents.[9]) Regardless, acquisition of *R. tsutsugamushi* by chiggers by means of ingestion can be of little true significance in the ecology of infection, unless one or both of two events follow: the rickettsiae eventually break through the gut barrier and enter the genital system, so that transovarian transmission can be effected, or the chiggers do not follow the usual course of events of parasitizing only a single vertebrate host but, instead, subsequently reattach to a second mammal or bird and transmit the infection to it, either by feeding or perhaps by scarification, after being crushed on the host.

The single successful isolation of *R. tsutsugamushi* (in 43 attempts) from the progeny of previously normal chiggers that had fed on rickettsemic mice may very well be a bona fide instance of transovarian transmission, but the possibility of error in the records cannot be excluded, although such an error is considered highly remote. It may be significant that this particular strain was a mild one, and therefore unique in our program on experimental infection, and certainly different in behavior from the Sialkot strain to which the parental generation had been exposed. However, it cannot be assumed that a truly acquired infection would retain all its characteristics after transovarian transmission. It is conceivable that this isolation really represents a strain of low virulence that existed undetected in our "normal" colony, but this would be exceedingly strange, because, despite intensive search, there has been no evidence of infection in our stock cultures. Further, none of the colonies used in these tests had ever been exposed to mice with *R. tsutsugamushi*. Regardless, comparison of the serotype of the F_1 isolate with that of the original strain is in progress to determine whether they are identical. Although the tissues of the mouse upon which these particular F_1 chiggers had fed failed to yield rickettsiae upon testing, this result may lack significance. For example, Davis et al.[29] reported results of 166 "paired isolation experiments" in which both host tissues and pools of chiggers from the same mammal were inoculated and noted that in 16 instances, the chigger pools were positive but not the mammal tissues, whereas the reverse was true in five instances. On only four occasions were the "pairs" positive.

Although it is now documented that *R. tsutsugamushi* has been isolated from inocula known to consist of purely *L. subintermedium, L. arenicola,* and *G. ligula,* it is stressed that they represent experimental "infections," not natural ones. It is noteworthy that all three species readily attach to and feed to repletion on man (as does *A. indica*), and though *L. arenicola* is now regarded as a major vector in Western Malaysia, nothing is really known about the vector capacity of the other three species.[5]

The relative ease with which *R. tsutsugamushi* can be acquired by pools of chiggers feeding on infected hosts lends credence to the suggestion [5, 33] that many of the reported isolations of *R. tsutsugamushi,* reported for nonvector species of chiggers, actually represent the transient presence of ingested rickettsiae rather than true infection.

The reattachment phenomenon is worth considering as a possible mechanism for replenishment of *R. tsutsugamushi* in nature, now that we realize that an appreciable number of chiggers may actually attempt to feed a second time, especially if the original host dies. Another reason is our evidence that rickettsiae may be acquired during a very brief feeding on the first mammal and yet persist long enough for detection at least 16 days later. It is true that there was only one such instance, but only a limited number of the complex laborious experiments was attempted. In view of the enormous chigger population supported by theraphions in endemic areas, the high rate of natural infection with *R. tsutsugamushi* and the normal attrition in the hosts caused by predation, and so on, reattachment may be of consequence in the field, even though it is only an occasional event in the laboratory. Nevertheless, the fact that no infection was ever noted in the "possibly infected" cultures indicates that any spontaneous reattachment that might have occurred after the routine 2-hr exposure to infected mice was insufficient to produce demonstrable transmission of *R. tsutsugamushi* under those special conditions.

The observations on the ability of larval and nymphal trombiculids to survive long periods of submersion are of epidemiologic significance. Outbreaks of chigger-borne rickettsiosis have been associated with flooding of rivers in Pakistan, Japan, and other countries so much that the disease was called Japanese River fever. On the Indian subcontinent, the endemic areas may be dry for months, and vast stretches of land along the rivers may then be submerged for days or weeks, as the rivers rise from the heavy rains in the hills. It was obvious that some stage of the trombiculid vector had to be able to survive under those conditions, but it had been speculated that the mites did so in rodent burrows in patches of higher ground, along with the mammals. Such an explanation was not very satisfactory, because the infected foci were too continuous and widespread to be accounted for by migration of chiggers from scattered refuges, especially in view of the extremely limited mobility of the mites. It makes much more sense for them to be able to survive prolonged submersion and to be washed by the waters to new foci.

As in the case of the naturally infected colonies of Audy [20, 30] and Krishnan *et al.*,[31] it was impossible to find any evidence of *R. tsutsugamushi* in our chiggers after a few generations were fed on normal mice, even though it had been easy to isolate rickettsiae from pools in the F_3 generation of our naturally infected lines, and even though the chiggers used as rearing stock came from pools of mites that transmitted infection by feeding. Perhaps, the failure was due to the small number of infected mites in the cultures and to the fact that they had been lost by chance selection, as in the course of colonization. Nevertheless, the question remains as to whether this may be the usual pattern when there is no "replenishment" of rickettsiae by feeding on infected hosts. Because every strain, except one, isolated was of standard virulence, the loss of the infected lines cannot be readily ascribed to low virulence.

Our data on the naturally infected lines raise another point, namely, whether there is a greater chance of acquiring scrub typhus when two or more infected chiggers bite than when only one does so. It would be otherwise difficult to see why the average number of chiggers per isolation was 1.8 times higher when small batches of chiggers (5–49) were fed on mice than when 50–199 were employed. Rapmund *et al.*[7] showed that the bite of a single infected chigger could result in the death of a white mouse, but, again, that strain may have been highly lethal.

Because transovarian transmission also occurs in tick-borne rickettsiosis, some comments thereon are pertinent, although one cannot necessarily validly extrapoláte from such observations to chigger-borne rickettsiosis. Burgdorfer [37] noted that infected female ticks passed rickettsiae to practically 100% of their progeny, which, in turn, transmitted the infection to 100% of their offspring. Later studies extended these observations to cover seven generations, still with 100% filial infection rates.[14] However, as Burgdorfer and Varma [14] emphasized, those tests had been conducted with susceptible guinea pigs used to feed the ticks, and it could be assumed that reinfection of the ticks occurred in every stage and in every generation of tick that fed, because the arthropods remain attached long enough for that phenomenon to transpire. To preclude such reinfection, additional experiments were undertaken in which immunized guinea pigs were used as hosts, for six generations of ticks. One of the two strains under study consistently produced 100% filial infection rates, but with the other, rickettsial antigen was encountered that was no longer infectious for guinea pigs. Other lines became negative in subsequent filial generations, but some persisted in being 100% infective.[14] The reasons for the loss in efficiency in transovarian transmission are not fully understood, but the immune state of the host may be a factor to consider. Other noteworthy observations on tick-borne rickettsiosis include the importance of new lines of infections in ticks that result from simultaneous feeding of infected and noninfected ticks on susceptible hosts and the infection of ova in ticks during fertilization by rickett-siae-bearing sperm.[17]

These points are of unknown relevance to the ecology of chigger-borne rickettsiosis. The notable investigations by Rapmund et al. on transovarian transmission involved tests by single chiggers feeding on susceptible hosts.[6,7] Thus, the complications imposed by nature were lacking, wherein the hosts may be infected, and even may have a rickettsemia, or already be immune, at the times the chiggers are feeding, and wherein hundreds of chiggers may simultaneously infest the host, some in one stage of engorgement, others in another, some of which may be infected and others not infected. It cannot be assumed that naturally infected chiggers feeding en masse on an immune host transmit the infection to their progeny in the same way as does a single female, with a virulent strain, attached to a susceptible host. Moreover, several different species of Leptotrombidium may be found on the same host, and because several serotypes have beeen known to be present in just one small field,[5] it is possible that the chiggers on a host may be transmitting more than one strain of R. tsutsugamushi to the mammal. Other probable relevant factors include the known occurrence of parthenogenesis in Leptotrombidium,[5] the fact that the progeny may normally be uniformly males or all females,[5] and the restriction of infection to just the female trombiculid in certain lines.[6] The course of transovarian transmission over generations under such circumstances in the field may be very different from that noted in the laboratory, where the picture is already confused by the apparent loss of strains over a period of generations, even when susceptible hosts, like normal white mice, were solely used. If immune animals are encountered in the wild, there may even be a greater loss in the efficiency of transovarian transmission of natural infection, but no data are available as to what is actually transpiring in nature.

There is yet another important factor that requires consideration and clarification, namely, the possibility that the studies in our laboratory and elsewhere have been affected by selection of certain genetic lines of chiggers for experimentation. In our case, we have worked with lines that tend to acquire rickettsiae by feeding and have used them for breeding stock. In early tests in Malaysia, others were doing just the opposite: rearing from cultures in which the members did *not* readily ingest rickettsiae. The results may not have been comparable for those reasons, but the main point is that in nature, there may very well be marked variability with respect to acquisition of rickettsiae, and of infection, by chiggers. It also seems highly probable that there are analogous differences in family lines of chiggers with respect to both virulence of the strain of *R. tsutsugamushi* they harbor and to the efficiency in transovarian transmission of rickettsiae.

From what has been stated above, it is clear that the role of theraphions as reservoirs of *R. tsutsugamushi* cannot be properly evaluated in the light of available information. On the other hand, the chiggers that are vectors of rickettsiosis undoubtedly also serve as true reservoirs, even if the mechanism of transovarian transmission may not be as uniformly effective over a period of generations, as the findings of Rapmund *et al.*[7, 16, 39] imply. If small mammals never do constitute a source of rickettsiae for chiggers, it must be axiomatic that in certain family lines of certain species of chiggers (and no others), either the infection has been successfully passed from one generation to another from time immemorial, or infective rickettsiae have sporadically appeared *de novo* within the mites, perhaps derived from symbionts or parasites. In either case, it would be difficult to comprehend the following points: a single serotype of *R. tsutsugamushi* occurs in several species of *Leptotrombidium;* there is one rickettsial strain that is found throughout the range of the rickettsiosis (even outstripping the range of *L. deliense,* which extends from southern China and Indochina through the Indonesian archipelagoes as far as New Guinea and Australia); there is no correlation between serotype, on the one hand, and, on the other, the species of vector chigger, a specific host theraphion, the geographic region, or the microhabitat in the endemic foci.[5, 38] Even at an extreme periphery of the range of chigger-borne rickettsiosis, in West Pakistan, where the infection occurs in unusual habitats and in the absence of known vectors, there was no evidence obtained for the existence of new serotypes that could be regarded as geographic variants that resulted from local, selective evolutionary pressure.[38] One possible explanation for these anomalies is that the differentiation into strains of *R. tsutsugamushi* preceded the speciation of *Leptotrombidium* in the course of evolution. Another one is that the taxonomy of rickettsiae is inadequately understood and that in reality there is a correlation of serotypes with species and distribution of trombiculids that cannot be discovered without new criteria. If, however, ground-dwelling rodents act as a source of rickettsiae for replenishing or supplementing the cycles in chiggers by means of acquisition of rickettsiae by ingestion or by reattachment, the problems posed by the serotypes are more readily explainable, at least in theory.

Wild or native forms of the subgenus *Rattus* are the most likely candidates for such a true primary reservoir of chigger-borne rickettsiosis, because this group of rats is intimately associated with the ecology of this infection wherever it occurs.[5] The distribution of wild *Rattus* thus coincides with that of one of the serotypes of *R. tsutsugamushi,* but it should not be inferred from this analogy that we are suggesting that this rickettsia evolved from a murine symbiont or parasite rather than from an acarine one. Microtines (voles) and tupaiids in endemic areas, which are also excellent hosts for the vector *Leptotrombidium,* could then be regarded as secondary reservoirs. Interaction by the rickettsiae with all such hosts and their characteristic trombiculid fauna could have assisted in the diversification of serotypes.

Rats are tolerant hosts of *R. tsutsugamushi*, in that, once infected, they harbor rickettsiae for very long periods, if not for life, but show no signs of illness,[5, 25] and this is the pattern exhibited by true reservoirs. Tree squirrels, in contrast, do not come into contact with vector mites and are scarcely involved in the ecology of this rickettsiosis,[5] and it is of interest that Walker *et al.*[25] have found them to be resistant to infection, that is, in the category of what we here term refractory hosts.

CONCLUSIONS

Although vector chiggers undoubtedly are important true reservoirs of chigger-borne rickettsiosis, the following reasons suggest that theraphions may also serve as a wellspring for maintenance of the rickettsial cycle in nature.

Uninfected chiggers may acquire rickettsiae while feeding on hosts with rickettsemia, and such ingested organisms may at least survive for weeks. Transovarian transmission to the next generation was demonstrated in one pool of chiggers with such acquired rickettsiae. An appreciable number of chiggers will detach from their original host, particularly if it dies prematurely, and successfully attach to a second host and develop normally thereafter. In one instance, the chiggers that detached from the second host still bore evidence of rickettsiae acquired by feeding on the first one, more than 1 week earlier. Natural infection with *R. tsutsugamushi* is often common in a variety of ground-dwelling theraphions in endemic areas. Vector species may be extremely abundant on such hosts. The geographic and ecologic distribution and host relationships of the known serotypes of *R. tsutsugamushi* do not correlate with those of the vector species of *Leptotrombidium*. There are conflicting laboratory data on the efficiency of the mechanism of transovarian transmission, even when the tests are limited to using susceptible hosts to feed naturally infected chiggers. There is no information available as to the course of natural infection in generations of chiggers in the field, where there are many complicating factors; for example, both immune and susceptible hosts may be infested with large numbers of chiggers in various stages of engorgement, representing several species of *Leptotrombidium*, and including both infected and uninfected individuals, with the possibility that more than one serotype of *R. tsutsugamushi* is present in the pools of chiggers. There may be marked genetic variability in chiggers with respect to the ability to acquire rickettsiae (and infection) by feeding. Similarly, there probably are significant differences in family lines of chiggers regarding the virulence of the *R. tsutsugamushi* they carry and in the efficiency of the mechanism of transovarian transmission.

More data are required on most of these points before the existing questions can be answered about the importance of theraphions as a source of rickettsiae to chiggers.

ACKNOWLEDGMENTS

We are grateful to Col. Garrison Rapmund, MC, and Col. Francis C. Cadigan, Jr., MC, with respect to our obtaining specimens of trombiculid mites from the U.S. Army Medical Research Unit (Malaysia). Mr. Lim Boo Liat and Mr. M. Nadchatram of the Institute for Medical Research, Kuala Lumpur, rendered great assistance in helping us collect such material or in sending us live specimens. Dr. Bennett L. Elisberg, formerly of the Walter Reed Army Institute of Research, and Major Jerry S. Walker, VC, then at USAMRU, who were engaged in research on other facets of these general problems, were most helpful and cooperative concerning the exchange of ideas and data.

REFERENCES

1. AUDY, J. R. 1968. Red Mites and Typhus. The Athlone Press. London, England.
2. MACKIE, T. T., G. E. DAVIS, H. S. FULLER, J. A. KNAPP, M. L. STEINACKER, K. F. STAGER, R. TRAUB, W. L. JELLISON, D. D. MILLSPAUGH, R. C. AUSTRIAN, E. J. BELL, G. M. KOHLS, W. HSI & J. A. V. GIRSHAM. 1946. Observations on tsutsugamushi disease (scrub typhus) in Assam and Burma. Preliminary report. Amer. J. Hyg. **43:** 195–218.
3. PHILIP, C. B. 1948. The reservoirs of infection in rickettsial diseases of man. *In* Rickettsial Diseases of Man. F. R. Moulton, Ed. : 97–112. American Association for the Advancement of Science. Washington, D.C.
4. TRAUB, R. & C. L. WISSEMAN, JR. 1968b. Ecological considerations in scrub typhus. 2. Vector species. Bull. World Health Org. **38:** 209–218.
5. TRAUB, R. & C. L. WISSEMAN, JR. 1974. The ecology of chigger-borne rickettsiosis (scrub typhus). J. Med. Entomol. **11:** 237–303.
6. RAPMUND, G., A. L. DOHANY, C. MANIKUMARAN & T. C. CHAN. 1972. Transovarial transmission of *Rickettsia tsutsugamushi* in *Leptotrombidium* (*Leptotrombidium*) *arenicola* Traub (Acarina: Trombiculidae). J. Med. Entomol. **9:** 71, 72.
7. RAPMUND, G., R. W. UPHAM, JR., W. D. KUNDIN, C. MANIKUMARAN & T. C. CHAN. 1969. Transovarian development of scrub typhus rickettsiae in a colony of vector mites. Trans. Roy. Soc. Trop. Med. Hyg. **63:** 251–258.
8. U. S. ARMY MEDICAL RESEARCH UNIT (MALAYA). 1969. Annual report; scrub typhus. *In* Annual Report of the Institute of Medical Research (Kuala Lumpur) for 1968. : 183–198.
9. TARASEVICH, I. V. & J. REHACEK. 1972. Cultivation of *Rickettsia tsutsugamushi* in ixodid ticks. Acta Virol. **16:** 168–170.
10. FUKUZUMI, S. 1953. The route of infection of scrub typhus. Jap. J. Bacteriol. **8:** 149–156.
11. TRAUB, R. & M. NADCHATRAM. 1967. New species of chiggers of the subgenus *Leptotrombidium* from the mountains of West Pakistan (Acarina: Trombiculidae). J. Med. Entomol. **4**(1): 1–11.
12. BOESE, J. L. 1972. 6. Tissue reactions at the site of attachment of chiggers. J. Med. Entomol. **9:** 591, 592.
13. KUCHERUK, V. V. 1965. On the paleogenesis of natural plague. *In* Theoretical Questions of Natural Foci of Diseases. B. Rosicky & K. Heyberger, Eds. : 379 394. Publishing House of Czechoslovak Academy of Science. Prague, Czechoslovakia.
14. BURGDORFER, W. & M. G. R. VARMA. 1967. Trans-stadial and transovarian development of disease agents in arthropods. Annu. Rev. Entomol. **12:** 347–376.
15. PHILIP, C. B. 1949. Scrub typhus, or tsutsugamushi disease. Sci. Monthly **69:** 281–289.
16. ROBERTS, L. W., D. M. ROBINSON, G. RAPMUND, J. S. WALKER, E. GAN & S. RAM. 1975. Distribution of *Rickettsia tsutsugamushi* in organs of *Leptotrombidium* (*Leptotrombidium*) *fletcheri* (Prostigmata: Trombiculidae). J. Med. Entomol. In press.

17. PHILIP, C. B. & W. BURGDORFER. 1961. Arthropod vectors as reservoirs of microbial disease agents. Annu. Rev. Entomol. **6:** 391–412.
18. TAMIYA, T. (Ed.) 1962. Recent Advances in Studies of Tsutsugamushi Disease in Japan. Medical Culture, Inc. Tokyo, Japan.
19. TOYOKAWA, K. 1972. 9. Transmission of *Rickettsia orientalis* from experimentally infected mice to vector mites. J. Med. Entomol. **9:** 593.
20. AUDY, J. R. 1961. The ecology of scrub typhus. *In* Studies in Disease Ecology. J. M. May, Ed. Chap. **12:** 389–432. Vol. II of Studies in Medical Geography. American Geographical Society, Hafner Publishing Co., Inc. New York, N.Y.
21. HARRISON, J. L. & J. R. AUDY. 1951a. Hosts of the mite vector of scrub typhus. I. A check list of the recorded hosts. Ann. Trop. Med. Parasitol. **45:** 171–185.
22. HARRISON, J. L. & J. R. AUDY. 1951b. Hosts of the mite vector of scrub typhus. II. An analysis of the list of recorded hosts. Ann. Trop. Med. Parasitol. **45:** 186–194.
23. WHARTON, G. W. & H. S. FULLER. 1952. A manual of the chiggers. Mem. Entomol. Soc. Wash. **4.**
24. LEARMONTH, A. T. A. 1972. 10. Atlases in medical geography 1950–70. A review. *In* Medical Geography. N. D. McGlashan, Ed. : 135–152. Methuen & Co., Ltd. London, England.
25. WALKER, J. S., E. GAN, C. T. CHYE & I. MUUL. 1973. Involvement of small mammals in the transmission of scrub typhus in Malaysia. Isolation and serological evidence. Trans. Roy. Soc. Trop. Med. Hyg. **67:** 838–845.
26. COMMISSION ON RICKETTSIAL DISEASES, ARMED FORCES EPIDEMIOLOGICAL BOARD, ANNUAL REPORT. 1970. Washington, D. C.
27. COMMISSION ON RICKETTSIAL DISEASES, ARMED FORCES EPIDEMIOLOGICAL BOARD, ANNUAL REPORT. 1971. Washington, D. C.
28. COMMISSION ON RICKETTSIAL DISEASES, ARMED FORCES EPIDEMIOLOGICAL BOARD, ANNUAL REPORT. 1972. Washington, D. C.
29. DAVIS, G. E., R. C. AUSTRIAN & E. J. BELL. 1947. Observations on tsutsugamushi disease (scrub typhus) in Assam and Burma. The recovery of strains of *Rickettsia orientalis.* Amer. J. Hyg. **46:** 268–286.
30. AUDY, J. R. 1958. The role of mite vectors in the natural history of scrub typhus. Proc. 10th. Int. Congr. Entomol. **3:** 639–649.
31. KRISHNAN, K. V., R. O. A. SMITH, P. N. BOSE, K. N. NEOGY, B. K. G. ROY & M. GOSH. 1949. Transmission of *Rickettsia orientalis* by the bite of the larvae of *Trombicula deliensis.* Indian Med. Gaz. **84:** 41–43.
32. TRAUB, R., C. L. WISSEMAN, JR. & N. AHMAD. 1967. The occurrence of scrub typhus infection in unusual habitats in West Pakistan. Trans. Roy. Soc. Trop. Med. Hyg. **61:** 23–57.
33. TRAUB, R. & C. L. WISSEMAN, JR. 1968a. Ecological considerations in scrub typhus. I. Emerging concepts. Bull. World Health Org. **39:** 209–218.
34. GISPEN, R. 1950. The role of rats and mites in the spread of endemic scrub typhus in Batavia. Med. Maandbl. **3:** 45–58.
35. BOVARNICK, M. P., J. C. MILLER & J. C. SNYDER. 1950. The influence of certain salts, amino acids, sugars and proteins upon the stability of rickettsiae. J. Bacteriol. **59:** 509–521.
36. KALRA, S. L. 1959. Progress in the knowledge of rickettsial diseases in India. Indian J. Med. Res. **47:** 477–483.
37. BURGDORFER, W. 1963. Investigation of *Rickettsia rickettsii* in the wood tick, *Dermacentor andersoni.* Exp. Parasitol. **14:** 152–159.
38. SHIRAI, A. & C. L. WISSEMAN, JR. 1975. Serologic classification of scrub typhus isolates from Pakistan. Amer. J. Trop. Med. Hyg. **24(1):** 145–153.
39. U. S. ARMY MEDICAL RESEARCH UNIT (MALAYA). 1971. Annual Report; Scrub typhus. *In* Annual Report of the Institute of Medical Research (Kuala Lumpur) for 1969. : 176–191.

INHERITED INFECTION IN THE EPIDEMIOLOGY OF DIPTERA-BORNE DISEASE: PERSPECTIVES AND AN INTRODUCTION *

Andrew Spielman

Department of Tropical Public Health
Harvard University School of Public Health
Boston, Massachusetts 02115

Historical Perspective

That vector-borne pathogens of vertebrates might, in part, be maintained by direct transgenerational passage in the vector was one of the possibilities considered by the earliest students of such disease entities. Smith's epochal [1] demonstration in 1893 of inherited protozoan infection in ticks was soon confirmed and extended by Koch, Ricketts, and others working with a variety of vertebrate pathogens in ticks.[1a] Protozoa, spirochaetes, rickettsiae, and viruses all are readily inherited both by successive generations of ticks and by other acarines.[2] Indeed, both one-host ticks and chiggers can transmit disease only when transgenerational passage is possible. Thus, there is a long history of solidly established work that demonstrates that pathogens of vertebrates commonly infect the descendents of infected acarine vectors.

Insects, too, may transmit certain microorganisms directly from generation to generation, and the history of these observations even precedes those of Smith. Wheeler, in 1889,[3] observed bacteroids in the eggs of roaches and ascribed their presence to transovarial transmission. These endosymbionts, which are remarkably widespread among insects,[4] were noted by Leydig, Huxley, Metschnikov, and others.[5] At least a third of all insect species harbor such "organism-like, intracellular particles . . . that are transmitted through the cytoplasm of the egg," for which Lanham resurrects Wheeler's term "Blochmann bodies." That these particles are transmitted via the egg has long been inferred and, more recently, rigorously demonstrated.[6, 7]

Tsetse flies are host to at least two kinds of symbiotic Blochmann bodies: a large bacterium-like agent, observed a half century ago by Roubaud and Wigglesworth, and a recently recognized smaller "rickettsia." [8] These agents, which are ubiquitous in tsetse, seem to provide a factor essential to development of these insects.

Symbionts of fruit flies, described as mycoplasma-like, are universally present in the gonads of *Drosophila paulistorum*.[9] The microorganism is associated with hybrid-male sterility, causing a reduction in the abundance of motile sperm when introduced into the testes of alien males. Some kind of "a discord between the hybrid host genotype and the symbiont" presumably affects the latter stage of spermatogenesis. A strong tissue affinity ensures that these microorganisms, present in oocytes (and trophocytes), are enclosed within the mature egg and enter the germ line once the germinal primordia differentiate.

* Supported by Grant AI10274 from the National Institute of Allergy and Infectious Diseases, National Institutes of Health.

Fruit flies are host to another such agent, a rhabdovirus, that is transmitted via the egg. l'Héritier and his colleagues discovered that carbon dioxide sensitivity of *Drosophila melanogaster* results from hereditary infection with a cytoplasmic particle.[10] As little as 20% of atmospheric carbon dioxide may induce irreversible paralysis in infected flies. Inherited infection is widespread among natural populations and can be transmitted to noninfected flies by injection of triturated tissues. Flies, infected in this manner, may acquire oogonial infection, in which case the virus becomes established in the germ line and is transmitted to all offspring. As in the case of the mycoplasma, these symbionts of fruit flies appear to bear a strong affinity for germ tissue. Seecof[10] speculates that infection with sigma virus may protect against superinfection with other more pathogenic agents, a suggestion fraught with possibilities for medical entomology. Fruit flies carry various other heritable agents, including a sterility virus, polyhedral viruses, spirochaetes, and an agent that causes distortion of sex ratio.[11]

In 1924, Hertig and Wolbach[12] discovered a rickettsia-like infection in the ovaries of the common house mosquito, *Culex pipiens,* and similar infections are now recognized in *Aedes scutelaris.*[12a] This condition appears to be universal among members of infected populations, but the rickettsiae are apparently highly restricted in distribution. These infected species are peculiar for another reason: both manifest "cytoplasmic incompatibility" when specimens from one location intermate with those from certain other sites. This nonreciprocal fertility is maternally inherited, which suggests an association with the rickettsia.[13] It is interesting that the ovaries of the two members of the *C. pipiens* complex endemic to Australia contain "similar virus-like particles" in place of these rickettsiae.[14]

Mosquitoes are host to iridescent viruses that require transgenerational passage for completion of the life cycle.[15, 16] Mature larval *Aedes taeniorhynchus* ingest the virus when exposed to diseased larvae. After infection, development proceeds normally and resultant females deposit viable eggs. However, virtually all of these eggs contain virus, and the first generation of progeny ultimately die late in the fourth larval instar. The cycle is completed when other larvae feed on the cadaver of one of these diseased larvae. Survival of the host through the adult instar is possible only when infection immediately precedes pupation. Younger larvae die before they can mature. Although adult mosquitoes do not seem to be affected by this agent, they can be infected by injection.[17]

Certain protozoan infections are sustained by transgenerational passage. An early record, published by 1906,[18] suggests transovarial transmission in the case of *Aedes aegypti* infected with the sporozoan, *Plistophora stegomyiae.* However, a long history of apparently contradictory observations followed.[19] Infection by various *Nosema, Thelohania,* and *Plistophora* resulted in such massive destruction of ovarian tissue that infected mosquitoes seemed invariably to be sterilized. Apparently, parasite and host become so exquisitely coadapted that production of infected viable eggs requires a highly specific relationship. *Culex tarsalis* infected with *Thelohania californica*[19] and *Anopheles quadrimaculatus* infected with *Thelohania legeri*[20] are two effective combinations. Such female mosquitoes seem able to suppress sporogony of the parasite, while maintaining virtually asymptomatic schizogonic infections. Males are destroyed during the fourth instar by fulminating sporogonic infections.

TRANSMISSION OF VERTEBRATE PATHOGENS

The early medical and veterinary entomologists were certainly alert to the possibilities of inherited infection in the vector. Viral diseases, in particular, provided fruitful ground for speculation, and yellow fever seemed a prime candidate. Some such special means of interepidemic survival was suggested by the sporadic manner in which yellow fever seemed to recur locally. Indeed, Marchoux and Simond [18] reported a laboratory demonstration of the agent in the progeny of infected *A. aegypti*. However, unlike their report of inherited microsporidian infection, this finding has not been confirmed, and subsequent attempts to systematically test the possibility of transovarial transmission have produced negative results. [21]

A series of classic studies on the epidemiology of dengue were conducted in the Philippines by Simmons *et al.* [22] They concluded "that dengue virus is not transmitted from infected female *A. aegypti* through the egg to the offspring."

In temperate regions, interepidemic survival of the mosquito-borne encephalitides requires special adaptations, presenting a set of problems that remain unanswered. Reintroduction in migrating birds and hibernation in mosquitoes, acarines, bats, local birds, and reptiles have been suggested as possible mechanisms for survival, [23, 24] but none seems to satisfy all of the epidemiologic requirements. Until recently, evidence for transgenerational passage was weak. Japanese encephalitis virus was recovered from larval *Culex tritaeniorhynchus* collected in an endemic situation in Japan and from seven lots of adult *Aedes albopictus* reared from larvae from an epidemic focus in China. [23] One pool of larval *Culiseta melanura* collected in December 1956 in southeastern Massachusetts contained the virus of Eastern equine encephalitis (EEE). [23a] However, these isolated observations have not generally been accepted. Particularly contradictory is the finding that in Massachusetts, EEE virus has never been recovered from the adult *C. melanura* emerging early in a given season. Of course, the total number of isolations is rather small for definitive statistical treatment.

Laboratory findings, recorded before the present decade, suggest that transgenerational passage generally might not apply to the epidemiology of mosquito-borne encephalitis virus. Particularly impressive were the findings recorded by Chamberlain *et al.*, [25] who tested more than 10,000 adult progeny of *C. pipiens* infected with St. Louis encephalitis (SLE) without finding evidence of inherited virus. Negative results were obtained also with Western equine encephalitis (WEE) in *C. tarsalis*, [26] Venezuelan equine encephalitis (VEE) in *A. aegypti*, [27] and West Nile virus in *A. aegypti*. [28] In unpublished work performed in my laboratory, no evidence could be adduced to support the possibility that Sindbis or vesicular stomatitis virus (Indiana serotype) might be present in the adult progeny of infected mosquitoes. On the other hand, the eggs of infected mosquitoes frequently seem to carry virus. More than 90% of the egg rafts of *C. pipiens* bore SLE virus, [25] and at least 10% of *C. tarsalis* egg rafts bore WEE virus. [26] It is problematic that adult mosquitoes reared from these eggs appear to be noninfected.

The concept of heritable transmission of arboviruses by hematophagous insects recently gained general acceptance. In 1972, investigators in Panama presented convincing data on VSV in the progeny of infected phlebotomine sand flies, [29, 29a] and in 1973, investigators in Wisconsin established that a California virus may be maintained vertically in mosquitoes. [30, 30a] Publication of these reports prompted general reexamination of earlier work on the subject.

Even serum hepatitis, in a recent report on propagation in mosquitoes, has been suggested as a candidate for transovarial passage.[31] However, this evidence is weak, because antigen was identified only in the eggs of one mosquito and only at 3 days after infection.

Thus, prevailing opinion has come full circle. Within the first decade of this century, inherited infection seemed a likely explanation for many problems that involved entomologic epidemiology. Masses of negative results obtained during the next half century reversed this attitude and seemed to limit vertical transmission to the realm of arachnology. Information developed during the last decade suggests that inheritance of infection may have considerable epidemiologic significance.

Penetration of the Egg

A prerequisite to effective study of transovarial passage is precise knowledge of the mode of infection of the ovum. This information is crucial, especially in the event of negative results. Ovaries of ticks differ fundamentally from those of insects and in a manner that suggests differences in vulnerability to infection of the oocyte. Bertram [32] suggests that three membranes protect the oocytes of insects, whereas only one membrane protects those of ticks. However, the limiting membranes of both the ovariole and of the ovary of *A. aegypti* are fenestrated; they are fully permeable to hemolymph-borne particles in the micron range.[33] Relatively coarse particles of colloidal carbon penetrate to the innermost membrane, the basement lamina of the follicular epithelium.

The presence of this epithelial envelope is another such point of distinction.[34] The highly organized channels between these cells would seem to mechanically filter particles larger than 25 nm,[33] and the minimum diameter of most viruses exceeds this value. Although Roth and Porter [35] report that these spaces greatly dilate during oogenesis, we could not confirm this finding.[33] In any case, such a relaxation of the barrier would be ephemeral, because the oocyte is soon protected by the developing chorion, deposited by the end of the first day after blood feeding. During this first day, any material that enters the periooocytic space is engulfed within micropinocytosis vesicles and incorporated into the ooplasm.

More distal follicles are at earlier stages of development and may differ in vulnerability to infection. Ovarioles are tubular structures, each of which comprises as many as four follicular compartments (in the case of *A. aegypti*). At the time that the egg in the basal primary follicle is mature, the neighboring secondary follicle has begun to develop, and a tertiary follicle has split off from the distal germarium. Oocytes and trophocytes are differentiated within these developing follicles, and each is enclosed by a complete follicular epithelium. Only the germarium lacks such a potentially protective layer of cells.

Because of these developmental features, the timing of ovarian exposure to the parasite becomes relevant. Timing may become crucial in the event that the microorganism in question resides in the hemolymph for only a limited period of time.

The pattern of development of viral infection suggests that mosquitoes become viremic only about 4 days or more after taking an infectious blood meal. During the first 3 or 4 days, virus can be recovered only from the gut.[26, 36, 37] Recovery from salivary glands follows a similar additional time lapse. When mosquitoes are infected by injection, the glands acquire virus in about half the total time. Taken together, these observations suggest an initial cycle of viral propagation in the gut, followed, at about Day 4, by dispersal to other tissues. The appendages of infected mosquitoes first contain Japanese B virus at this time, and this fact suggests viremia.[26, 36] However, attempts to directly measure circulation of Uganda S[38] and Whataroa[39] virus produced contradictory results. The former report claimed direct cannulation of the dorsal aorta, while the latter describes insertion of capillary tubes into the hemocoel. In both studies, the presence of virus was recorded within 1 hr of the infectious blood meal and persisted thereafter. This extraordinary observation, which implies apparent "leakage" from the gut lumen, requires confirmation. Preliminary results in my laboratory that employed perfusion techniques suggest that Sindbis virus is most abundant in the hemolymph of *A. aegypti* around Day 4.

Published descriptions of attempts to accomplish transovarial transmission of togavirus, in general, follow other rationales. Most report extensive analyses based on the clutch of eggs that is induced by the infectious blood meal. For these eggs to become infected, viremia during the first day after infection would be required. LaMotte's[36] observation that virus titer of the ovaries of infected mosquitoes increases with the passage of time influenced the design of at least two of these studies. Chamberlain *et al.*[25] cited this observation as the basis for sampling successive batches of eggs from infected mosquitoes. However, the timing of each blood meal appeared to be arbitrary, without regard to possible periods of viremia. Furthermore, only three batches of eggs from the fourth ovarian cycle were tested. In a simultaneous study based on similar reasoning, Nir[28] reported on smaller samples of mosquitoes, but only from the first three egg batches after infection. Both studies recorded essentially negative results.

Surprisingly, establishment of any germ line infection, even of Blochmann bodies, seems difficult. After the natural symbionts present in roaches are destroyed by antibiotics, somatic infection can be reestablished through hemocoelic injection.[7] However, the progeny of these roaches do not acquire infection in the normal manner and remain devoid of symbionts. Similarly, injection of spotted fever rickettsiae into adult ticks does not seem to result in heritable infection.[36a] Infection of the germ line requires exposure of the ovary during some specific nymphal stage of development. On the other hand, somatic infection is readily established. This difficulty in producing heritable infections prevents fulfillment of Koch's postulates in the case of the cytoplasmic incompatibility factor of *C. pipiens* mosquitoes.[12a] Here again, oocytes seem to be protected against infection, even by obligate symbionts, and this applies to some extent for ticks.

It might be useful, at this point, to review the manner in which the germ line differentiates during dipteran embryogenesis. The egg is fertilized during deposition. After syngamy, the nucleus divides, the daughter nuclei migrating toward the periphery of the yolk mass. Eventually, cellular membranes form around each nucleus, including a group of special nuclei located posteriorly, which are destined to form the germ cells. Thus, the cytoplasm of both oogonial and somatic cells is derived from a common pool. But, at the very beginning of embryogenesis, germ tissues differentiate, remaining apart, and, in female flies, eventually form the oogonium. Accordingly, microorganisms may enter the germ line by passive inclusion at the time that cell membranes initially form. The alternative is invasion at some later developmental stage.

A considerable body of information has become available regarding invasion of *Drosophila* oocytes by sigma virus (reviewed by Seecof [10]). Flies that inherit the infection from the maternal parent sustain, themselves, a low titer of virus but transmit the virus to all of their offspring. When initial infection is by injection of adult female flies, much higher somatic titers are attained, but only occasional daughters sustain infection. However, once this oogonial infection occurs, the virus becomes "stabilized," infecting a high proportion of individuals in successive generations. Furthermore, virus strains differ in their ability to invade the oocyte. It seems likely that this demonstration of continuity of "germ line infections" may apply more generally to include other infections of epidemiologic significance.

At least in the case of a protozoan, *T. legeri,* a special device appears to be employed for invasion of the oocyte.[20] "Blood cells containing these plasmodia enter the ovaries and some become cysts of cylindrical spores between the ovarioles . . . the spores become pressed between the developing eggs. This produces pressure on the spores which could extrude the polar filament releasing the sporoplasm." Such an adaptation might provide another organism, secondarily parasitizing the insect, with access to the germ line.

Transgenerational infection is not limited to passage of microorganisms that invade oocytes or oogonia, and, here again, sigma virus in *D. melanogaster* serves as a prime model (reviewed by Seecof[10]). The progeny of noninfected females may sustain somatic infection inherited from infected fathers but not a germ-line infection. It is as though the zygote becomes infected after the germarium is no longer vulnerable. Virus is apparently present within the sperm themselves, as is suggested by experiments that involved multiple insemination by genetically marked males. This finding indicates that the term "transovarial transmission" is too specific for use as a generic term to describe inherited infection. Passage by invasion of oocytes must not be assumed. The mature egg may be penetrated during fertilization, and even this need not be limited to particles within the sperm. Agents present in the spermathecal or atrial fluids might accompany sperm into the ooplasm.

In this regard, it is noteworthy that SLE virus is frequently present on the surface of freshly deposited eggs.[25] As many as 92% of egg rafts may carry surface virus that is presumably derived from fluids present in the genital tract. That this "infection" is generally self-limiting is problematic. However, virus occasionally is present in larvae. Of 4000 larvae tested, four contained SLE virus, and three of them were in the last larval instar. One came from eggs that had been surface sterilized. About the same number of adult as larval progeny of infected mosquitoes were tested, but without finding infection. Although transstadial transmission is well documented, this finding prompted the suggestion that such transmission must be so inefficient that inherited infection "is not a significant means of [virus] persistence in nature." This conclusion is quantitative, and different statistics may be applicable in other virus-vector combinations.

INTRODUCTION TO SESSION

At least in the case of certain Diptera-borne diseases of vertebrates, there is no longer doubt that transgenerational passage plays a role in the maintenance of infection. The crucial question that remains is one of degree. How important is this vertical aspect of transmission as compared to the more conventional pattern, which requires that infection alternate between vector and reservoir? Several of the papers presented in the preceding session provide us with a point of departure, as they deal with transgenerational passage of acarine-borne rickettsioses. Burgdorfer and Brinton even question the epidemiologic requirement for a reservoir in the case of spotted fever. They suggest that the tick vector may serve as a reservoir. Past confusion on this point resulted from failure to recognize that infection of ova requires that the oocyte be infected at a specific early developmental stage. Under optimum conditions, germ-line infection is highly efficient. Traub *et al.* describe parallel findings for scrub typhus infection carried by chiggers. They report that continuous inherited infection is efficient but that it is difficult to establish a new germ-line infection. Thus, these two rickettsioses appear to be "enzootic" in a peculiar manner. An important part of the discussion that follows relates to this question for disease transmitted to Diptera.

Tesh and Chaniotis begin the discussion of Diptera-transmitted agents by bringing together and analyzing the several reports that have accumulated which suggest inherited infection in phlebotomine sandflies. Viruses of at least three diverse groupings appear to readily infect the ovaries of these insects. This suggests that phlebotomine ovaries might possess some unique anatomic vulnerability to infection, or perhaps that the duration of the viremic period might favor ovarial infection. Other possibilities are suggested, but no definitive physiologic information is available. In spite of a rather poor efficiency of transgenerational passage, Tesh and Chaniotis cite evidence that sandflies, like ticks and chiggers, may serve both as vector and reservoir for agents of vertebrate disease.

Watts *et al.* extend their landmark findings on the epidemiology of LaCrosse virus in *Aedes triseriatus*. This is the first human pathogen shown to readily be inherited by vector mosquitoes. As with sandflies, the efficiency of transgenerational passage is poor (30%). However, convincing evidence is cited to support the conclusion that vertically infected treehole mosquitoes are responsible for the winter survival of this California encephalitis virus.

LeDuc *et al.* present their epidemiologic studies on Keystone virus, another member of the California encephalitis group. These studies confirm that transgenerational transmission must be important in interepidemic survival of California group viruses, but they carry the problem a step further. They query whether vertebrate hosts may "amplify" transmission. These preliminary studies prepare the way for further work on this recently recognized disease of man.

Yen discusses a complementary aspect of inherited infection of mosquitoes and one that has recently attracted the attention of medical entomologists. Although the role of rickettsiae in mosquito reproduction appears to be complex, it is clear that the presence of these microorganisms may be associated with pathology. This may provide a potential point of vulnerability exploitable for genetic control of these vectors of disease.

Denlinger and Ma describe an alternative mechanism for transgenerational passage that would be peculiar to tsetse and to pupiperous flies. Because the larvae of these insects dwell *in utero* after hatching, there is opportunity for maternal infection to circumvent the ovum. Recently, several investigators, interested in reproduction in tsetse, have renewed our interest in the bacteroid symbionts of these insects, and Denlinger and Ma bring this work together.

A symbiotic dependence between insects and certain microorganisms implies that there be a highly efficient mechanism for transgenerational transfer of infection. Brooks discusses the various problems implicit to this relationship, with emphasis on how insects control the location and rate of multiplication of the symbiotes. Survival of infected progeny is obviously prerequisite to the effectiveness of transgenerational passage.

Fine directly approaches the central problem of this Conference by devising a system for quantifying vertical and horizontal aspects of transmission. The model is greatly complicated by the possibility that the microorganism may affect the fitness of both the vector and of the reservoir. Thus, in evaluating the epidemiologic importance of heritability of infection, attenuation becomes as important a concern as is efficiency of transgenerational passage. Fine's synthesis provides a unifying element for this Conference.

REFERENCES

1. SMITH, J. & F. L. KILBOURNE. 1893. Investigations into the nature, causation and prevention of southern cattle fever. Bull. U.S. Bureau Animal Ind. No. 1.
1a. FINE, P. E. M. This monograph.
2. BURGDORFER, W. & M. G. R. VARMA. 1967. Trans-stadial and transovarial development of disease agents in arthropods. Annu. Rev. Entomol. **12:** 347–376.
3. WHEELER, W. M. 1889. The embryology of *Blatta germanica* and *Doryphora decimlineata*. J. Morphol. **3:** 291–386.
4. BUCHNER, P. 1965. Endosymbiosis of Animals with Plant Microorganisms. Interscience Publishers. New York, N.Y.
5. LANHAM, V. N. 1968. The Blochmann bodies: hereditary intracellular symbionts of insects. Biol. Rev. **43:** 269–286.
6. BROOKS, M. A. & A. G. RICHARDS. 1955. Intracellular symbiosis in cockroaches. I. Production of aposymbiotic cockroaches. Biol. Bull. **109:** 22–39.
7. BROOKS, M. A. & A. G. RICHARDS. 1956. Intracellular symbiosis in cockroaches. III. Reinfection of aposymbiotic cockroaches. J. Exp. Zool. **132:** 447–465.
8. PINNOCK, D. E. & R. T. HESS. 1974. The occurrence of intracellular rickettsialike organisms in the tsetse flies, *Glossina morsitans, G. fuscipes, G. brevipalpus* and *G. pallidipes*. Acta Trop. **31:** 70–79.
9. EHRMAN, L. & R. P. KERNAGHAN. 1972. Infectious heredity in *Drosophila paulistorum*. *In* Pathogenic Mycoplasmas. : 227–250. Elsevier. Amsterdam, The Netherlands.
10. SEECOF, R. 1968. The sigma virus infection of *Drosophila melanogaster*. Curr. Topics Microbiol. Immunol. **42:** 59–93.
11. LEVENTHAL, E. A. 1971. The SR condition in *Drosophila bifasciata: in vivo* and *in vitro* growth. Curr. Topics Microbiol. Immunol. **55:** 233–240.
12. HERTIG, M. & S. B. WOLBACH. 1924. Studies on rickettsia-like microorganisms in insects. J. Med. Res. **44:** 329–374.
12a. YEN, J. H. This monograph.
13. YEN, J. H. & A. R. BARR. 1973. The etiological agent of cytoplasmic incompatibility in *Culex pipiens*. J. Invert. Pathol. **22:** 242–250.
14. IRVING-BELL, R. J. 1974. Cytoplasmic factors in the gonads of *Culex pipiens* complex mosquitoes. Life Sci. **14:** 1149–1151.
15. LINLEY, J. R. & H. T. NIELSEN. 1968. Transmission of a mosquito iridescent virus in *Aedes taeniorhynchus*. I. Laboratory experiments. J. Invert. Pathol. **12:** 7–16.
16. LINLEY, J. R. & H. T. NIELSEN. 1968. Transmission of a mosquito iridescent virus in *Aedes taeniorhynchus*. II. Experiments related to transmission in nature. J. Invert. Pathol. **12:** 17–24.
17. FUKUDA, T. & T. B. CLARK. 1975. Transmission of the mosquito iridescent virus (RMIV) by adult mosquitoes of *Aedes taeniorhynchus* to their progeny. J. Invert. Pathol. **25:** 275, 276.

18. Marchoux, E. & P. L. Simond. 1906. Etudes sur la fièvre jaune, deuxième mémoire de la mission francaise à Rio de Janeiro. Ann. Inst. Pasteur **20**: 16–40.
19. Kellen, W. R. & W. Wills. 1962. The transovarian transmission of *Thelohania californica* Kellen and Lipa in *Culex tarsalis* Coquillett. J. Insect Pathol. **4**: 321–326.
20. Hazard, E. I. & J. Weiser. 1968. Spores of *Thelohania* in adult female *Anopheles:* development and transovarial transmission, and rediscriptions of *T. legeri* Hesse and *T. obesa* Kudo. J. Protozool. **15**: 817–823.
21. Gillett, J. D., R. W. Ross, G. W. A. Dick, A. J. Haddow & L. E. Hewitt. 1950. Experiments to test the possibility of transovarial transmission of yellow fever virus in the mosquito *Aedes (Stegomyia) africanus.* Ann. Trop. Med. Parasitol. **44**: 342–350.
22. Simmons, J. S., J. H. St. John & F. H. K. Reynolds. 1931. Experimental studies of Dengue. Philippine J. Sci. **44**: 1–247.
23. Miles, J. A. R. 1960. Epidemiology of the arthropod-borne encephalitides. Bull. World Health Org. **22**: 339–371.
23a. Institute of Laboratories, Commonwealth of Massachusetts. 1956. Unpublished observations.
24. Reeves, W. C. 1961. Overwintering of arthropod-borne viruses. Progr. Med. Virol. **3**: 59–78.
25. Chamberlain, R. W., W. D. Sudia & R. H. Gogel. 1964. Studies on transovarial transmission of St. Louis encephalitis virus by *Culex quinquefasciatus.* Amer. J. Hyg. **80**: 254–265.
26. Thomas, L. A. 1963. Distribution of the virus of western equine encephalomyelitis in the mosquito vector, *Culex tarsalis.* Amer. J. Hyg. **78**: 150–165.
27. Mussgay, M. 1964. Growth cycle of arboviruses in vertebrate and arthropod cells. Progr. Med. Virol. **6**: 193–267.
28. Nir, Y. 1963. Failure to obtain experimental transovarian transmission of West Nile virus by *Aedes aegypti.* Ann. Trop. Med. Parasitol. **57**: 428, 429.
29. Tesh, R. B., B. N. Chaniotis & K. M. Johnson. 1972. Vesicular stomatitis virus (Indiana serotype): transovarial transmission by phlebotomine sandflies. Science **175**: 1477–1479.
29a. Tesh, R. B. & B. N. Chaniotis. This monograph.
30. Watts, D. M., S. Pantuwatana, G. E. DeFoliart, T. M. Yuill & W. H. Thompson. 1973. Transovarial transmission of LaCrosse Virus (California encephalitis group) in the mosquito, *Aedes triseriatus.* Science **182**: 1140, 1141.
30a. Watts, D. M., S. Pantuwatana, T. M. Yuill, G. R. DeFoliart, W. H. Thompson & R. P. Hanson. This monograph.
31. Blumberg, B. S., W. Wills, I. Millman & W. T. London. 1973. Australia antigen in mosquitoes: feeding experiments and field studies. Res. Commun. Chem. Pathol. Pharmacol. **6**: 719–731.
32. Bertram, D. S. 1960. Contribution to the discussion of the symposium on the evolution of arbovirus diseases. Trans. Roy. Soc. Trop. Med. Hyg. **54**: 130, 131.
33. Anderson, W. A. & A. Spielman. 1971. Permeability of the ovarian follicle of *Aedes aegypti* mosquitoes. J. Cell Biol. **50**: 201–221.
34. Hecker, H. & A. Aeschlimann. 1970. Ultrastrukturelle Aspekte der Eibildung bei *Rhipicephalus bursa.* Z. Tropenmed. Parasitol. **21**: 31–45.
35. Roth, T. F. & K. R. Porter. 1964. Yolk protein uptake in the oocyte of the mosquito *Aedes aegypti* L. J. Cell Biol. **20**: 313–332.
36. LaMotte, L. C., Jr. 1960. Japanese B encephalitis virus in the organs of infected mosquitoes. Amer. J. Hyg. **72**: 73–87.
36a. Burgdorfer, W. & L. P. Brinton. This monograph.
37. Doi, R., A. Shirasaka & M. Sasa. 1967. The mode of development of Japanese encephalitis virus in the mosquito *Culex tritaeniorhynchus summorosus*

as observed by the fluorescent antibody technique. Jap. J. Exp. Med. **37:** 227–238.

38. BOORMAN, J. 1960. Observations on the amount of virus present in the haemo-lymph of *Aedes aegypti* infected with Uganda S, yellow fever and Simliki Forest viruses. Trans. Roy. Soc. Trop. Med. Hyg. **54:** 362–365.

39. MILES, J. A. R., J. S. PILLAE & T. MAGUIRE. 1973. Multiplication of Whataroa virus in mosquitoes. J. Med. Entomol. **10:** 176–185.

TRANSOVARIAL TRANSMISSION OF VIRUSES BY PHLEBOTOMINE SANDFLIES

Robert B. Tesh and Byron N. Chaniotis

Pacific Research Section
Laboratory of Parasitic Diseases
National Institute of Allergy and Infectious Diseases
National Institutes of Health
Honolulu, Hawaii 96806

INTRODUCTION

Vertebrate viruses isolated from phlebotomine sandflies belong to three distinct arbovirus serogroups: [1-5] vesicular stomatitis, Phlebotomus fever, and Changuinola.* In addition to their antigenic dissimilarities, the physicochemical properties and morphologic characteristics of these sandfly-associated viruses are also quite different.[7-10] However, one feature that they share in common, in contrast to most other vertebrate arboviruses, is their apparent inability to produce a significant viremia in infected animals or man. This characteristic suggests that vertebrates may be dead-end hosts for most sandfly viruses and that a maintenance mechanism other than the classic vertebrate-insect cycle must be postulated to explain their biologic survival. Accumulating evidence indicates that insect-to-insect (transovarial) transmission is the maintenance mechanism. In the present paper, we shall examine the field and laboratory evidence in support of this hypothesis and will present new data on the transovarial transmission of vesicular stomatitis virus, Indiana serotype (VSV-Indiana), by sandflies.

SANDFLY BIONOMICS

Before considering viruses transmitted by phlebotomine sandflies, it might be informative to briefly review the biology of these insects. More detailed reviews of this subject have recently been published by Lewis.[11, 12] Sandflies belong to the family Psychodidae but differ from other psychodids in that they possess biting mouthparts and are obligatory bloodsuckers. Only the female takes blood. More than 500 different species are known.[11] These species are divided into six genera: *Phlebotomus* and *Sergentomyia* in the Old World and *Lutzomyia, Brumptomyia, Warileya,* and *Hertigia* in the New World. Sandflies are most abundant in the tropics and subtropics but also occur in temperate regions of Europe, Asia, and North America.[11, 12] They inhabit diverse biotypes that range from arid areas of the Middle East to tropical rainforests of South America. They are vectors of three types of diseases that affect man: leishmaniasis (both cutaneous and visceral forms), bartonellosis, and several viral diseases, the most important of which is sandfly (pappataci) fever.

---

* One additional ungrouped virus (Charleville) has also been isolated from sandflies in Australia [6] but will not be included in this discussion.

Sandflies are terrestrial insects. Their life cycle consists of egg, four larval instars, pupa, and adult. The entire life cycle takes from 5 to 10 weeks, depending on species and the ambient temperature.[13-15] The larvae develop in soil in warm, moist, shaded microhabitats protected from direct sunlight and rainfall, such as tree buttresses, animal burrows, caves, and crevices in rocks and masonry.[11, 12, 16, 17] The larvae feed on decomposing organic matter, including dead insects, animal feces, leaf litter, and other rotting vegetation.[13-17] Both immature stages and adults are very susceptible to desiccation and require high humidity and constant moisture to survive.[13, 18] During periods of adverse climate, such as prolonged dry periods or cold, some species diapause as fourth instar larvae.[14, 17] In temperate areas, it is the diapausing larvae that survive the winter months and emerge as adults the following spring. Most sandfly species are crepuscular and nocturnal in their biting activity.[19-21]

Three aspects of sandfly biology, particularly relevant to this discussion, are flight range, longevity, and size of the blood meal. Sandflies commonly move in short hops and rarely travel more than a few hundred meters from their resting and breeding sites.[11, 20-23] This characteristic obviously limits host availability. The lifetime of sandflies under natural conditions is not precisely known, but laboratory data suggest that it is relatively short (2–5 weeks).[11, 13-15] Because each gonadotrophic cycle lasts 4–7 days, this small duration limits both their opportunities to become infected and their vector potential.[11, 13-15] Studies of the quantity of blood ingested by *Phlebotomus papatasi*, an important vector of sandfly fever, indicate that this sandfly species ingests approximately 0.0003–0.0005 ml of blood per feeding.[18] Theoretically, this means that a viremic host would require a blood virus level of at least $10^{4.0}$ infectious units per milliliter to infect a biting sandfly.

Transmission of VSV-Group Viruses

Serologic surveys in Panama, in an endemic area of VSV-Indiana activity, indicated that this virus naturally infects a broad spectrum of animal species, including man.[24] Repeated isolations of VSV-Indiana from wild sandflies in the same area[3] and evidence of virus multiplication in, and bite transmission by, experimentally infected sandflies[25] implicated these insects as vectors of the virus. However, a susceptible vertebrate species that developed a viremia sufficient to infect a biting arthropod was not found. Studies of VSV-Indiana experimental infections in a variety of animals and in man indicate that the viremia associated with VSV infection is low level and transient.[26] Thus, we were unable to explain how sandflies acquired the virus in nature. This led us to investigate the possibility of transovarial virus transmission.

These studies focused on four anthropophilic sandfly species (*Lutzomyia trapidoi, L. ylephilator, L. sanguinaria,* and *L. gomezi*). VSV-Indiana vertical transmission occurred in *L. trapidoi* and *L. ylephilator* but not in *L. sanguinaria* or *L. gomezi*,[27] a result that indicates species differences in the ability to transmit the agent. Transovarial transmission rates in the former two species varied from 20 to 27%. The procedures of these experiments have been described previously.[27] TABLE 1 lists the infection rates and virus titers obtained in F_1 progeny of experimentally infected *L. trapidoi* females. Virus was recovered from all developmental stages. Mean virus titers of infected F_1 adult females were about 10^4 higher than those observed in infected eggs and first instar larvae, which indicates that virus multiplication occurred during development of the sandflies. VSV-Indiana was recovered from F_1 adults of both sexes. Virus titers of 36 infected *L. trapidoi* F_1 adult females ranged from $10^{2.8}$ to $10^{6.1}$ (mean $10^{5.1}$) tissue culture ID_{50}, titers comparable to those found in wild and experimentally infected sandflies. These infected F_1 female sandflies transmitted VSV-Indiana by bite to susceptible animals and also transmitted the virus transovarially to 34% of their offspring (F_2 generation). These results demonstrated that the virus can be passed from generation to generation.

We also investigated whether VSV-Indiana infection affected the fertility of female sandflies or if it was deleterious to their progeny. TABLE 2 summarizes the results of an experiment that compared the development of offspring and the fecundity of VSV-Indiana infected and control (noninfected) *L. trapidoi*. The number of eggs laid by both groups was similar, as was the period of development and sex ratio of their respective progeny. The number of F_1 adults pro-

TABLE 1

INFECTION RATES AND VIRUS TITERS OF VSV-INDIANA IN F_1 PROGENY OF EXPERIMENTALLY INFECTED *L. trapidoi* *

Developmental Stage	No. Positive/ No. Tested	Positive (%)	Virus Titers of Positive Insects †		
			No. Tested	Range	Mean
Egg	10/154	6.5	7	0.3–0.8	0.7
First instar	25/108	23.1	22	0.3–2.3	1.1
Second instar	23/143	16.1	15	1.3–3.6	2.2
Third instar	28/142	19.7	20	1.3–2.8	2.3
Fourth instar	24/132	18.2	22	1.6–4.8	3.2
Pupa	56/154	36.4	19	1.8–4.0	2.5
F_1 adult male	48/225	21.3	27	2.0–4.0	3.0
F_1 adult female	61/248	24.6	36	2.8 6.1	5.1

* After Tesh *et al.*[27]
† Titers expressed as $\log_{10}$ of $TCID_{50}$ units per insect.

duced by the infected parents was actually slightly higher, even though 26.5% of the offspring were infected. These data indicated that VSV-Indiana is innocuous to the insect. Interestingly, VSV-Indiana also replicated in *Drosophila melanogaster*, after inoculation.[28] In this abnormal host, however, the virus caused a reduction in both the longevity of adult flies and the fertility of females.[28]

In the experiment summarized in TABLE 2, vertical transmission rates for each of the infected parent sandflies were determined. Of the 40 VSV-Indiana infected females in this experiment, 27 (68%) produced infected progeny. Individual transovarial virus transmission rates among these 27 sandflies varied from 6 to 100%. Infection rates among F_1 generation offspring of representative females from this group are shown in TABLE 3. From these data, it is apparent that there are marked differences in the ability to transmit VSV-Indiana among individual *L. trapidoi*. Because of the difficulties in rearing sandflies in

TABLE 2

COMPARATIVE FECUNDITY AND DEVELOPMENT OF OFFSPRING OF VSV-INDIANA
INFECTED AND CONTROL *L. trapidoi*

	Control	Infected
Number parent females	38	40
Total eggs laid	1161	1163
Mean number of eggs	30.6	29.1
Number F_1 adults produced	457	562 *
Emergence, % (F_1 adults/eggs)	39.4	48.3
Life cycle range (days)	40–73	38–73
Sex ratio (females/males)	233/220	283/256
Mean longevity of F_1 adults (days)		
Female	11.4 (100) †	9.3 (28)
Male	9.6 (82)	7.7 (25)

* One hundred and fourty nine (26.5%) of these F_1 adults were infected.
† Sample size is listed within parentheses.

captivity, we were unable to carry this experiment further and determine whether these differences were genetically controlled.

Chandipura, a second member of the VSV serologic group,[2] was originally isolated from sick persons in India during a dengue-like epidemic.[29] Neutralization tests on sera of humans and domestic animals living in the area indicated a high prevalence of Chandipura virus infection,[29] similar to the patterns observed in endemic areas of VSV-Indiana activity.[24] Although only a few studies have been reported on the behavior of Chandipura virus in vertebrates, the available data suggest that infection does not produce a sufficient viremia to infect a biting arthropod.[29] Recent recovery of Chandipura virus from wild sandflies in India [5] thus completes the analogy with VSV-Indiana. Obviously, experiments are now needed to determine whether Chandipura transovarial transmission also occurs in sandflies.

TABLE 3

VSV-INDIANA TRANSOVARIAL TRANSMISSION RATES BY INDIVIDUAL
L. trapidoi FEMALES TO THEIR F_1 GENERATION PROGENY

No. Infected Offspring/Total Tested	Infected (%)
5/5	100
4/5	80
10/16	63
8/13	62
12/22	54
14/29	48
12/32	38
6/21	29
5/22	23
1/10	10
1/18	6

TRANSMISSION OF PHLEBOTOMUS FEVER-GROUP VIRUSES

The Phlebotomus fever serologic group currently includes 22 antigenically related virus serotypes isolated in Europe, Africa, Central Asia, and tropical America.[4] Fifteen of these agents have been recovered from sandflies,[4] their presumed insect vector. Five of the 22 agents have been recovered from persons with illnesses indistinguishable from classic sandfly fever, which indicates that the disease is caused by several different virus serotypes.[4]

Epidemiologic studies in areas where sandfly fever occurs annually indicate that new cases of the disease begin each spring with the first appearance of sandflies.[30–32] This phenomenon has led several investigators to postulate that the virus overwinters in the insect.[30, 32] Presumptive evidence of vertical transmission of "sandfly fever virus" was first reported by Whittingham [33] in 1924 and again in 1937–38 by two groups of Russian workers.[30, 34] Basically, these studies consisted of feeding P. papatasi on sandfly fever patients, collecting the subsequent eggs and rearing the offspring under laboratory conditions, and inoculating pools of the F_1 generation offspring into, or feeding them on, human subjects to reproduce the disease. Because these studies were conducted before techniques for isolation and identification of Phlebotomus fever group viruses were available, the serotypes used were unknown. However, despite the lack of virologic confirmation, in retrospect, the methods used were sound, and the results appear valid. In each of these experiments, sandflies were fed in groups or inoculated in pools, but it is apparent from the results that the transovarial transmission rates were low (probably less than 5%).[30, 33, 34]

In one set of experiments, Petrischeva and Alymov [30] demonstrated transovarial transmission by naturally infected P. papatasi. They also reported vertical transmission of virus by laboratory-reared F_1 generation females to their offspring (F_2 generation).[30] The same workers showed that the virus survived for 7 months in transovarially infected, diapausing fourth instar larvae kept in a cold chamber under simulated winter conditions.[30] On the basis of these studies, they first suggested the possibility that sandflies might be the natural reservoir of "sandfly fever virus" and that the agent was transmitted from generation to generation.[30]

Recent studies of the level and duration of viremia in sandfly fever patients support this hypothesis. Detectable blood virus titers of volunteers infected with the Sicilian Phlebotomus fever serotype were of relatively short duration (less than 48 hr) and did not exceed $10^{3.4}$/ml, as assayed in tissue culture and in human subjects.[35, 36] After infection, however, the volunteers developed specific neutralizing antibodies, which suggested permanent immunity.[35, 36] In view of the minute quantity of blood ingested by P. papatasi (0.0003–0.0005 ml),[18] the amount of virus present in the serum of a sandfly fever patient is barely at the theoretic threshold level ($\pm 10^{4.0}$/ml) necessary to infect the insect. These data suggest that few sandflies would be infected by feeding on a viremic person. They also fail to explain how the virus survives during the winter season, when adult sandflies are absent. Unless an animal species that develops a prolonged and high-titered viremia can be identified, one must assume that vertical transmission is the maintenance mechanism.

Additional evidence for transovarial transmission of Phlebotomus fever-group viruses is provided by the frequency of isolates from male sandflies. Seven of the 15 sandfly-associated virus serotypes have been recovered from male and from female sandflies.[3] As shown in TABLE 4, from a collection that yielded comparable numbers of male and female insects in Panama, sex isolation rates for three of the viruses were similar. Because male sandflies do not suck blood, these isolations were interpreted as indicating that transovarial virus transmission occurs in nature.[3]

CHANGUINOLA-GROUP VIRUSES

This arbovirus group consists of several antigenically closely related serotypes.[3] Approximately 200 isolates of Changuinola-group agents have been obtained from sandflies collected in Central and South America.[1-3, 37-39] In contrast to the Phlebotomus fever group, only a single Changuinola isolate has been made from male sandflies.[3] A wild rodent (*Oryzomys* sp.) and man have yielded two additional isolates,[2] but little is known about the ecology of this virus group or the possibility of vertebrate reservoirs. Field studies in Panama indicated that the virus infection rate among sandflies was maintained at a fairly

TABLE 4

SANDFLY VIRUS ISOLATION BY SEX FROM TWO LOCALITIES IN PANAMA *

Sex	No. Sandflies	No. Pools	Punta Toro-CoAr 3319	Agua-cate	Cacao
El Aguacate-mixed species from tree buttresses (ground)					
Male	39,463	193	2	3	0
Female	26,217	381	3	1	3
Limbo-*L. trapidoi* from canopy platform (30 m)					
Male	8683	58	3	4	1
Female	9754	191	5	1	3

* From Tesh *et al.*[3]

constant level from season to season, which suggested low-level endemic activity.[3] Limited studies of laboratory animals experimentally infected with Changuinola-group agents demonstrated that they failed to develop detectable virus levels in their blood. Newborn mice and hamsters inoculated intracerebrally with these agents did not develop detectable viremia, although large quantities of virus were present in the brain at death.[40] A similar phenomenon has been observed with several Phlebotomus fever-group agents.[40] Though there is no solid evidence yet to suggest transovarial transmission of Changuinola-group viruses, the analogies with other sandfly-associated agents still raise this possibility.

DISCUSSION

The aforementioned data suggest that the ecology of sandfly-transmitted viruses may be quite different from the conventional vertebrate-insect cycle presumed for most other arthropod-borne viruses. This observation, if true, has important epidemiologic implications, because it provides an efficient mechanism for overwintering of the viruses and for ensuring their survival in the absence of susceptible vertebrate hosts. In view of the very limited flight range of sandflies and of their relatively short life as adults, vertical transmission may be essential for survival of the viruses. Studies of the epidemiology of leishmaniasis,[41-43] a protozoan disease transmitted by sandflies, indicate that the vertebrate host develops a chronic infection, which thus ensures survival of the parasite during periods of sandfly inactivity. There is no evidence to suggest that this mechanism occurs with sandfly-transmitted viruses. In contrast, the available data suggest that vertebrate hosts of these viruses play a nominal role in their maintenance and may actually be dead-end hosts. Transovarial virus transmission by the insect appears to be the principal maintenance mechanism.

Studies of VSV-Indiana infected sandflies (TABLE 2) indicate that the virus is innocuous to the insect. One would also expect this to be the case with other sandfly-transmitted viruses. In view of the apparent symbiotic relationship between virus and insect host, it is interesting to speculate on the evolutionary origin of these viruses. Maramorosch[44] has suggested that such agents were originally arthropod viruses and, because of the long association between host and parasite, developed a symbiont-like relationship. Additional support for this view is provided by evidence that several of the agents have the capacity of passing directly through the egg of the vector to the progeny and of being thus maintained indefinitely in sandflies without the necessity of alternating vertebrate hosts.

One obvious question raised by the aforementioned data is how can these viruses sustain themselves in the sandfly population with such low transovarial transmission rates? Vertical transmission rates for VSV-Indiana in *L. trapidoi* and *L. ylephilator* varied from 20 to 27%, whereas those of "sandfly fever virus" in *P. papatasi* appear to be less than 5%. With these transmission rates, the viruses could not survive for long in the insect population without one or more of the following: selective survival of infected sandflies, the existence of another virus source that occasionally replenishes the transovarial cycle, virus transmission to females during insemination by infected males, or genetic control of transovarial transmission, which would result in strains or individuals that infect most of their progeny.

The data provided in TABLE 2 indicate that VSV-Indiana infection does not increase the fecundity or survival of *L. trapidoi*. Thus, the first possibility seems unlikely, at least for VSV-Indiana. The existence of a vertebrate reservoir of virus that occasionally replenishes the transovarial cycle has not been identified for VSV-Indiana, despite considerable experimental work.[26] The existence of an animal reservoir for viruses of the Phlebotomus fever group has not been adequately investigated.

The possibility of virus transmission to females during insemination by infected males is intriguing and worthy of further investigation. Sexual transmission of sigma virus (a rhabdovirus of insects) has been reported in *D. melanogaster*.[45] Recently, Plowright et al.[46] demonstrated male to female transmission of African swine fever (ASF) virus by the tick, *Ornithodoros moubata porcinus*. Experimentally infected male *O. moubata* sexually transmitted ASF virus to 88% of female contacts.[46] Actually, the situation with ASF virus is not unlike that for VSV-Indiana and other sandfly-transmitted viruses. ASF virus has been isolated repeatedly from naturally infected *O. moubata* in East Africa.[46] In many areas of East Africa, the only known reservoir of ASF virus is the warthog (*Phacochoerus aethiopicus*); however, experimental studies indicate that this animal does not develop a viremia adequate to infect ticks.[46] Transovarial transmission of ASF virus also occurs in *O. moubata* but at low rates.[46, 47] Transovarially and sexually infected females subsequently transmitted the virus by bite to susceptible pigs.[47] In view of the ease and frequency with which sexual transmission occurs, this mechanism appears to be an important factor in ASF virus maintenance and amplification.[46, 47]

The fourth possibility, genetic control of transovarial transmission, has been reported with two plant viruses and their insect vectors. Transovarial transmission of European wheat striate mosaic virus and wound tumor virus occurs in the leafhoppers, *Delphacodes pellucida* and *Agallis constricta,* respectively.[48-50] Studies indicate that genetic mechanisms control the efficiency of transovarial virus passage in both leafhopper species, and races (strains) with high and low vertical transmission rates have been developed.[48-50] A similar phenomenon has been observed in the transovarial transmission rates of *Rickettsia tsutsugamushi,* the etiologic agent of scrub typhus, by various strains of trombiculid mites.[51] If a similar genetic mechanism occurred in sandflies and a few insects transmitted virus to a high percentage of their progeny, a virus could theoretically be maintained at a constant level in this subpopulation, although the overall infection and vertical transmission rates in the total sandfly population would remain quite low. The data listed in TABLE 3 on VSV-Indiana transovarial transmission rates by individual *L. trapidoi* females might be compatible with this hypothesis. Obviously, additional work is needed before we can fully understand the maintenance mechanisms of the various sandfly-associated viruses, but their ecology clearly appears to be quite different from most mosquito-borne viruses, which, until recently, have been considered models of arthropod-borne vertebrate viruses.

REFERENCES

1. TAYLOR, R. M. 1967. Catalogue of Arthropod-Borne Viruses of the World. U.S. Government Printing Office. Washington, D.C.
2. THEILER, M. & W. G. DOWNS. 1973. The Arthropod-Borne Viruses of Vertebrates. : 281–290. Yale University Press. New Haven, Conn.
3. TESH, R. B., B. N. CHANIOTIS, P. H. PERALTA & K. M. JOHNSON. 1974. Ecology of viruses isolated from Panamanian phlebotomine sandflies. Amer. J. Trop. Med. Hyg. 23: 258–269.
4. TESH, R. B., P. H. PERALTA, R. E. SHOPE, B. N. CHANIOTIS & K. M. JOHNSON. 1975. Antigenic relationships among Phlebotomus fever group arboviruses and their implications for the epidemiology of sandfly fever. Amer. J. Trop. Med. Hyg. 24: 135–144.
5. DHONDA, V., F. M. RODRIGUES & S. N. GHOSH. 1970. Isolation of Chandipura virus from sandflies in Aurangabad. Indian J. Med. Res. 58: 179, 180.
6. DOHERTY, R. L. 1972. Arboviruses of Australia. Australian Vet. J. 48: 172–180.
7. MURPHY, F. A., A. K. HARRISON & S. G. WHITFIELD. 1973. Bunyaviridae: morphologic and morphogenetic similarities of Bunyamwera serologic supergroup viruses and several other arthropod-borne viruses. Intervirology 1: 297–316.
8. KNUDSON, D. L. 1973. Rhabdoviruses. J. Gen. Virol. 20: 105–130.
9. BORDEN, E. C., R. E. SHOPE & F. A. MURPHY. 1971. Physicochemical and morphological relationships of some arthropod-borne viruses to bluetongue virus—a new taxonomic group. Physicochemical and serological studies. J. Gen. Virol. 13: 261–271.

10. MURPHY, F. A., E. C. BORDEN, R. E. SHOPE & A. HARRISON. 1971. Physico-chemical and morphological relationships of some arthropod-borne viruses to bluetongue virus—a new taxonomic group. Electron microscopic studies. J. Gen. Virol. **13**: 273–288.

11. LEWIS, D. J. 1971. Phlebotomid sandflies. Bull. World Health Org. **44**: 535–551.

12. LEWIS, D. J. 1974. The biology of Phlebotomidae in relation to leishmaniasis. Annu. Rev. Entomol. **19**: 363–384.

13. JOHNSON, P. T. & M. HERTIG. 1961. The rearing of Phlebotomus sandflies (Diptera: Psychodidae). 2. Development and behavior of Panamanian sand-flies in laboratory culture. Ann. Entomol. Soc. Amer. **54**: 764–766.

14. CHANIOTIS, B. N. 1967. The biology of California Phlebotomus (Diptera: Psychodidae) under laboratory conditions. J. Med. Entomol. **4**: 221–233.

15. FOSTER, W. A., T. M. TESFA-YOHANNES & T. TECLE. 1970. Studies on leishmaniasis in Ethiopia. 2. Laboratory culture and biology of *Phlebotomus longipes*. Ann. Trop. Med. Parasitol. **64**: 403–409.

16. HANSON, W. J. 1961. The breeding places of Phlebotomus in Panama (Diptera, Psychodidae). Ann. Entomol. Soc. Amer. **54**: 317–322.

17. ADLER, S. & O. THEODOR. 1957. Transmission of disease agents by phlebotomine sandflies. Annu. Rev. Entomol. '**2**: 203–226.

18. THEODOR, O. 1936. On the relation of *Phlebotomus papatasii* to the temperature and humidity of the environment. Bull. Entomol. Res. **27**: 653–671.

19. CHANIOTIS, B. N., M. A. CORREA, R. B. TESH & K. M. JOHNSON. 1971. Daily and seasonal man-biting activity of phlebotomine sandflies in Panama. J. Med. Entomol. **8**: 415–420.

20. FOSTER, W. A. 1972. Studies on leishmaniasis in Ethiopia. 3. Resting and breeding sites, flight behavior, and seasonal abundance of *Phlebotomus longipes* (Diptera: Psychodidae). Ann. Trop. Med. Parasitol. **66**: 313–328.

21. QUATE, L. W. 1964. *Phlebotomus* sandflies of the Paloich area in the Sudan. J. Med. Entomol. **1**: 213–268.

22. CHANIOTIS, B. N. & M. A. CORREA. 1974. Comparative flying and biting activity of Panamanian phlebotomine sandflies in a mature forest and adjacent open space. J. Med. Entomol. **11**: 115, 116.

23. CHANIOTIS, B. N., M. A. CORREA, R. B. TESH & K. M. JOHNSON. 1974. Horizontal and vertical movements of phlebotomine sandflies in a Panamanian rain forest. J. Med. Entomol. **11**: 369–375.

24. TESH, R. B., P. H. PERALTA & K. M. JOHNSON. 1969. Ecologic studies of vesicular stomatitis virus. 1. Prevalence of infection among animals and humans living in an area of endemic VSV activity. Amer. J. Epidemiol. **90**: 255–261.

25. TESH, R. B., B. N. CHANIOTIS & K. M. JOHNSON. 1971. Vesicular stomatitis virus, Indiana serotype: multiplication in and transmission by experimentally infected phlebotomine sandflies (*L. trapidoi*). Amer. J. Epidemiol. **93**: 491–495.

26. TESH, R. B., P. H. PERALTA & K. M. JOHNSON. 1970. Ecologic studies of vesicular stomatitis virus. 2. Resutls of experimental infection in Panamanian wild animals. Amer. J. Epidemiol. **91**: 216–224.

27. TESH, R. B., B. N. CHANIOTIS & K. M. JOHNSON. 1972. Vesicular stomatitis virus (Indiana serotype): transovarial transmission by phlebotomine sandflies. Science **175**: 1477–1479.

28. PRINTZ, P. 1973. Relationship of sigma virus to vesicular stomatitis virus. Advan. Virus Res. **18**: 143–157.

29. BHATT, P. N. & F. M. RODRIGUES. 1967. Chandipura: a new arbovirus isolated in India from patients with febrile illness. Indian J. Med. Res. **55**: 1295–1305.

30. PETRISCHEVA, P. A. & A. Y. ALYMOV. 1938. On transovarial transmission of virus of pappataci fever by sandflies. Arch. Biol. Sci. (Moscow) **53**: 138–144.

31. BRIT, C. 1910. Phlebotomus fever in Malta and Crete. J. Roy. Army Med. Corps **14:** 236–258.
32. ALYMOV, A. Y. 1961. Phlebotomus (sand-fly) fever. *In* A Course in Epidemiology. I. I. Elkin Ed. : 431–434. Pergamon Press, Ltd. London, England.
33. WHITTINGHAM, H. E. 1924. The etiology of Phlebotomus fever. J. State Med. **32:** 461–469.
34. MOCHKOVSKI, S. D., N. A. DIOMINA, V. D. NOSSINA, E. A. PAVLOVA, J. L. LIVCHITZ, H. J. PELS & V. P. ROUBTZOVA. 1937. Researches on sandfly fever. 8. Transmission of sandfly fever virus by sandflies hatched from eggs laid by infected females. Med. Parazitol. Parazitarn. Bolezni **6:** 922–937.
35. EDDY, G. A. 1974. Personal communication.
36. BARTELLONI, P. J. & R. B. TESH. 1975. Clinical and serologic responses of volunteers infected with Phlebotomus fever virus (Sicilian type). Amer. J. Trop. Med. Hyg. In press.
37. PERALTA, P. H. & A. SHELOKOV. 1966. Isolation and characterization of arboviruses from Almirante, Republic of Panama. Amer. J. Trop. Med. Hyg. **15:** 369–378.
38. GALINDO, P., S. SRIHONGSE, E. DE RODANICHE & M. A. GRAYSON. 1966. An ecological survey for arboviruses in Almirante, Panama, 1959–1962. Amer. J. Trop. Med. Hyg. **15:** 385–400.
39. WOODALL, J. P. 1967. Atas do Simpósio sôbre a Biota Amozônica, **6:** 31–63.
40. TESH, R. B. Unpublished data.
41. PETRISCHEVA, P. A., D. N. ZASUKHIM & V. M. SAF'YANOVA. 1963. The leishmaniases. *In* Natural Foci of Human Infections. E. N. Pavlovskii, Ed. : 164–201. Israel Program for Scientific Translations. Jerusalem, Israel.
42. LAINSON, R. & J. J. SHAW. 1970. Epidemiological considerations of the leishmanias with particular reference to the New Worlrd. *In* Ecology and Physiology of Parasites. A. M. Fallis, Ed. : 21–56. University of Toronto Press. Toronto, Ontario, Canada.
43. HERRER, A., S. R. TELFORD & H. A. CHRISTENSEN. 1971. Enzootic cutaneous leishmaniasis in eastern Panama. I. Investigation of the infection among forest mammals. Ann. Trop. Med. Parasitol. **65:** 349–358.
44. MARAMOROSCH, K. 1955. Multiplication of plant viruses in insect vectors. Advan. Virus Res. **3:** 221–249.
45. SEECOF, R. 1968. The sigma virus infection of *Drosophila melanogaster.* Curr. Top. Microbiol. Immunol. **42:** 59–93.
46. PLOWRIGHT, W., C. T. PERRY & A. GREIG. 1974. Sexual transmission of African swine fever virus in the tick, *Ornithodoros moubata porcinus,* Walton. Res. Vet. Sci. **17:** 106–113.
47. PLOWRIGHT, W., C. T. PERRY & M. A. PEIRCE. 1970. Transovarial infection with African swine fever virus in the argasid tick, *Ornithodoros moubata porcinus,* Walton. Res. Vet. Sci. **11:** 582–584.
48. NAGARAJ, A. N. & L. M. BLACK. 1962. Hereditary variation in the ability of a leafhopper to transmit two unrelated plant viruses. Virology **16:** 152–162.
49. SINHA, R. C. & S. SHELLEY. 1965. The transovarial transmission of wound tumor virus. Phytopathology **55:** 324–327.
50. WATSON, M. A. & R. C. SINHA. 1959. Studies on the transmission of European wheat striate mosaic virus by *Delphacodes pellucida* Fabricius. Virology **8:** 139–163.
51. TRAUB, R. & C. L. WISSEMAN. 1974. The ecology of chigger-borne rickettsiosis (scrub typhus). J. Med. Entomol. **11:** 237–303.

TRANSOVARIAL TRANSMISSION OF LACROSSE VIRUS IN *AEDES TRISERIATUS* *

D. M. Watts,† S. Pantuwatana,‡ T. M. Yuill,§ G. R. DeFoliart,||
W. H. Thompson,¶ and R. P. Hanson §

University of Wisconsin
Madison, Wisconsin 53706

INTRODUCTION

The concept of an arbovirus being transmitted transovarially in an arthropod evolved primarily from knowledge accumulated on the endemicity of these viruses. In this context, this virus-host relationship has been considered mainly as a survival mechanism for arboviruses in which the natural transmission cycle is periodically interrupted by adverse climatic conditions. In temperate zones, continuous viral transmission is precluded by winter temperatures that result in the cessation of adult vector activity. These vectors survive in the adult and immature stage of their life cycle. The consistent finding of virus, especially in species that overwinter as eggs or larvae, suggested the hypothesis that certain arboviruses remain endemic in the population as a result of transovarial transmission.[1]

A considerable amount of investigation has been conducted in an attempt to demonstrate transovarial transmission of arboviruses in their respective natural vectors; however, conclusive evidence is available only for some tick-borne viruses [2-4] and *Phlebotomus*-transmitted viruses.[5, 6] Studies that involved several mosquito species and different arboviruses have produced contradictory results, as indicated in reviews by Chamberlain and Sudia [7] and, more recently, by Reeves.[8] Thus, until our recent studies on LaCrosse (LAC) virus and *Aedes triseriatus* mosquitoes, transovarial transmission of an arbovirus in a mosquito was considered to be unlikely.

LAC virus is one of the California group arboviruses that for the most part have been discovered during the past two decades in North America and other countries.[9] Despite recent recognition of the California viruses, their association with human disease [10] has stimulated intensive and widespread investigation on their epidemiology and ecology. Observations made during these studies have revealed several salient features that appear to be common to all members of this group of viruses.[10, 11] Each tends to be endemic in a specific geographic zone; however, considerable overlap is evident from viral and serologic sur-

* Supported in part by National Institutes of Health Grants 5-ROI-00771, AI 07453, and AI 11547 and by Center for Disease Control Grant CC 00203.

† Present address: Department of Entomology, Walter Reed Army Institute of Research, Washington, D.C. 20012.

‡ Present address: Department of Microbiology, Mahidol University, Bangkok 4, Thailand.

§ Department of Veterinary Science.

|| Department of Entomology.

¶ Department of Preventive Medicine.

veillance studies. The natural transmission cycle involves mosquitoes, primarily of the genus *Aedes* and various sedentary mammalian species. Both a primary vector species and a primary vertebrate host species have been implicated for the more intensively studied California-group viruses. Circulation of these viruses tends to be restricted to forest areas, where tangential infection of man is most likely to occur. Viral transmission ceases with the disappearance of the arthropod vector in the fall and winter in temperate zones.

Since the original isolation of LAC virus from man in Wisconsin in 1964,[12] its natural transmission cycle has been studied intensively. These studies show that the virus circulates during the summer season in deciduous forests of the southwestern and western parts of this state.[13, 14] The mosquito, *A. triseriatus*, has been fully incriminated as the primary vector,[14-16] and the primary vertebrate hosts include chipmunks and, to a lesser extent, gray squirrels.[17-19] Man frequently becomes infected on entering LAC virus enzootic areas.[20]

DEMONSTRATION OF TRANSOVARIAL TRANSMISSION OF LAC VIRUS IN COLONIZED *A. triseriatus*

Evidence accumulated on the summer season maintenance cycle of LAC virus strongly suggested that it remained endemic in Wisconsin during the winter season. Considering the virus's narrow host range, either the vector and/or the vertebrate host could account for the continuous endemicity. Experiments aimed at demonstrating latent infection in chipmunks after experimental inoculation with LAC virus were negative.[21] However, the isolation of the virus from field-collected *A. triseriatus* larvae during the summer and fall of 1972[22] prompted laboratory investigation to explore the possibility of transovarial transmission of LAC virus in *A. triseriatus*. A more detailed description of this investigation has been presented elsewhere.[23]

Materials and Methods

In laboratory experiments, colony *A. triseriatus* were allowed to ingest LAC virus in guinea pig defibrinated blood through an artificial membrane. The amount of virus ingested by the mosquitoes was determined by an infectivity assay that employed suckling mice.

After the first ovarian cycle eggs were laid, mosquitoes were allowed to feed at various intervals on mice and hamsters. These animals served as a source of blood for subsequent egg production and as an indicator of infection in parent mosquitoes.

A portion of the eggs from each ovarian cycle, except the first one, were assayed for virus, and some of them were hatched to provide larvae and adults. The larvae were assayed for virus in pools of 10, and the F_1 adults were tested individually. Also, some of the female mosquitoes were allowed to feed on mice to determine if viral transmission was possible.

Eggs, larvae, and adults were assayed for virus by intracerebral inoculation into suckling mice. Viral infectivity endpoints were calculated according to the methods of Reed and Muench.[24]

Mosquitoes were maintained on a 5% sucrose-water diet at 27° C in 80% relative humidity under a 16-hr photoperiod.

Results

A group of 30 adult female mosquitoes became infected after ingesting a LAC virus-blood mixture that contained $10^{6.4}$ $SMLD_{50}$ (suckling mouse lethal dose, 50% effective) per 0.03 ml. Most of these mosquitoes survived for 43 days, during which time they fed on hamsters or suckling mice at 10- to 12-day intervals. The eggs laid after each blood meal were considered to represent the first, second, third, and fourth ovarian cycles, respectively.

Eggs of the first ovarian cycle were not assayed for virus, and virus was not recovered from a suspension made from 35 eggs of the second ovarian cycle. LAC virus was, however, detected in suspensions made from each of two pools of 75 eggs of the third and fourth ovarian cycles.

LAC virus was recovered from *A. triseriatus* larvae and adults that originated from each of the four ovarian cycles. Of 177 adult mosquitoes tested, virus was detected in 39% (33/85) of males and in 30% (28/92) of females. Of the 28 infected females, 21 were capable of transmitting virus to mice. No attempt was made to recover virus from pupae.

The recovery of virus from larvae and F_1 adults that originated from eggs of ovarian cycle two, from which virus was not recovered, suggests that these eggs contained a nondetectable level of virus. Subsequent findings tend to support this suggestion, because virus quantities detected in five groups of eggs have never exceeded $10^{0.5} SMLD_{50}/0.03$ ml. Virus titers obtained for individual third and fourth instar larvae ranged from $10^{1.5}$ to $10^{2.5} SMLD_{50}/0.03$ ml, whereas titers for individual males and females were slightly higher; the latter ranged from $10^{2.5} SMLD_{50}/0.03$ ml to $10^{3.5} SMLD_{50}/0.03$ ml.

After discovering that LAC virus was vertically transmitted in *A. triseriatus,* an experiment was conducted to determine whether the virus was transmitted on the surface or within the eggs. First, eggs were obtained from an *A. triseriatus* mosquito in which we had confirmed vertical transmission of LAC virus. One half of the eggs were surface sterilized, whereas the other half were not treated. After inoculation of suspensions of these eggs into mice, virus was recovered from both groups of eggs, thus indicating that LAC virus was transmitted within the eggs.

OBSERVATIONS ON TRANSOVARIAL TRANSMISSION OF LAC VIRUS IN FIELD POPULATIONS OF *A. triseriatus*

The demonstration in the laboratory of transovarial transmission of LAC virus in *A. triseriatus* [23] and isolation of the virus from field-collected *A. triseriatus* larvae [22] strongly indicated that transovarial transmission of the virus occurs in nature. To explore this possibility, an investigation was conducted that tested the hypothesis that transovarial transmission was the overwintering mechanism for LAC virus in Wisconsin. The details of these experiments have been presented elsewhere and are summarized below.[25]

A brief description of the biology of the vector, *A. triseriatus*, will make the approach employed in this part of the study more easily understood. The geographic distribution of this mosquito species extends throughout much of the North American continent east of the Rocky Mountains.[26] *A. triseriatus* breeds primarily in water retained in basal treeholes, and in the northern part of its range, it is active as an adult from June until the late fall months.[27, 28] The adults are incapable of surviving during the winter, but the eggs of this species remain viable in a diapaused state until spring.[29] Thus, LAC virus transovarially transmitted to the eggs of *A. triseriatus* survives during the winter season.

Materials and Methods

A. triseriatus larvae were collected prior to the emergence of adult mosquitoes from water of basal treehole breeding sites located in unglaciated areas of southwestern Wisconsin during the spring of 1973. The treehole breeding sites were located in the Pinnacle Farm (PF) and Davis Farm (DF) study areas of Iowa County and in the Greenwald Coulee (GW), Grandad Bluff (GB), and Farnum Drive (FD) study areas in LaCrosse County. Larvae were also collected on one occasion from automobile tires located near State Road Coulee (SRC) in LaCrosse County. Serologic evidence of recent infection in man and small mammals and the isolation of the virus from mosquitoes indicated that LAC virus was enzootic in this area.

Mosquito larvae were identified, and some were pooled for virus isolation attempts. Larvae not sacrificed were reared to adults for virus assay and for viral transmission attempts to mice. Male mosquitoes were sacrificed 1–5 days after emergence and stored at −70° C in pools of one to 12 mosquitoes. Females were retained for 1–13 days, during which time they were allowed to feed on mice. These mosquitoes were then sacrificed and stored at −70° C for virus assay. Suckling mice were used to assay larvae and mosquitoes for virus.

Results

As shown in TABLE 1, a total of 125 pools that contained 1422 third and fourth instar *A. triseriatus* larvae were assayed for virus. LAC virus was first

TABLE 1

ISOLATIONS OF LaCROSSE VIRUS FROM FIELD-COLLECTED *A. triseriatus* LARVAE

Breeding Site	April 20–26	May 10–17	May 23–June 7	Total
PF-11	1/7 (140) *	0/5 (50)	— †	1/12 (190)
GW-15	0/2 (20)	1/3 (30) *	1/9 (90) *	2/14 (140)
SRC tires	—	—	5/10 (100) *	5/10 (100)
Other sites	0/65 (748)	0/20 (200)	0/4 (44)	0/89 (992)
Total	1/74 (908)	1/28 (280)	6/23 (234)	8/125 (1422)

* Pools that yielded LAC virus/number pools tested (total number individual larvae).

† Larvae either not collected or allowed to develop to adults.

TABLE 2

LaCrosse Virus Isolations from Adult *A. triseriatus* Originating
from Field-Collected Larvae

Breeding Site	+ Pools/Pools (no. individuals)		Total Both Sexes
	Males	Females	
PF-11	1/09 (41) *	0/20 (50)	1/29 (91)
SRC-tires	4/11 (108)	1/29 (110)	5/40 (218)
Other sites	0/52 (269)	0/79 (205)	0/131 (474)
Total	5/72 (418)	1/128 (365)	6/200 (783)

* Total number of pools that yielded LAC virus/total number pools tested (total number individuals per breeding site).

isolated from a pool of 20 larvae collected on April 26 from the PF-11 breeding site. Virus was also isolated from two pools of 10 larvae each collected on May 17 and 23 from the GW-15 breeding site and from five pools that contained 10 larvae each collected on May 23 from the tire breeding site. Virus isolation attempts from larvae collected from six other breeding sites were unsuccessful, even though comparable numbers of specimens were assayed. The minimum field infection rate (MFIR) based on one infected specimen per pool was one per 110 larvae tested from the PF-11 and GW-15 breeding sites and one per 20 larvae obtained from the tires.

A total of 72 pools that contained 418 male mosquitoes and 128 pools that contained 365 female mosquitoes that were reared from field-collected *A. triseriatus* larvae were assayed for virus (TABLE 2). From the eight treehole breeding sites, LAC virus was isolated from only one pool of 10 male mosquitoes that originated from the PF-11 breeding site. Attempts to isolate virus from 255 female mosquitoes that originated from treehole breeding sites were unsuccessful. Virus isolations were successful from four pools of males that contained five, 10, 10, and 11 mosquitoes, respectively, that originated from the tire breeding site. Also, LAC virus was isolated from a pool of two female mosquitoes that were reared from larvae collected from the tires. The MFIR was one per 41 male mosquitoes of the PF-11 breeding site and one per 27 male mosquitoes from the tire breeding site. A MFIR of one per 110 females was observed for mosquitoes from the tire breeding site.

A total of 241 mosquitoes that represented the nine breeding sites fed on mice as groups of two to six mosquitoes per mouse. None of the 165 mosquitoes that originated from treehole breeding sites transmitted virus to mice. Of 76 mosquitoes that originated from the tire breeding site, LAC virus was transmitted to a mouse by one or two 13-day-old mosquitoes.

As mentioned earlier, LAC virus was isolated from *A. triseriatus* larvae and adults that originated from the tire breeding site. After initial removal of the larvae, the water and debris found in the tire was transferred to plastic containers in the laboratory. After approximately 4 weeks, the water had evaporated from the containers. On adding water to the dry debris, several *A. triseriatus* larvae hatched within 16–24 hr. Of 57 individual larvae assayed, 13 yielded isolations of LAC virus. Also, virus was isolated from nine of 18 female and from four of 23 male mosquitoes. Viral transmission was accomplished to mice by four of eight infected mosquitoes.

Approximately 1 month after hatching *A. triseriatus* eggs, a third brood of larvae was obtained by adding water to the tire debris. LAC virus was isolated from two of 11 female and from one of 10 male mosquitoes.

In summarizing the data for the tire breeding site, we find LAC virus infection rates to be 23% (13/57) for larvae, 38% (11/29) for females, and 15% (5/33) for males.

DISCUSSION

Laboratory findings suggest that LAC virus circulated in ovarian tissue of *A. triseriatus* within a few days after ingestion of the infectious blood meal. This is supported by the recovery of the virus from progeny derived from first ovarian cycle eggs, which are usually deposited by colony mosquitoes 3–5 days after ingesting a blood meal. Apparently, infection persisted in the ovaries, because LAC virus was detected in either eggs or progeny that originated from the second, third, and fourth ovarian cycles of the infected mosquitoes. These findings are consistent with those observed for western equine encephalitis (WEE) virus and *Culex tarsalis*.[30] This virus was detected in ovarian tissue of infected mosquitoes 4 days after ingestion of the infectious blood meal, and infection persisted throughout the life of the mosquito. However, the failure to demonstrate transovarial transmission of WEE virus in *C. tarsalis* suggests that factors other than the time and duration of infection of the ovaries may influence transovarial transmission of an arbovirus in a mosquito.

As reported for vesicular stomatitis virus (VSV), Indiana serotype,[31] and for some tick-borne arboviruses,[32] LAC virus was shown to be transstadially transmitted in *A. triseriatus*. Virus concentration increased during metamorphosis from very low levels in the eggs, $10^{0.5}SMLD_{50}/0.03$ ml or less, to titers of $10^{3.5}SMLD_{50}/0.03$ ml in adult mosquitoes. No difference in virus titer was noted between male and female mosquitoes. A similar pattern of virus propagation was observed in experiments that involved *Lutzomyia trapidoi* and VSV, Indiana serotype.[30]

The transovarial infection and accompanying filial infection rates for *A. triseriatus* mosquitoes infected with LAC virus cannot be determined from the data obtained in the present study. However, preliminary findings of an investigation not presented in this report suggest that not all infected mosquitoes support this route of transmission. With regard to filial infection rates, data based on progeny from two mosquitoes suggest rates that approach 100%. These experiments were hampered by high infertility rates in eggs of infected *A. triseriatus* mosquitoes and problems encountered in hatching eggs that were fertile.

The results of field investigation clearly showed that LAC virus relies on transovarial transmission as an overwintering mechanism. Additional studies, however, will be necessary to assess the role of this transmission route during periods of vector activity. Evidence accumulated strongly implies that infection of chipmunks serves to amplify virus circulation;[23] however, the necessity of infection of a vertebrate host in regard to the perpetuation of the virus remains to be determined. In addition, amplification of virus circulation by male mosquitoes must not be excluded, because it is conceivable that infection could be transmitted to female mosquitoes during copulation.

Finally, the phenomenon of installment hatching of *A. triseriatus* eggs may prove to be important for the maintenance of LAC virus. Such a mechanism would result in the hatching of only a portion of the infected eggs after rainfalls during the yearly warm season. As a result, the unhatched portion of the infected eggs could ensure the persistence of LAC virus in situations of high larval or adult mortality and other pitfalls to virus persistence, such as the failure of mosquitoes to make contact with a vertebrate host or when mosquitoes fed on a vertebrate that failed to develop a viremia of sufficient magnitude to infect other mosquitoes.

Summary

As part of a continuing investigation on the ecology of LaCrosse virus in Wisconsin, field and laboratory studies we're conducted to explore the possibility that the virus is transmitted transovarially in *A. triseriatus* mosquitoes. In laboratory experiments, *A. triseriatus* mosquitoes were infected by ingesting LaCrosse virus in defibrinated blood. LaCrosse virus was recovered from F_1 eggs, larvae, and adults that originated from the infected parent mosquitoes. In a subsequent field study aimed at determining if transovarial transmission accounted for the survival of LaCrosse virus during the winter season, larvae that originated from overwintering *A. triseriatus* eggs were collected from a LaCrosse virus enzootic area in southwestern Wisconsin. LaCrosse virus was isolated from these larvae and from adult *A. triseriatus* that were reared from field-collected larvae. These findings strongly imply that *A. triseriatus* is the reservoir of LaCrosse virus and that transovarial transmission is the mechanism responsible for the maintenance of the virus during the winter season in the north central region of the United States.

Acknowledgments

We appreciate the technical assistance of Mrs. Joan Schallern and Mrs. Dianne Fisher. We also thank Dr. Cameron B. Gundersen, Gundersen Clinic, LaCrosse, Wisconsin and Dr. W. D. Sudia, Center for Disease Control, Atlanta, Georgia for consultation and assistance during this study.

References

1. REEVES, W. C. 1961. Overwintering of arthropod-borne viruses. Progr. Med. Virol. **3:** 59–78.
2. HOOGSTRAAL, H. 1966. Ticks in relation to human diseases caused by viruses. Annu. Rev. Entomol. **11:** 261–308.
3. BLASKOVEC, D. & J. NOSEK. 1972. The ecological approach to the study of tickborne encephalitis. Progr. Med. Virol. **14:** 215–320.
4. BALASLOV, Y. S. 1972. Bloodsucking ticks (Ixodoidea) vectors of diseases of man and animals. Misc. Publ. Entomol. Soc. Amer. **8:** 159–376.

5. BARNETT, H. C. & W. SUYEMOTO. 1961. Field studies on sandfly fever and Kala-azar in Pakistan, in Iran, and in Baltistan (Little Tibet) Kashmir. Ann. N.Y. Acad. Sci. **23:** 609–617.
6. SCHMIDT, J. R., M. L. SCHMIDT & M. I. SAID. 1971. Phlebotomos fever in Egypt: Isolation of Phlebotomos fever viruses from *Phlebotomos* papatasi. Amer. J. Trop. Med. Hyg. **20:** 483–490.
7. CHAMBERLAIN, R. W. & W. D. SUDIA. 1961. Mechanism of transmission of viruses by mosquitoes. Annu. Rev. Entomol. **6:** 371–390.
8. REEVES, W. E. 1974. Overwintering of arboviruses. Progr. Med. Virol. **17:** 193–220.
9. PARKIN, W. E., W. McD. HAMMON & G. E. SATHER. 1972. Review of current epidemiological literature on viruses of the California arbovirus group. Amer. J. Trop. Med. Hyg. **21:** 964–978.
10. HENDERSON, B. E. & P. H. COLEMAN. 1971. The growing importance of California arboviruses in the etiology of human disease. Progr. Med. Virol. **13:** 401–461.
11. SUDIA, W. D., V. F. NEWHOUSE, C. H. CALLISHER & R. W. CHAMBERLAIN. 1971. California group arboviruses isolations from mosquitoes in North America. Mosquito News **31:** 576–600.
12. THOMPSON, W. H., B. KALFAYAN & R. O. ANSLOW. 1965. Isolation of California encephalitis group virus from a fatal human illness. Amer. J. Epidemiol. **81:** 245–253.
13. THOMPSON, W. H. & S. L. INHORN. 1967. Arthropod-borne California group viral encephalitis in Wisconsin. Wisc. Med. J. **66:** 250–253.
14. THOMPSON, W. H., R. O. ANSLOW, R. P. HANSON & G. R. DEFOLIART. 1972. LaCrosse virus isolations from mosquitoes in Wisconsin, 1964–1968. Amer. J. Trop. Med. Hyg. **21:** 90–96.
15. WATTS, D. M., C. D. MORRIS, R. E. WRIGHT, G. R. DEFOLIART & R. P. HANSON. 1972. Transmission of LaCrosse virus (California encephalitis group) by the mosquito *Aedes triseriatus*. J. Med. Entomol. **9:** 125–127.
16. WATTS, D. M., R. R. GRIMSTAD, G. R. DEFOLIART, T. M. YUILL & R. P. HANSON. 1973. Laboratory transmission of LaCrosse encephalitis virus by several species of mosquitoes. J. Med. Entomol. **10:** 583–586.
17. MOULTON, D. W. & W. H. THOMPSON. 1971. California group virus infection in small forest-dwelling mammals of Wisconsin. Some ecological considerations. Amer. J. Trop. Med. Hyg. **20:** 474–482.
18. PANTUWATANA, S., W. H. THOMPSON, D. M. WATTS & R. P. HANSON. 1972. Experimental infection of chipmunks and squirrels with LaCrosse and trivittatus viruses and biological transmission of LaCrosse by *Aedes triseriatus*. Amer. J. Trop. Med. Hyg. **21:** 476–481.
19. GAULD, L. W., R. P. HANSON, W. H. THOMPSON & S. K. SINHA. 1974. Observations on a natural cycle of LaCrosse virus (California group) in southwestern Wisconsin. Amer. J. Trop. Med. Hyg. **23:** 983–992.
20. THOMPSON, W. H. & A. S. EVANS. 1965. California encephalitis virus studies in Wisconsin. Amer. J. Epidemiol. **81:** 230–244.
21. PANTUWATANA, S. 1973. Epizootiological studies on the viruses of the California encephalitis group in Wisconsin. Ph.D. Thesis. University of Wisconsin. Madison, Wisc.
22. PANTUWATANA, S., W. H. THOMPSON, D. M. WATTS, T. M. YUILL & R. P. HANSON. 1973. Isolation of LaCrosse virus from field collected *Aedes triseriatus* larvae. Amer. J. Trop. Med. Hyg. **23:** 246–250.
23. WATTS, D. M., S. PANTUWATANA, G. R. DEFOLIART, T. M. YUILL & W. H. THOMPSON. 1973. Transovarial transmission of LaCrosse virus (California encephalitis group) in the mosquito, *Aedes triseriatus*. Science **182:** 1140, 1141.
24. REED, L. J. & H. MUENCH. 1938. A simple method of estimating fifty percent endpoints. Amer. J. Hyg. **27:** 493–497.

25. WATTS, D. M., W. H. THOMPSON, T. M. YUILL, G. R. DEFOLIART & R. P. HANSON. 1974. Overwintering of LaCrosse virus in *Aedes triseriatus*. Amer. J. Trop. Med. Hyg. **23:** 694–700.

26. ZAVORTINK, T. J. 1972. XXVIII. The New World species formerly placed in *Aedes* (Finlaya). Contrib. Amer. Entomol. Inst. (Ann Arbor) **8:** 30.

27. CARPENTER, S. J. & W. LA CASSE. 1955. Mosquitoes of North America (North of Mexico). : 255–257. University of California Press. Berkeley, Calif.

28. LOOR, K. A. & G. R. DEFOLIART. 1970. Field observations on the biology of *Aedes triseriatus*. Mosquito News **30:** 60–64.

29. BAKER, F. C. 1935. The effect of photoperiodism on resting treehole mosquitoes larvae. Can. Entomol. **67:** 149–153.

30. THOMAS, L. A. 1963. Distribution of the virus of western equine encephalomyelitis in the mosquito vector, *Culex tarsalis*. Amer. J. Hyg. **78:** 150–165.

31. TESH, R. B., B. N. CHANIOTIS & K. M. JOHNSON. 1972. Vesicular stomatitis virus (Indiana serotype): transovarial transmission by Phlebotomine sandflies. Science **176:** 1477, 1478.

32. BURGDORFER, W. & M. A. R. VARMA. 1967. Trans-stadial and transovarial development of disease agents in arthropods. Annu. Rev. Entomol. **12:** 347–376.

ECOLOGY OF KEYSTONE VIRUS, A TRANSOVARIALLY MAINTAINED ARBOVIRUS *

James W. LeDuc, John F. Burger,
Bruce F. Eldridge, and Philip K. Russell

*Walter Reed Army Institute of Research
Washington, D.C. 20012*

INTRODUCTION

For the past several years, we have studied the ecology of the Keystone (KEY) strain of California encephalitis (CE) in the Pocomoke Cypress Swamp in Worcester County, Maryland. Our study area consists of a disturbed fresh water swamp and the surrounding coastal pine forest. Part of the swamp is covered by a thick mat of interwoven tree roots and duff, while the remainder is open water. The surrounding forest is a relatively flat area of land that has reverted to pines and some hardwoods from farmland over the past 40–50 years. Several arboviruses are known to occur in the swamp, including eastern and western equine encephalitis (EEE, WEE) [1] and Jamestown Canyon (JC) and KEY strains of CE. [2]

COMPARISON OF EEE/WEE AND KEY ECOLOGY

One aspect of the ecology of arboviruses in the swamp that has occupied our attention is the mechanism of interepizootic survival of the various arboviruses. The possible mechanisms for EEE and WEE have been discussed previously. [3] After the beginning of our studies of KEY virus in the swamp, we noted two important differences between the ecology of KEY and WEE/EEE. First, a floodwater mosquito, *Aedes atlanticus* Dyar and Knab, was found to be the source of virtually all KEY virus isolations from mosquitoes. [2] Nearly all EEE and WEE isolates were from *Culiseta melanura* (Coquillett). [1] The former species overwinters in the egg stage, whereas the latter overwinters as a larva. Second, a comparison of several years' population curves of the two species along with the occurrence of virus isolates showed two basically different patterns. FIGURE 1 presents a typical year's data for each vector-virus system. [1,2] The pattern for *C. melanura* is typical of several arboviruses, including EEE, WEE, and Japanese encephalitis (JE) in Japan. [4] Numbers of vectors begin a gradual buildup as warm weather approaches, reaching a peak in mid-summer. Virus isolations are obtained from mosquitoes only after the vector population of adults has achieved substantial numbers. The last isolate from mosquitoes usually occurs after the population peak has subsided but before the adult

* In conducting the research described in this report, the investigators adhered to the *Guide for Laboratory Animal Facilities and Care,* as promulgated by the Committee on the Guide for Laboratory Animal Facilities and Care of the Institute of Laboratory Animal Resources, National Academy of Sciences, National Research Council.

population has disappeared. In our 1969 collections, more than 21,000 adult *C. melanura* were tested for virus with negative results before the first virus isolate; almost 10,000 were tested after the last isolate.

We found, in examining the 1971 data for KEY (FIGURE 1), a completely different situation. As is typical for floodwater mosquito species, the duration of adult activity was much shorter than that for *C. melanura,* and the population peak was thus much sharper. The first KEY isolate, however, was early in the season; it occurred virtually at the very start of the appearance of adults. The last isolate, moreover, coincided with the disappearance of adults. We concluded that in the case of EEE/WEE, the vector population became infected in significant numbers only after the level of virus activity had become amplified through vector-vertebrate interchange of virus, whereas in KEY, the vector population must be infected in substantial numbers at the time of the initial emergence of

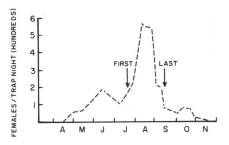

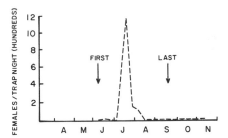

FIGURE 1. Population curves based on light trap samples and first and last virus isolates from mosquitoes for *C. melanura* and eastern and western equine encephalitis, 1969 (*top*), and for *A. atlanticus* and the Keystone strain of California encephalitis, 1971 (*bottom*), both in Pocomoke Cypress Swamp, Worcester County, Md.

adult females. The population dynamics and infection pattern suggested to us the strong possibility of transovarial transmission, a phenomenon that had yet to be confirmed for mosquitoes at that time.

Transovarial Transmission of KEY Virus

In the spring of 1973, we learned of the outstanding discovery made by Watts *et al.* at the University of Wisconsin.[5] This finding spurred our efforts to collect *A. atlanticus* larvae for the purpose of attempting virus isolations of KEY. We isolated KEY virus several times, both from field-collected larvae and from males and females that had been reared from field-collected larvae maintained in virus-free laboratories.[6] The isolation rate was found to be approximately the same in larvae, males, and females and comparable to field isolation rates in wild-trapped females (approximately 1:300). Interestingly, from field-collected and laboratory-reared pupae tested, we have obtained no virus isolates. The frequency of transovarial transmission among infected female mosquitoes and the proportion of infected eggs that arises from an infected ovary are problems that we are presently attempting to solve, as is the transmission rate of KEY virus in transovarially infected females.

THE ROLE OF VERTEBRATES

FIGURE 2 is a hypothetic vector diagram for KEY virus circulation in nature. Arrows that lead away from "infected" blocks designate factors that tend to increase the ratio of uninfected/infected individuals; the opposite is true for arrows that lead toward "infected" blocks. Factors for which we have no experimental evidence are indicated by a question mark. One can envision a model in which mosquitoes become infected only through vertical (transstadial) transmission and where vertebrates, if they do become infected by bites of infected mosquitoes, do so only accidentally and serve as dead-end hosts. The field data that we have collected since 1971 plus an examination of FIGURE 2 argue, on theoretic grounds, against such a situation. For all 4 years of our KEY studies, the field infection rate in both adults and larvae has been approximately 1:300. Because, as can be seen in FIGURE 2, the only vector arrow that leads *toward* the infected compartment of the mosquito cycle is from infected vertebrates and because one may assume, at least on theoretic grounds, several arrows that lead *away* from the infected compartment of the mosquito cycle, a vertebrate source of virus for mosquitoes is necessary to maintain a relatively stable uninfected/infected ratio from year to year.

Although serologic studies indicate that vertebrates, including man, become infected with KEY virus in nature,[7] detailed studies of viremia levels in potential vertebrate hosts, in addition to infection and transmission parameters in mos-

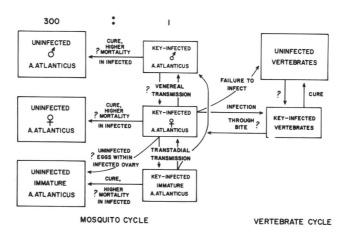

FIGURE 2. Hypothetic vector diagram for the circulation of the Keystone strain of California encephalitis virus in nature.

TABLE 1

EVALUATION OF POTENTIAL VERTEBRATE HOSTS OF KEYSTONE VIRUS

Host	Engorged *A. atlanticus* (%) *	Neutralizing Aby to Keystone Virus (pos/tested)	Viremia After Experimental Infection
Whitetail deer	34	12/121 †	ND ‡
Turtles	15	0/227	ND
Rabbit	12	1/3	+ §
Gray squirrel	6	8/27	+
Raccoon	4	7/39	+ (low)
Opossum	2	0/18	—
Others	27	ND	ND

* Total of 436 blood meals.
† 75/121 contained Aby to Jamestown Canyon.
‡ Not done.
§ Domestic rabbit.

quitoes, are needed to establish probable roles of vertebrates in the virus cycle. In 1973, we demonstrated KEY infection in vertebrates by the exposure of sentinel rabbits in the swamp. We were able to correlate dates of seroconversions in sentinel rabbits with dates of *A. atlanticus* activity. We also were aware that rabbits would be bitten by *A. atlanticus,* based on earlier results of attractiveness studies with caged animals. Thus, we concluded that *A. atlanticus* probably did transmit KEY virus to vertebrates in nature, and probably at the time of their initial blood meal.

Next, we considered the role in the amplification of KEY virus of various vertebrates that live in the swamp. Two criteria should be met by potential vertebrate hosts to incriminate them as being involved in the virus cycle. First, vector mosquitoes must feed on them regularly; second, they must be susceptible to infection by the virus and must produce a viremia of sufficient titer to infect feeding mosquitoes. These parameters may be measured by serologic identification of blood meals of randomly collected engorged vector mosquitoes, serologic profiles of wild-caught vertebrates to KEY virus, and by viremia produced by each species after infection with KEY virus. We have gathered data on the feeding patterns of *A. atlanticus* based on several years' collections and serologic profiles to KEY virus of common vertebrates of southern Maryland. We also have some data on viremia levels in experimentally infected animals. TABLE 1 summarizes our research to date on these factors. Whitetail deer probably represent the greatest biomass of the potential hosts in the swamp, and they are frequently fed upon by *A. atlanticus.* Only a few deer had detectable neutralizing antibody to KEY virus, although about 60% of those tested had antibody against the JC strain of CE. We have not yet attempted experimental infection of whitetail deer and are aware of only one such experiment in the literature.[8] In that instance, only trace amounts of virus were detected on Days 2 and 3 postinoculation (pi), although infection was confirmed by the presence of antibody on Day 21 pi. Additional studies along these lines are needed.

Turtles and opossums do not appear to act as amplifying hosts of KEY virus, and even though cottontail rabbits may exhibit a viremia of sufficient titer to infect feeding mosquitoes, it is difficult to assess their importance, because attempts to live-trap them have been unsuccessful, and the amount of feeding on them by *A. atlanticus* is masked by the presence of sentinel rabbits. The gray squirrel appears to be a good candidate for an important vertebrate host, primarily because, experimentally, it has been shown to produce viremias to 10^5 PFU/ml and is readily fed upon by *A. atlanticus* adults. Raccoons may also be involved if only low levels of viremia are needed to infect vector mosquitoes. The cotton rat, implicated in KEY virus cycles elsewhere, does not inhabit our study area.

Vector Biology

The true significance of transovarial transmission can be assessed only after a thorough study of vector biology and of vertebrate-host-virus interactions. Our studies on the blood-feeding habits of adult females have been summarized above. We have also conducted studies on adult behavior similar to those by Roberts,[9] who found that *A. atlanticus* in the area of Houston, Texas remains in shaded forests during the daytime and migrates to adjacent open grassland near dusk. Most animals active in the forest are attacked anytime during the day, but grassland-inhabiting animals, such as cotton rats and cottontail rabbits, are not bitten until evening. There are no naturally occurring grasslands adjacent to the upland forests in our study area, but extensive logging has resulted in large openings that have been invaded by grasses. We have found that the behavior of *A. atlanticus* in our area is comparable to that described by Roberts for Houston. Whereas no cotton rats are present in our area, deer frequently browse in the forest openings in the evening and roam in wooded areas during the day. This situation may explain the high frequency of deer feeding by *A. atlanticus.*

A significant aspect of the ecology of *A. atlanticus* is the fact that adult activity is restricted to a very small part of the year, in spite of apparently favorable weather conditions of much greater duration. We are gradually discovering the factors that control the hatching of eggs and thus produce the distinctive population curve of the species. We have observed in the field that two conditions must be met before the bulk of the eggs of this species will hatch. First, there must be a period of several weeks of warm ($>25°$ C) weather; second, a heavy sustained rain must occur, sufficient to flood fully the forest depressions where *A. atlanticus* eggs have been deposited. The upland forest soil is almost pure sand, so that precipitation of medium or light intensity or duration drains off too rapidly to permit hatching and larval development. We have found, furthermore, that eggs are laid only in fairly deep troughs or depressions, usually at least 0.5 m or more in depth. Because of soil porosity, eggs deposited in shallower depressions would not remain flooded long enough to permit larval development. This situation may not pertain to areas further inland, where the clay content of the soil is greater. We have confirmed the necessity of exposure of the eggs to prolonged warm temperature through laboratory studies. We have found that eggs from soil samples collected at various times of the year will hatch promptly if they have been exposed to a period of warm temperature of several week's duration either in the field (summer collections) or in the laboratory (winter collections). We have also found no evidence of a true diapause that requires a period of egg chilling or a long photoperiod exposure of some life cycle stage for egg hatching. This type of response to winter conditions is consistent with the generally southern temperate zone distribution of *A. atlanticus*. FIGURE 3 illustrates the approximate geographic distribution of this species. It is probably limited on the north by the 0° C January isotherm and on the west by the 100-cm precipitation line. Our study area is approaching the northern limit of its range. Generally, where the greatest area of a species' range occurs in areas that have a mild winter, that species does not undergo a true diapause along its northern range limit.[10, 11]

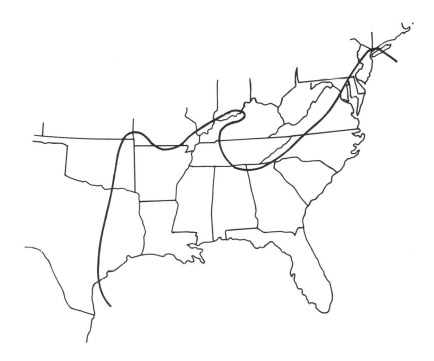

FIGURE 3. Approximate range of *A. atlanticus* Dyar and Knab, based on published and unpublished collection records.

The technique of vector age grading has assumed an increasingly important role in epidemiologic studies since its development and description by Detinova.[12] Unfortunately, this technique, which was originally used with *Anopheles* mosquitoes, does not work well with all mosquito species. After working with laboratory-reared females of known oviposition history, however, we found that dilations of the ovarian pedicel were easily detected in *A. atlanticus*. Therefore, during the 1974 period of adult activity, we dissected a sample of females from each day's collection to determine the physiologic state of the ovaries. During 1974, the period of adult activity, as determined by light trapping and daily monitoring of larval breeding sites, lasted only 2 weeks. All females trapped during the first 4 days after emergence of the first females were nulliparous. Uniparous females appeared on the fifth day, and by the 13th day, the last day a substantial number of females was trapped, all females dissected were uniparous. We found no females that we could classify as multiparous.

These data must be considered preliminary, because the 1974 period of adult activity was abnormally short. For this year, however, certain conclusions seem justified. Apparently, the period of adult activity was long enough only for females to ingest a single blood meal. If this is true, susceptible vertebrates would be infected, but there would be no significant infection of uninfected vectors. KEY infection of vertebrates was, in fact, confirmed by the sero-conversion of two of eight sentinel rabbits sometime between August 28 and September 20, a period that overlaps the period of adult *A. atlanticus* activity (August 20 to September 1). Thus, for 1974, this evidence suggests that there is no vector arrow that leads toward the infected compartment of the mosquito cycle of the virus (FIGURE 2). This conclusion assumes that the bulk of the vector population emerged within the first few days of the period of adult activity, and our observations indicate that this assumption is valid. Further-more, the appearance of uniparous females on the fifth day of the trapping period strongly suggests the occurrence of autogeny in the vector population. This phenomenon would further complicate the dynamics of virus transmission. Additional studies of these factors are planned, both in the laboratory and in the field. Again, the fact that we are studying this mosquito near the northern limit of its range must be emphasized. One would expect the population dynamics, and therefore the transmission pattern of KEY, to be different further south, where adult mosquitoes are active for a longer period of time.

Summary and Conclusions

Our studies in the Pocomoke Cypress Swamp of Maryland have shown that KEY strain of CE is endemic and is carried by the floodwater mosquito *A. atlanticus*. The virus is transmitted transstadially in nature, as evidenced by our recovery of virus from larvae and males of this species. Serologic evidence, both here and elsewhere, indicates that vertebrates are infected with KEY, but their role in the transmission cycle remains unknown. We have found several animals, for example, the gray squirrel, that are potential vertebrate reservoirs for the virus. Gray squirrels possess antibodies to KEY in nature, are known to be fed upon by *A. atlanticus* females, and have been shown to circulate a high-titered viremia after experimental inoculation. Evidence from 1974 collections, however, indicates that *A. atlanticus* females ingested only a single blood meal during the period when adults were active. We will not be able to assess the relative importance of the vertebrate and mosquito cycles until much more work has been performed on vector-reservoir-virus dynamics.

References

1. SAUGSTAD, E. S., J. M. DALRYMPLE & B. F. ELDRIDGE. 1972. Ecology of arbo-viruses in a Maryland freshwater swamp. I. Population dynamics and habitat distribution of potential mosquito vectors. Amer. J. Epidemiol. **93**: 114–122.
2. LeDuc, J. R., W. SUYEMOTO, T. J. KEEFE, J. F. BURGER, B. F. ELDRIDGE & P. K. RUSSELL. 1975. Ecology of California encephalitis viruses on the Del

Mar Va Peninsula. I. Virus isolations. Amer. J. Trop. Med. Hyg. **24:** 118–123.

3. DALRYMPLE, J. M., O. P. YOUNG, B. F. ELDRIDGE & P. K. RUSSELL. 1972. Ecology of arboviruses in a Maryland freshwater swamp. III. Vertebrate hosts and summary. Amer. J. Epidemiol. **96:** 129–140.

4. BUESCHER, E. L., W. F. SCHERER, M. Z. ROSENBERG, I. GRESSER, J. L. HARDY & H. R. BULLOCK. 1959. Ecologic studies of Japanese encephalitis virus in Japan. II. Mosquito infection. Amer. J. Trop. Med. Hyg. **8:** 651–664.

5. WATTS, D. M., S. PANTUWATANA, G. DE FOLIART, T. M. YUILL & W. H. THOMPSON. 1973. Transovarial transmission of LaCrosse virus (California encephalitis group) in the mosquito, *Aedes triseriatus*. Science 182: 1140, 1141.

6. LeDUC, J. W., W. SUYEMOTO, B. F. ELDRIDGE, P. K. RUSSELL & A. R. BARR. 1975. Ecology of California encephalitis viruses on the Del Mar Va Peninsula. II. Demonstration of transovarial transmission. Amer. J. Trop. Med. Hyg. **24:** 124–126.

7. PARKIN, W. E., W. McD. HAMMON & G. E. SATHER. 1972. Review of current epidemiological literature on viruses of the California arbovirus group. Amer. J. Trop. Med. Hyg. **21:** 964–978.

8. COOK, R. S. & D. O. TRAINER. 1969. Experimental exposure of deer to California encephalitis virus. Bull. Wildlife Disease Ass. **5:** 3–7.

9. ROBERTS, D. R. 1973. Studies on the biologies of mosquito species incriminated as vectors of Keystone virus in Houston, Texas. Ph.D. Dissertation. University of Texas at Houston. Houston, Texas.

10. ELDRIDGE, B. F. 1968. The effect of temperature and photoperiod on blood-feeding and ovarian development in mosquitoes of the *Culex pipiens* complex. Amer. J. Trop. Med. Hyg. **17:** 133–140.

11. ELDRIDGE, B. F., C. L. BAILEY & M. D. JOHNSON. 1972. A preliminary study of the seasonal geographic distribution and overwintering of *Culex restuans* Theobald and *Culex salinarius* Coquillett. J. Med. Entomol. **9:** 233–238.

12. DETINOVA, T. S. 1962. Age grouping methods in Diptera of medical importance with special reference to some vectors of malaria. World Health Org. Mon. Ser. **47:** 1–216.

TRANSOVARIAL TRANSMISSION OF *RICKETTSIA*-LIKE MICROORGANISMS IN MOSQUITOES *

Janice H. Yen

Department of Epidemiology
School of Public Health
University of California
Los Angeles, California 90025

INTRODUCTION

Most mosquitoes reportedly do not have transovarially transmitted *Rickettsia*. There are, however, two exceptions. Hertig and Wolbach[1] provided the first complete description of a vertically transmitted rickettsia-like microorganism, and now, over 50 years later, a second one has been found.[2] The two microorganisms are *Wolbachia pipientis*, found in the mosquito, *Culex pipiens*, and a still unnamed *Wolbachia* in a member of the *Aedes scutellaris* group. This aedine mosquito, presently called the Tafahi strain, has not yet been assigned a species rank.

C. pipiens is a widely distributed mosquito found throughout the temperate and tropical zones of the Old and New Worlds. *Wolbachia* has been found without exception in every member of the *C. pipiens* complex examined. The Tafahi strain was obtained from Tafahi, one of the islands of the Tongan archipelago, and the wolbachiae are apparently limited to the Tafahi strain. However, some important members of the *Aedes scutellaris* group have not been examined at all and others only cursorily.

A phenomenon called cytoplasmic incompatibility is also found in only two species complexes of mosquitoes, the same two groups, *C. pipiens* and *A. scutellaris*, that possess microorganisms. Incompatibility is the name given to a type of cross from which no hybrid offspring are produced, and it is called cytoplasmic because the factors responsible for the incompatibility are transmitted from one generation to the next through the maternal cytoplasm.[3]

This paper describes the microorganisms found in the two different species of mosquito and the biologic mechanisms that they influence.

MATERIALS AND METHODS

C. pipiens strains were obtained from various geographic locations and rendered autogenous and stengamous by genetic selection. Two strains, designated *1* and *3* for convenience, were extensively used for the experiments, because they are nonreciprocally incompatible; that is, when *3* females are crossed with *1* males, the cross is incompatible, but when *1* females are crossed with

* Supported by Research Grant CC 00367-05 from the Center for Disease Control, Atlanta, Georgia and by United States Public Health Service Training Grant TI-AI00132-11.

3 males, the cross is compatible and normal hatches are seen. The characteristics of the two strains are as follows:

Strain 1. This strain is from Dixon, California and is marked with ruby eye, a recessive, fully penetrant gene in the second linkage group.

Strain 3. Originally from Hamburg, Germany, this strain is marked with yellow fat body, an autosomal recessive in the second linkage group.

A third strain (*10*) was also used because of its incompatibility with several strains. It is marked with white eye, a sex-linked recessive in the first linkage group.

Aedes polynesiensis is an unmarked anautogenous aedine from one of the islands of Polynesia; the Tafahi strain is autogenous, has several phenotypic markers, and was obtained by Dr. James Hitchcock from Tonga.

Specimens for electron microscopy were fixed in glutaraldehyde, postfixed in osmium, and dehydrated in increasing concentrations of ethanol.[4] Strains of *C. pipiens* were rendered free of rickettsiae by treating eggs or larvae with tetracycline.[5, 6]

MICROORGANISMS AND THEIR LIFE CYCLE IN THE HOST

The morphologic features of *W. pipientis* have been examined by light microscopy [1, 7] and by electron microscopy.[4, 5, 8, 9] The organisms found in *C. pipiens* are small pleomorphic rods and cocci about 0.3 μm in diameter and 1.5 μm in length. Enlarged coccoid forms as large as 2 μm or more in diameter can occasionally be seen. A mixture of rods and cocci is almost always found in each infected cell (FIGURE 1). They are found in abundance in both the male and female reproductive cells but are found in greater numbers per unit area in the female. Like true rickettsiae, they are gram negative and stain red with Giemsa's stain. They divide by binary fission, multiply only in the cytoplasm of the cell, and are found almost exclusively in the cells of the testis and ovary. Occasionally, Malpighian tubule cells are also infected.

Ultrastructural studies show that *Wolbachia* has two membranes, an outer cell wall and an inner plasma membrane, and, in addition, is surrounded by a third membrane of host origin. Often 10–20 microorganisms can be seen clumped together in a vacuole. Small ribosome-like particles and strands of DNA are present in the cytoplasm.

Wolbachiae have been found in all life cycle stages of *C. pipiens,* from the newly laid egg to the adult male and female. They are concentrated just beneath the micropyle in the egg (FIGURE 2) and presumably move to the cells of the gonads during embryonic development. *Wolbachia* is present in all its structural forms in the egg, but the rods and cocci predominate. Occasionally, greatly enlarged cocci can also be seen.

In first instar larvae, which have been removed from the egg, wolbachiae are present in only moderate numbers in the germ cells. They are much less pleomorphic, and none of the greatly enlarged cocci or the clumps of wolbachiae can be seen. The pathologic cells, which are often observed in later mosquito stages, appear to be absent or extremely rare in the embryo. Nuclei and cell organelles are apparently normal in cells infected with microorganisms. Although several organs, such as the brain, fat body, and gut, were surveyed, *W. pipientis* was found only in the cells of the gonads.

In third and fourth instars, the microorganisms multiply rapidly, and some

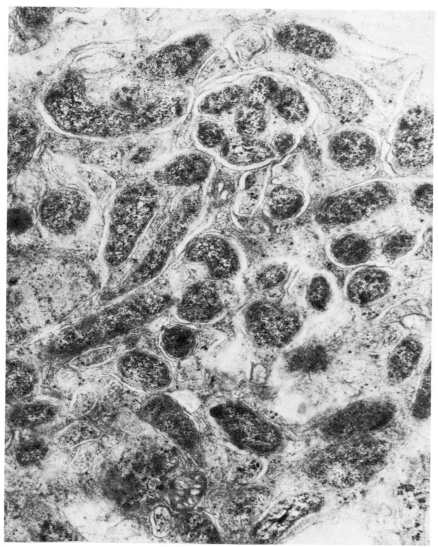

FIGURE 1. *W. pipientis* in a *C. pipiens* pupal testis cell. × 36,300.

pathologic cells can be seen. These pathologic cells contain a degenerating pycnotic nucleus, many cytoplasmic vacuoles, and show disorganization of cell organelles. The pupae and adults are very heavily infected, particularly the females, whose oocyte and nurse cells are always infected. Organisms have not been found in intracellular spaces of the ovary or in the follicular epithelium. Some of the cells that contain *Wolbachia* exhibit the pathologic features mentioned before (pycnotic, degenerating nucleus and disorganized cytoplasm), and whether the microorganism causes the pathologic condition has been the subject of much discussion.[5, 7, 9] This question may be answered through observations made in the male mosquito.

Serial electron microscopic sections of pupal testis reveal that some spermatocytes are not infected, others have some wolbachiae, and that still others contain large numbers of microorganisms.[10] It is of interest that not all pathologic cells contain microorganisms.[10] Serial sections show that some cells have

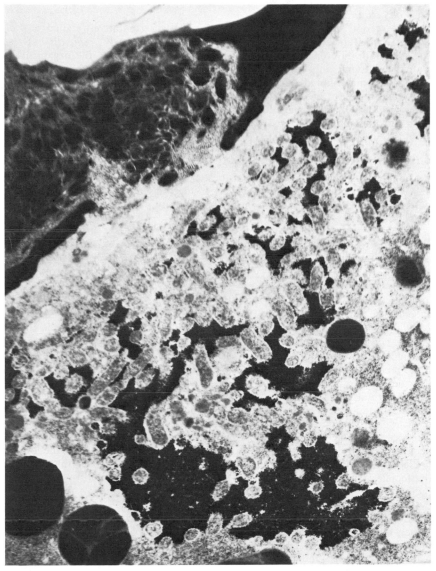

FIGURE 2. *W. pipientis* present in large numbers beneath the micropyle of a recently oviposited egg. $\times$ 12,100.

typical degenerate pycnotic nuclei, cytoplasmic vacuoles, and disorganization of cytoplasmic organelles but contain not one *Wolbachia* within them! Other cells are filled with the organism but exhibit no obvious pathologic characteristics. Thus, microorganisms probably do not produce pathologic cells; instead, the cell, once it starts to degenerate, may become very "susceptible" to infection, and the organisms might then multiply rapidly to fill the cytoplasm. As in the female, the wolbachiae in the male are found only in the cytoplasm. As the spermatocytes differentiate into spermatids and the cytoplasm is shed, the microorganisms, too, are removed with the cytoplasm, and the mature sperms contain no *Wolbachia*.

The second transovarially transmitted rickettsia (tentatively called a *Wolbachia*) in Tafahi has some of the same characteristics as *W. pipientis* but also shows certain differences.[2] Like the *Wolbachia* in *C. pipiens,* the organisms in Tafahi are found only in the cytoplasm. They are present in the cells of the male and female gonads (specifically in the germ cells; never in the epithelial cells) and have not been found in any other tissue of the mosquito. Similar to *W. pipientis*, it is gram negative, possesses two membranes, and is surrounded by a third membrane of host origin. It also has ribosome-like particles and strands of DNA in its cytoplasm (FIGURE 3).

It is larger than *W. pipientis*, with an average length of 1.5–2 μm, and it is refractory to Giemsa stain. It also does not appear to cause as heavy an infection of the host cell as *W. pipientis* does, nor are there as many degenerating cells filled with microorganisms. The egg stage has not yet been examined to determine if the organisms are concentrated in any particular region of the egg cytoplasm.

Wolbachia AND CYTOPLASMIC INCOMPATIBILITY

For years, the symbiont of *C. pipiens* has been known to entomologists studying the *C. pipiens* complex.[1, 7, 11, 12] Because it caused no human disease and apparently affected its host very little, it was, however, the object of much speculation but not of intensive investigation. Little was it known that *Wolbachia* plays a profound role in its host's reproductive processes, a role that is still not completely understood today.

Interest was rekindled in *Wolbachia* during our studies of incompatibility in *C. pipiens*. Incompatibility is seen when females of certain strains are mated to males of certain other strains. Mating and insemination of the female appear to be normal, because sperm are found in the female's spermatheca. The females produce eggs that are fertilized by entrance of sperm into the egg, but no karyogamy occurs. About half of the eggs produced from incompatible crosses contain dead haploid embryos, but a diploid parthenogenetic female is occasionally produced by fusion of one of the polar bodies with the oocyte nucleus.[3] From extensive backcrossing experiments, it is known that most of the female genome can be replaced with no loss of incompatibility.[13] Thus, the factor(s) responsible for the incompatibility is not chromosomal; rather, it is a cytoplasmic transovarially transmitted factor(s).

Because it had been reported that the sperm in incompatible eggs are adversely affected,[14] eggs from incompatible and compatible crosses were examined by electron microscopy. Furthermore, because large numbers of *Wolbachia* were present beneath the micropyle, it was immediately suspected that *Wolbachia* was Laven's "cytoplasmic factor."[15]

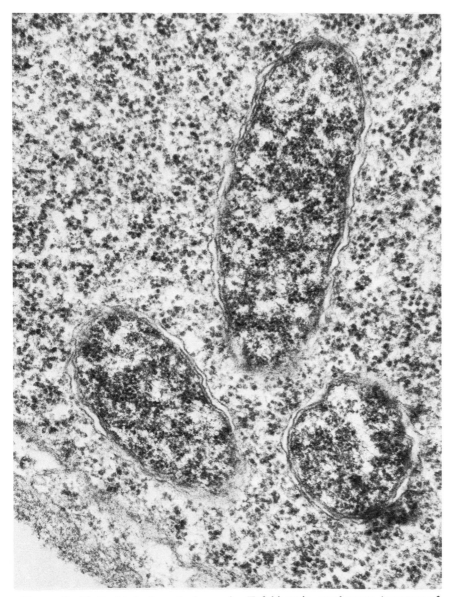

FIGURE 3. *Wolbachia* in the cytoplasm of a Tafahi-strain pupal ovary (courtesy of J. Wright, University of California at Los Angeles). × 48,100.

TABLE 1
CROSSES WITH APOSYMBIOTIC STRAINS

Cross	Egg Rafts	Average Size	Average Larvae	Average Dead	Average Infertile	Proportion Hatched
Compatible Crosses						
Aposymbiotic Strains						
1. 1A×1A	45	56.3	29.5	11.8	15.1	0.524
2. 1A×3A	49	65.6	55.3	3.7	6.6	0.844
3. 3A×1A	71	50.7	30.8	3.6	16.3	0.608
4. 3A×3A	50	64.4	47.6	7.2	9.6	0.738
Aposymbiotic Males						
5. 1×1A	27	47.7	27.5	7.7	12.5	0.577
6. 1×3A	45	45.7	27.6	7.0	11.1	0.605
7. 3×1A	66	54.9	40.6	1.3	13.1	0.738
8. 3×1A	6	43.3	15.5	0.8	25.3	0.357
9. 3×3A	43	44.8	17.6	4.6	22.6	0.393
10. 6×3A	15	70.1	60.8	2.4	6.9	0.867
11. 9×1A	27	54.7	22.3	10.5	21.9	0.408
12. 9×3A	30	64.8	13.6	3.5	47.7	0.210
13. 10×1A	24	40.5	8.2	0.9	31.4	0.202
14. 10×3A	31	55.2	40.9	6.9	7.4	0.741
15. 11×1A	25	49.2	28.8	6.1	14.3	0.585
16. 11×3A	34	42.5	8.4	3.8	30.3	0.198
17. 21×3A	24	46.4	27.8	4.0	14.7	0.597
18. 24×3A	10	74.6	49.6	1.2	23.8	0.665
Incompatible Crosses						
19. 1×9	29	62.3	0.4	9.1	52.8	0.001
20. 1×11	23	57.4	0.0	25.3	32.1	0.000
21. 3×1	45	47.7	0.0	18.8	28.9	0.000
22. 3×9	31	67.6	0.0	38.2	29.4	0.000
23. 3×10	29	52.3	0.0	23.4	28.9	0.000
24. 3×11	37	66.5	0.0	15.4	51.1	0.000
25. 11×1	18	49.8	0.1	29.8	19.9	0.002
Infertile Crosses						
26. 1A×1	31	48.5	0.0	0.8	47.7	0.000
27. 1A×3	40	57.0	0.0	0.0	57.0	0.000
28. 1A×10	20	43.7	0.0	0.0	43.7	0.000
29. 1A×11	37	68.5	0.0	0.3	68.2	0.000
30. 3A×1	88	59.7	0.0	0.8	58.9	0.000
31. 3A×3	43	61.6	0.0	0.0	61.6	0.000
32. 3A×9	23	66.4	0.0	0.1	66.3	0.000
33. 3A×10	25	46.4	0.0	0.1	46.3	0.000
34. 3A×11	16	59.4	0.0	0.1	59.3	0.000
Control Crosses						
35. 1×1	27	42.6	9.4	14.3	18.9	0.221
36. 1×1 *	45	69.5	61.2	2.8	5.5	0.881
37. 1×3	23	48.6	20.9	4.8	22.9	0.524
38. 1×10	35	74.8	68.4	0.9	5.5	0.914
39. 3×3	34	44.2	22.2	7.4	14.6	0.502
40. 3×3 *	49	64.3	53.9	4.0	6.4	0.838
41. 9×1	19	50.1	22.6	7.8	19.7	0.451
42. 9×3	47	56.8	41.6	2.6	12.6	0.732
43. 9×9	14	53.9	15.4	18.5	20.0	0.286
44. 10×1	33	50.1	36.5	2.3	11.3	0.729
45. 10×3	11	54.4	31.7	3.4	19.3	0.583
46. 10×10	35	47.4	31.3	2.8	13.3	0.660
47. 11×3	48	49.2	39.0	3.4	6.8	0.793
48. 11×11	19	48.1	21.3	5.8	21.0	0.443

* Crosses that utilized recently outcrossed males and females.

To prove that the wolbachiae were the causative agents of incompatibility, certain mutually incompatible strains were rendered free of *Wolbachia* by treating them with tetracycline.[6, 16] Three strains, for convenience numbered *1, 3,* and *10,* were treated with tetracycline. Strains *1* and *3* were treated at the same time, and strain *10* was independently treated 2 years later. Once the organisms had been eliminated from the parent generation of mosquito, subsequent generations of mosquitoes remained aposymbiotic. Strains treated 4 years ago are still free of wolbachiae. Strains *1* and *3* are nonreciprocally incompatible, with the *3* female × *1* male cross incompatible and the reverse cross, the *1* female × *3* male, compatible.† The strain-*10* males are incompatible with several different strains. The strains used, their geographic origin, and genetic markers and linkage group, respectively, are as follows: *1,* Dixon, Calif., ruby eye II recessive; *3,* Hamburg, Germany, yellow body II recessive; *6,* Orange Co., Calif., white eye I recessive; *9,* Paris, France, yellow body II recessive; *10,* ?, white eye I recessive; *11,* Scauri, Italy, wild-type; *21,* Dixon, Calif., wild-type; *24,* Boston, Mass., wild-type.

As can be seen from TABLE 1, in every cross in which aposymbiotic males were used, live larvae hatched from the egg rafts. Thus, the incompatible *3* × *1* cross became compatible when aposymbiotic males were mated to normal *3* females. As expected, when aposymbiotic males were mated to aposymbiotic females, the crosses were also compatible, and the progeny were true hybrids. When aposymbiotic females were crossed with males with symbionts, however, no progeny were produced. The eggs that were laid were undeveloped and resembled eggs that are unfertilized. Thus, although the females mated normally and stored sperm in their spermathecae, they produced no viable progeny.

As mentioned before, incompatibility has been observed in only two groups of mosquitoes, the *C. pipiens* complex and the *A. scutellaris* group. In 1954, it was reported that *A. scutellaris scutellaris* and *A. scutellaris katherinensis* were nonreciprocally fertile.[17] Because incompatibility, at that time, was thought to be due to genetic factors, *A. scutellaris* and *A. katherinensis* were not examined for microorganisms, and now, the two subspecies used in the crossing experiments are unavailable for examination. Thus, when crossing experiments with Tafahi and *A. polynesiensis* revealed a high degree of nonreciprocal incompatibility, an excellent opportunity arose to determine if an infectious agent was in some way involved with the incompatibility.

In crosses with *A. polynesiensis* and Tafahi, the P × T (*polynesiensis* female × Tafahi male) cross is incompatible, whereas the reverse cross (T × P) is compatible. Eggs are laid by the incompatible female, but most of the eggs do not hatch to produce live progeny. A small proportion of the eggs, however, do hatch and produce offspring that are true hybrids. The Tafahi females, when mated to *A. polynesiensis* males, produce large numbers of perfectly normal hybrids.

Both *A. polynesiensis* and Tafahi were examined for rickettsia-like microorganisms, and they were found only in Tafahi.[2] As concluded previously, the incompatibility in *C. pipiens* was believed to be due to the symbionts in the male, because males freed of their organisms became compatible, and now, significantly, it is the male in the incompatible P × T cross that has the *Wolbachia.* It is expected that after the Tafahi are treated to render them aposymbiotic, they will become compatible with *A. polynesiensis.*

---

† By convention, in all crosses, the female is given first and the male last, so that *3* × *1* is strain *3* female crossed with strain *1* male.

The precise mechanism by which the wolbachiae affect the sperm in such a way to render them incompatible in some egg cytoplasms has not been elucidated. The incompatible sperm apparently are unable to either penetrate deeply into the egg cytoplasm or to unite with the oocyte nucleus. It is reasonable to assume that strains of C. pipiens have their own strains of microorganisms. The microorganisms may in some way determine the "antigenicity" of the sperm. In a compatible egg, the sperm are accepted and can continue the normal process of penetration and zygote formation. In an incompatible egg, the sperm are somehow rejected. In aposymbiotic males, the sperm are "nonantigenic" and can complete their task in the egg. Electron micrographs of sperm in incompatible eggs were closely examined for some type of egg-sperm reaction. Some sperm in incompatible eggs have a clear area around their head that may be a precipitate (or perhaps only an artifact of fixation).[4]

Studies of the role of Wolbachia in its hosts are badly needed. Why, for example, do aposymbiotic females produce no progeny when mated to males with symbionts? The presence of Staphylococcus sp. in eggs of the beetle, Xyleborus ferrugineus, is thought to be necessary for normal meiosis to occur,[18] and this may be true of Wolbachia in C. pipiens. If this belief is true, however, why do aposymbiotic females produce offspring when mated to aposymbiotic males? As is often the case, one question (what causes incompatibility?) has been answered, but, as a result, many more have been created.

SUMMARY

The wolbachiae found in Culex pipiens and the Tafahi strain of the A. scutellaris group are small rickettsia-like symbionts of the gonads. They are extrachromosomal self-replicating units that are vertically transmitted through the ovaries. Their presence in the only two groups of mosquitoes known to exhibit incompatibility, the fact that they are found in only the Tafahi strain, and the loss of incompatibility after removal of Wolbachia in C. pipiens are compelling evidence for the role that Wolbachia plays in incompatibility.

ACKNOWLEDGMENTS

I thank J. Wright and J. Potaro for allowing their work on Aedes and Culex to be included and Dr. A. R. Barr who provided invaluable guidance and encouragement during this research.

REFERENCES

1. HERTIG, M. & S. B. WOLBACH. 1924. Studies on rickettsia-like microorganisms in insects. J. Med. Res. 44: 329–374.
2. WRIGHT, J. 1975. Personal communication.
3. LAVEN, H. 1967. Speciation and evolution in Culex pipiens. In Genetics of Insect Vectors of Disease. J. W. Wright & R. Pal, Eds. : 251–275. Elsevier. Amsterdam, The Netherlands.
4. YEN, J. H. & A. R. BARR. 1974. Incompatibility in Culex pipiens. In The Use of Genetics in Insect Control. R. Pal & M. J. Whitten, Eds. : 97–118. Elsevier. Amsterdam, The Netherlands.

5. YEN, J. H. & A. R. BARR. 1973. The etiological agent of cytoplasmic incompatibility in *Culex pipiens*. J. Invert. Pathol. **22:** 242–250.

6. POTARO, J. 1975. Curing *Wolbachia* infections. J. Med. Entomol. In press.

7. HERTIG, M. 1936. The rickettsia, *Wolbachia pipientis* (gen. et. sp. n.) and associated inclusions of the mosquito, *Culex pipiens*. Parasitology **28:** 453–486.

8. BYERS, J. R. & A. WILKES. 1970. A rickettsia-like microorganism in *Dahlbominus fuscipennis* (Zett.) (Hymenoptera, Eulophidae). Observations on its occurrence and ultrastructure. Can. J. Zool. **48:** 959–964.

9. IRVING-BELL, R. J. 1974. Cytoplasmic factors in the gonads of *Culex pipiens* complex mosquitoes. Life Sci. **14:** 1149–1151.

10. POTARO, J. 1975. Personal communication.

11. CALLOT, J. 1950. Sur *Wolbachia pipientis* Hertig 1936. Ann. Parasitol. Hum. Comp. **25:** 354.

12. ZULUETA, J. 1965. The rickettsia *Wolbachia pipientis* in *C. pipiens* and *C. fatigans*. WHO/VBC/125.65: 69–70.

13. LAVEN, H. 1957. Vererbung durch Kerngene und das Problem der ausserkaryotischen Vererbung bei *Culex pipiens*. II. Ausserkaryotische Vererbung. Z. Induktive Abstammungs- Vererbungslehre **88:** 478–516.

14. JOST, E. 1970. Untersuchungen zur Kreuzungssterilität im *Culex-pipiens*-Komplex. Arch. Entwicklungsmech. Organ. **166:** 173–188.

15. YEN, J. H. & A. R. BARR. 1971. New hypothesis of the cause of cytoplasmic incompatibility in *Culex pipiens* L. Nature (London) **232:** 657, 658.

16. YEN, J. H. 1972. The microorganismal basis of cytoplasmic incompatibility in the *Culex pipiens* complex. Ph.D. Dissertation. University of California. Los Angeles, Calif.

17. SMITH-WHITE, S. & A. R. WOODHILL. 1954. The nature and significance of nonreciprocal fertility in *Aedes scutellaris* and other mosquitoes. Proc. Linnean Soc. N.S.W. **79:** 163–176.

18. PELEG, B. & D. M. NORRIS. 1972. Bacterial symbiote activation of insect parthenogenetic reproduction. Nature [New Biol.] **236:** 111, 112.

MATERNAL NUTRITIVE SECRETIONS AS POSSIBLE CHANNELS FOR VERTICAL TRANSMISSION OF MICROORGANISMS IN INSECTS: THE TSETSE FLY EXAMPLE *

David L. Denlinger

The Biological Laboratories
Harvard University
Cambridge, Massachusetts 02138

Wei-Chun Ma

International Centre of Insect Physiology and Ecology
Nairobi, Kenya

The nutritive commitment of a female insect to her progeny is usually limited to the deposition of sufficient yolk for completion of embryogenesis. After chorionation and fertilization, the egg is deposited, and the progeny begins an independent existence. In several groups of insects, however, females have undergone structural and physiologic modifications that permit nutrient transfer during later stages of development. In one direction, this evolution has resulted in the production of ova that are devoid of yolk. A maternal secretory structure transfers nutriment to the developing embryos, and at the completion of embryogenesis, the progeny are expelled from the female. This form of viviparity is known in two families of the order Dermaptera and in the cockroach *Diploptera punctata.*[1] In *D. punctata,* the maternal secretion is produced by the brood sac, an integumentary gland that encloses the embryos.[2,3] In another direction, glandular secretions from the mother are used, not as nutriment for embryogenesis, but as the source of larval food. Two fly taxa of major medical and veterinary importance are involved in this form of viviparity: the tsetse flies (Glossinidae) and the Pupipara (Hippoboscidae, Nycteribiidae, and Streblidae). These flies mature only one egg at a time, the egg hatches inside the uterus of the female, and the progeny feeds throughout its larval life on a secretion from a modified female accessory gland called the milk gland. The female gives birth to a fully grown third instar that pupariates within 1–2 hr after parturition. That the newly deposited larva can weigh more than its mother[4] vouches for the massive volume of secretion that passes from the milk gland to the larva.

The transfer of nutritive secretions from the mother to her progeny could serve as a convenient conveyor of microorganisms between mother and progeny. We know nothing about vertical transfer of microorganisms in Dermaptera or in *D. punctata,* but the economic importance of the tsetse fly and sheep ked has provided the impetus needed for investigation. In a major study of symbiosis in Pupipara, Zacharias[5] found the milk gland lumen of the sheep ked *Melophagus ovinus* and several other species to be inhabited by bacteria. The lumen of the tsetse fly milk gland is likewise occupied by bacteria. Although Roubaud[6]

* Publication 23 from the International Centre of Insect Physiology and Ecology, Nairobi, Kenya.

and Wigglesworth [7] suggested that the tsetse milk gland may be involved in transmission of bacteria between mother and progeny, the existence of bacteria in the milk gland lumen has been verified only recently.[8]

Our knowledge of the bacteria in the tsetse fly is still too fragmentary to permit construction of a definitive cycle of transmission. We know that bacteria exist in several distinct localities, but the interaction between these sites is not clear. In the anterior portion of the adult midgut, a distinct region of giant cells (the mycetome) contains intracellular symbionts [6, 9, 10] described by Wigglesworth [7] as Gram-negative bacteroids. In the larva, Roubaud [6] found bacteroids inhabiting a special region of midgut cells adjacent to the proventriculus, and from his account, we can construct the path of the gut bacteroids from the larva to the adult. During metamorphosis, a layer of new adult epithelial cells surrounds the larval gut in a "sac within a sac" arrangement. Clusters of larval cells that contain the symbionts become dissociated from neighboring cells and rupture, releasing the symbionts between the new and old epithelial layers. As the adult gut differentiates, the cells destined to form the giant cell region enlarge and are colonized by the symbionts. As this mycetome continues to differentiate, the intracellular bacteroids multiply rapidly and form a dense mass within these specialized cells. Ultrastructural details of the bacteroids in the mycetome of the adult midgut are known from recent work by Reinhardt et al.,[10] Huebner and Davey,[11] and Pinnock and Hess.[12]

The transition that Roubaud proposes from the larval to the adult mycetome seems quite tenable, but the actual transfer mechanism from mother to offspring is still unclear. Bacteria are found in both the milk gland and the ovaries of the female, but we still have to determine which, if either, of these two groups of bacteria are the progenitors of the bacteria in the larval mycetome.

Roubaud, who actually saw free bacteria within the gut lumen of the in utero larva, was convinced that the milk gland was involved in the transmission. In our ultrastructural examination of the milk gland,[8, 13] we found an abundance of Gram-negative bacteria in the lumen of the gland. The milk gland, similar to other female accessory glands, is an integumentary gland with a cuticular lining. The walls of the milk gland tubules consist of two layers of cells: an epidermal cell with a cuticular intima and a secretory cell.[8] The secretion from each glandular cell is first released into a storage space that is separated from the lumen of the gland by a porous, but dense, cuticular rete. At the rete, the intima is invaginated to form a cup-shaped indentation in the wall of the milk gland tubule. Although the bacteria are dispersed throughout the lumen, one bacterium frequently occupies each invagination. Even though the cuticular rete permits the outflow of milk, it is much too dense to allow the large bacteria to pass freely into the cell's secretion reservoir. We have never observed the bacteria within the secretion reservoir or within the cells of the milk gland. We have examined 64 tsetse females (including *Glossina morsitans morsitans, G. austeni,* and *G. longipalpis pallidipes*), and milk gland bacteria are universally present. Their existence in *G. austeni* has also recently been reported by Bonnanfant-Jaïs.[14] There is, of course, no physical barrier that could prevent the transfer of bacteria from the milk gland lumen to the larva feeding in the uterus.

Vertical transfer of microorganisms in the tsetse fly, however, need not be restricted to transfer through the mother's milk. The more conventional channels of transovarial passage can also operate in these viviparous flies. In *Glossina,* bacteroids have recently been found in the cytoplasm of oocytes and nurse cells and occasionally in follicle cells and the sheath cells of the ovary.[11, 12] These bacteroids, rather than the milk gland bacteria, could prove to be the source of the symbionts in the larval gut.

It is quite possible that the milk gland bacteria are not merely a free form of bacteria in transit from the adult mycetome to the larval mycetome but, instead, are performing a vital function within the lumen of the milk gland. It is easy to imagine that the very specialized diet of the tsetse larva may be supplemented with nutrients supplied by symbiotic bacteria. Regardless of their function, because they constitute a normal component of the adult milk gland, the bacteria must be transmitted from one generation to the next. If they are not part of the adult mycetome → larval mycetome sequence, they may go through a parallel cycle of vertical transfer: adult milk gland → larval gut → primordial milk gland tissue. An ultrastructural study of the ontogeny of the milk gland could be extremely helpful in understanding the bacterial invasion of the milk gland. Several invasion routes are possible: directly into the differentiating milk gland, penetration through the ovary or other reproductive structures and migration through the ducts that are continuous with the milk gland, or infection of the milk gland by bacteria from the first larva that enters the uterus. The last possibility seems unlikely but could easily be tested by examining females prior to their first pregnancy.

The Pupipara, although not thought to be closely related to tsetse flies,[15] closely parallel the tsetse in adult feeding habits and reproductive strategy. The adults feed on the blood of vertebrates, and the larvae are nurtured from the female's milk gland. The Pupipara milk gland secretion has been considered as the medium of transfer between bacteria in the adult mycetome and the larval mycetome.[5, 16, 17] In many species of Pupipara, bacteria have been seen in the lumen of the milk gland. With the light microscope, the progression of the bacteria has been traced from the milk gland → larval mycetome → adult mycetome. Bacteria found in the hemocoel are presumed to close the link between the adult midgut and the young milk gland. Channels of transovarial passage are also possible in these flies, and Aschner [16] reports that *Rickettsia* are being vertically transferred through the ovary in *Lynchia maura*.

Maternal nutritive secretions pose an interesting dimension to mechanisms of vertical transfer of microorganisms. Although very few insect species have access to this curious channel of transfer, the economic impact of the species involved will hopefully stimulate researchers to determine the function of the microorganisms and the cycle of transmission. The problem captured the interest of outstanding biologists, such as Roubaud and Wigglesworth, at the beginning of the century, but the problem has largely been ignored in the intervening years. Hopefully, the appearance of several papers on tsetse bacteria in 1974 marks the renewal of such research effort.

[NOTE ADDED IN PROOF: After submission of this manuscript, P. E. Pell and D. I. Southern published a paper (1975. Experientia **13**: 650, 651) entitled Symbionts in the female tsetse fly *Glossina morsitans morsitans*. This contribution adds to our knowledge of vertical transfer in the tsetse fly by describing symbionts in the embryo that appear to be identical to the forms observed in the ovaries. These authors doubt that the microorganisms found in the embryo and ovary are related to the vertical transmission of the large intracellular bacteria of the adult mycetome.]

REFERENCES

1. HAGAN, H. R. 1951. Embryology of the Viviparous Insects. The Ronald Press Company. New York, N.Y.
2. ROTH, L. M. & E. R. WILLIS. 1958. An analysis of oviparity and viviparity in Blattaria. Trans. Amer. Entomol. Soc. **83:** 221–238.
3. STAY, B. & A. C. COOP. 1974. 'Milk' secretion for embryogenesis in a viviparous cockroach. Tissue Cell **6:** 669–693.
4. DENLINGER, D. L. & W.-C. MA. 1974. Dynamics of the pregnancy cycle in the tsetse *Glossina morsitans*. J. Insect Physiol. **20:** 1015–1026.
5. ZACHARIAS, A. 1928. Untersuchungen über die intracellulare Symbiose bei den Pupiparen. Z. Morphol. Ökol. Tiere **10:** 676–737.
6. ROUBAUD, E. 1919. Les particularites de la nutrition et la vie symbiontique chez les mouches tsetses. Ann. Inst. Pasteur **33:** 489–537.
7. WIGGLESWORTH, V. B. 1929. Digestion in the tsetse-fly: a study of structure and function. Parasitology **21:** 288–321.
8. MA, W.-C. & D. L. DENLINGER. 1974. Secretory discharge and microflora of milk gland in tsetse flies. Nature (London) **247:** 301–303.
9. STUHLMANN, F. 1907. Beiträge zur Kenntnis der Tsetsefliege. Arb. Gesundhamt. **26:** 301–383.
10. REINHARDT, C., R. STEIGER & H. HECKER. 1972. Ultrastructural study of the midgut mycetome bacteroids of the tsetse flies *Glossina morsitans*, *G. fuscipes*, and *G. brevipalpis* (Diptera, Brachycera). Acta Trop. **29:** 280–288.
11. HUEBNER, E. & K. G. DAVEY. 1974. Bacteroids in the ovaries of a tsetse fly. Nature (London) **249:** 260, 261.
12. PINNOCK, D. E. & R. T. HESS. 1974. The occurrence of intracellular rickettsialike organisms in the tsetse flies, *Glossina morsitans*, *G. fuscipes*, *G. brevipalpis* and *G. pallidipes*. Acta Trop. **31:** 70–79.
13. MA, W.-C., D. L. DENLINGER, U. JÄRLFORS & D. S. SMITH. 1975. Structural modulations in the tsetse fly milk gland during a pregnancy cycle. Tissue Cell **7:** 319–330.
14. BONNANFANT-JAÏS, M.-L. 1974. Morphologie de la glande lactee d'une Glossine, *Glossina austeni* Newst, au cours du cycle de gestation. I. Aspects ultrastructuraux en periode de gestation. J. Microsc. **19:** 265–284.
15. POLLOCK, J. N. 1971. Origin of the tsetse flies: a new theory. J. Entomol. (B) **40:** 101–109.
16. ASCHNER, M. 1931. Die Bakterienflora der Pupiparen (Diptera). Eine Symbiosestudie an blutsaugenden Insekten. Z. Morphol. Ökol. Tiere **20:** 368–442.
17. BUCHNER, P. 1965. Endosymbiosis of Animals with Plant Microorganisms. John Wiley & Sons, Inc. New York, N.Y.

SYMBIOSIS AND ATTENUATION *

Marion A. Brooks

Department of Entomology, Fisheries, and Wildlife
University of Minnesota
St. Paul, Minnesota 55108

INTRODUCTION

In microbiology, the term attenuation refers to reducing virulence; in other fields, attenuation expresses the concept of weakening or diluting. I shall use the word in both senses, that is, attenuating the virulence of a pathogen or weakening the beneficial effects of a mutualist. Arthropods are associated with a vast array of microorganisms, encompassing viruses, bacteria and rickettsiae, mycoplasmas, protozoa, fungi, and nematodes. The relationships of the microorganisms to the hosts cover a wide spectrum of symbiosis, from pathologic, through commensalism to mutualism, and, finally, to a vector relationship in which the arthropod host is (usually) unharmed. Destruction of the gut epithelium of the human louse by *Rickettsia prowazeki* is one of the notable exceptions to this rule. More than 80% of the infectious diseases of the world are transmitted by arthropod vectors.[1] We may ask why the vectors are not harmed by microorganisms that infect the definitive host, causing pathologic conditions and often death. To reply that this is a matter of host specificity is not satisfactory. By some reaction, the virulence of the parasites is attenuated while they reside in the arthropod host. In the following discussion, the term symbiosis will include only those relationships that, in nature, are constant, with every individual of the host species being infected or inhabited by members of the reciprocal species.

OBSERVATIONS

The orders of insects and ticks that are inhabited by mutualistic symbiotes are relatively nonsusceptible to pathogenic microorganisms of any kind; cockroaches and flies are prime examples. On the other hand, the orders that have no symbiotes are highly susceptible to pathogens, particularly viruses and microsporida. The Lepidoptera exemplify this condition. The possible relationship between the presence of symbiotes and the evolution of a nonspecific immune reaction is a speculative topic.

Insects are not considered to be immunocompetent.[2, 3] There is very little evidence for their ability to produce antibodies similar to those of vertebrates, and when they are induced to produce antibacterial substances, the latter are nonspecific. A lysozyme-like principle is the active agent in many insects.[4-8] Mohrig and Messner[6] reported that the injection of gram-positive bacteria and nonspecific substances into the hemocoel of insects raises the lysozyme value in

* Supported in part by Research Grant AI 09914 from the National Institute of Allergy and Infectious Diseases, National Institutes of Health. This is Paper 9067, Scientific Journal Series, Minnesota Agricultural Experiment Station.

the blood; lysozyme reaches a maximum in 24 hr and their declines. Mohrig and Messner feel that this increase explains all the phenomena of natural and acquired immunity so far observed in insects. Bakula[9] isolated an acid-soluble substance from the lysosomal fraction of *Drosophila* larvae cells that was trypsin sensitive, but it was not lysozyme. The antibacterial agent from *Samia cynthia*, characterized by Boman *et al.*,[10] was trypsin sensitive and protected by reducing agents, but it also was considered not to be a lysozyme.

Insects have a very effective means of protecting themselves from parasites and almost any kind of foreign body (except intraspecific tissue transplants) by encapsulation and melanization.[3, 11] It is generally believed that hemocytes first surround the foreign body and that phenolic substances released from certain cells then melanize the capsule. Götz and Vey,[11] however, found that melanin is formed in both cellular and humoral encapsulation as a primary activity of phenoloxidases and causes formation of the capsule substance.

Such spectacular processes do not occur in the case of parasitic protozoa in insects and ticks, which are intermediate hosts. From the literature of helminthology, we learn of the concept of "eclipsed antigens," which refers to antigenic determinants of parasite origin that resemble antigenic determinants of the host.[12] The sharing of antigenic determinants is called "molecular mimicry." This term implies that "the host will not recognize an eclipsed antigen as being foreign and thus will not produce antibodies against it." This idea has been useful in explaining the tolerance of hosts to parasites, such as helminths, although there is evidence that bacteria may also contain heterogenetic antigens.[12] Eclipsed antigens presumably arose through selection and mutation operating on antigens that were similar in the two partners.

The concept of sharing between vectors and parasites may be inferred from the work of Fromentin *et al.*[13] They immunized mice against *Trypanosoma cruzi* by injecting homogenized intestines of the flagellate's host, *Triatoma infestans*. In this case, the insect intestine contained an antigen in common with the flagellate. A nonspecific protection against *Pasteurella pestis* evidently was conferred upon a rabbit.[14] The rabbit had been fed upon first by uninfected ticks, and later, after it had been fed upon again by hundreds of infected ticks, it survived, contrary to expectation. This result may be explained as an example of an antigen common to both the tick and the plague organism. The coevolution and selection of similar antigens is offered as an explanation of the ability of a host to tolerate parasites through lack of recognition of foreignness. From the viewpoint of attenuation, this explanation is equivalent to a weakening of the parasite's effect on the host.

In insects living symbiotically with microorganisms, there is considerable evidence that some host factor operates to control both the location and the rate of multiplication of the symbiotes. Noda[15] has calculated changes in the population of yeastlike symbiotes in the smaller brown planthopper, *Laodelphax striatellus*. The number of organisms is strictly regulated throughout the entire life cycle of the insect; that is, there is no rampant increase, as might be encountered with a pathogen. This is one of the characteristics of symbiosis, and the mechanism for its regulation has been sought in numerous cases. Bacterial symbiotes transmitted ovarially by cockroaches undergo a burst of doubling only during terminal stages of vitellogenesis.[16] Growth and differentiation of membranes in these bacteria were indicated by aggregation of protein particles.[17] The changes were regulated by juvenile hormone from the corpora allata of host insects.

Symbiotes that are confined to particular cells or organs (mycetocytes or mycetomes) perish if they are exposed to hemolymph or are injected into other tissue types. A factor in this control is said to be a lysozyme-like substance, found in fat body cells and in hemolymph.[18-20] This agent supposedly lyses all symbiotes not protected by the specialized mycetocytes. If this is so, it represents a striking example of the regulation of the symbiote population. After the injection of lysozyme in a sodium chloride solution, into the hemocoel of cockroaches, the symbiotes in mycetocytes and around oocytes are lysed.[4, 19-25] However, perhaps the regulation is not simply a direct effect of lysozyme on the symbiote cell wall. Wharton and Lola[26, 27] demonstrated that the injection of lysozyme into cockroaches is followed by increased levels of sodium, calcium, and magnesium ions in the blood. Daniel and Brooks[21] suggested that the elevated lysozyme level has far-reaching effects on the host membranes, permitting physiologic alterations in blood chemistry to result in lysis of the bacterial symbiotes.

Landureau and Jollès[28] noticed that a cell line from a cockroach has a high resistance to infection in vitro. They tested the spent tissue culture medium in which the cockroach cells had grown and found significant activity against polymers of N-acetylglucosamine and N-acetylmuramic acid, constituents of bacterial cell walls. The enzyme produced by the cells was active against the standard assay organism, Micrococcus lysodeikticus, but it was 20 times as active as hen egg-white lysozyme against low-molecular-weight polymers of N-acetylglucosamine. With purification of the enzymes from cultured cells and from hemolymph, Bernier et al.[29] separated two chitinases from insect serum. These serum chitinases had no lytic activity against M. lysodeikticus; if hemocytes were lysed, however, they released lytic activity that corresponded to about 25 μg lysozyme/ml of hemolymph, which was comparable to the activity of hen egg-white lysozyme. The metabolized culture medium of the cockroach cell line also contained similar chitinases.

The chitinase activity of hemolymph was systematically determined in the different stages of development of the insects.[29] No chitinase activity was recovered from Periplaneta americana females carrying oothecae. This depression of chitinase activity should be experimentally compared with our measurements of symbiote growth in Blattella germanica that occur in the extracellular spaces around the terminal oocytes. It is very significant that there seems to be no chitinase activity in the hemolymph at this time.

Deutsch and Landureau[30] have studied the fine structure of cultured cockroach cells that produce chitinase. Electron micrographs reveal crystalline granules in the cells that increase with time between changes of medium and that could be correlated with an increase in enzymatic activity in the medium. The crystalline structures were interpreted as aggregates of chitinase molecules or as an inactive form of the enzyme held in reserve in the cells. Two days after replenishment of the culture medium, the enzymatic activity reached an almost optimum level, and there were no crystalline inclusions in the cells.

Some of the difficulties in propagating symbiotes and parasites in insect cell cultures may be caused by the release of lytic enzymes from injured cells, which would inhibit the growth of the microorganisms.[31]

Crystalline inclusion bodies with unknown function have been reported for parasitic protozoa and symbiotic bacteria during certain stages in their life cycles. The stages of parasites known to contain such paracrystalline bodies are those found in the invertebrate host, whereas symbiotes that contain paracrystalline bodies are transitional stages. Molyneux[32] described cytoplasmic inclusions in the promastigote form of an isolate of *Leishmania hertigi* cultured in the laboratory. The particles were passed to the daughter cells during binary longitudinal fission. Because these inclusions had not been observed in previous studies, the inclusions were interpreted as being virus-like particles, and it was unknown if they were acquired from the sandfly vector. The motile stages, that is, the ookinetes of *Parahaemoproteus, Leucocytozoon,* and *Plasmodium,* possess crystalline bodies as a regular feature.[33-35] These bodies have been interpreted as lipoprotein reserve food material for sustenance during the time the parasite passes through the midgut cells of the mosquito vector.[34] Körner and Feldhege[36] have described paracrystalline inclusions in the intracellular symbiotic bacteria of the small cicadellid, *Euscelis plebejus.* The inclusions are digestible with pronase or chymotrypsin. Other periodic formations have been described in symbiotes of the scale insect, *Icerya purchasi,*[37] of a leafhopper, *Helochara communis,*[38] and of several other homopterous species.[39] All of the foregoing symbiotes are transmitted vertically. Although no function has been ascertained for the crystalline bodies, conceivably they are utilized during the penetration of insect cells or contain factors that protect the symbiotes against adverse actions of the insect cells.

Ball[40] has cataloged many kinds of microorganisms that live on and in protozoa, in addition to some "structures of uncertain nature." An unusual structure, the diplosome, which is an elongate intracytoplasmic body with a characteristic bipolar appearance, is found in the trypanosomatid flagellate, *Blastocrithidia culicis.* Brueske[41] found that the diplosome was antibiotic sensitive, and he was able to produce adiplosomic strains by employing chloramphenicol in the culture medium. The adiplosomic strains were unable to infect the normal mosquito host. Thus, the loss of an apparent endosymbiote from a protozoan was followed by attenuation of infectivity of the protozoan host. Chang and Trager[42] demonstrated that in the absence of the symbiote, this flagellate has a requirement for hemin, which makes it comparable in its nutrition to certain other flagellates that do not have symbiotes. Loss of infectivity by the adiplosomic strain must reflect the fact that the mosquito host cannot provide hemin.

The transmission of symbiotes from generation to generation, and from cell to cell within a single individual insect, is always strictly regulated, and symbiologists frequently discuss this fact. Vertically transmitted symbiotes are usually intracellular for most of the life cycle; the symbiotes of cockroaches in the extra egg space is one clearly demonstrable case of a brief sojourn extracellularly. In this connection, it has been pointed out above that the cyclic decline in hemolymph chitinase and lysozyme[29] may be correlated with this period in the life cycle of the symbiotes. Hinde[43] has observed that symbiotes of aphids are occasionally seen in the hemocoel, probably released by chance from mycetocytes. The released symbiotes are phagocytosed by hemocytes and are destroyed. Hinde proposed that while within the mycetocytes, the symbiotes are protected from the normal immune and bactericidal responses of the insect. Whereas hemocytes react to symbiotes as if they were foreign material, the mycetocytes are adapted to take up organisms that are recognized as foreign by the rest of the insect, and protect them.

To recapitulate, there is abundant evidence that insects possess lysozymes, lysozyme-like substances, or chitinases in tissue cells, hemocytes, and serum. Nonspecific antibacterial substances can be induced by the injection of lysozyme, bacteria, salt solutions,[2, 10] and other nonspecific agents. The induced substances confer short-term immunity against a variety of bacteria. Symbiotic microorganisms are protected from destruction by the normal lytic agents by remaining inside special cells that have lost the ability to recognize the symbiotes as "nonself." There is evidence that during transmission extracellularly, the symbiotes are protected by an endocrine repression of hemolymph lytic agents. The importance of metallic ions in these processes should be examined.

Hutner[44] has reviewed the requirements of microorganisms for trace elements. The symbiotes of cockroaches fail to be transmitted through the ovaries if an unfavorable ratio of calcium to manganese is fed to the developing insect.[45] Weinberg[46] has emphasized the necessity for certain divalent metallic ions in the attachment of parasites to host cell membranes. He has also pointed out that the susceptibility or resistance of a cell to a parasite may be governed by ligands that sequester metallic ions and keep them from the parasite. Perhaps, the peaceful coexistence of parasites within insect and tick hosts and vectors is accomplished in part by the salt composition of the hemolymph, which is much different from that encountered in the vertebrate host.

Sterile salt solution injected into insects provokes a nonspecific antibacterial reaction[10] and also raises the lysozyme level.[6, 26] This finding indicates that the ions are affecting permeability of the membranes of hemocytes and other cells, which permits leaking of the cellular lytic agents. In the presence of high concentrations of lysozyme, one would expect that the membranes of mycetocytes would be altered and ionic regulation disturbed. The mycetocytes could no longer sequester the symbiotes nor protect them from the lytic effects of the serum. If this should prove to be the mechanism for lysis of symbiotes, it would constitute recognition by the host of symbiotes as "nonself."

Summary

Parasitic protozoa and bacteria transmitted by vector insects and ticks resist destruction in the intermediate host, possibly through the possession of antigens similar to those of the host. There is no evidence that symbiotic microorganisms have evolved similar eclipsed antigens. Symbiotes are protected from destruction by the natural lytic agents in the host, because they remain for the most part inside special cells that have lost the ability to recognize the symbiotes as "nonself." Metallic ions may play an important role in attenuation through their effect on cell membranes and on the release of lytic agents. The symbiotes of insects are useful and interesting subjects for studying attenuation.

References

1. Soulsby, E. J. L. & W. R. Harvey. 1972. Disease transmission by arthropods. Science 176: 1153–1155.
2. Götz, P. 1973. Immunreaktionen bei Insekten. Naturw. Rundschau 26: 367–375.
3. Nappi, A. J. 1974. Insect hemocytes and the problem of host recognition of foreignness. In Contemporary Topics in Immunobiology. E. L. Cooper, Ed. Vol. 4: 207–224. Plenum Publishing Corporation. New York, N.Y.
4. Malke, H. 1965. Über das Vorkommen von Lysozym in Insekten. Z. Allgem. Mikrobiol. 5: 42–47.

5. MOHRIG, W. & B. MESSNER. 1968a. Lysozym als antibakterielles Agens im Bienenhonig und Bienengift. Acta Biol. Med. Germ. **21:** 85–95.
6. MOHRIG, W. & B. MESSNER. 1968b. Immunreaktionen bei Insekten. I. Lysozym als grundlegender antibakterieller Faktor im humoralen Abwehrmechanismus der Insekten. Biol. Zentr. **87:** 439–470.
7. POWNING, R. F. & W. J. DAVIDSON. 1973. Studies on insect bacteriolytic enzymes. I. Lysozyme in haemolymph of *Galleria mellonella* and *Bombyx mori.* Comp. Biochem. Physiol. **45B:** 669–686.
8. POWNING, R. F. & H. IRZYKIEWICZ. 1967. Lysozyme-like action of enzymes from the cockroach *Periplaneta americana* and from some other sources. J. Insect Physiol. **13:** 1293–1299.
9. BAKULA, M. 1971. The isolation of intracellular antibacterial activity from *Drosophila melanogaster* larvae. J. Insect Physiol. **17:** 313–319.
10. BOMAN, H. G., I. NILSSON-FAYE, K. PAUL & T. RASMUSON, JR. 1974. Insect immunity. I. Characteristics of an inducible cell-free antibacterial reaction in hemolymph of *Samia cynthia* pupae. Infect. Immunity **10:** 136–145.
11. GÖTZ, P. & A. VEY. 1974. Humoral encapsulation in Diptera (Insecta): defence reactions of *Chironomus* larvae against fungi. Parasitology **68:** 193–205.
12. DAMIAN, R. T. 1964. Molecular mimicry: antigen sharing by parasite and host and its consequences. Amer. Naturalist **98:** 129–149.
13. FROMENTIN, H., A. DODIN & P. DESTOMBES. 1967. Essai d'immunisation de la souris (hôte vertébré) contre *Trypanosoma cruzi,* par une suspension de tissu de triatome (hôte invertébré). Acta Trop. **24:** 261 265.
14. BELL, J. F. 1942. Some factors concerned in the infection of ticks with *Pasteurella pestis.* Ph.D. Thesis. University of Minnesota. Minneapolis, Minn.
15. NODA, H. 1974. Preliminary histological observation and population dynamics of intracellular yeast-like symbiotes in the smaller brown planthopper, *Laodelphax striatellus* (Homptera: Delphacidae). Appl. Entomol. Zool. **9:** 275–277.
16. KURTTI, T. J. & M. A. BROOKS. Unpublished results.
17. LIU, T. P. 1974. The effect of corpora allata on the plasma membrane of the symbiotic bacteria of the oocyte surface of *Periplaneta americana* L. Gen. Comp. Endocrinol. **23:** 118–123.
18. EHRHARDT, P. 1966. Wirkung von Lysozym-injektionen auf Aphiden und deren Symbionten. Z. Vergleich. Physiol. **53:** 130–141.
19. MALKE, H. & W. SCHWARTZ. 1966a. Untersuchungen über die Symbiose von Tieren mit Pilzen und Bakterien. XI. Die Rolle des Wirtslysozyms in der Blattidensymbiose. Arch. Mikrobiol. **53:** 17–32.
20. MALKE, H. & W. SCHWARTZ. 1966b. Untersuchungen über die Symbiose von Tieren mit Pilzen und Bakterien. XII. Die Bedeutung der Blattiden-Symbiose. Z. Allgem. Mikrobiol. **6:** 34–68.
21. DANIEL, R. S. & M. A. BROOKS. 1972. Intracellular bacteroids: electron miroscopy of *Periplaneta americana* injected with lysozyme. Exp. Parasitol. **31:** 232–246.
22. MALKE, H. 1964a. Wirkung von Lysozym auf die Symbionten der Blattiden. Z. Allgem. Mikrobiol. **4:** 88–91.
23. MALKE, H. 1964b. Production of aposymbiotic cockroaches by means of lysozyme. Nature (London) **204:** 1223, 1224.
24. MALKE, H. & G. BARTSCH. 1966. Elektronenoptische Untersuchung zur intracellulären Bakteriensymbiose von *Nauphoeta cinerea* (Olivier) (Blattariae). Z. Allgem. Mikrobiol. **6:** 163–176.
25. WHARTON, D. R. A. & J. E. LOLA. 1969a. Lysozyme action on the cockroach, *Periplaneta americana,* and its intracellular symbionts. J. Insect Physiol. **15:** 1647–1658.
26. WHARTON, D. R. A. & J. E. LOLA. 1969b. Lysozyme action in the cockroach—blood changes. J. Insect Physiol. **15:** 1877–1886.
27. WHARTON, D. R. A. & J. E. LOLA. 1970. Blood conditions and lysozyme action in the aposymbiotic cockroach. J. Insect Physiol. **16:** 199–209.

28. LANDUREAU, J. C. & P. JOLLÈS. 1970. Lytic enzyme produced *in vitro* by insect cells: lysozyme or chitinase? Nature (London) **225:** 968, 969.
29. BERNIER, I., J. C. LANDUREAU, P. GRELLET & P. JOLLÈS. 1974. Characterization of chitinases from haemolymph and cell cultures of cockroach (*Periplaneta americana*). Comp. Biochem. Physiol. **47B:** 41–44.
30. DEUTSCH, V. & J. C. LANDUREAU. 1970. Caractéristiques ultrastructurales de cellules d'insectes produisant une chitinase en culture *in vitro*. Compt. Rend. **270**(Ser. D): 1491–1494.
31. BROOKS, M. A. Applications of insect tissue culture to an elucidation of parasite transmission. *In* Invertebrate Tissue Culture: Research Applications. K. Maramorosch, Ed. Academic Press, Inc. New York, N.Y. In press.
32. MOLYNEUX, D. H. 1974. Virus-like particles in *Leishmania* parasites. Nature (London) **249:** 588, 589.
33. DESSER, S. S. 1972. The fine structure of the ookinete of *Parahaemoproteus velans* (=*Haemoproteus velans* Coatney and Roudabush) (Haemosporidia: Haemoproteidae). Can. J. Zool. **50:** 477–480.
34. DESSER, S. S. & W. D. TREFIAK. 1971. Crystalline inclusions in *Leucocytozoon simondi*. Can. J. Zool. **49:** 134, 135.
35. GARNHAM, P. C. C., R. G. BIRD & J. R. BAKER. 1962. Electron microscope studies of motile stages of malaria parasites. III. The ookinetes of *Haemamoeba* and *Plasmodium*. Trans. Roy. Soc. Trop. Med. Hyg. **56:** 116–120.
36. KÖRNER, H. K. & A. FELDHEGE. 1970. Einschlusskörper in symbiontischen Bakterien einer Kleinzikade (*Euscelis plebejus* Fall.). Cytobiologie **1:** 203–207.
37. LOUIS, C. 1969. Histochimie et ultrastructure des mycétomes et symbiotes d'*Icerya purchasi* Mask. (Homoptera-Coccoidea-Monophlebinae). (Note.) Compt. Rend. **268**(Ser. D): 445–448.
38. CHANG, K. P. & A. J. MUSGRAVE. 1972. Multiple symbiosis in a leafhopper, *Helochara communis* Fitch (Cicadellidae: Homoptera): envelopes, nucleoids and inclusions of the symbiotes. J. Cell Sci. **11:** 275–293.
39. HAMON, C. 1971. Etude au microscope électronique des symbiontes à transmission héréditaire chez quelques insectes Homoptères auchénorhynques femelles. Z. Zellforsch. **119:** 244–256.
40. BALL, G. H. 1968. Organisms living on and in protozoa. *In* Research in Protozoologie. T. T. Chen, Ed. Vol. **3:** 565–718. Pergamon Press, Inc. New York, N.Y.
41. BRUESKE, W. A. 1967. The diplosome of *Blastocrithidia culicis* (Novy, MacNeal, and Torrey, 1907) (Mastigophora: Trypanosomatidae). Ph.D. Thesis. University of Minnesota. Minneapolis, Minn.
42. CHANG, K. P. & W. TRAGER. 1974. Nutritional significance of symbiotic bacteria in two species of hemoflagellates. Science **183:** 531, 532.
43. HINDE, R. 1971. The control of the mycetome symbiotes of the aphids *Brevicoryne brassicae, Myzus persicae,* and *Macrosiphum rosae*. J. Insect Physiol. **17:** 1791–1800.
44. HUTNER, S. H. 1972. Inorganic nutrition. Annu. Rev. Microbiol. **26:** 313–346.
45. BROOKS, M. A. 1960. Some dietary factors that affect ovarial transmission of symbiotes. Proc. Helminthol. Soc. Wash., D.C. **27:** 212–220.
46. WEINBERG, E. D. 1966. Roles of metallic ions in host-parasite interactions. Bacteriol. Rev. **30:** 136–151.

VECTORS AND VERTICAL TRANSMISSION:
AN EPIDEMIOLOGIC PERSPECTIVE

Paul E. M. Fine

Department of Medical Protozoology
London School of Hygiene and Tropical Medicine
London WC1E 7HT, England

The inheritance of infection is a widespread phenomenon; it occurs at every level of biologic organization. The congenital (e.g., transplacental) and trans-mammary infections of man and other mammals, the egg-borne infections of poultry, the seed-borne infections of plants, and the transovarial and transovum infections of invertebrates are all well-known examples of inherited infections. Furthermore, the cytoplasmic inheritance of various microorganisms, which occurs within populations of single cells, would seem to be a logical extension of this general concept.[27, 48]

Students of vector-borne diseases of animals and plants have long been familiar with examples of the inheritance of microorganisms in invertebrate vector populations. The classic papers cited in TABLE 1 indicate the extent of the literature on this subject and the variety of biologic contexts in which this type of transmission is known to play a role. Several pathogens of great social and economic importance are involved, a factor that gives the problem not only theoretic but also practical significance.

The inheritance of vertebrate and plant pathogens, in their invertebrate vectors, presents a highly complex problem in infectious disease epidemiology. Infectious agents that are transmitted solely by one-host vectors (e.g., *Rickettsia tsutsugamushi* in *Leptotrombidium akamushi* or *Babesia bigemina* in *Boophilus annulatus*) clearly depend for their survival upon some hereditary transfer in the vector. It can be shown that this is a logical necessity. Otherwise, however, the epidemiologic role of such transmission in the maintenance of disease in natural communities is less certain. It is a quantitative problem, the solution of which depends upon consideration of the relative and absolute amounts of the different kinds of transmission occurring in nature.

There is now a growing literature on the rates of egg transmission of various infections in invertebrate vector species, but as yet, there has been no attempt to fully assess the contribution of this transmission modality to the maintenance of disease agents in nature. The elegant quantitative models developed for the description of such vector-borne infections as malaria [10, 33] and schistosomia-sis [20, 39] have not had to include hereditary transmission, because it plays no part in their epidemiology. On the other hand, there have been several attempts to construct mathematic models of vector-borne disease systems in which some transovarial transmission is known to occur in the invertebrate host, but these models have failed to examine the interrelationship between the *rates* of such hereditary transfer and other parameters of the systems.[35, 49, 56] An understanding of this interrelationship is essential if we are to assess the epidemiologic significance of this transmission modality.

This paper outlines a general approach to the epidemiology of hereditary

TABLE 1

MAJOR GROUPS OF VERTEBRATE AND PLANT PATHOGENS KNOWN TO UNDERGO HEREDITARY TRANSMISSION THROUGH THEIR INVERTEBRATE VECTORS *

	Pathogen	Invertebrate Vector	Reference
Infections of vertebrates	Protozoon *Babesia bigemina*	arthropod (tick) *Boophilus annulatus*	Smith & Kilborne [60]
	Spirochaete *Borrelia duttoni*	arthropod (tick) *Ornithodorus moubata*	Dutton & Todd [11] & Koch [25]
	Rickettsia *Rickettsia rickettsii*	arthropod (tick) *Dermacentor andersoni*	Ricketts [54]
	Virus Nairobi sheep disease virus	arthropod (tick) *Rhipicephalus appendi- culatus*	Montgomery [38]
	Protozoon *Histomonas melea- gridis*	helminth (nematode) *Heterakis gallinarum*	Graybill & Smith [17]
	Virus Swine influenza virus	helminth (nematode) *Metastrongylus* spp.	Shope [57]
	Rickettsia *Neorickettsia helmin- thoeca*	helminth (trematode) *Nanophyetus salmincola*	Cordy & Gorham [9]
Infections of plants	Virus Rice dwarf virus	arthropod (hemiptera) *Nephotettix cincticeps*	Fukushi [14]

* Cited herein is the first published confirmation of this transmission phenomenon, for each of the given pathogen-vector combinations.

infections, with particular reference to vertebrate and plant pathogens that are inherited in their invertebrate vector species.

THE CONCEPT OF "VERTICAL" TRANSMISSION

Most of the terms used in discussions of the hereditary transmission of infection are descriptive of specific biologic mechanisms responsible for the transfer, for example: transplacental, transmammary, transovarial, transovum, and seed-borne transmission. The common denominator for all these types of transmission is clear when we consider them in an epidemiologic context. This fact was recognized during the 1940s, by Gross and others, and led to the formulation of the concept of "vertical" transmission to cover all these contingencies.[3, 18] Following these authors, vertical transmission can be defined as *the direct transfer of infection from a parent organism to his, her, or its progeny.* The logical complement to vertical transmission is then "horizontal" transmission, which may be defined as *any transfer of infection between host species individuals, except that which occurs directly from parent to progeny.* (Andrewes [3] added a further term to this lexicon, "zig-zag" transmission, which is defined as the indirect vector-mediated transmission between animal or plant organisms. For purposes of the present discussion, however, such vector-mediated transfer may be interpreted as a form of indirect horizontal transmission between hosts.)

The distinction between these terms is clarified in FIGURE 1, which illustrates the two fundamental types of transmission as manifested in asexually (*left*) or sexually (*right*) reproducing populations. It should be noted that horizontal transfer of infection can occur either within or between generations of the host species, but not directly from parent to progeny. The pedigree diagram in FIGURE 1 (*right*) may be considered to represent a family history of some invertebrate vector species. The solid line, then, represents the vertical transmission of some infectious agent from parent to progeny, and the broken lines represent the indirect horizontal (or "zig-zag") transfer of the agent that occurs through the plant or vertebrate hosts of the vector species.

CLASSIFICATION OF VERTICAL TRANSMISSION SYSTEMS

Although several workers have recognized analogies between different forms of vertical transmission phenomena, there has been no attempt to categorize the epidemiologic and ecologic similarities between the many examples. What is required is a conceptual framework that is at once epidemiologic in orientation, manageable in size, and yet inclusive of all hereditary transmission phenomena. Such a framework is embodied in the classification described below and illustrated in TABLE 2.

A few words of explanation about the diagrams used in TABLE 2 should help the reader in understanding this classification. The basic structure of the diagrams is illustrated in FIGURE 2. The square boxes represent *populations* of successive *generations* of some host species (called B), set along a time axis that runs from left to right. Each of these boxes is drawn schematically as an age-prevalence graph, depicting infection rates with some agent (called A) in the host species (B). Vertical transmission, which serves to transfer the agent (A) from the parents in one host generation to their progeny in the next generation, is represented by the solid arrows drawn between successive boxes. Horizontal transmission of the infectious agent (A) is represented by broken

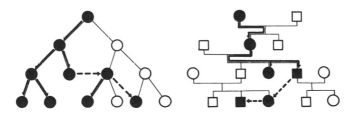

FIGURE 1. Patterns of vertical (——→) and horizontal (- - -→) transmission as manifested in asexually (*left*) and sexually (*right*) reproducing populations. The populations are represented as pedigree diagrams that cover four successive generations of the host species. Conventional symbols are used on the right-hand side: circles for females and squares for males. Shaded symbols represent infected individuals.

TABLE 2

CLASSIFICATION OF VERTICAL TRANSMISSION SYSTEMS *

Type	Diagram	Definition	Examples	Rates	References
Ia		no horizontal transfer	bipolar body (A) in *Crithidia oncopelti* (B)		19
			Theileria spp. (A) in cultured lymphocytes (B)		22, 36
Ib		with horizontal transfer	kappa (A) in *Paramecium aurelia* (B)		47, 61
			Leishmania spp. (A) in vertebrate tissue cells (B)		26

Single-cell hosts

Two-species systems

IIa	no horizontal transfer	sigma virus (A) in Drosophila melanogaster (B)	$r \simeq 0.99$ $v > 0.0$	28, **29**, 30
		cytoplasmic SR (sex ratio) (A) in Drosophila bifasciata (B)	$r \simeq 0.95$	34, **46**
		Wolbachia pipientis (A) in Culex pipiens (B)	$r > 0.99$	**68**
IIb	horizontal transfer within generations	Nosema bombycis (A) in Bombyx mori (B)		41
IIc	horizontal transfer within and between generations	polyhedrosis viruses (A) in many arthropod species (B)		2, 21, 58
		Thelohania spp. (A) in mosquitoes (B)		23, 24
		Nocardia rhodnii (A) in triatomine bugs (B)		40

* Boldface reference numbers designate the sources of the quoted vertical transmission rates (r=maternal vertical transmission rate; v=paternal vertical transmission rate).

TABLE 2 (cont'd.)

Three-species systems

Type	Diagram	Definition	Examples	Rates	References
IIIa		one-host vectors (B) no direct transfer between vertebrates or plants (C)	Rickettsia tsutsugamushi (A) in Leptotrombidium akamushi (B) + vertebrates (C)	$r \simeq 0.98$	4, **50**
			Babesia bigemina (A) in Boophilus spp. (B) + cattle (C)	$r = 0.05$– 0.8	35, **55**, 56 60
IIIb		one-host vectors (B) with direct transfer between vertebrates or plants (C)	swine influenza virus (A) in Metastrongylus spp. (B) + swine (C)		57
			Histomonas meleagridis (A) in Heterakis gallinarum (B) + birds (C)	$r \simeq 0.005$	17, **31**
			Parahistomonas wenrichi (A) in Heterakis gallinarum (B) + birds (C)	$r \simeq 0.25$	**13**
IIIc		multihost vectors (B) no direct transfer between vertebrates or plants (C)	Rickettsia rickettsii (A) in Dermacentor andersoni (B) + vertebrates (C)	$r \simeq 0.99$ $v > 0.0$	**7**, 43, 54
			Borrelia duttoni (A) in Ornithodorus moubata (B) + vertebrates (C)	$r = 0.02$– 0.43 $v > 0.0$	1, 11, **16**, 25, **66**
			rice dwarf virus (A) in Nephotettix cincticeps (B) + rice		
			clover club leaf virus (A) in Agalliopsis novella (B) + clover (C)	$r > 0.99$	14, **37**
IIId		multihost vectors (B) with direct transfer between vertebrates or plants (C)	African swine fever virus (A) in Ornithodorus moubata (B) + swine (C)	$r \simeq 0.98$	**5**
			Brucella melitensis (A) in Haemaphysalis warburtoni (B) + goats (C)	$r = 0.55$– 0.81	44
					65

arrows. The longer arrows, which join adjacent boxes, represent horizontal transmission between individuals of different generations. The shorter arrows signify transfer of infection between individual members of the same generation.

The classification in TABLE 2 comprises nine general transmission types, or patterns, and should cover all known and likely examples of the vertical transmission of infection. These nine patterns fall into three major groups, numbered I, II, and III.

Type I (a and b) patterns describe biologic systems in which the host organisms are single cells. The supplementary drawings in TABLE 2 illustrate this feature. The inclusion of these single-cell host systems is essential for the classification as a whole, because much of the general literature on hereditary infections is devoted to them.[27, 48] Their allocation to a separate group is necessary because of the special nature of the "microepidemiologic" problems that

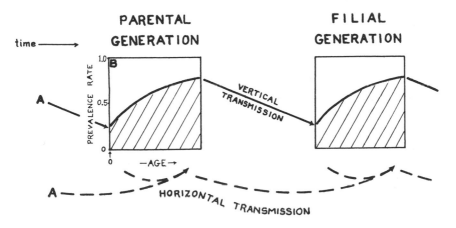

FIGURE 2. General diagram that illustrates vertical and horizontal transmission of an infectious agent (A) over two successive generations of a host (B) population. Each generation of hosts is represented as an age-prevalence graph. Several variations of this diagram appear in TABLE 2.

they pose and the special analytic techniques appropriate for their mathematic description.[32, 47, 52] They will not be discussed further in this paper.

The type-II (a, b, and c) and type-III (a, b, c, and d) transmission groups include those systems in which the hosts are metazoan or metaphytan organisms. They include all examples of vertical transmission in invertebrates and are the major concern of this paper. The type-II group covers the simple associations between an infectious agent (A) and a single host species (B). Type III describes the more complicated associations, which involve three species: infectious agent (A), invertebrate vector (B), and vertebrate or plant host (called C).

In the diagrams for the type-III patterns (TABLE 2), large rectangles have been introduced to represent the populations of vertebrates or plants (C) that serve as hosts of both the vertically transmitting invertebrate species (B) and the infectious agent (A). They are drawn as schematic age-prevalence graphs, which depict prevalence rates of infection with the agent (A) in the plant or vertebrate population (C). Transfer of infection between the vector species (B) and the vertebrate or plant species (C) is represented by broken lines, as a form of indirect horizontal transmission (*vide supra*).

A few comments on each of the patterns classified within types II and III will highlight their epidemiologic implications. It should be emphasized that although the present discussion is restricted to examples in which the species (B) host is an invertebrate, these transmission patterns serve equally well to describe other kinds of vertical transmission phenomena, for example, the congenital infections of mammals, egg-borne infections of poultry, and seed-borne infections of plants. Indeed, much may be gained through a recognition of the widespread occurrence of such epidemiologic patterns in nature. The reader is referred to TABLE 2 for examples and literature citations throughout the following discussion.

Type IIa

Type IIa includes all infections that are maintained in the host population by vertical transmission alone. Many varieties of microorganisms are thought to be maintained in this manner. The best known examples are the various bacteroid "mutualist" symbiotes of arthropods, which are so intimately associated with their hosts that they never need escape the confines of the host organism. The extensive literature on these symbiotic associations has been reviewed by Buchner.[6] Two groups of *Drosophila* infections are also included in type IIa: the so-called sigma (CO_2 sensitivity) virus and the SR (sex ratio) agents. These *Drosophila* examples deserve special mention because of the excellent epidemiologic work that has been performed on them, some of which will be referred to below. In addition, several invertebrate vectors of disease maintain these type-IIa infections; for example, most populations of the *Culex pipiens* complex are thought to maintain rickettsial agents classified as *Wolbachia pipientis*.[68]

The outstanding epidemiologic characteristic of the type-IIa systems is their absolute dependence on vertical transmission. In most examples, this transmission occurs mainly through the female line. In some cases, transmission is entirely matroclinal. It can be shown that such strictly matroclinal infections must impart some selective advantage to the host if they are to persist. The proof of this statement will be presented in the quantitative section below.

Type IIb

The type-IIb pattern describes infections that are transmitted *between* generations by vertical transmission alone but in which some horizontal transmission occurs *within* host generations. Such a transmission pattern is likely to apply only to host species in which generations are distinctly separate in time. (Several infections of annual plants are maintained in this manner; the infectious agents are carried over from year to year on seed.) The pattern may describe some infections of invertebrate species that overwinter as ova and in which infectious agents are carried over from one year to the next either on or inside the eggs. In addition, there is some evidence that *Nosema bombycis* infections are maintained in this manner in silkworm colonies; the infection is introduced into each generation of caterpillars via the ova. Pasteur's [41] regimen for the control of this disease ("pébrine") was based upon an assumption that the infections were maintained according to this type-IIb pattern.

Some species of invertebrates in the temperate zone may go through several generations each year, yet always pass the winter in the egg stage. If specific infectious agents rely upon association with these diapause ova for carriage from one year to the next, they might be classified within this type-IIb pattern. In such situations, the diagram boxes might be best interpreted as entire annual populations of the (B) hosts rather than as just single generations.

Vertical transmission is clearly essential for the maintenance of these type-IIb infections.

Type IIc

The type-IIc pattern describes the more common situation in which horizontal transmission occurs both within and between generations of the host species. It covers the majority of inherited infections of vertebrates and plants, in addition to those of invertebrates. Many polyhedrosis virus and microsporidan infections of arthropods are known to be transmitted vertically, at least to some extent, in their host species and would fit this pattern.

In type IIc, vertical transmission is not qualitatively essential for the maintenance of the infectious agent within the host population, because there is the added option of intergenerational horizontal transmission. Any requirement for vertical transmission would be quantitative only and dependent upon the actual amount of horizontal transmission that occurs within the system. If vertical transmission alone were insufficient for the maintenance of infection in the population, the balance would have to be contributed by horizontal transfer of the agent. The relationship between these two types of transmission will be further explored below.

It should be noted that this type-IIc diagram is, in effect, a skeletal form for all of the more complex patterns included under type III, in which the horizontal transmission between species-B individuals is mediated via some animal or plant organisms upon which they (the invertebrate vectors) feed.

Type IIIa

The type-IIIa pattern is characterized by two specific criteria: the species-B vector feeds upon only a single host in its lifetime (these are thus the so-called one-host vector systems), and the infection is transmitted between the vertebrate or plant hosts exclusively by the species-B vectors. The abrupt rise in the prevalence curve in the diagrams of the vector (B) population may not be strictly correct in a temporal sense but is meant to signify the single opportunity that these vectors have, in a lifetime, to pick up the infection. Vertical transmission is clearly obligatory for the maintenance of infections transmitted in this manner, because the only way in which a one-host vector can be capable of infecting its vertebrate host is by first receiving the infection vertically from one of its parents.

The most important groups of invertebrate vectors that fit this type-IIIa pattern are the trombiculid mites (vectors of *R. tsutsugamushi*)[4] and the boophilid ticks (vectors of *B. bigemina*).[55] The diseases they transmit, scrub typhus of man and redwater fever of cattle, respectively, are of considerable social and economic importance over wide areas of the world. It is worth pointing out that the association between *B. bigemina* and *B. annulatus,* discovered by Smith and Kilborne in 1893, was the first recognized example of the vertical transmission of a vertebrate pathogen in an arthropod vector.

Type IIIb

As in type IIIa, the vectors in type-IIIb systems contact only a single host during their lifetime. The pattern is distinguished from the preceding in that there is an additional option of direct horizontal transfer of the infectious agent between vertebrate hosts. Because of this option, vertical transfer through the vector species is not absolutely essential for short-term maintenance of the agent in nature.

It is interesting to note that most, if not all, of the vectors (B) classifiable in type IIIb are helminths.

Type IIIc

In type IIIc, the vectors normally feed upon more than a single vertebrate or plant host in their lifetime. They are thus called "multihost" vectors. In addition, the type-IIIc pattern stipulates that all transmission of infection between vertebrate (or plant) hosts is mediated by the species-B vectors.

This pattern includes the majority of vector-borne infections of plants and animals in which vertical transmission within the vector species has been reported. Examples include most of the group-B arbovirus, *Rickettsia, Borrelia,* and *Babesia* infections of vertebrates. Most of the relevant vectors are acarines. There are a few reports of the vertical transmission of vertebrate-infecting viruses through dipterans (sandflies and mosquitoes), which would also be included in type IIIc.[42, 64, 67] Most of the plant infections included in this group are transmitted by hemipteran bugs (e.g., leafhoppers).[5, 14, 37, 45]

Many of the invertebrate vectors that appear to fall naturally within this group are two-host or three-host ixodid ticks. Some of these ticks normally feed, at different stages in their life histories, upon different vertebrate species (e.g., the larval and nymphal stages may feed upon small rodents, and the adult ticks feed upon larger mammals). If only a single blood meal were normally taken from the vertebrate species (C) that harbors the agent (A), the system would be effectively one-host in this context and might be better classified within type IIIa.

Vertical transmission is not essential for the short-term maintenance of type-IIIc agents within their host populations because of the repeated opportunity for indirect horizontal transmission, through the vertebrate or plant hosts, within each vector generation. Several examples of this transmission pattern have been studied extensively, for example, *Rickettsia rickettsii* and *Borrelia duttoni* infections. It might be possible to assess the relative and absolute contributions of the different transmission modalities, for these examples, from data available in the literature.

Type IIId

The type-IIId pattern is characterized by multihost vectors and by the additional availability of some direct horizontal transfer of infection between the vertebrate or plant hosts. There are rather few recorded examples. The inclusion of *Brucella melitensis* in this category is highly debatable, because there is little evidence that ticks play a significant role in its maintenance in nature. (On the other hand, direct vertical, transplacental or transmammary, transmission in the *vertebrate* host is undeniably important in the epidemiology of *B. melitensis*. It might thus be best considered as an example of type-IIc transmission; the B-level host would be the goat.[53]) The other example of type-IIId transmission cited in TABLE 2, African swine fever, poses an extremely complicated epidemiologic problem and is not fully understood.[44]

THE MEASUREMENT OF VERTICAL TRANSMISSION

Vertical transmission is clearly essential for even the short-term maintenance of the agents included within types Ia, IIa, IIb, and IIIa of the classification just described. In the other transmission patterns, however, the contribution of vertical transmission can only be assessed quantitatively, in terms of the relative contributions of vertical and horizontal transmission that occur within specific systems.

The need to quantify vertical transmission in invertebrate vectors has been evident to many workers in the past. In their 1967 review of the literature on this subject, Burgdorfer and Varma recognized the need for standard rates, which would allow comparisons between work performed by different authors and on different systems. They proposed the following definitions: [8] *"Transovarial infection rates:* the percentage of females that pass microorganisms to their progeny." *"Filial infection rates:* the percentage of infected progeny derived from an infected female."* These defined rates have since been used by several authors.[44, 50]

Certain difficulties arise, however, when these definitions are applied in general epidemiologic analyses. The first definition is of a "transovarial" transmission rate. It might be better to use the general term "vertical" here, because this term avoids the narrow mechanistic connotations of "transovarial." The use of this more general term is especially necessary now that invertebrate pathologists have begun to distinguish "transovarial transmission" (defined as transmission that occurs within the ovary) from "transovum transmission" (defined as transmission that occurs on the surface of the egg).[62] Second, both of the definitions specify the female as the source parent. This specification is sufficient for the description of many systems in nature but is inadequate for several in which transmission by the male is known to occur (e.g., sigma virus,[28] *R. rickettsii,*[43] and *B. duttoni*[66]). Third, it is not clear whether the filial infection rate may relate to populations, as opposed to individual females, and, if so, whether it should apply only to females that transmit the infection to at least some of their progeny.

When analyzing the epidemiologic implication of vertical transmission, it is easier to use a different set of basic definitions from those given above. The alternative definitions, as proposed here, are analogous to the set used by l'Heritier in his studies of sigma virus infections in *Drosophila meleanogaster* populations: [29] r = *maternal vertical transmission rate,* the prevalence rate of infection among the progeny of infected females when mated with uninfected males; v = *paternal vertical transmission rate,* the prevalence rate of infection among the progeny of infected males when mated with uninfected females. These definitions are directly applicable to all vertical transmission systems classified within types II and III above. Some published values for these rates have been included in TABLE 2.

To assess the contribution of vertical transmission to the prevalence of infection in a population, it is also necessary to take into account the effect of the infection upon the hereditary host. For example, if the infection were to depress the fertility of its host, the contribution of inherited infections to the prevalence rate among members of the next generation would be correspondingly reduced. It is suggested that the following parameters, which are, again, consistent with those used by l'Heritier,[29] be adopted for general use in this context. α = relative fertility (number of progeny) of infected adults when compared with their uninfected peers; β = relative survival potential (to reproductive age) of congenitally infected young when compared with uninfected young. Unfortunately, there are relatively few data available that relate to these parameters.

Assessing the Contribution of Vertical Transmission

The fundamental epidemiologic question that underlies studies of vertical transmission is that of its contribution to the maintenance of infection in host populations. An important corollary is the question of whether vertical transmission by itself might not be sufficient, in some cases, for the continued maintenance of an infectious agent in nature.

Some authors have presumed that because vertical transmission can maintain an infection over several generations in a selected population of vectors in the laboratory, it could maintain the agents indefinitely in the field. Comments such as the following (which refers to the transovarial transmission of *Rickettsia conori* in *Haemaphysalis leachi*) are found in the literature: [15] ". . . there is hereditary transmission of the rickettsiae through the egg to the succeeding generations. Apparently this hereditary transmission may continue indefinitely. . . . No mammalian reservoir is therefore necessary for preserving the infection in nature." There is a fallacy in such an argument, if the evidence in its favor is based upon experiments that involve the conscious selection of infected individuals at each generation and neglects implications of such artificial selection procedures for prevalence rates that would prevail in natural populations.

This problem is analogous to that faced by population geneticists when they predict the prevalence rate of some gene in subsequent generations of a carrier species or population. In fact, a technique used in the analysis of such genetic problems may be adapted to the present context. (For a discussion of the diagrammatic approach used below, as applied to a genetic problem, see Smith,[59] p. 202.)

We now construct a model to describe the quantitative contribution of vertical transmission to the prevalence of infection in a host population, by first investigating the situation in which such transmission is itself sufficient for the maintenance of infection. The following assumptions and definitions underlie this basic model. We assume some infection (A) to be present in a proportion

B_a of the adult members of a sexually reproducing population (B). This infection is assumed to be maintained by vertical transmission alone and to persist throughout the entire lifetime of hereditarily infected individuals. Mating occurs at random in the host population. The infection is assumed to have similar effects on both males and females of the host species. The basic parameters r, v, α, and β are as defined above.

Because a proportion B_a of the adult females are infected, the complementary proportion $(1 - B_a)$ must be free of infection. According to the definition of α, which describes the effect of infection on host fertility, each infected female has on the average α times as many progeny as does an uninfected female. Therefore, the numbers of progeny born to infected and uninfected females, respec-

PATERNAL PARENT

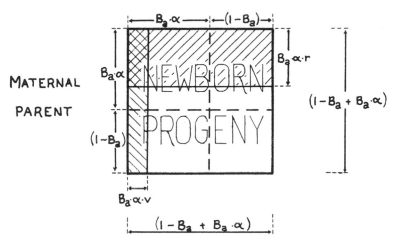

FIGURE 3. Dimensioned Venn diagram square [59] that illustrates the relationship between infection rates among parents and their newborn (or newly hatched) progeny. The prevalence rate of infection among both males and females of the parental generation is B_a. The shaded area corresponds to progeny that receive the infection from at least one parent.

tively, will be in the ratio of $B_a\alpha/(1 - B_a)$. An identical argument applies to the adult males in the population. We can now investigate the implications of these relationships for the infection rates among newborn progeny.

Consider a dimensioned Venn diagram square, constructed so as to represent the parentage probabilities of newborn hosts (FIGURE 3). The female parent is represented along the vertical margin of the square, and the male parent is represented along the horizontal margin. Each of these margins is marked off with distances that correspond to the relative proportions of progeny produced by infected and uninfected parents, that is, $B_a\alpha$ and $(1 - B_a)$, respectively. It is important to note that these margins are each $(1 - B_a + B_a\alpha)$ in length and thus are not equivalent to unity unless $\alpha = 1$. The total area of the square is $(1 - B_a + B_a\alpha)^2$ and represents the total number of newborn progeny.

Dotted lines have been drawn orthogonally across the square, at the points that separate infected from uninfected parentage. These dotted lines divide up the progeny population (area) according to the infection status of the parents. Only the progeny represented by the relative area below and to the right of the dotted lines had parents both of whom were not infected. However, not all of the progeny born to infected parents necessarily receive the infection from them. Only a proportion r of the progeny produced by infected females receive the infection from the maternal parent; a proportion v of the progeny of infected males receive the infection from the father. These proportions have been measured off along the regions of the square margins referable to progeny from infected female and male parents, respectively. The solid lines drawn across the square at these points thus divide up the progeny according to whether they actually receive the infection from one or another parent. The shaded area within the total square, then, represents the proportion of the total progeny to which the infection is transmitted by at least one parent.

By inspection, we see that the proportion infected among newborn progeny, given by the shaded area divided by the total area of the square, is:

$$\text{proportion of newborn progeny infected} = \frac{B_a \alpha r(1 - B_a + B_a \alpha) + B_a \alpha v(1 - B_a + B_a \alpha - B_a \alpha r)}{(1 - B_a + B_a \alpha)^2}.$$

The proportion of progeny uninfected is the complement to this expression:

$$\text{proportion of newborn progeny not infected} = \frac{(1 - B_a + B_a \alpha - B_a \alpha r)(1 - B_a + B_a \alpha - B_a \alpha v)}{(1 - B_a + B_a \alpha)^2}.$$

These proportions may not refer to the adult members of the progeny population, however, because there may be differential mortality between the infected and uninfected individuals. The relative survival rate to maturity, of infected to uninfected individuals, has been defined as β. Therefore, if we define B_a' as the prevalence rate of inherited infections among adults of the progeny generation, we have the following relationship:

$$B_a' = \frac{\beta[B_a \alpha r(1 - B_a + B_a \alpha) + B_a \alpha v(1 - B_a + B_a \alpha - B_a \alpha r)]}{\beta[B_a \alpha r(1 - B_a + B_a \alpha) + B_a \alpha v(1 - B_a + B_a \alpha - B_a \alpha r)] +}{(1 - B_a + B_a \alpha - B_a \alpha r)(1 - B_a + B_a \alpha - B_a \alpha v)}.$$

This equation proves to be extremely important in the general analysis of hereditary infections and will be called the *fundamental vertical transmission equation*. It provides an initial solution to the fundamental problem, that of the quantitative contribution of vertical transmission to the prevalence rates of infection in subsequent generations.

Given any set of values for B_a, r, v, α, and β, the solution of the fundamental equation is straightforward. By repeatedly substituting the solution B_a' into the right-hand side for B_a, one can iterate the calculation, determining the prevalence rates of infection that would be found in successive generations of hosts, as long as the assumptions held. Results of two such iterations are illustrated in FIGURE 4.

The values used in the first simulation, represented by the dotted line, were as follows: initial prevalence rate $B_a = 0.5$, $r = 0.95$, $v = 0.05$, $\alpha = 1.0$, and $\beta = 1.25$. It is evident that the prevalence rate under these circumstances would stabilize at approximately 0.83. These parameter values are therefore compatible with a type-IIa vertical transmission system, in which the infection can be maintained persistently by the vertical transmission mode alone.

The solid line in FIGURE 4 represents another iterated solution of the fundamental equation. The initial prevalence was again set at $B_a = 0.5$, but here, $r = 0.8$, $v = 0.05$, $\alpha = 0.9$, and $\beta = 0.9$. The prevalence rate is seen to drop off steadily, ultimately to zero. In other words, these parameter values are not compatible with type-IIa transmission, because they are incapable of supporting the infection indefinitely in the host population. Such will be the case with most, if not all, of the vertical transmission systems included within types IIb, IIc, IIIa, IIIb, IIIc, and IIId of the above classification.

The latter condition of "incompetent" vertical transmission is typical of almost all of the vector-borne infections of animals and plants that are trans-

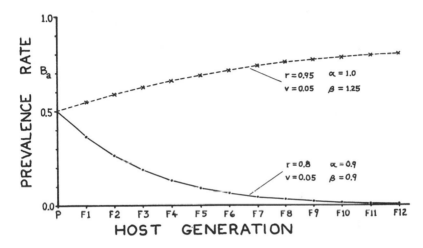

FIGURE 4. Two results obtained by iteration of the *fundamental vertical transmission equation,* which illustrate prevalence rates of infection that would be maintained over 12 successive generations of hosts, if no horizontal transmission occurred. In each case, the initial prevalence rate in the P generation is set at $B_a = 0.5$. The r, v, α, and β parameters are as specified.

mitted at times vertically through their invertebrate vectors. There is as yet insufficient evidence to assert that any of these infectious agents could be maintained in perpetuity within the invertebrate host by vertical transmission alone. As mentioned above, most of the laboratory demonstrations of repeated vertical transmission of infectious agents in invertebrate vectors have involved the selection of hereditarily infected individuals at each generation. This procedure is tantamount to creating artificially high α and β parameters for the system and therefore has little bearing upon the situation that would obtain in nature.

It is possible to predict directly, on the basis of the "fundamental equation," whether any set of r, v, α, and β values is compatible with the continued maintenance of infection in a population by vertical transmission alone (i.e., type-IIa transmission). If such persistence were possible, repeated iteration of the fundamental equation should demonstrate that the prevalence converges to some asymptote greater than zero, at which B_a would equal B_a'. The existence of such an asymptote can be investigated directly, by substituting B_a for B_a' in the fundamental equation and solving for B_a. A quadratic equation is obtained:

$$B_a{}^2[(\beta\alpha^2 - \alpha^2)(r + v - rv) - (\beta\alpha - \alpha)(r + v) + (\alpha - 1)^2]$$
$$+ B_a[(2\beta\alpha - \alpha)(r + v) - \beta\alpha^2(r + v - rv) + 2\alpha - 2]$$
$$+ 1 - \beta\alpha r - \beta\alpha v = 0.$$

Any set of r, v, α, and β values may be substituted into this equation. If these values are compatible with type-IIa transmission, there will be at least one root, B_a, between 0 and 1. If there are no such roots, the parameter values are not compatible with maintenance of infection by vertical transmission alone.

Derivation of a Symbiote Fitness Criterion

There is a more elegant method of predicting whether any given set of r, v, α, and β values is compatible with type-IIa transmission. It is evident that one root of the above quadratic equation must be zero, if the constant term $(1 - \alpha\beta r - \alpha\beta v)$ should equal zero. In this condition, $1 - \alpha\beta r - \alpha\beta v = 0$, so $\alpha\beta(r + v) = 1$. Any increase in the value of this product, $\alpha\beta(r + v)$, so that it exceeds unity is equivalent to moving one root of the quadratic equation, B_a, above zero. This product term thus informs us of a sufficient condition for the maintenance of a type-IIa vertical transmission system in nature, and is defined here as the fitness of a symbiote $= \alpha\beta(r + v)$. ("Symbiote" is used here in its broadest sense, as referring to any infecting agent within a host. It is inclusive of mutualism, commensalism, and parasitism.[51, 62]) Just as a chromosomal allele should be maintained in a population if its fitness (defined as the relative reproductive success attributable to the allele) exceeds unity, so should an agent be maintained by vertical transmission alone if $\alpha\beta(r + v) > 1$. It should be emphasized that this criterion, herein defined as the symbiote fitness, provides a *sufficient* condition for the maintenance of infection by vertical transmission alone. The condition is not absolutely necessary, however, because it can be demonstrated that there are situations in which $\alpha\beta(r + v) < 1$, yet which are still compatible with roots B_a in the range 0–1. It can be shown that these exceptional conditions do not seriously affect the usefulness of the symbiote fitness criterion as defined above. The exceptional circumstances occur in a narrow range of parameter values and are associated with extremely high vertical transmission rates (e.g., $r + v > 1.65$). Such exceptional conditions rarely, if ever, obtain in nature. This property of the symbiote fitness criterion will be discussed at length in a future publication.

As an illustration of this fitness criterion, we examine the value of $\alpha\beta(r + v)$ for the two sets of parameters discussed above and illustrated in Figure 4 . For the first set, represented by the dotted line in Figure 4, $\alpha\beta(r + v) = 1.25$, which indicates that vertical transmission is sufficient for maintenance under these circumstances. For the second set of parameters, represented by the solid line in Figure 4, $\alpha\beta(r + v) = 0.6885$, which indicates incompetent vertical transmission. These conclusions are consistent with those arrived at by iteration of the fundamental equation.

It should also be noted that this symbiote fitness criterion is fully consistent with l'Heritier's published work.[29] l'Heritier based his discussion of fitness upon

an assumption of strict matroclinal inheritance ($v = 0$), in which case the
fitness criterion becomes $\alpha\beta r > 1$. It can be proven that this criterion is both
sufficient and necessary for matroclinal systems.[12]

The fitness criterion defined above has a profound implication. It stipulates
that an infectious agent may be maintained in a host population by vertical
transmission alone, even if it imparts some selective disadvantage to its hereditary host (i.e., $\alpha < 1$ and/or $\beta < 1$). This is valid, *provided* that there is sufficient vertical transmission by both parents to bring the product $\alpha\beta(r + v)$ above
unity. This surprising capacity of vertical transmission mechanisms was pointed
out by l'Heritier[30] in his discussion of the maintenance of sigma virus infections
in *Drosophila* populations.

The implications of the fitness criterion are summarized diagrammatically in

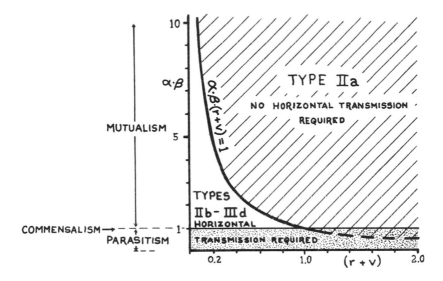

FIGURE 5. Graphic representation of the symbiote fitness criterion, which shows
$\alpha\beta$ plotted against $(r+v)$. The curved line is the equation: $\alpha\beta \, (r+v) = 1$.

FIGURE 5. The vertical axis in this Figure represents the product $\alpha\beta$, which
describes the net effect of the infection upon both the fertility and the survival
potential of the host. This product is closely analogous to the Wrightian fitness
parameter used by population geneticists to describe the net effect of a gene
upon its carrier.[63] In the present context, it may be interpreted as a quantitative
definition of symbiotic relationships. If this product exceeds unity, the infection
is providing some net selective advantage to its host, and the agent involved may
be termed a "mutual." If the product $\alpha\beta$ were exactly equivalent to unity, the
infection has no selective effect on its hereditary host, and the agent may be
termed a "commensal." On the other hand, if the $\alpha\beta$ product were less than
unity, the infected hosts are at a selective disadvantage when compared with
uninfected ones, and the infecting agent may thus be termed a "parasite" in
its hereditary host. It is considered that these quantitative definitions, which

are compatible with widely accepted qualitative definitions of these terms,[51, 62] may be helpful when describing the nature of hereditary symbiotic associations.

Along the horizontal axis of FIGURE 5 is set the sum of the maternal and paternal vertical transmission rates. This sum can never exceed 2 and in only a few systems surpasses 1.1.

The heavy curved line represents the fitness criterion, $\alpha\beta(r + v) = 1$. The fact that the criterion becomes less robust as $(r + v) \to 2$ is indicated by the broken curve in the region that corresponds to the higher abscissa values.

The region to the right of the curve, which implies that $\alpha\beta(r + v) > 1$, covers the parameter combinations that are compatible with the maintenance of infection by vertical transmission alone. This area, with diagonal shading on the diagram, includes virtually all of the type-IIa vertical transmission systems. Exceptions are considered unlikely, as mentioned above.

The area to the left of the curve, which implies that $\alpha\beta(r + v) < 1$, covers all circumstances in which the vertical transmission modality is in itself insufficient for the long-term maintenance of the infection. Within this area lie the examples of vertical transmission classified within types IIb, IIc, IIIa, IIIb, IIIc, and IIId, above.

This graphic representation may prove useful as a general guideline for studies on the vertical transmission of infection. The distribution of points that represent specific known examples of vertical transmission, on this diagram, is of some theoretic interest. Some clustering of points, according to both transmission type and phylogenetic affiliation, would not be surprising. Unfortunately, there is at present insufficient information to allow many systems to be plotted precisely in such a Figure.

THE RELATIONSHIP BETWEEN VERTICAL AND HORIZONTAL TRANSMISSION

The above discussion has outlined a method of assessing the quantitative contribution of vertical transmission to prevalence rates of infection in subsequent generations of hosts. In most of the medically and agriculturally important examples of vertical transmission, this transmission modality is in itself not sufficient for the long-term maintenance of infection in the host (B) species. In these examples, some alternative types of transmission, namely, direct or indirect horizontal transfer, must compensate for the incompetence of vertical transmission.

The extent of the contribution made by horizontal transmission can be assessed from the "fundamental equation" described above. If some reasonable value is substituted in the equation for B_a (i.e., some value that approximates the magnitude found in field situations), one can calculate an expected prevalence rate of *inherited* infections among the adults of the subsequent generation (B_a'). The difference between the prevalence rate in the parental generation and that predicted for the progeny generation (i.e., $B_a - B_a'$) is a measure of the deficit in prevalence rate that must be made up by horizontal transmission modalities. This may be formulated in terms of a net incidence rate of (horizontal) infections during the period of one generation: net incidence rate per generation $= (B_a - B_a')/(1 - B_a')$. (The denominator here is the proportion of adults that do not carry inherited infections and measures the "population at risk" in this situation.)

It is possible to continue with this analysis and to construct a series of algebraic statements that describe the horizontal transmission component of each of the transmission types IIb, IIc, IIIa, IIIb, IIIc, and IIId. Each of these arguments requires further precision of the biologic processes involved and a stipulation of appropriate assumptions. These developments deserve extended discussion, however, and will not be treated in this paper. The structures of several such models have been outlined by Fine.[12]

Summary and Conclusions

The vertical transmission of infectious agents in invertebrate vectors can be considered within the context of a general theory of hereditary symbiosis (inclusive of "mutualism," "commensalism," and "parasitism"). It is proposed that all hereditary infections be classified within a system of nine epidemiologic types, according to the nature of the organisms involved and the availability of alternative transmission pathways. The contribution of vertical transmission to the maintenance of infectious agents can be assessed by an extension of methods used by l'Heritier in studies of sigma virus in *Drosophila*. It is shown that a sufficient condition for the maintenance of infection by vertical transmission alone is $\alpha\beta(r + v) > 1$, where r and v are defined as the maternal and paternal vertical transmission rates, and α and β are the relative fertility and survival potential of infected to uninfected hosts, respectively. The amount of horizontal (or "zig-zag") transmission required, as a supplement to the vertical transmission contribution, to maintain an infectious agent can also be estimated by this approach. The investigation of examples of vertical transmission, in the light of this classification and analytic system, should facilitate objective assessment of the epidemiologic importance of this transmission modality vis-à-vis the maintenance, and possible control, of infections in nature.

Acknowledgments

I appreciate the encouragement and criticism of Dr. James Renwick, Professor W. H. R. Lumsden, Dr. Brian Southgate, and Dr. Valerie Beral during the work described herein.

Addendum

Two terms used in the above discussion deserve clarification. First, the symbol r, here defined as the "maternal vertical transmission rate," has nothing to do with the so-called intrinsic rate of natural increase, which is frequently given the same symbol by demographers, population geneticists, and ecologists. To avoid confusion on this issue, it might be better to use another symbol (e.g., l'Heritier's d) for the maternal vertical transmission rate parameter. Second, α is here defined as a "relative fertility" parameter, in the sense of the relative *number of progeny* of infected as compared with uninfected hosts. This reflects a common usage of the term "fertility" by anglophone demographers. Many geneticists prefer to use the word "fecundity" in this context, however, and l'Heritier[29] uses "fecundity" in his original definition of the α parameter. It should be emphasized that the α, as defined in this paper, is absolutely equivalent to that of l'Heritier.

The author is indebted to Dr. Lee Ehrman for having pointed out these foci of confusion in the present discussion.

REFERENCES

1. AESCHLIMANN, A. 1958. Développement embryonnaire d'*Ornithodorus moubata* (Murray) et transmission transovarienne de *Borrelia duttoni*. Acta Trop. **15:** 15–64.
2. AIZAWA, K. 1963. The nature of infections caused by nuclear-polyhedrosis viruses. *In* Insect Pathology—An Advanced Treatise. E. A. Steinhaus, Ed. : 381–412. Academic Press, Inc. New York and London.
3. ANDREWES, C. H. 1957. Factors in virus evolution. Advan. Virus Res. **4:** 1–24.
4. AUDY, J. R. 1968. Red Mites and Typhus. The Athlone Press. London, England.
5. BLACK, L. M. 1953. Transmission of plant viruses by cicadellids. Advan. Virus Res. **1:** 69–89.
6. BUCHNER, P. 1965. Endosynmbiosis of Animals with Plant Microorganisms. Interscience Publishers. New York, N.Y.
7. BURGDORFER, W. 1963. Investigation of "transovarial transmission" of *Rickettsia rickettsii* in the wood tick, *Dermacentor andersoni*. Exp. Parasitol. **14:** 152–159.
8. BURGDORFER, W. & M. G. R. VARMA. 1967. Trans-stadial and transovarial development of disease agents in arthropods. Annu. Rev. Entomol. **12:** 347–376.
9. CORDY, D. R. & J. R. GORHAM. 1950. The pathology and etiology of salmon disease in the dog and fox. Amer. J. Pathol. **26:** 617–637.
10. DIETZ, K., L. MOLINEAUX & A. THOMAS. 1974. A malaria model tested in the African Savannah. Bull. World Health Org. **50:** 347–357.
11. DUTTON, J. E. & J. L. TODD. 1905. The nature of human tick fever in the eastern part of the Congo Free State. Mem. Liverpool School Trop. Med. **17:** 1–18.
12. FINE, P. E. M. 1974. The epidemiological implications of vertical transmission. Ph.D. Thesis. University of London. London, England.
13. FINE, P. E. M. 1975. Quantitative studies on the transmission of *Parahistomonas wenrichi* by ova of *Heterakis gallinarum*. Parasitology **70:** In press.
14. FUKUSHI, T. 1933. Transmission of virus through the eggs of an insect vector. Proc. Imp. Acad. Tokyo **9:** 457–460.
15. GEAR, J. 1954. The rickettsial diseases of southern Africa. S. African J. Clin. Sci. **5:** 158–175.
16. GEIGY, R. & A. AESCHLIMANN. 1964. Langfristige Beobachtungen über transovarielle Übertragung von *Borrelia duttoni* durch *Ornithodorus moubata*. Acta Trop. **21:** 87–91.
17. GRAYBILL, H. W. & T. SMITH. 1920. Production of fatal blackhead in turkeys by feeding embryonated eggs of *Heterakis papillosa*. J. Exp. Med. **31:** 647–655.
18. GROSS, L. 1949. The "vertical epidemic" of mammary carcinoma in mice—its possible implications for the problem of cancer in general. Surg. Gynecol. Obstet. **88:** 295–308.
19. GUTTERIDGE, W. E. & R. F. MACADAM. 1971. An electron microscopic study of the bipolar bodies in *Crithidia oncopelti*. J. Protozool. **18:** 637–640.
20. HAIRSTON, N. G. 1962. Population ecology and epidemiological problems. *In* Ciba Foundation Symposium on Bilharziasis. G. E. W. Wolstenholme & M. O'Conner, Eds. : 36–62. Little, Brown and Company. Boston, Mass.
21. HUKUHARA, T. 1962. Generation to generation transmission of the cytoplasmic polyhedrosis virus of the silkworm, *Bombyx mori* (Linnaeus). J. Insect Pathol. **4:** 132–135.
22. HULLIGER, L. 1965. Cultivation of three species of *Theileria* in lymphoid cells *in vitro*. J. Protozool. **12:** 649–655.
23. KELLEN, W. R., H. C. CHAPMAN, T. B. CLARK & J. E. LINDEGREN. 1965. Host-

parasite relationships of some *Thelohania* from mosquitoes (Nosematidae: Microsporidia). J. Invert. Pathol. **7:** 161–166.

24. KELLEN, W. R., H. C. CHAPMAN, T. B. CLARK & J. E. LINDEGREN. 1966. Transovarian transmission of some *Thelohania* (Nosematidae: Microsporidia) in mosquitoes of California and Louisiana. J. Invert. Pathol. **8:** 355–359.

25. KOCH, R. 1905. Vorläufige Mitteilungen über die Ergebnisse einer Forschungsreise nach Ostafrika. Deut. Med. Wochschr. **47:** 1865–1871.

26. LAMY, L. H. 1972. Protozoaires intracellulaires en culture cellulaire. Intérêt-possibilités-limites. Ann. Biol. **11** (Fasc. 3–4): 145–183.

27. LEDERBERG, J. 1952. Cell genetics and hereditary symbiosis. Physiol. Rev. **32:** 403–430.

28. L'HERITIER, P. 1958. The hereditary virus of *Drosophila*. Advan. Virus Res. **5:** 195–245.

29. L'HERITIER, P. 1970. *Drosophila* viruses and their role as evolutionary factors. Evolution Biol. **4:** 185–209.

30. L'HERITIER, P. 1971. Les relations du virus héréditaire de la drosophile avec son hôte. Ann. Parasitol. Hum. Comp. **46:** 173–178.

31. LUND, E. E. & R. H. BURTNER. 1957. Infectivity of *Heterakis gallinae* eggs with *Histomonas meleagridis*. Exp. Parasitol. **6:** 189–193.

32. LURIA, S. E. 1951. The frequency distribution of spontaneous bacteriophage mutants as evidence for the exponential rate of phage reproduction. Cold Spring Harbor Symp. Quant. Biol. **16:** 463–470.

33. MACDONALD, G. 1957. The Epidemiology and Control of Malaria. Oxford University Press. London, England.

34. MAGNI, G. E. 1959. Il carattere sex-ratio in popolazioni naturali ed artificiali di *Drosophila bifasciata*. Rend. Ist. Lombardo Sci. Lett. B. **93:** 103–116.

35. MAHONEY, D. F. & D. R. ROSS. 1972. Epizootiological factors in the control of bovine babesiosis. Australian Vet. J. **48:** 292–298.

36. MALMQUIST, W. A., M. B. A. NYINDO & C. G. D. BROWN. 1970. East coast fever: cultivation *in vitro* of bovine spleen cell lines infected and transformed by *Theileria parva*. Trop. Anim. Health Prod. **2:** 139–145.

37. MARAMOROSCH, K. & D. D. JENSEN. 1963. Harmful and beneficial effects of plant viruses in insects. Annu. Rev. Microbiol. **17:** 495–530.

38. MONTGOMERY, E. 1917. On a tick-borne gastro-enteritis of sheep and goats occurring in British East Africa. J. Comp. Pathol. Ther. **30:** 28–57.

39. NÅSELL, I. & W. M. HIRSCH. 1971. Mathematical Models of Some Parasitic Diseases Involving an Intermediate Host. Courant Inst. Math. Sci. New York University. New York, N.Y.

40. NYIRADY, S. A. 1973. The germfree culture of three species of Triatominae: *Triatoma protracta* (Uhler), *Triatoma rubida* (Uhler) and *Rhodnius prolixus* (Stal). J. Med. Entomol. **10:** 417–448.

41. PASTEUR, L. 1870. Études sur la Maladie des Vers à Soie. Paris, France.

42. PETRISCHEVA, P. A. & A. J. ALYMOV. 1938. On transovarial transmission of virus of papataci fever by sandflies. Arch. Biol. Sci. **53:** 138–144 (in Russian); Transl. No. 80, Dept. Med. Zool. U.S. NAMRU 3 (in English).

43. PHILIP, C. B. & R. R. PARKER. 1933. Rocky Mountain spotted fever: investigation of sexual transmission in the wood tick *Dermacentor andersoni*. Publ. Health Rep. **48:** 266–272.

44. PLOWRIGHT, W., C. T. PERRY & M. A. PIERCE. 1970. Transovarial infection with African swine fever virus in the argasid tick *Ornithodorus moubata porcinus,* Walton. Res. Vet. Sci. **11:** 582–584.

45. POSNETTE, A. F. & C. E. ELLENBERGER. 1963. Further studies of green petal and other leafhopper-transmitted viruses infecting strawberry and clover. Ann. Appl. Biol. **51:** 69–83.

46. POULSON, D. F. 1963. Cytoplasmic inheritance and hereditary infections in *Drosophila. In* Methodology in Basic Genetics. W. J. Burdette, Ed. : 404–424. Holden-Day, Inc. San Francisco, Calif.

47. PREER, J. R. 1948. The killer cytoplasmic factor kappa: its rate of reproduc-

tion, the number of particles per cell, and its size. Amer. Naturalist **82:** 35–42.
48. PREER, J. R. 1971. Extrachromosomal inheritance: hereditary symbionts, mito-chondria, chloroplasts. Annu. Rev. Genetics **5:** 361–406.
49. PRETZMANN, G., J. LOEW & A. RADDA. 1963. Untersuchungen in einem Natur-herd der Fruhsommer-Meningoenkephalitis (FSME) in Neiderosterreich. Zentr. Bakteriol. Parasitenk. Abt. I Ref. **190:** 299–312.
50. RAPMUND, G., R. W. UPHAM, W. D. KUNDIN, C. MANIKUMARAN & T. C. CHAN. 1969. Transovarial development of scrub typhus rickettsiae in a colony of vector mites. Trans. Roy. Soc. Trop. Med. Hyg. **63:** 251–258.
51. READ, C. P. 1970. Parasitism and Symbiology. The Ronald Press Company. New York, N.Y.
52. REEVE, E. C. R. & G. J. S. ROSS. 1963. Mate killer (mu) particles in *Parame-cium aurelia:* further mathematical models for metagon distribution. Genetic Res. **4:** 158–161.
53. RENOUX, G. 1957. Brucellosis in goats and sheep. Advan. Vet. Sci. **3:** 241–273.
54. RICKETTS, H. T. 1907. Further experiments with the wood tick in relation to Rocky Mountain spotted fever. J. Amer. Med. Ass. **12:** 1278–1281.
55. RIEK, R. F. 1964. The development of *Babesia bigemina* (Smith and Kilborne, 1893) in the tick *Boophilus microplus* (Canes). Australian J. Agr. Res. **15:** 802–821.
56. ROSS, D. R. D. F. MAHONEY. 1974. Bovine babesiasis: computer simulation of *Babesia argentina* rates in *Bos taurus* cattle. Ann. Trop. Med. Parasitol. **68:** 385–392.
57. SHOPE, R. E. 1941. The swine lungworm as a reservoir and intermediate host for swine influenza virus. II. The transmission of swine influenza virus by the swine lungworm. J. Exp. Med. **74:** 49–68.
58. SMIRNOFF, W. A. 1962. Trans-ovum transmission of virus of *Neodiprion swainei* Middleton (Hymenoptera, Tenthredinidae). J. Insect Pathol. **4:** 192–200.
59. SMITH, C. A. B. 1969. Biomathematics. Vol. 2. Charles Griffin & Co. Ltd. London, England.
60. SMITH, T. & F. L. KILBORNE. 1893. Investigations into the nature, causation, and prevention of Texas or southern cattle fever. U.S. Dept. Agr. Bur. Anim. Ind. Bull. No. 1. U.S. Government Printing Office. Washington, D.C.
61. SONNEBORN, T. M. 1959. Kappa and related particles in *Paramecium.* Advan. Virus Res. **6:** 229–356.
62. STEINHAUS, E. A. & M. E. MARTIGNONI. 1970. An Abridged Glossary of Terms Used in Invertebrate Pathology. 2nd edit. Pacific Northwest Forest & Range Experiment Station. U.S. Department of Agriculture, Agr. Forest Service. U.S. Government Printing Office. Washington, D.C.
63. STRICKBERGER, M. W. 1968. Genetics. Collier-Macmillan, Ltd. London, Eng-land.
64. TESH, R. B., B. N. CHANIOTIS & K. M. JOHNSON. 1972. Vesicular stomatitis virus (Indiana serotype): transovarial transmission by phlebotomine sandflies. Science **175:** 1437–1479.
65. VOLKOVA, A. A., R. V. GREBENYUK, A. F. TIMOFEEV & R. S. GALIYEV. 1960. Study on the role of ticks of the genera *Dermacentor* and *Haemaphysalis* in transmission of brucellosis. Isv. Akad. Nauk. Kirg. SSR Ser. Biol. Nauk. **2(3):** 5–24 (in Russian); Transl. No. 134, Dept. Med. Zool. U.S. NAMRU 3 (in English).
66. WAGNER-JEVSEENSKO, O. 1958. Fortpflanzung bei *Ornithodorus moubata* und genitale Ubertragung von *Borrelia duttoni.* Acta Trop. **15:** 118–168.
67. WATTS, D. M., S. PANTUWATANA, G. R. DEFOLIART & W. H. THOMSON. 1973. Transovarial transmission of LaCross virus (California encephalitis group) in the mosquito *Aedes triseriatus.* Science **182:** 1140, 1141.
68. YEN, J. H. & A. R. BARR. 1973. The etiological agent of cytoplasmic incom-patibility in *Culex pipiens.* J. Invert. Pathol. **22:** 242–250.

COMPARATIVE EFFECTS OF VIRUSES ON ARTHROPOD AND VERTEBRATE CELLS: AN INTRODUCTION

John A. Wise

Department of Pathobiology
School of Public Health and Community Medicine
University of Washington
Seattle, Washington 98195

This Conference encompasses a very large and diverse area of biology. However, one of the unifying themes involves studies on parasites that infect both invertebrate and vertebrate or plant hosts. An understanding of mechanisms by which an organism can parasitize two hosts as taxonomically distinct as mosquito and man will ultimately result in knowledge of the most fundamental biologic principles. This session addresses the problem at the cellular level and involves experiments that were made possible only quite recently by the availability of a variety of invertebrate cell cultures.

One of the interesting findings to emerge from studies on arboviruses in cell culture is that exposure of invertebrate cells to virus results in a chronic infection. Togavirus-infected mosquito cells continue to divide indefinitely, produce large amounts of virus, yet appear normal with no apparent pathologic effects. In contrast, vertebrate cells undergo acute infection with pronounced cytopathology. This situation is similar to *in vivo* infections, as shown by the elegant work of Murphy *et al.* at the Communicable Disease Center in Atlanta. They found that the infection of mosquitoes by group-A or -B togaviruses resulted in progressive infections with massive virus shedding and involved virtually every organ in the mosquito, yet there were no noticeable pathologic features and no apparent effect on feeding habits or life-span of the mosquito. The same virus infecting a mouse caused acute infection, noticeable pathology, and commonly resulted in death.

Although many types of nonarboviruses can establish a persistent infection in vertebrate cell cultures, usually some selective process for surviving cells is necessary, or, more commonly, a temperature-sensitive viral mutant is employed at nonpermissive temperatures. It would appear that this is due to a difference in the intrinsic properties of vertebrate and invertebrate cells. However, recent studies by Holland indicate that persistently infected cell cultures can result from defective interfering virus particles that arise from high-multiplicity passage of virus. These and other possible mechanisms of persistent infection are examined in two interesting papers by Peleg and by Stollar *et al.* with studies on BHK cells chronically infected with Sindbis virus.

The results of these studies have implications beyond the arboviruses and their invertebrate hosts. Recent evidence suggests that some chronic diseases of man, such as multiple sclerosis, are due to a persistent infection of brain tissues by measles virus, but the mechanisms may be much easier to elucidate in an invertebrate where a "natural" persistence occurs.

One impetus for studying viral diseases of insects is their potential use in the control of insect pests, and Kurstak and Garzon explored the possibility of

195

amplifying the pathogenicity of virus for insects by examining the effects of mixed virus infection in invertebrate cells. The possible use of such insecticides should be approached with extreme caution, as the authors carefully point out. These studies, however, are also an important first step in examining dual infections of vertebrate arboviruses and strictly invertebrate viruses, an event that is not unlikely to occur in nature. The effects of phenotypic mixing in such an infection could have sobering implications for human diseases, especially when one considers an earlier report by Kurstak of an insect (densonucleosis) virus that causes transformation of vertebrate cells.

One of the most intriguing aspects of viral biology is the mechanisms that determine host cell specificity. Such specificity is one of the most characteristic properties of viruses. Yet, the arboviruses and plant pathogens that also multiply in invertebrate hosts show a remarkable lack of specificity. Buckley presents evidence that arboviruses and nonarboviruses compose a serologically related rabies serogroup in which a spectrum of biologic specificity is represented, with viruses that grow only in vertebrate cells, viruses that multiply in both vertebrate and invertebrate cell cultures, and viruses that reproduce only in the latter cell type. Such a virus group may represent an ideal model for examining the mechanism of virus specificity at the genetic level, because a similar rhabdovirus, vesicular stomatitis virus, has proven very amenable to genetic studies.

Buckley's observation that some of these viruses can be adapted to vertebrate cells after cocultivation with infected invertebrate cells also suggests the interesting possibility that host-induced modifications could play a role in specificity. One type of modification involves the variations in the lipid membrane of the viral envelope that is derived from the host cell. Studies by Jenkin have shown the existence of substantial differences in lipid composition of invertebrate and vertebrate cells. In addition, the pattern of lipid synthesis is altered by viral infection. Because the viral envelope is derived from the host cell membrane, mosquito-propagated virus may have altered infectivity for heterologous host cells and vice versa. Likewise, the carbohydrate composition of the glycoprotein is host specified and may also alter viral infectivity in heterologous cells. However, Stollar et al. present evidence that the presence or absence of sialic acid on the Sindbis virus glycoprotein (obtained by growth in vertebrate and invertebrate cells, respectively) has no effect on efficiency of infection.

In my discussion on virus receptors, I point out that any restriction on the host range or tissue tropism exhibited by arboviruses may not be due to the failure of virus to absorb to cells. Certainly, cells have intracellular mechanisms for limiting viral growth, as indicated by the failure of infectious poliovirus RNA to productively infect invertebrate cells.[1] That resistance to arboviruses probably occurs intracellularly rather than at the surface is even more convincingly demonstrated by Murphy. In his studies on togavirus-infected mosquitoes, only one in five gut cells or one in 20 salivary gland epithelial cells were infected, despite the presence of high concentrations of extracellular virus. Murphy discusses possible mechanisms of this cellular resistance to arboviruses and the limitation of virus spread.

REFERENCE

1. PELEG, J. 1969. Inapparent persistent virus infection in continuously grown Aedes aegypti mosquito cells. J. Gen. Virol. 5: 463–471.

CELLULAR RESISTANCE TO ARBOVIRUS INFECTION

Frederick A. Murphy

Public Health Service
Center for Disease Control
United States Department of Health, Education, and Welfare
Atlanta, Georgia 30333

INTRODUCTION

Arboviruses have evolved a remarkable capacity to complete their life cycles alternately under conditions as diverse as those in the organs and tissues of arthropods and vertebrates. Perhaps even more remarkable than this capacity to adapt such differing cell materials for virus replicative functions is their success in overcoming or circumventing the diverse specific mechanisms and environmental conditions involved in host resistance. In considering resistance, we tend to focus on the environment generated by the complex machinery of vertebrate inflammation and immunity, but the environment faced by a virus in the arthropod may be no less hostile.[1]

To complete its life cycle, an arbovirus must invade arthropod tissues and survive anatomic, physiologic, and biochemical barriers in several organs before progeny virus is delivered to salivary secretions for injection into the vertebrate host. The infectious processes that must occur in arthropod tissues and organs for successful perpetuation of virus seem, on the one hand, to reflect highly developed, highly productive adaptive patterns that are well entrenched in nature. The widespread occurrence and importance of arboviruses argues this point. On the other hand, these infectious processes in arthropods seem to involve the most tenuous aspects of life cycle continuity. An impasse in the processes of viral spread or proliferation in the earliest stages of infection in an arthropod host can be most effective because the fewest infectious units are available. During these earliest stages of infection, the relatively few virus particles must survive the most adverse extracellular conditions within the host body before being able to initiate replication.

ABSOLUTE REFRACTORINESS

Failures in the establishment of arthropod infections most often result from impasses at the earliest stages of viral invasion. Such intrinsic failures have been attributed to the presence of a "gut barrier" or "threshold," although whether these occur as physiologic or anatomic impasses to the movement of virus from an infected blood meal in the gut lumen or as impasses in viral adsorption, penetration, or infection of gut epithelium is not known.[2] Absolute refractoriness may be an expression of either active destruction of virus by means unknown or of the gradual dying off of ingested virus in the absence of favorable environmental requirements. In particular, such factors as toxicity of digestive fluids, impermeability of a peritropic membrane, physicochemical deficiencies of gut cell membranes, and activities of arthropod "surface defense mechanisms" of unknown nature have been considered.[3, 4] In view of more recent knowledge, the fundamental contributions of host factors in the replication of arboviruses in arthropods seem to be more subtle than previously thought. The failure of poliovirus RNA to initiate infection in mosquito cell cultures, which are quite susceptible to togavirus RNA,[5] exemplifies the need for a more comprehensive understanding of the biochemical parameters of viral replication. In this case, viral RNAs with similar replication, transcription, and translation mechanisms behave differently in a system where viral surface functions (adsorption, penetration, and so on) are not factors. The expression of intrinsic defense mechanisms may be genetically determined, and being so, these mechanisms probably have had predominant roles in the evolution of vector-borne infections and in their positions in nature.[6] In other words, it is the narrow range of competence and the widespread occurrence of refractoriness of potential vectors [7] that keep us from literally being overrun by viruses that use invertebrate hosts indiscriminately.

MODULATION OF ARTHROPOD INFECTION

Mechanisms that cause absolute arthropod refractoriness must be different from those that quantitatively limit or modulate virus yield within an effective arthropod vector species. There is a wide variation in the resistance of vertebrate hosts to particular arboviruses; this variation in the probability of vertebrate infection is often directly related to the amount of infectious virus delivered by the biting arthropod. Therefore, the quantal modulation in the productivity of infection in arthropod tissues, particularly in salivary glands, has an important role in nature.[8] An understanding of the mechanisms of this modulation may provide a key to future human intervention and disease control.

Infectious processes in arthropods have primarily been studied by sequential assay of viral transmissibility and sequential titration of arthropod organs and tissues.[2, 9] These approaches have been complemented by immunofluorescence [10-12] and, more recently, by electron microscopy of arthropod tissues.[13-17] In general, such studies have shown early infection of midgut epithelium and later invasion of salivary glands.[2, 4] In each of these organs, a rapid rise in virus infectivity, virus antigen accumulation, and virus particle concentration has been followed by either a "plateau" phase or a gradual decline through the remainder of the life-span of the arthropod host. Electron microscopic studies performed in our laboratory on *Aedes triseriatus* mosquitoes infected with eastern equine encephalitis (EEE; an alphavirus) virus [14] and of *Culex pipiens* mosquitoes infected with St. Louis encephalitis (SLE; a flavivirus) virus [15] clearly showed that the plateau and decline in the proportion of gut cells infected occurred before theoretic limits were reached. The yield of virus particles was also low relative to the potential of the available cell population through the time course studied. For example, SLE virus never infected more than one of every five gut cells, and EEE virus plateaued after infecting one of every three cells. In the salivary glands of *A. triseriatus,* EEE virus cumulatively reached high concentrations late in infection, and in *C. pipiens,* SLE virus became so concentrated that particles formed paracrystalline arrays (see FIGURE 1); however, there was no instance where more than one in every 20

FIGURE 1. Electron micrograph of St. Louis encephalitis virus in salivary gland of a *C. pipiens* mosquito 25 days after infection. Virus concentration in a luminal diverticulum is so great that a paracrystalline array is formed. $\times$ 41,000.

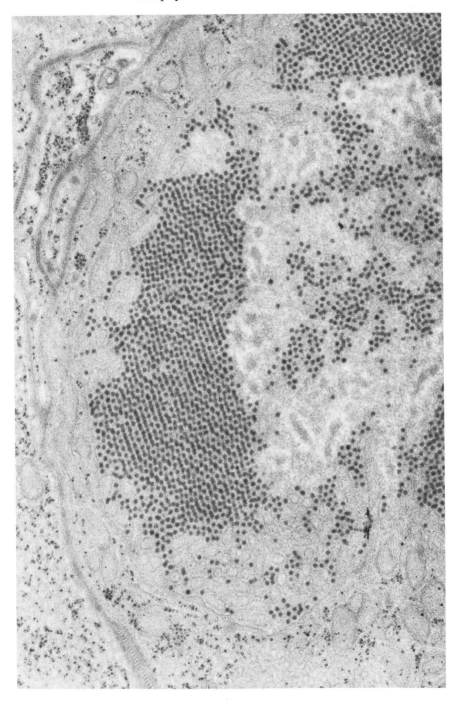

salivary gland epithelial cells was infected. No morphologic evidence to explain this homeostatic condition was found, and no cytopathic effect of infection was ever identified.

MECHANISMS OF INFECTION MODULATION

As with infectivity titration and immunofluorescence studies, the electron microscopic studies performed in our laboratory have not indicated any one hypothetic modulating mechanism, nor have any of these studies localized the mechanism to the arthropod, the virus, or the arthropod-virus interaction. There has been no evidence of hemocytic migration, proliferation, or accumulation in arthropod tissues that carry the highest infectivity titers. We found no evidence of physical degradation of progeny virus in arthropod tissues. This result must be contrasted with one study of *Aedes albopictus* cells grown in culture and infected with Ross River virus (an alphavirus).[18] After a virus proliferation phase, these mosquito cells "cured" themselves of residual infection via a unique endophagocytic process; this phenomenon needs to be studied further.

Because we cannot explain arbovirus modulation as a function of arthropods themselves (other than to associate it with a limitation in the proportion of potential host cells actually productively infected), the several general virus-limiting mechanisms known in vertebrates need to be examined for appropriate analogies. These vertebrate cell mechanisms also act by limiting virus spread and may be considered "primitive," in that they are active in undifferentiated cells and cells in culture. First, a defense elicited by the vertebrate host itself but triggered by virus infection, namely, interferon synthesis, may effectively prevent continuing virus replication cycles. There is preliminary evidence of interferon-like activity in mosquitoes and mosquito cells in culture,[19, 20] but the suspected suppressor of viral replication must be further characterized physicochemically before we can conclude that arthropods make and use interferon.

Another general mechanism that can be effective in restricting viral spread is homologous autointerference.[21, 22] Homologous autointerference may be mediated by the progeny of infecting virus in several ways: progeny viral constituents indistinguishable from those of parental type (wild type) may mediate interference; mutants of the parental virus that can still replicate under some conditions may interfere with wild-type replication; defective-interfering viral progeny or constituents, which can only replicate in the presence of intact virus, may competitively interfere with wild-type replication; and, finally, the distinct phenomenon called "intrinsic interference" may be operative in arthropods.

Wild-Type Virus Autointerference

Regulation failure that results in a shortage of virion constituents would favor a buildup of progeny RNA and double-stranded replicative intermediate species; the latter are known in several circumstances to be inhibitory to further RNA replication. This sort of feedback inhibition acting at the level of viral RNA replication might be particularly effective in arthropod cells in the absence of cytopathology; it might also be active over the long course of infection in arthropods. A further inhibitory effect could be associated with normal wild virus replication; the continuing translation from viral RNA messenger species might yield concentrations of viral products that would affect further transcription and even further replication of viral RNA. The "toxic" properties of accumulated viral proteins are now being widely considered as a mechanism of terminating infection. Experimental proof of viral protein buildup in arthropod tissues is minimal,[10, 12] but viral protein buildup seems to occur in mosquito cell cultures.[18]

Mutant Virus Interference

Temperature-sensitive mutants, small-plaque-sized mutants, virus particle surface antigenicity mutants, and heat-labile mutants have been commonly isolated from mosquito cell cultures infected persistently with several arboviruses.[23-28] Such mutations are often associated with a decrease in vertebrate host virulence and a decrease in progeny virus yield. These RNA[+] mutants can replicate under permissive conditions, and there is evidence that they may interfere with wild-type virus replication.[29] If these mutations are also related to failures in the regulation of viral synthetic processes or in viral constituent formation, the buildup of double-stranded RNA species would inhibit further synthesis, just as was described for wild-type virus interference. Alternatively, if mutations reflect sublethal quantitative or qualitative deficiencies in viral constituents, infection cycles might be affected directly.

Defective Interference

This type of modulation is a property of virus particles with defective RNA content that competes successfully for replication of viral RNA but yields noninfectious virus. Defective interference is a special case of mutation in which multiplication of mutant RNA is amplified.[22] It is commonly seen in some infections, such as influenza, parainfluenza, rhabdovirus, and arenavirus.[21, 30] Recently, defective-interfering particles with abnormal RNA have been found in two alphaviruses in cell culture; they are Sindbis [31-33] and Semliki Forest viruses.[34] These in vitro findings should now be tested in intact mosquitoes by sequential assays of infectious:defective particle ratios. In an infected arthropod, the yield of defective virus particles from an initial infection site could seed other cells in the same organ or even elsewhere in the body and competitively inhibit normal viral RNA synthesis.

Intrinsic Interference

The initial observation of this phenomenon was that cells in culture infected with rubella virus (a togavirus) were refractory to superinfection with Newcastle disease virus but could be productively infected with several other viruses.[35] The phenomenon does not require new cellular synthesis (as does the interferon response) but depends upon viral proteins blocking early steps in the replication of the superinfecting virus. This mechanism should be further considered in the modulation of arbovirus infections in arthropods; it may also have a role in the heterologous interference exhibited when two related arboviruses infect the same arthropod.[36] This mechanism and others may also play a role in interference between endogenous arthropod viruses and superinfecting arboviruses.

Conclusions

The likelihood that any or all of these modulating mechanisms might be active in arbovirus-infected arthropods may not warrant consideration, because experimental evidence is not available. Nevertheless, modulation is a real phenomenon, and the mechanisms described could, in the absence of real immune mechanisms, greatly affect infectious virus titers and transmissibility. From the standpoint of the natural history of arboviruses, the mechanisms under consideration might keep viral burdens within bounds that are physiologically tolerable to the vector species involved and at the same time provide a survival advantage to vector and virus alike. From another standpoint, we must consider means of intentional genetic manipulations of modulating mechanisms. With further understanding of their modes of action, we may be able to introduce variant characteristics into wild vector populations and, in doing so, make poor virus vectors out of good ones.

Summary

When an arbovirus enters an arthropod in an infected blood meal, several mechanisms may interact to affect its life cycle and ultimate transmissibility. Intrinsic absolute failure in the establishment of infection must be contrasted with infection that is successfully established but is variably modulated in its viral yield throughout the vector's life-span. Degrees of vertebrate host resistance make this modulation a central factor in determining whether an arthropod is an important vector in nature; moreover, human intervention that affects modulating mechanisms may become a basis for disease control. In the absence of evidence of real immune resistance to arbovirus infections in arthropods, other more primitive modulating mechanisms must be considered: interferon-like substances may be formed in arthropod cells; arthropod cells may "cure" themselves by a unique endophagocytic digestion of their virus burden; homologous interference with viral replicative processes may be mediated via wild or mutant viral RNA species acting to shut down further RNA synthesis; and homologous interference may be mediated by RNA of defective-interfering virus formed earlier in infection.

Acknowledgments

The author thanks Drs. Roy W. Chamberlain and John F. Obijeski for their thoughtful contributions to this topic. The experimental work reviewed was performed in collaboration with Miss Sylvia G. Whitfield and Dr. W. Daniel Sudia.

REFERENCES

1. MURPHY, F. A., S. G. WHITFIELD, W. D. SUDIA & R. W. CHAMBERLAIN. 1975. *In* Invertebrate Immunology. Mechanisms of Invertebrate Vector/Parasite Relations. K. Maramorosch, Ed. : 25–48. Academic Press, Inc. New York, N.Y.
2. CHAMBERLAIN, R. W. & W. D. SUDIA. 1961. Ann. Rev. Entomol. **6:** 371–390.
3. CHAMBERLAIN, R. W., D. B. NELSON & W. D. SUDIA. 1954. Amer. J. Hyg. **60:** 278–285.
4. CHAMBERLAIN, R. W. 1968. Curr. Topics Microbiol. Immunol. **42:** 38–58.
5. PELEG, J. 1969. Nature (London) **221:** 193, 194.
6. SCHLESINGER, R. W. 1971. Curr. Topics Microbiol. Immunol. **55:** 241–252.
7. VARMA, M. G. R. 1972. *In* Moving Frontiers in Invertebrate Virology. J. L. Melnick, Ed. : 49–56. S. Karger. Basel, Switzerland.
8. SCHAEFFER, M. & E. H. ARNOLD. 1954. Amer. J. Hyg. **60:** 231–236.
9. LaMOTTE, L. C. 1960. Amer. J. Hyg. **72:** 73–87.
10. DOI, R. 1970. Jap. J. Exp. Med. **40:** 101–115.
11. MAGUIRE, T. 1973. Personal communication.
12. GAIDAMOVICH, S. Y., N. V. KHUTORETSKAYA, A. I. LVOVA & N. J. SVESHNIKOVA. 1973. Intervirology **1:** 193–200.
13. BERGOLD, G. H. & J. WEIBEL. 1962. Virology **17:** 554–562.
14. WHITFIELD, S. G., F. A. MURPHY & W. D. SUDIA. 1971. Virology **43:** 110–122.
15. WHITFIELD, S. G., F. A. MURPHY & W. D. SUDIA. 1973. Virology **56:** 70–87.
16. JANZEN, H. G. & K. A. WRIGHT. 1971. Can. J. Zool. **49:** 1343–1345.
17. LARSEN, J. R. & R. F. ASHLEY. 1971. Amer. J. Trop. Med. Hyg. **20:** 754–760.
18. RAGHOW, R. S., T. D. C. GRACE, B. K. FILSHIE, W. BARTLEY & L. DALGARNO. 1973. J. Gen. Virol. **21:** 109–122.
19. BERGOLD, G. H. & N. RAMIREZ. 1972. *In* Moving Frontiers in Invertebrate Virology. J. L. Melnick, Ed. : 56–59. S. Karger. Basel, Switzerland.
20. ENZMANN, P.-J. 1973. Arch. Ges. Virusforsch. **41:** 382–389.
21. HUANG, A. & D. BALTIMORE. 1970. Nature (London) **226:** 325–327.
22. HUANG, A. 1973. Annu. Rev. Microbiol. **27:** 101–117.
23. SHENK, T. E., K. A. KOSHELNYK & V. STOLLAR. 1974. J. Virol. **13:** 439–447.
24. SIMARACHATANANT, P. L. C. OLSEN. 1973. J. Virol. **12:** 275–283.
25. SINGH, K. R. P. 1971. Curr. Topics Microbiol. Immunol. **55:** 127–133.
26. PELEG, J. 1971. Curr. Topics Microbiol. Immunol. **55:** 155–161.
27. SIMIZU, B. & N. TAKAYAMA. 1971. Arch. Ges. Virusforsch. **35:** 242–250.
28. MUDD, J. A., R. W. LEAVITT, D. T. KINGSBURY & J. J. HOLLAND. 1973. J. Gen. Virol. **20:** 341–351.
29. STOLLAR, V., J. PELEG & T. E. SHENK. 1974. Intervirology **2:** 337–344.
30. PFAU, C. J., R. M. WELSH & R. S. TROWBRIDGE. 1973. *In* Lymphocytic Choriomeningitis Virus and Other Arenaviruses. F. Lehmann-Grube, Ed. : 101–111. Springer-Verlag. Berlin, Federal Republic of Germany.
31. SCHLESINGER, S., M. SCHLESINGER & B. W. BURGE. 1972. Virology **48:** 615–617.
32. SHENK, T. E. & V. STOLLAR. 1972. Biochem. Biophys. Res. Commun. **49:** 60–67.
33. EATON, B. T. & P. FAULKNER. 1973. Virology **51:** 85–93.
34. LEVIN, J. G., J. M. RAMSEUR & P. M. GRIMLEY. 1973. J. Virol. **12:** 1401–1406.
35. MARCUS, P. I. H. L. ZUCKERBRAUN. 1970. Ann. N.Y. Acad. Sci. **173:** 185–198.
36. LAM, K. S. K. & I. D. MARSHALL. 1968. Amer. J. Trop. Med. Hyg. **17:** 625–636, 637–644.

IN VIVO BEHAVIOR OF A SINDBIS VIRUS MUTANT ISOLATED FROM PERSISTENTLY INFECTED AEDES AEGYPTI CELL CULTURES

J. Peleg

Department of Virology
Israel Institute for Biological Research
Ness-Ziona, Israel

Sindbis virus, like other mosquito-borne viruses, multiplies both in mosquitoes and in mice. However, whereas infection in mosquitoes is inapparent and lifelong, in mice it is short term and lethal.[1] The reason for these differences in the outcome of infection by the same virus is unknown. In an attempt to investigate these host-virus relationships, we applied information gained from experiments *in vitro* to *in vivo* studies in mosquitoes and mice. This information was concerned with homologous interference and its suggested causative agent observed in *Aedes aegypti* cell cultures infected by Sindbis virus.[2] Such an approach seemed appropriate, because it had been shown previously that infection in mosquito cells *in vitro* mimicked infection in intact mosquitoes.[3-8] Some observations on homologous interference in *A. aegypti* cell cultures infected by Sindbis virus will be briefly recapitulated.

In *A. aegypti* cell cultures infected with Togaviruses, there is first a rapid growth phase that culminates in peak titers of the virus. Then, after a gradual decline and leveling off in virus titers, infection enters into a persistent stage that is characterized by a constant low yield of cell-associated and released virus.[4, 5, 9] Cells in persistently infected cultures or after being subcultured are indistinguishable from cells in uninfected cultures of the same age with respect to morphologic characteristics and growth capacity. These cells are, however, resistant to superinfection by the homologous virus but not by heterologous viruses.[2, 9-11] Although this phenomenon has been studied by us since it was first observed, progress on its cause was achieved only recently. In collaboration with Dr. Stollar, the present author found that the transition to a state of cellular resistance in Sindbis virus-infected *A. aegypti* cultures coincided with the appearance in the culture of a small plaque-forming mutant, which was designated SV-S. The plaque-purified SV-S was shown to interfere with the growth of the wild strain of Sindbis virus SV-W in several invertebrate and vertebrate cell cultures.[2]

Regarding its significance for protection, at present there is no evidence to prove or disprove the role of homologous interference in protecting cells against the deleterious effects of viruses. Assuming, however, that any mechanism that arrests the spread of virus could also have a sparing effect on the host, this might apply also to homologous interference. Furthermore, its regular appearance in mosquito cell cultures at the late stage of infection appears also to strengthen such a suggestion.[2, 9-11] Following this line of reasoning, one could assume that because of the resemblance between the *in vitro* and *in vivo* behavior of Togaviruses in *A. aegypti,* the course of infection in both cases is controlled by the same mechanism, and that the absence of homologous interference in virus-infected mice might be one of the reasons for the lethality of the infection. As a first step in testing these assumptions, we studied the behavior of SV-S in *A. aegypti* mosquitoes and in mice.

Behavior of SV-S in *A. aegypti* Mosquitoes

The mosquitoes used were derived from a laboratory-reared colony maintained since 1952. The same mosquitoes also served as sources for the establishment of two cell lines in which the studies on persistent viral infection were performed. Unless otherwise indicated, the mosquitoes were infected 5–6 days after emergence either by feeding on viremic suckling mice or through membranes. In the latter case, 1 mg ATP and 0.1 ml of a lysate that was prepared from a concentrated suspension of goose erythrocytes were added per milliliter of virus suspension. ATP served to enhance feeding;[12] the lysate facilitated separation of mosquitoes that engorged from those that did not, so that we could use in all experiments only the engorged mosquitoes. A constant feeding temperature of 35° C was maintained by a thermostat-controlled incubator.

SV-S was tested in mosquitoes with respect to growth capacity and transmissibility and to its effect on the growth and transmissibility of SV-W. The growth of virus was determined by grinding groups of 20 mosquitoes in 2 ml of physiologic saline that contained 10% normal inactivated rabbit serum. The suspensions were centrifuged and passed through a 0.45 millipore filter and then were assayed on BHK cells. The capacity to transmit the virus was determined by exposing 2–3-day-old suckling mice to the bites of the infected mosquitoes. For SV-W, death of mice after symptoms and an incubation period that are characteristic for this virus indicated a positive transmission. SV-S inoculated peripherally in suckling mice produces an inapparent infection; therefore, development of resistance to challenge by SV-W subsequent to mosquito bites was considered an indication of positive virus transmission.

Comparative Growth of SV-S and SV-W in *A. aegypti* and Their Transmissibility

SV-S was acquired by mosquitoes through membrane feeding, because the virus level in the bloodstream of suckling mice was below the threshold dose required to infect mosquitoes. Infection with SV-W was performed on viremic suckling mice that had been inoculated with this virus 26 hr earlier. The growth of these viruses is illustrated in Figure 1. SV-S, like SV-W, replicated in the mosquitoes to high titers, and infection in both cases was lifelong. Regarding transmissibility, whereas SV-W was transmitted regularly up to about 30 days after infection and irregularly thereafter, SV-S was never transmitted by the infected mosquitoes (Table 1). The negative transmission of SV-S could be attributed to several factors. One of them, which currently is being investigated, is the possibility that the salivary glands are not invaded by this virus or that its level therein is so low that the amount of virus that the mosquitoes inject into the suckling mice is insufficient to initiate infection. In this context, we tested the minimal dose of SV-S that is capable to elicit protection in mice. It was found that 10–50 plaque-forming units (PFU) of SV-S inoculated subcutaneously (sc) was sufficient to confer protection against 100 mouse $LD_{50}(MLD_{50})$ of SV-W inoculated intracerebrally (ic).

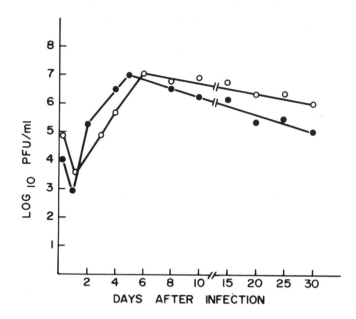

FIGURE 1. Growth of SV-S and SV-W in *A. aegypti.* Mosquitoes were infected with 10^5 PFU of SV-S (○) or SV-W (●). At the times indicated, 20 mosquitoes were triturated in 2 ml of diluting medium and subsequently titrated on BHK cells.

TABLE 1

TRANSMISSION OF VIRUSES TO SUCKLING MICE BY *A. aegypti*

Days	SV-S			SV-W	
	Mosquitoes *	Mice †	Challenge ‡	Mosquitoes	Mice
7	40	0/8	8/8	35	5/8
12	55	0/8	8/8	48	8/8
15	39	0/7	8/8	27	7/7
20	54	0/8	8/8	38	7/7
25	40	0/8	8/8	32	8/8
30	35	0/8	8/8	22	6/6

   * Number of mosquitoes fed on mice.

   † Numerator denotes number of mice that died; denominator denotes number of mice exposed to mosquito bites.

   ‡ Mice that survived after exposure to mosquito bites were challenged ic with 100–500 MLD_{50} of SV-W.

Effect of SV-S on the Growth and Transmissibility of SV-W

Mosquitoes were infected with SV-S or were mock infected with a suspension that contained all the ingredients, except the virus. Subsequently, the engorged mosquitoes were divided into two groups. In mosquitoes of the first group, the growth of SV-S was followed as long as 30 days, and these mosquitoes served as controls. The mosquitoes in the second group and those that were mock infected were superinfected with SV-W 6 days later. The growth of SV-W in the presence of SV-S is shown in FIGURE 2, and the transmission experiments are summarized in TABLE 2. The titer of SV-W in doubly infected mosquitoes was lower than that in singly infected mosquitoes of the same age.

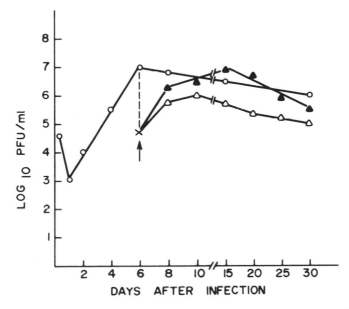

FIGURE 2. Growth of SV-W in the presence of SV-S. Mosquitoes were initially infected with SV-S (○). Six days later, some of them were superinfected with SV-W (△); controls were infected with SV-W (▲). At the times indicated, 20 mosquitoes were triturated in 2 ml of diluting medium and subsequently titrated on BHK cells.

With respect to transmission, neither of the viruses was transmitted by the doubly infected mosquitoes. This result could be due to interference in the mice or in the mosquitoes. Interference in the mice after simultaneous injection of the two viruses by mosquitoes appears to be very unlikely. We found that after simultaneous inoculation of mice with SV-S and SV-W, even when the former virus had a quantitative advantage over SV-W of a magnitude of 10^4 PFU, the outcome of infection was still determined by the latter. Interference in mosquitoes seems to be more likely; this phenomenon could occur either in the salivary glands, provided that they are invaded by SV-S, or in some other organ outside the salivary glands.

TABLE 2

TRANSMISSION OF VIRUSES TO SUCKLING MICE BY DOUBLE-INFECTED *A. aegypti*

| | First Feeding SV-S | | Second Feeding | | | | |
| | | | SV-S and SV-W | | | NMBS* and SV-W | |
Days	Mosquitoes †	Mice ‡	Mosquitoes	Mice	Challenge §	Mosquitoes	Mice
5			49	0/8	7/7		
6			40	0/7	7/7	35	3/5
7	52	0/8	60	0/8	8/8		
10	43	0/8	41	0/8	7/7	28	7/7
15	28	0/6	24	0/5	4/4		
20	32	0/8	40	0/7	7/7	30	6/8
25	41	0/8	37	0/7	6/6	16	2/4
32	37	0/7					

* Normal mouse brain suspension.

† Number of mosquitoes fed on mice.

‡ Numerator denotes number of mice that died; denominator denotes number of mice exposed to mosquito bites.

§ Mice that survived after exposure to mosquito bites were challenged ic with 100–500 MLD$_{50}$ of SV-W.

BEHAVIOR OF SV-S IN MICE

Most of the experiments were performed in suckling mice 2–3 days old. We used suckling mice instead of adults, because the outcome of infection, at least up to a certain age, was not affected by neutralizing antibodies. SV-S in mice was studied with respect to growth and virulence and to its effect on the course of infection by SV-W.

Comparative Growth and Virulence of SV-S and SV-W in Suckling Mice

Mice were inoculated either sc or intracerebrally (ic) with both viruses. At various time intervals, groups of four litters were sacrificed, their brains were harvested, and the suspensions thus obtained were titrated on BHK cells. The brain titers after inoculation of 10^5 PFU of both viruses are shown in FIGURE 3. SV-W, regardless of the routes of inoculation, always grew rapidly, and the infection produced killed the mice within 2–3 days after inoculation. SV-S, however, was lethal only after ic inoculation. The difference between the outcome of infection in sc and ic inoculated mice seems to reflect the difference in the process of infection. In sc inoculated mice, the virus multiplies slowly; maximum titers are reached only 6–7 days after inoculation, and the brain titers finally decline to undetectable levels.

Effect of Infection by SV-S on the Course of Infection by SV-W

In these experiments, the early response of suckling mice inoculated by SV-S toward superinfection by SV-W was investigated. Groups of mice were inoculated sc with 10^6 PFU of SV-S or were mock infected with phosphate-buffered saline. Subsequently, infected and control mice were divided into three groups. Mice in the first two groups were superinfected either sc or ic with 100–500 MLD_{50} of SV-W. Mice in the third group served as serum donors for neutralization experiments. The results of these experiments are presented in TABLE 3. Mice that were challenged immediately after inoculation by SV-S succumbed to infection, as did those inoculated only with SV-W. In these experiments, the route of challenge or excess dose of SV-S over that of SV-W did not affect the course of infection. Thereafter, the route and time of challenge became decisive factors in the infection outcome. Forty, 75, and 100% of the mice survived after sc challenge on Days 1, 2, and 3, respectively, after inoculation by SV-S. However, in ic challenged mice, the first signs of protection were manifested on the sixth day after inoculation by SV-S. The level of neutralizing antibodies was determined by inoculating suckling mice sc with serial dilutions

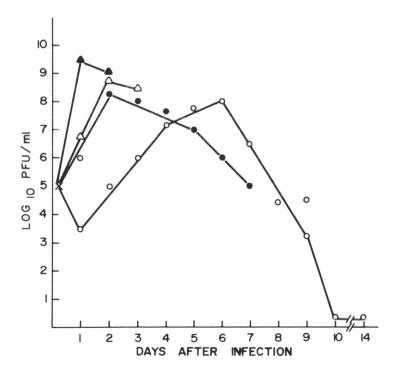

FIGURE 3. Growth of SV-S and SV-W in the brains of suckling mice. Mice were inoculated with SV-S sc (○), SV-S ic (●), SV-W sc (△), and SV-W ic (▲). At the times indicated, four litters were sacrificed, and their brain virus titers were determined on BHK cells.

TABLE 3

PROTECTION OF SUCKLING MICE BY SV-S AGAINST LETHAL DOSES OF SV-W:
EFFECT OF THE ROUTES AND TIME OF CHALLENGE BY SV-W *

| | Challenge | | | | NI | Control | |
Days	sc †	% ‡	ic	% ‡	Log §	sc	ic
0	12/12	0	10/10	0		8/8	8/8
1	7/12	40	10/10	0			
2	4/16	75	12/12	0			
3	0/16	100	16/16	0		8/8	8/8
4	0/16	100	10/10	0	UD ¶	8/8	8/8
5	0/10	100	15/15	0		8/8	8/8
6	0/15	100	12/16	25		8/8	
7			10/15	34	1.2		8/8
8			8/24	67	2.0		
9			0/12	100			8/8
10			0/16	100			16/16

* Mice were inoculated sc with SV-S. On the days indicated in column 1, they were challenged sc or ic with 100–500 MLD$_{50}$ of SV-W.

† Numerator denotes number of mice that died; denominator denotes number of mice challenged.

‡ Percent protected.

§ Mice inoculated with SV-S were bled, and their sera were tested for neutralizing antibodies, expressed as a neutralization index (NI).

¶ Undetectable.

of SV-W mixed with a constant 1:5 dilution of sera from SV-S inoculated mice and was expressed as the log neutralizing index. Neutralizing antibodies were first detected in the sera of suckling mice that were inoculated with SV-S 7 days earlier. Consequently, the early protection against sc challenge by SV-W was afforded in the absence of detectable neutralizing antibodies.

MECHANISM OF PROTECTION

The above results prompted us to test whether protection could be attributed to an acid-resistant antiviral substance or to interference by SV-S with the growth of SV-W, which would be analogous to the protection demonstrated in cultured mosquito cells [2] and to a lesser degree in intact *A. aegypti* mosquitoes (FIGURE 2 and TABLE 2).

Test for an Acid-Resistant Antiviral Substance

Mice were inoculated with SV-S or were mock infected as before. Three and 14 days later, when the brain titers were high or had decreased to undetectable levels, respectively, eight to 10 mice were sacrificed, and the harvested brain suspensions were then divided into three portions. The first portion was titrated for its virus content; the two other portions, one of which was not treated further and the other, which was then acidified, were inoculated sc into suckling mice. The mice thus inoculated were challenged sc 3 days later with 100–500 MLD$_{50}$ of SV-W. As shown in TABLE 4, only brain suspensions that contained the virus conferred protection, whereas the same suspension after being inactivated failed to do so. Therefore, protection due to an acid-resistant substance could be excluded.

TABLE 4

PROTECTION OF MICE BY UNTREATED OR ACID-TREATED BRAIN SUSPENSIONS
FROM SV-S-INOCULATED MICE AGAINST LETHAL DOSES OF SV-W *

Days	SV-S PFU/ml	Challenge After Inoculation with: †			
		UIMBS	TIMBS	UNMBS	TNMBS
3	6.0	2/16 ‡	16/16	16/16	16/16
14	<1.0	16/16	16/16	16/16	16/16

* Mice were inoculated with SV-S, their brains were harvested, and their virus content was titrated, as indicated in columns 1 and 2, respectively. Subsequently, the suspensions were inoculated into suckling mice sc, which 14 days later were challenged with 100–500 MLD$_{50}$ of SV-W.

† UIMBS and TIMBS, untreated and acid-treated infectious mouse brain suspensions, respectively; UNMBS and TNMBS, untreated and acid-treated normal mouse brain suspensions, respectively.

‡ Numerator denotes number of mice that died; denominator denotes number of mice challenged.

Protection Due to Growth Interference

Mice were inoculated with SV-S or were mock infected as before. Three days later, when infection was already well established, the mice were superinfected either sc or ic with 1000–5000 MLD$_{50}$ of SV-W. Subsequently, at various time intervals, four litters from each of the infected groups were sacrificed, and the virus titers in their brains were determined on BHK cells. The results of these experiments are shown in FIGURE 4. Superinfection by the sc route resulted in suppression of the growth of SV-W to levels undetectable by the method employed in these experiments. Consequently, the outcome of infection was the same as that in mice inoculated only with SV-S, that is, nonlethal. On the other hand, in ic challenged mice, SV-S was outgrown by SV-W; therefore, the outcome of infection was determined by the latter; that is, it was lethal.

These results show that the early protection by SV-S against lethal doses of SV W inoculated sc (TABLE 3) was due to interference by the former virus with the growth of SV-W.

SUMMARY

A mutant of the Sindbis virus SV-S was found to interfere with the regular course of infection by the wild strain of the virus SV-W in *A. aegypti* mosquitoes and in suckling mice. In mosquitoes, this result was manifested by a reduced titer of SV-W in the presence of SV-S and by a failure of the mosquitoes

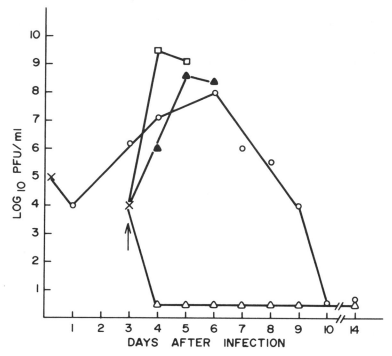

FIGURE 4. Growth of SV-W in the brains of suckling mice in the presence of SV-S. Mice were initially inoculated sc with 10^5 PFU of SV-S ($\bigcirc$). Three days later, some of them were superinfected with 5000 MLD_{50} of SV-W sc ($\triangle$) or ic ($\square$). Control mice were infected sc with SV-W ($\blacktriangle$). At the times indicated, four litters were sacrificed, and their brain virus titers were determined on BHK cells.

to transmit SV-W. In the brains of suckling mice, in the presence of SV-S, the growth of sc inoculated SV-W was suppressed, and as a result, the usually lethal course of infection by this virus was converted into a nonlethal one.

REFERENCES

1. CASALS, J. 1957. The arthropod-borne group of animal viruses. Trans. N.Y. Acad. Sci. 19(3): 219–231.
2. PELEG, J. & V. STOLLAR. 1974. Homologous interference in Aedes aegypti cell cultures infected with Sindbis virus. Arch. Ges. Virusforsch. 45: 309–318.
3. FILSHIE, B. K. & J. REHACEK. 1968. Studies of the morphology of Murray Valley encephalitis and Japanese encephalitis viruses growing in cultured mosquito cells. Virology 34: 435–443.
4. PELEG, J. 1968. Growth of arboviruses in monolayers from subcultured mosquito embryo cells. Virology 35: 617–619.
5. PELEG, J. 1969. Inapparent persistent virus infection in continuously grown Aedes aegypti mosquito cells. J. Gen. Virol. 5: 463–471.
6. STEVENS, T. M. 1970. Arbovirus replication in mosquito cell lines (Singh) grown in monolayer or suspension culture. Proc. Soc. Exp. Biol. Med. 134: 356–361.

7. RAGHOW, R. S., T. D. C. GRACE, B. K. FILSHIE, W. BARTLEY & L. DALGARNO. 1973. Ross River virus replication in cultured mosquito and mammalian cells: virus growth and correlated ultrastructural changes. J. Gen. Virol. **21:** 109–122.

8. DAVEY, M. W. & L. DALGARNO. 1974. Semliki Forest virus replication in cultured Aedes albopictus cells: studies on the establishment of persistence. J. Gen. Virol. **24:** 453–463.

9. ARTSOB, H. & L. SPENCE. 1974. Persistent infection of mosquito cell lines with vesicular stomatitis virus. Acta Virol. **18:** 331–340.

10. PELEG, J. 1972. Studies on the behaviour of arboviruses in an Aedes aegypti mosquito cell line (Peleg). Arch. Ges. Virusforsch. **37:** 54–61.

11. STOLLAR, V. & T. E. SHENK. 1973. Homologous viral interference in Aedes albopictus culture chronically infected with Sindbis virus. J. Virol. **11:** 592–595.

12. GALUN, R. 1967. Feeding stimuli and artificial feeding. Bull. World Health Org. **36:** 590–593.

OBSERVATIONS ON *AEDES ALBOPICTUS* CELL CULTURES PERSISTENTLY INFECTED WITH SINDBIS VIRUS *

Victor Stollar, Thomas E. Shenk,† Rose Koo,
Akira Igarashi, and R. Walter Schlesinger

*Department of Microbiology
College of Medicine and Dentistry of New Jersey
Rutgers Medical School
Piscataway, New Jersey 08854*

INTRODUCTION

The insect-transmitted togaviruses are remarkable and differ from most other viruses that can cause disease in man in that they can replicate in host organisms as widely apart phylogenetically as mosquitos and man. In turn, many of these viruses are important pathogenic agents for man and other mammalian species but apparently not for the mosquito. In attempts to understand the properties of these viruses and how they replicate, many studies have been performed with togaviruses in cell culture, generally of vertebrate cells, such as chick or hamster. In view of the fact that an important part of their "life cycle" occurs in the insect vector, our knowledge of these viruses will necessarily remain incomplete until we know much more about their relationship to the insect host. This point seems especially important, because, at least with the alphaviruses (group-A togaviruses), the outcome of infection is generally very different in mosquito and vertebrate cells. Whereas most vertebrate cells are rapidly killed by alphaviruses, such as Sindbis or Semliki Forest viruses, infected mosquito cultures, in the face of high yields, fail to show any cytopathic effect. Furthermore, it seems likely that important phenotypic host modifications of the virus occur in the insect host, the vertebrate host, or both, which might conceivably influence the properties of the virus for the alternate host. Finally, one or the other host may select for certain types of genetic variants, which, again, might influence the outcome of virus infection in the alternate host.

With the availability of established lines of mosquito cells, togaviruses can now be examined readily both in insect cells and in vertebrate cells, which thus makes the entire life cycle of the togaviruses accessible to study, at least if one speaks of *in vitro* systems.

The system we have chosen to study is that of Sindbis virus in the *Aedes albopictus* cell line of Singh. In these experiments, we address ourselves to some comparative aspects of Sindbis virus replication in mosquito and vertebrate cells and to the characterization of the *A. albopictus* cells, which are chronically infected with Sindbis virus-*A. albopictus* (SV-C).

* Supported by Grant GB37707 from the National Science Foundation, by Grant AI-11290 from the National Institute of Allergy and Infectious Diseases, and by the United States-Japan Cooperative Medical Science Program through United States Public Health Service Grant AI-05920.

† Present address: Department of Biochemistry, Stanford University School of Medicine, Stanford University Medical Center, Stanford, Calif. 94305.

214

MATERIALS AND METHODS

The primary chick fibroblasts, the BHK-21 cells, and the *A. albopictus* (Singh) cell cultures have all been previously described,[1] as have the plaque-purified stocks of Sindbis virus (SV-W) and eastern equine encephalitis virus (EEEV).[2] SV-BP-18 is a stock obtained after 18 serial undiluted passages in BHK cells.[3] Uncloned Sindbis virus obtained from chronically infected cultures is referred to as SV-C and was taken several months after the initial infection. Chronically infected cultures of *A. albopictus* cells are referred to as *A. albopictus* (SV-C). Cloned virus was derived from SV-C by plaque purification followed by growth of small stocks, in each instance on BHK cell monolayers at 34° C. Plaque assays of SV and EEEV were performed on BHK-21 cells at 34° C, unless otherwise indicated.[4]

The assays for sialic acid and for sialyl transferase activity are according to Warren [5] and Grimes and Burge,[6] respectively. Sucrose-D_2O gradients were used for isopycnic centrifugation of virus.[3] Labeling of viral RNA was with [3H]uridine, performed in the presence of actinomycin D, and double-stranded RNA was identified by resistance to RNase.[1] Further details and the procedures used for sucrose gradient analysis of the viral RNA have been provided elsewhere.[1, 3]

The methods used for preparation of viral antiserum, for virus neutralization, and for the complementation tests with temperature-sensitive mutants have already been described.[4] Identification of *ts* mutants as RNA+ was based on the ability to synthesize viral RNA at 39.5° C.[4, 7]

RESULTS

Growth of Sindbis Virus in Cultured A. albopictus Cells

Cultured *A. albopictus* cells have been shown to support the replication of several group-A togaviruses, including Sindbis, Semliki Forest, Ross River, and Chikungunya viruses.[8-11] With both Sindbis and Semliki Forest viruses, the kinetics of viral replication in mosquito cells at 28° C were similar to those observed in vertebrate cell cultures at 37° C, and for each virus, yields of 10^8 PFU/ml or higher have been reported. FIGURE 1 illustrates a typical growth curve of SV in *A. albopictus* cells. In no case was any cytopathic effect observed in the infected mosquito cell cultures; instead, virus production continued, although at a slower rate than that observed initially, and chronically infected cultures were produced.[2]

Comparisons of Sindbis Virus Grown in Chick Embryo Cells and in Mosquito Cells

Interest in the comparative study of togaviruses in mosquito and vertebrate cells derives from two main considerations. First, the outcome of infection is very different in the two systems. Second, such studies might be useful for examining the role and influence of host modifications on viral properties and functions.

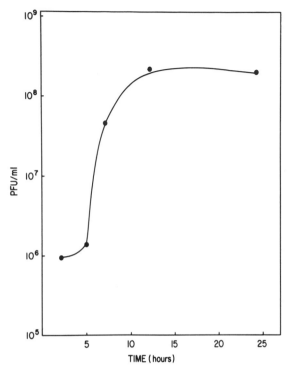

FIGURE 1. Growth of Sindbis virus in *A. albopictus* cells at 28° C. The input multiplicity was approximately 30 PFU/cell.

A recent report has shown that several days after *A. albopictus* cells were infected with Sindbis virus, the virus population obtained from such cultures was distinctly heterogeneous with respect to size.[12] At 5 days, not only were normal-sized particles (62 nm in diameter) found, but also two other classes of smaller particles (52 and 39 nm in diameter) were found. By that time, in fact, the smaller particles were far more numerous than the larger or normal-sized particles. Apart from size, the shape and general morphologic features of the smaller particles resembled those of the normal virions.

Experiments in our laboratory have provided further evidence for a physically heterogeneous virus population from infected *A. albopictus* cells again increasing with time after infection. In these experiments, medium was harvested, clarified by low-speed centrifugation, and centrifuged to equilibrium on sucrose-D$_2$O gradients. Fractions were collected and assayed for infective virus. Whereas virus from infected chick or BHK cells uniformly banded at a density close to 1.20 g/cc, virus from mosquito cells was distributed in a much more heterogeneous fashion throughout the gradient (FIGURE 2). Virus released between 1 and 18 hr after infection showed a main peak at 1.20 g/cc, along with heavier and lighter peaks at 1.23 and 1.17 g/cc, respectively. Virus released from cells between 22 and 40 hr exhibited a basically similar pattern. The last part of FIGURE 2 illustrates the gradient pattern of virus released from

54 to 72 hr after infection. In this case, the 1.20-g/cc peak was much smaller, and a band between 1.16 and 1.17 g/cc was the predominant one.

In other experiments, the exact banding pattern of virus from mosquito cells has varied from those shown in FIGURE 2, but in each case, the distribution of virus, in contrast to virus from vertebrate cells, has been disperse and heterogeneous.

Although there is not yet any direct evidence, it appears likely that some relationship exists between the variability in the density of virus particles that we have seen and the variability in size described by Brown and Gliedman [12] and referred to above. How these changes in size and density of viral particles

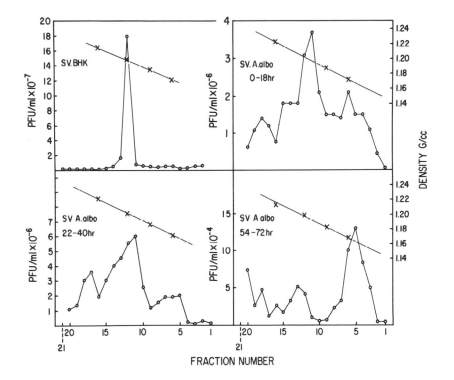

FIGURE 2. Sucrose-D_2O equilibrium gradients of Sindbis virus from BHK cells and *A. albopictus* cells.

BHK cells were infected at an input multiplicity of approximately 50 PFU/cell and maintained at 37° C. Culture medium was harvested after 22 hr.

A. albopictus cells were also infected with an input multiplicity of 50 PFU/cell, but the medium was changed several times so as to collect the virus yields between 1 and 18 hr, 22 and 40 hr, and 54 and 72 hr.

All virus samples were extracted once with Genesolv-D® (trichlorotrifluoroethane) and clarified by low-speed centrifugation.

A sample (0.8 ml) of each preparation was then layered over 11.2 ml of 14–40% sucrose (w/w) in TNE buffer [3] made up in D_2O. Centrifugation was in the SW-41 rotor at 10° C for 15 hr at 31,000 rpm. Fractions were then collected (0.6 ml) and assayed for plaque formation on BHK-21 cell monolayers.

occur is not clear, nor is it evident at this time if and to what degree such changes might affect various biologic properties of the virus.

Another approach we have employed in comparative studies with Sindbis virus has been to examine the sialic acid content of SV grown in vertebrate and mosquito cells. In contrast to the viral RNA and polypeptides, there is good evidence that certain viral envelope components (lipid and the carbohydrate residues of glycoproteins) are specified not by the viral genome but, instead, by the infected host cells.[13, 14] For example, it is thought that the sugar residues are added to viral glycoproteins by preexisting or normal host glycosyl transferase enzymes. Because it is known that most invertebrate cells lack sialic acid,[15, 16] its absence in virus grown in mosquito cells could be considered a strong confirmation of the above hypothesis.

TABLE 1

SIALIC ACID CONTENT OF MEDIA AND CELLS

Material Assayed *	Medium or Packed Cells (μM/ml)
Fetal calf serum	
Not dialyzed	5.5
Dialyzed	4.8
4% Bovine serum albumin (BSA)	0.01
MM medium with 5% fetal calf serum (FCS)	0.32
	0.37
MM medium † without serum	<0.01
BHK cells grown with 10% serum	0.37
Overnight with 0.1% serum	0.37
Overnight with 0.2% BSA	0.32
A. albopictus cells grown with 5% FCS	0.17
Overnight with 0.2% FCS	0.09
A. albopictus cells grown without serum	
In suspension cultures	<0.01
As monolayers	<0.01

* Cells to be assayed for sialic acid were harvested by scraping, then washed three to five times in PBS, and finally pelleted at 1200 rpm for 5 min.
† Medium of Mitsuhashi and Maramorosch.[26]

The data in TABLE 1 show that normal cultured A. albopictus cells lack sialic acid. Some uncertainty arose in the initial experiments, which appeared to indicate, even after thorough washing with phosphate-buffered saline, that the A. albopictus cell pellets generally contained some sialic acid. A likely explanation appeared to be that its presence was due to contamination by glycoproteins from the serum component of the medium. This idea was supported by the observation that the apparent sialic acid level of the A. albopictus cells was reduced if the serum content of the medium was lowered. However, our finding that A. albopictus cells would multiply for several weeks in medium that did not contain serum (although more slowly) enabled us to demonstrate even more convincingly that these cells contained no sialic acid.

The lack of covalently bound sialic acid in mosquito cells might be attributed to, or associated with, the absence of sialyl transferase, the enzyme

TABLE 2

SIALYL TRANSFERASE ACTIVITY IN CHICK AND MOSQUITO CELLS *

Incubation Mixture	Source of Enzyme and Incubation Temperature		
	CEF, 37° C	Λ. albopictus, 37° C	Λ. albopictus, 28° C
Complete	5422 †	29	11
—Acceptor	607	37	25
—Enzyme	0	NT ‡	78

* The enzyme preparation from chick or *A. albopictus* cells was as described by Grimes and Burge.[6] The enzyme reaction was prepared as described by Grimes[27] and contained [³H]CMP sialic acid and desialylated fetuin as the acceptor. After a 2-hr incubation, the trichloroacetic acid- (TCA) precipitable counts ([³H]sialic acid in the form of glycoprotein) were measured.

† Numbers represent acid precipitable cpm.

‡ Not tested.

that transfers the sialic acid moiety onto the terminal position of many glycoproteins. TABLE 2 demonstrates that this enzyme activity, which was found in chick cells, could not be found in mosquito cells whether the assay was performed at 28 or 37° C. Because neither sialic acid nor sialyl transferase could be found in *A. albopictus* cells, it appeared likely that SV grown in these cells would also lack sialic acid.

The approach used to test for viral sialic acid content was to grow virus in the presence of [1-¹⁴C]glucosamine (a precursor of sialic acid in vertebrate cells),[17] purify the virus, then treat it with neuraminidase, and finally measure the release of trichloroacetic acid (TCA) -soluble radioactivity. Sialic acid residues in glycoproteins would be TCA precipitable, but, after release by neuraminidase, they would be acid soluble.

TABLE 3 shows that in glucosamine labeled SV grown in chick or BHK cells,

TABLE 3

RELEASE OF ACID-SOLUBLE RADIOACTIVITY FROM GLUCOSAMINE-LABELED SINDBIS VIRUS

Virus Origin	BHK Cells		Chick Embryo Fibroblasts		*A. albopictus* Cells	
Neuraminidase used	C *	P †	C	P	C	P
TCA-precipitable cpm added	3014	3147	3074	3354	5623	6212
Acid soluble + enzyme cpm Released	307	422	312	378	38	86
— enzyme	50	49	42	47	35	31
Δ	257	373	270	331	3	55
Input cpm released (%)	8.3	11.9	8.8	9.9	<0.1	0.9

* *Vibrio cholerae* neuraminidase.

† *Clostridium perfringens* neuraminidase.

neuraminidase treatment released about 9% of the input TCA-precipitable radioactivity as acid-soluble counts. Two different neuraminidases (from *Clostridium perfringens* and *Vibrio cholerae*) gave quite similar results. In contrast, little, if any acid-soluble radioactivity was released from SV labeled in a similar fashion but grown in mosquito cells. Again, the result was similar with the two neuraminidase preparations.

We are currently examining the possible biologic implications of sialic acid absence. Kennedy has already reported that 99% of the sialic acid can be removed from Semliki Forest virus without any loss of hemagglutinating or infectious activity.[18] In studies that compared the antigenic properties of SV grown in mosquito cells with that grown in chick cells,[19] we could not detect any significant differences. The available evidence thus indicates that the presence or absence of sialic acid has no demonstrable effect on any biologic properties of the alphaviruses. In view of the strong negative charge of sialic acid moieties, this observation appears to be rather surprising.

Cultures of A. albopictus Cells Persistently Infected with Sindbis Virus

As already noted, infection of cultured *A. albopictus* cells with Sindbis virus does not lead to cell death, as occurs with vertebrate cells, but, instead, to chronically infected cultures. The following section describes experiments that have resulted from studies on such cultures.

Cell cultures chronically infected with Sindbis virus (*A. albopictus,* SV-C) were assayed periodically for infectious virus in the medium, and one of the first and rather striking observations was that after a period of several months, the virus from these cultures gave rise to small plaques easily distinguishable from those made by wild-type virus (FIGURE 3).

Confirmation that the virus that caused the small plaques was, indeed, Sindbis virus and not a contaminant was sought by serologic tests with an antiserum produced in a rabbit against wild-type SV (SV-W). A neutralization test that employed the plaque reduction method revealed effective neutralization of the SV-C, although the concentration of serum needed to reduce the number of plaques by 50% was higher than that needed for SV-W (FIGURE 4).

Peleg has studied *A. aegypti* cells persistently infected with Semliki Forest virus (SFV) and has shown that such cultures are resistant to superinfection with the homologous virus but will support the replication of a related but heterologous virus (eastern equine encephalitis virus, another group-A togavirus). In a similar system, with cultures of *A. aegypti* chronically infected with Sindbis virus, evidence was presented to suggest that SV-S, a small plaque mutant derived from the chronically infected cultures, plays an important role in the resistance to superinfection with the wild-type Sindbis virus.[20]

The phenomenon of homologous interference to superinfection was also found in cultures of *A. albopictus* (SV-C) and is illustrated in FIGURE 5. Whereas normal cultures of *A. albopictus* supported the replication of EEEV and SV, cultures of *A. albopictus* (SV-C) supported only the growth of EEEV. Because the SV-C cultures gave rise to small plaque virus, the endogenously produced virus (SV-C) could easily be distinguished from the superinfecting virus. We thus were able to show that in cultures of *A. albopictus* (SV-C),

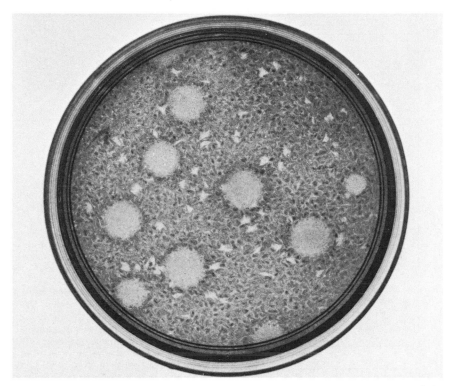

FIGURE 3. Plaques produced on a BHK-21 cell monolayer by SV-W and by Sindbis virus from a chronically infected culture of *A. albopictus* (SV-C). SV-W produces large round plaques that average 8 mm in diameter. SV-C produces irregularly shaped plaques that measure 1–2 mm. Monolayers were stained with neutral red 72 hr after addition of virus.

FIGURE 4. Neutralization of SV-C, SV-W, and eastern equine encephalitis virus (EEEV) with antiserum produced against SV-W. Percentage of surviving PFU is the ratio of the PFU remaining after treatment with immune serum to that present after treatment with the same dilution of preimmune serum. One hundred percent survival at a 5^{-6} dilution of serum was 438 PFU for SV-W, 169 PFU for SV-C, and 166 PFU for EEEV. ○, SV-W; ●, SV-C; ×, EEEV.

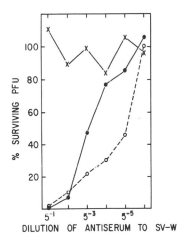

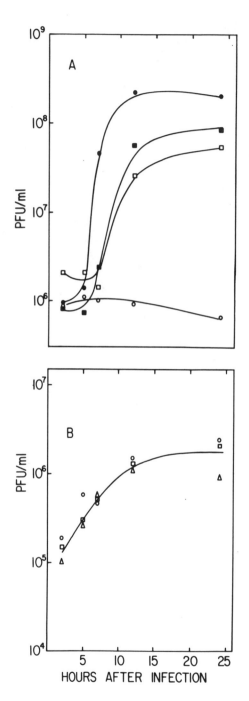

FIGURE 5. Growth of SV-W and EEE in normal and SV-C cultures of *A. albopictus* cells and the effect of superinfection on the production of SV-C.

A: Monolayer cultures of normal *A. albopictus* cells were infected with SV-W (●) or EEE (■) at input multiplicities of 20 and 80 PFU/cell, respectively. Chronically infected cultures were infected with either SV-W (○) or EEE (□) at the same input multiplicities. Virus was adsorbed for 1 hr at room temperature, after which time the cultures were washed three times with phosphate-buffered saline. Medium was added, the cultures were incubated at 28° C, and samples were taken at the indicated times for plaque assay. Plaque assays were performed at 34° C on monolayers of BHK-21 cells.

B: The production of SV-C in SV-C cultures of *A. albopictus* cells was monitored. ○, not superinfected; □, superinfected with SV-W; △, superinfected with EEE; at input multiplicities of 0.02 and 0.08 PFU/cell, respectively.

there was absolutely no increase in the titer of SV-W after superinfection with this virus.

Next, the question could be asked, "At which stage in viral replication is the superinfecting virus blocked?" We, therefore, examined the synthesis of viral double-stranded RNA (dsRNA) in normal *A. albopictus* cells and in cultures of *A. albopictus* (SV-C) after infection (or superinfection) with SV-W or with EEEV. Normal *A. albopictus* cell cultures infected with SV-W or with EEEV contained, as expected, a single peak of dsRNA, at 22S (FIGURE 6). In contrast, the SV-C cells, which had not been superinfected, contained hetero-geneous dsRNA, with only a small peak at 22S and with the major peak at about 12S (FIGURE 7). Superinfection with SV-W did not alter this pattern at all, which suggests that the interference occurs at an early stage or at least prior to viral RNA replication. We have not yet, however, ruled out a block at the

FIGURE 6. Double-stranded RNA in normal cultures of *A. albopictus* cells infected with SV-W or EEE. Uninfected cultures (●) or cultures infected with SV-W (○) or EEE (□) (input multiplicities of 20 and 80 PFU/cell, respectively) were la-beled with [5-³H]uridine (26.5 Ci/mM, 10 μCi/ml) in the presence of actinomycin D (4 μg/ml) from 6 to 11 hr after infection. Cells were then harvested, and RNA was extracted. The RNA species were resolved by centrifugation in 5–20% linear sucrose gradients (27,000 rpm, 18.5 hr, 4° C, Spinco SW-27 rotor). Each fraction was then treated with ribonuclease A, and the residual acid-precipitable ra-dioactivity was measured. These preparations were centrifuged at the same time in different gradients and were drawn together by superimpos-ing their marker RNA.

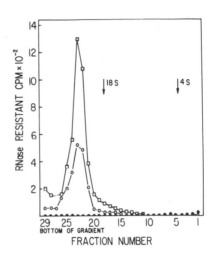

adsorption stage. When *A. albopictus* cells (SV-C) were superinfected with EEEV, we noted with interest an increase not only in 22S dsRNA but also in 12S dsRNA.

The Small Plaque Mutants of Sindbis Virus from Cultures of A. albopictus (SV-C) Are Temperature Sensitive

Further study of SV-C showed not only that it was mutant with respect to plaque size but also that it was temperature sensitive.

Whereas SV-W formed plaques equally well at 39.5, 34, and 28° C, SV-C with a titer of more than 4×10^6 PFU/ml at 28 or 34° C had a titer of 8.2×10^4 when plaqued at 37° C and less than 10 at 39.5° C (TABLE 4). Furthermore, as shown in FIGURE 8, SV-C, which grew more slowly in chick

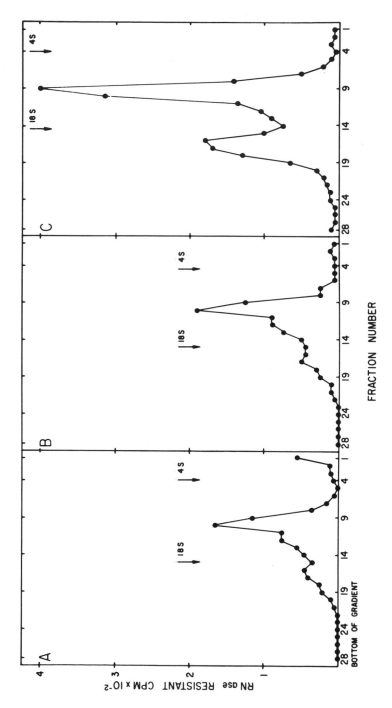

FIGURE 7. Double-standed RNA in SV-C cultures not superinfected (A) or superinfected with SV-W (B) or EEEV (C). All procedures were as described in the legend to FIGURE 6.

FIGURE 8. Growth curves of SV-W and SV-C in chicken cells incubated at 28, 34, 37, and 39.5° C. Prior to infection, phosphate-buffered saline and viral inocula were heated to 42° C. The viral inocula were warmed for only 2 min to prevent inactivation. The chicken monolayers were washed once with PBS and then were infected with either SV-C or SV-W at a multiplicity of infection of 1 PFU/cell. After adsorption for 1 hr at 39.5° C, the inocula were removed, the plates were washed three times with prewarmed PBS, and prewarmed medium was added. Plates were then incubated at the appropriate temperatures, and samples for plaque assay were taken at the times indicated. SV-W: ○, 28° C; □, 34° C; △, 37° C; ◇, 39.5° C. SV-C: ●, 28° C; ■, 34° C; ▲, 37° C; ◆, 39.5° C.

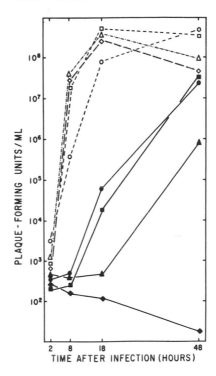

embryo cells than SV-W at all temperatures and gave yields at 48 hr of more than 10^7 PFU/ml at either 28 or 34° C, gave no yield at 39.5° C. In contrast, the yields of SV-W from infected chick cells were similar at all temperatures tested.

It was possible, however, that cells infected with SV-C and maintained at 39.5° C did produce progeny viral particles but that they were noninfectious.

TABLE 4

TEMPERATURE-SENSITIVE PLAQUE FORMATION ON BHK CELL MONOLAYERS BY SINDBIS VIRUS FROM CHRONICALLY INFECTED CULTURES OF *A. albopictus* *

Incubation Temperature ° C	SV-C (PFU/ml)	EOP †	SV-W † (PFU/ml)	EOP †
28	4.1×10^6	1.0	1.6×10^8	1.0
34	4.4×10^6	1.1	1.7×10^8	1.1
37	8.2×10^4	2.0×10^{-2}	1.7×10^8	1.1
39.5	< 10	$< 2.4 \times 10^{-6}$	1.6×10^8	1.0

* Adsorption was at 28° C, after which the cultures were incubated at the temperatures indicated for 48 hr.

† Values represent the titer at the indicated temperature divided by the titer at 28° C.

TABLE 5

FREQUENCY OF REVERTANTS IN STOCKS OF SINDBIS VIRUS MUTANT CLONES *

SV-C Clone	Frequency of Revertants
SV-C-2	$< 10^{-7}$
SV-C-4	$< 10^{-5}$
SV-C-8	6.7×10^{-5}
SV-C-13	3×10^{-6}
SV-C-16	$< 10^{-6}$
SV-C-19	$< 10^{-6}$

* Cloned virus was obtained from well-isolated plaques, and a portion of this virus was then grown to a stock. Both the initial plaque purification and the growth of the stock were in BHK-21 cells at 34° C.

† Frequency of ts^+ revertants is the ratio of the titer measured at 39.5° C to that measured at 34° C.

To test this hypothesis, BHK cells infected with SV-W or SV-C were maintained at permissive and nonpermissive temperatures, and the culture medium was tested after 24 hr for viral hemagglutinin. SV-W produced viral hemagglutinin equally well at both temperatures, whereas SV-C produced hemagglutinin only at 34° C, the permissive temperature. Thus, if any particles were produced by cells infected with SV-C and maintained at 39.5° C, they must have lacked both infectivity and hemagglutinating activity.

To obtain further information about the temperature-sensitive block in SV-C, 20 plaque isolates derived from SV-C were selected and grown to stocks in BHK cells. These individual virus clones were designated SV-C-1, SV-C-2, and so on. Like the uncloned SV-C, all stocks of the SV-C clones exhibited a low frequency of ts^+ revertants (ratio of titer measured at 39.5° C to that measured at 34° C). In some cases, there was no detectable plaque formation at 34° C, and in all cases, the frequency of revertants was less than 7×10^{-5}. Representative results are shown in TABLE 5. However, after serial undiluted passage several times in BHK cells, there was a significant rise in the frequency of ts^+ revertants, which increased in several cases up to 10^{-2} or even higher (TABLE 6). In most cases, the ts^+ revertants remained mutant with respect to plaque size; that is, they continued to produce only small plaques.

TABLE 6

ACCUMULATION OF REVERTANTS BY SERIAL UNDILUTED PASSAGE
IN BHK CELLS AT 34° C

SV-C Clone	Frequency of Revertants *	
	Passage 2	Passage 4
SV-C-2	4.4×10^{-6}	1.6×10^{-4}
SV-C-4	5.0×10^{-3}	5.9×10^{-2}
SV-C-8	7.5×10^{-4}	6.3×10^{-2}
SV-C-13	8.5×10^{-4}	1.0×10^{-3}
SV-C-16	1.9×10^{-4}	7.7×10^{-2}
SV-C-19	5.6×10^{-4}	8.5×10^{-2}

* Frequency of revertants is as described in the footnote to TABLE 5.

Next, complementation tests were performed with various combinations of the SV-C clones. In no case was complementation demonstrated between any of the SV-C clones (not shown here, but see Reference 4). Two *ts* mutants of Sindbis virus (*ts*-4 and *ts*-10), kindly sent to us by Dr. Elmer Pfefferkorn, did exhibit complementation, as expected. The failure to detect complementation with the SV-C clones could be explained if each of the clones tested were mutant in the same cistron or if each of these clones were mutant in more than one cistron.

Each of the 20 SV-C clones was then tested for its ability to make viral RNA at the nonpermissive temperature. Nineteen of them were able to do so and thus were designated RNA+. Representative results are provided in TABLE 7. The one exception was SV-C-2.

Further study of several SV-C clones showed that each one tested was much more thermally labile at 60° C than was SV-W. This finding was true of three RNA+ *ts* mutants (SV-C-8, SV-C-13, SV-C-16) and of SV-C-2, which was RNA− (FIGURE 9). If increased thermal lability is considered an indication

TABLE 7

RNA SYNTHESIS PHENOTYPE OF SINDBIS VIRUS VARIANTS

Sindbis Virus	SA * at 39.5° C: SA at 34° C	RNA Synthesis Phenotype
SV-W	0.84	+
SV-C-2	<0.01	−
SV-C-4	0.34	+
SV-C-8	0.39	+
SV-C-13	0.52	+
SV-C-16	0.53	+
SV-C-19	1.03	+

* Specific activity (SA) is expressed as counts per minute per absorbancy at 260 nm. The experimental details are described in MATERIALS AND METHODS.

of an alteration in one of the structural proteins, at least in SV-C-2, it seems likely that there are mutations in at least two different cistrons, one that involves a structural protein and one that involves a protein essential for viral RNA synthesis.

Defective-Interfering Particles of Sindbis Virus

It has now been demonstrated in several laboratories that serial undiluted passage of SV in BHK-21 cells or in chick embryo fibroblasts leads to the generation of defective-interfering (DI) viral particles.[21-23] Their presence may be signaled by a progressive fall or a cyclic variation in the titer of infectious virus and/or by the appearance of smaller species of intracellular viral RNA (both single stranded and double stranded) than are seen in cells infected with the wild-type virus (SV-W).[22]

Evidence was sought for the similar production of DI particles of SV in *A. albopictus* cells. However, even after more than 20–30 undiluted passages,

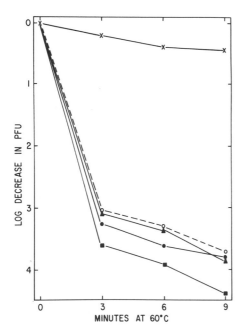

FIGURE 9. Inactivation kinetics of wild-type Sindbis virus (SV-W) ($\times$) and Sindbis virus mutant (SV-C) clones at 60° C. Undiluted 0.6-ml portions of SV-W and selected SV-C clones were heated in a 60° C water bath. Samples were withdrawn at the indicated times, rapidly chilled, and assayed for surviving PFU. $\bigcirc$, SV-C-2; $\blacktriangle$, SV-C-16; $\bullet$, SV-C-8; $\blacksquare$, SV-C-13.

there was no significant fall in the level of infectious virus, no cyclic variation in the yield, and no consistent sign of viral dsRNA (RNase resistant) smaller than the 22S dsRNA found in *A. albopictus* cells infected with SV-W (FIGURE 6).

Nevertheless, some indirect evidence for the presence of defective particles in mosquito cells has already been presented in FIGURE 7, in which it was shown that chronically infected cultures of *A. albopictus* cells contain not only 22S dsRNA but also the 12S species. Other experiments with *A. albopictus* (SV-C) cultures suggest that the amount of 12S relative to the 22S species tends to increase with time after the initial infection. If one can extrapolate from the experimental findings in BHK-21 and chick cells, the appearance of smaller dsRNA strongly suggests either the presence of defective particles or at least of defective but replicating viral genomes; the latter would perhaps be maintained by passage from mother to daughter cell.

Some extremely interesting results have been obtained recently in experiments conducted to compare the effects of SV-DI particles in vertebrate and mosquito cells. BHK-21 or *A. albopictus* cells were infected with SV-W or SV-BP-18 (obtained after 18 serial undiluted passages of SV-W in BHK-21 cells), and the viral dsRNA was examined. As expected, when either BHK or *A. albopictus* cells were infected with SV-W, only 22S dsRNA was found. Also, as shown elsewhere,[22, 24] when BHK cells were infected with SV-BP-18 or similar stocks, both 22S and 12S dsRNA were demonstrated. However, the finding that *A. albopictus* cells infected with SV-BP-18 contained only 22S dsRNA and no 12S dsRNA (FIGURE 10) was surprising. This result, however, did correlate with other experiments that showed that although BHK-21 cells infected with SV-W gave significantly higher yields of infectious virus than did SV-BP-18, *A. albopictus* cells infected with SV-W or SV-BP-18 gave similar yields (not shown). Thus, it appears that perhaps the DI particles present in SV-BP-18 are inert and perform no functions in mosquito cells. Alternatively, the lesion responsible for the defectiveness in hamster cells might be repaired at some point during the infection of the mosquito cell or perhaps the genome that is defective in the BHK-21 cell is seen as normal in the new environment of the mosquito cell.

DISCUSSION

The observations above provide evidence that the mosquito cell plays an important role in the "life cycle" of Sindbis virus. Virus obtained from infected cultures of mosquito cells is not only heterogeneous with respect to size and particle density but also lacks sialic acid. If the sialic acid moiety is not replaced by some other residue with a similar negative charge, it would be predicted that the net electrostatic charge of virus grown in mosquito cells would be quite different from that of virus grown in vertebrate cells. To date, however, experimental results have failed to demonstrate that the presence or absence of sialic acid influences any measurable biologic property of alphaviruses.

Of greater interest, however, may be the observations made on the chronically infected mosquito cell cultures. Such cultures are somehow able to exclude

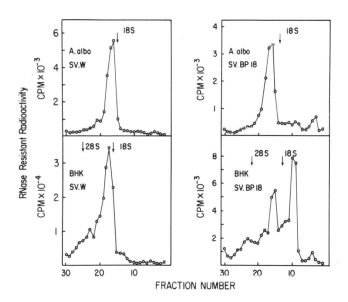

FIGURE 10. dsRNA in BHK-21 or *A. albopictus* cells infected with SV-W or SV-BP-18.

Cultures were infected with the indicated virus stock at an input multiplicity of approximately 25 PFU/cell. BHK-21 cells were maintained at 37° C and *A. albopictus* cells at 28° C. Cultures were labeled with [³H]uridine from 3 to 8·hr after infection and in the presence of actinomycin D (1 µg/ml). RNA was extracted from the infected cultures and fractionated on sucrose velocity gradients. Individual fractions were then assayed for RNase-resistant TCA-precipitable radioactivity.

superinfecting homologous virus but can still support the replication of a different or heterologous alphavirus. The mechanism involved requires further clarification but may involve either defective or mutant viral particles or both.

Furthermore, the *A. albopictus* (SV-C) cultures are of considerable importance, in that they eventually generate genetic variants of the original virus. The evidence that there are defective particles in the chronically infected cultures is only indirect and is based on a shift in the size of viral dsRNA found in the infected cell. However, true viral mutants can be obtained from the chronically infected cultures, and we have shown that they are temperature sensitive, are more thermolabile (measured at 60° C) than the wild-type virus, and that they form small plaques. We are now in the process of studying the evolution of these mutants and their properties in greater detail.

Experiments performed in cultured mosquito cells are still a large step away from an understanding of the behavior of these viruses in the intact mosquito as it lives and breeds in nature. Nevertheless, we believe that our findings have important implications at the level of the whole organism. For example, if infected mosquitos, like cultured mosquito cells, give rise to temperature-sensitive viral mutants, and if such mutants represent an increasing proportion of the total virus with increasing time after infection, this result would certainly influence the outcome of infection in species that have different body temperatures, for example, cold-blooded vertebrates, various mammalian species, and various avian species.

Our experiments were undertaken in an attempt to study that segment of the "life cycle" of togaviruses, still poorly understood, that occurs in the invertebrate, in this case the insect host. It is our hope that such studies can be extended not only in other *in vitro* systems but also at the level of the intact insect host.

REFERENCES

1. STOLLAR, V., T. E. SHENK & B. D. STOLLAR. 1972. Double-stranded RNA in hamster, chick, and mosquito cells infected with Sindbis virus. Virology **47:** 122–132.
2. STOLLAR, V. & T. E. SHENK. 1973. Homologous viral interference in *Aedes albopictus* cultures chronically infected with Sindbis virus. J. Virol. **11:** 592–595.
3. SHENK, T. E. & V. STOLLAR. 1973. Defective-interfering particles of Sindbis virus. 1. Isolation and some chemical and biological properties. Virology **53:** 162–173.
4. SHENK, T. E., K. A. KOSHELNYK & V. STOLLAR. 1974. Temperature-sensitive virus from *Aedes albopictus* cells chronically infected with Sindbis virus. J. Virol. **13:** 439–447.
5. WARREN, L. 1959. The thiobarbituric acid assay of sialic acids. J. Biol. Chem. **234:** 1971–1975.
6. GRIMES, W. J. & B. W. BURGE. 1971. Modification of Sindbis virus glycoprotein by host-specified glycosyl transferases. J. Virol. **7:** 309–313.
7. BURGE, B. W. & E. R. PFEFFERKORN. 1966. Isolation and characterization of conditional-lethal mutants of Sindbis virus. Virology **30:** 204–213.
8. SINGH, K. R. P. 1971. Growth of arboviruses in *Aedes albopictus* and *A. aegypti* cell ines. *In* Current Topics in Microbiology and Immunology. E. Weiss, Ed. Vol. **55:** 127–133. Springer-Verlag New York Inc. New York, N.Y.
9. DAVEY, M. W., D. P. DENNET & L. DALGARNO. 1973. The growth of 2 togaviruses in cultured mosquito and vertebrate cells. J. Gen. Virol. **20:** 225–232.

10. STEVENS, T. M. 1970. Arbovirus replication in mosquito cell lines (Singh) grown in monolayer or suspension culture. Proc. Soc. Exp. Biol. Med. **134:** 356–361.
11. RAGHOW, R. S., T. D. C. GRACE, B. K. FILSHIE, W. BARTLEY & L. DALGARNO. 1973. Ross River virus replication in cultured mosquito and mammalian cells: virus growth and correlated ultrastructural changes. J. Gen. Virol. **21:** 109–122.
12. BROWN, D. T. & J. B. GLIEDMAN. 1973. Morphological variants of Sindbis virus obtained from infected mosquito tissue culture cells. J. Virol. **12:** 1534–1539.
13. PFEFFERKORN, E. R. & H. S. HUNTER. 1963. The source of the ribonucleic acid and phospholipid of Sindbis virus. Virology **20:** 446–456.
14. STRAUSS, J. H., B. W. BURGE & J. E. DARNELL. 1970. Carbohydrate content of the membrane protein of Sindbis virus. J. Mol. Biol. **47:** 437–448.
15. WARREN, L. 1963. The distribution of sialic acids in nature. Comp. Biochem. Physiol. **10:** 153–171.
16. SCHLESINGER, R. W., T. M. STEVENS & E. J. MILLER. 1961. Interaction of influenza virus with sialic acid-containing substrates in extracts of marine organisms. Bacteriol. Proc.
17. KRAEMER, P. M. 1967. Regeneration of sialic acid on the surface of Chinese hamster cells in culture. II. Incorporation of radioactivity from glucosamine-1-^{14}C. J. Cell. Physiol. **69:** 199–208.
18. KENNEDY, S. I. T. 1974. The effect of enzymes on structural and biological properties of Semliki forest virus. J. Gen. Virol. **23:** 129–143.
19. STOLLAR, V., B. D. STOLLAR, R. KOO, K. A. HARRAP & R. W. SCHLESINGER. 1975. Sialic acid contents of Sindbis virus from vertebrate and mosquito cells: equivalence of biological and immunological viral properties. Virology. In press.
20. PELEG, J. & V. STOLLAR. 1974. Homologous interference in *Aedes aegypti* cell cultures infected with Sindbis virus. Arch. Ges. Virusforsch. **45:** 309–318.
21. PELEG, J. 1972. Studies on the behavior of arboviruses in an *Aedes aegypti* mosquito cell line (Peleg). Arch. Ges. Virusforsch. **37:** 54–61.
22. SCHLESINGER, S., M. SCHLESINGER & B. W. BURGE. Defective virus particles from Sindbis virus. Virology **48:** 615–617.
23. SHENK, T. E. & V. STOLLAR. 1972. Viral RNA species in BHK-21 cells infected with Sindbis virus serially passaged at high multiplicity of infection. Biochem. Biophys. Res. Commun. **49:** 60–67.
24. EATON, B. T. & P. FAULKNER. 1973. Altered pattern of viral RNA synthesis in cells infected with standard and defective Sindbis virus. Virology **51:** 85–93.
25. GUILD, G. M. & V. STOLLAR. 1975. Defective interfering particles of Sindbis virus. III. Intracellular viral RNA species in chick embryo cell cultures. Virology. In press.
26. MITSUHASHI, J. & K. MARAMOROSCH. 1964. Cell cultures derived from larvae of *Aedes albopictus* (Skuse) and *A. aegypti* (Singh). Contrib. Boyce Thompson Inst. **22:** 435.
27. GRIMES, W. J. 1970. Sialic acid transferases and sialic acid levels in normal and transformed cells. Biochmeistry **9:** 5083–5092.

MULTIPLE INFECTIONS OF INVERTEBRATE CELLS BY VIRUSES *

Edouard Kurstak and Simon Garzon

Laboratory of Comparative Virology
Department of Microbiology and Immunology
Faculty of Medicine
University of Montreal
Montreal, Quebec, Canada

INTRODUCTION

Multiple viral infections of vertebrate cells have been reported earlier,[1-5] but very little is known about such infections of invertebrate cells.[6-9] Multiple virosis in the same host can lead, as in the case of vertebrate animals or cells, to the following different responses: phenotypic mixing, viral stimulation, viral interference, or simultaneous replication without apparent mutual effect. The mechanisms of these responses, however, are still not well established.

The present study on multiple infections of larvae of the insect *Galleria mellonella* by three DNA viruses revealed some interesting cases of simultaneous infections and a case of viral interference at the cellular level. The densonucleosis virus (DNV), tipula iridescent virus (TIV), and nuclear polyhedrosis virus (NPV) were shown to replicate simultaneously or separately in this host. After infection of the larvae at 26 or 30° C, this replication was observed to occur either in adjacent cells, where NPV and DNV are implicated, or within the same cells, where the DNV or NPV is synthesized in the nucleus and the TIV in the cytoplasm.

HISTOCHEMICAL AND ELECTRON MICROSCOPIC STUDIES

The inoculum, administered intraperitoneally or perorally at a dose of 0.01 ml per larvae L_5 G. *mellonella* (Lepidoptera) consisted of a purified and concentrated suspension of virions (5×10^7 virions and polyhedra per milliliter for NPV and 10^2–10^7 virions per milliliter for TIV or DNV). The same preparations were also used for infecting ovarian cells or hemocytes *in vitro*, at a dose of 0.2 ml per Leighton tube. These experiments were performed at 26 or 30° C. The cultures were examined at 2-hr intervals during the first 24 hr and daily thereafter.

Observations were made by light microscopy after staining with Giemsa, by fluorescent microscopy after staining with acridine orange at pH 3.8, or by electron microscopy. For the latter, the samples were fixed with 0.4% paraformaldehyde and 0.5% glutaraldehyde in 0.067 M phosphate buffer (pH 7.2) for 2 hr at 4° C. After washing with phosphate buffer, the preparations were postfixed with 2% osmic acid for 45 min and embedded in Epon® 812. After

* Supported by Grants A-3746 from the National Research Council of Canada and MA-2385 from the Medical Research Council of Canada.

staining 500-Å sections with uranyl acetate and lead citrate, they were examined with a Philips 300 electron microscope.

DUAL INFECTION OF SINGLE CELLS

With TIV and DNV

Staining with acridine orange revealed the progressive and simultaneous accumulation of cytoplasmic double-stranded DNA of TIV and of nuclear

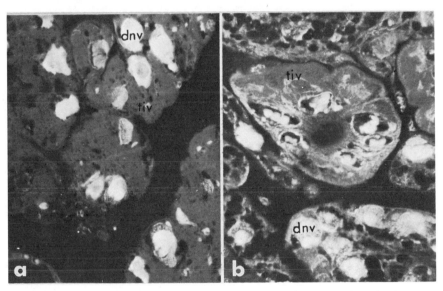

FIGURE 1. Viral DNA synthesis in the cytoplasm and nucleus after simultaneous infection with TIV and DNV; a, adipose tissue; b, silk gland duct. The cytoplasm shows green fluorescence (TIV), whereas the nucleus is yellow-green (DNA replicative forms) with red plaques (DNA mature virions with single-stranded DNA). Stained with acridine orange (pH 3.8). ×1000.

double-stranded and single-stranded DNA, which correspond to the replicative form and to the mature virions of DNV, respectively (FIGURE 1).

By electron microscopy, the simultaneous production of DNV and TIV virions in the nucleus and cytoplasm of the same cells can be readily observed (FIGURE 2). However, an oversynthesis of TIV viral proteins in the cytoplasm and of DNV DNA in the nucleus brings an end to the accumulation of viral structural material and reduces the yield of mature virions, particularly for DNV. Many DNV virions appear empty in the nucleus, probably because of the limited supply of the enzymes necessary for their assembly (FIGURE 7c).

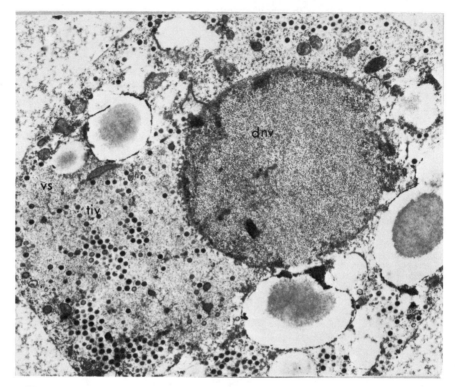

FIGURE 2. Dual infection of a hemocyte with TIV and DNV. Note the large numbers of virions of DNV in the nucleus and of TIV in the cytoplasm. ×12,400.

With NPV and TIV

The cells infected with these two viruses show nuclear hypertrophy, accompanied by the formation of virogenic stroma from which the NPV viral particles become detached and later by the accumulation of polyhedra. The latter can be observed to engulf mature virions or viral material with some abnormalities (FIGURES 3–6). Intracytoplasmic fibrous material, which is characteristic of NPV infection, is also present, although in a smaller amount and limited to the periphery of the nucleus (FIGURE 4, a & b).

The cells also exhibit considerable hypertrophy of the cytoplasm, which is due to the progressive invasion and broadening of viral material in the center of which the TIV virions are assembled. The RNA-rich cytoplasm and the remaining mitochondria are pushed back to the periphery of the nucleus (FIGURE 4). One of the consequences of double infection with TIV and NPV is a decreased production and assembly of NPV virions in the nucleus and, in some cases, their deficient incorporation into polyhedra (FIGURES 4 & 6). This phenomenon is particularly evident when there is an oversynthesis of TIV components in the cytoplasm. The mode of replication of neither virus is changed. Nevertheless, this dual infection causes certain abnormalities, possibly due to metabolic competition. Thus, the accumulation of TIV viral proteins manifests itself in the cytoplasm by the formation of hollow viral particles and of empty viral envelopes of variable lengths and with a diameter of 80 nm (FIGURE 7b). Depending on the degree of invasion of the cytoplasm by TIV, in the nucleus one can observe a strong production of NPV virions with few or no polyhedra (FIGURE 4a), an accumulation of intimate and developmental membranes, with a disproportional DNA synthesis, and an accumulation of membrane-like and nuclear fibrous material without the synthesis and assembly of NPV virions (FIGURE 5).

The morphology of the polyhedra and the virions also undergoes some modifications. The polyhedra become irregular in form, and numerous polyhedra completely cease incorporating enveloped virions. The incorporation of empty developmental membranes into certain polyhedra can also be observed (FIGURE 6). Some enveloped virions are longer than normal, sometimes reaching 80–100 nm (FIGURE 7a).

With DNV and NPV

This dual infection manifests itself either as viral interference or as independent replication of the two viruses in adjacent cells or tissues. Although these two viruses have the same nuclear affinity and invade similar types of cells, so far they have never been observed together in the same nucleus in thin sections.

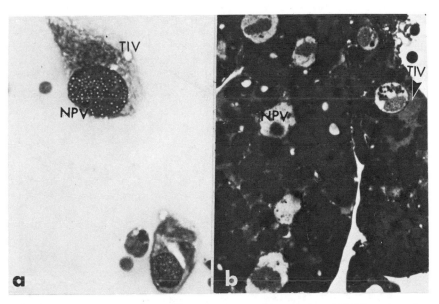

FIGURE 3. Dual infection of the same cells, with cytoplasmic TIV and nuclear NPV producing characteristic polyhedra. a, Hemocytes stained with Giemsa; b, adipose tissue stained with toluidine blue. ×2200.

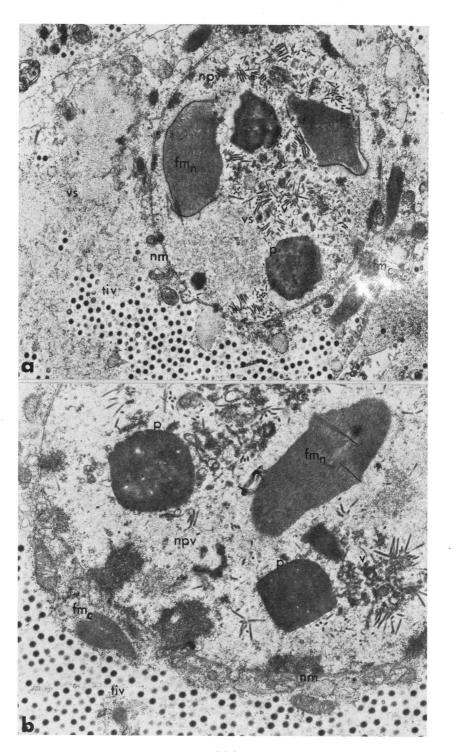

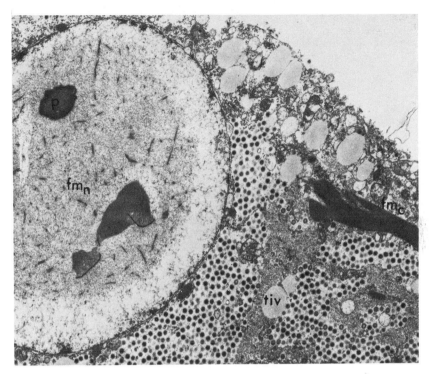

FIGURE 5. Anomaly observed in a dual viral infection with NPV and TIV: excess of production of intranuclear fibrous material (fm_n). ×9000.

Viral interference is best obtained when the revealing virus (DNV) is injected 24–36 hr after the inducing virus (NPV). In this case, only the lesions characteristic for NPV infection can be observed. These results suggested to us the possible production of an interferon-like factor by arthropod cells.[10] However, after the induction of viral interference, further investigations revealed the presence of lesions characteristic of DNV in some tissues of the larvae that are normally insensitive to NPV, such as the anterior and posterior gut. On the other hand, at an advanced stage of the infection, the regenerating hemocytes and lobes of adipose tissue become infected by the DNV. Because these new cells are exposed simultaneously to the two viruses, the more virulent DNV excludes the NPV. The results of electron microscopic studies suggested that this viral interference was not necessarily mediated by a chemical factor but could be due to competition at the level of nucleolar integrity. In fact, the replication of DNV depends on the nucleolus, which, however, is rapidly destroyed during the replication of NPV.[11]

FIGURE 4. Ultrastructural aspect of the dual infection of hemocytes with NPV and TIV. Note the production of intracytoplasmic fibrous material, the invagination of the nuclear membrane, and the different stages of polyhedra formation. fm_c, Intracytoplasmic fibrous material; fm_n, intranuclear fibrous material ;nm, nuclear membrane; p, polyhedra; v, virion; vs, virogenic stroma. a, ×7400; b, ×12,300.

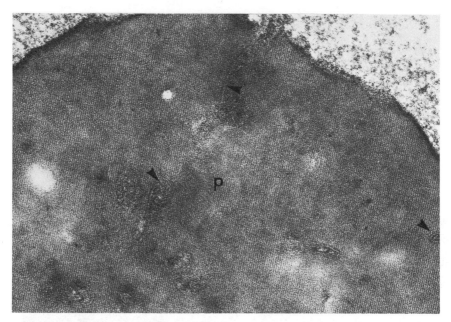

FIGURE 6. Aspect of certain polyhedra in dual infection with NPV and TIV. Note the absence of virions and the incorporation of developmental membranes (▶) in the polyhedra. ×93,900.

MULTIPLE VIRAL INFECTIONS AND MULTICOMPONENT VIRAL INSECTICIDES

In light of the results obtained with multiple viral infections, one has to consider that multicomponent viral insecticides may present some advantages over single viral insecticides. They avoid the selection of strains of virus-resistant insects and possess a maximum efficiency and a larger spectrum of virulence.

However, such systems release large amounts of abnormal viral particles and free viral nucleic acids. The possible role of these products is not yet known.

The hazards of such insecticides, multicomponent or single, must be considered in view of their possible ability to infect vertebrate cells. Recombination between this virus and a vertebrate virus genome may indeed be remotely possible. For example, if poxviruses of insects and vertebrates could be induced to replicate in the same cell system, these possibilities might be studied. It is well known that several arthropod viruses, namely, arboviruses, replicate in insects, such as mosquitos, which transmit these viruses to man, sometimes causing fatal diseases.

CONCLUSIONS

These studies of multiple viral infection of single cells indicated that the type of infection depends on the titers and time of inoculation of the infecting and superinfecting viruses. The manifestation of viral interference or synergism of viral pathogenesis depends mainly on these parameters. In general, multiple infections are induced successfully when the virulence of the superinfecting virus is adjusted by appropriate dilution so as to permit the penetration of the infecting virus and its expression. In such cases, the synergism of viral pathogenesis is revealed through an earlier and more elevated mortality of the hosts, which exhibit the combined symptoms of both diseases.

Histochemical and biochemical studies of the viral DNA, and of the morphogenesis of the DNV, TIV, and NPV virions, by electron microscopy indicated

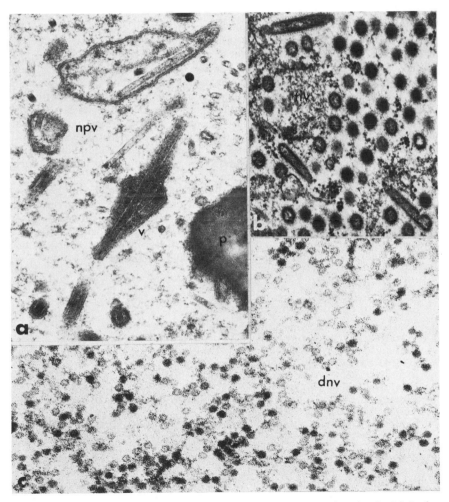

FIGURE 7. Anomalies in the structure of virions observed during the dual infection of adipose tissue with NPV or DNV and TIV. a, NPV particle of unusual length ($\times 42,000$); b, viral envelopes of TIV of tubular shape ($\times 26,500$); c, large number of hollow particles of DNV ($\times 100,800$).

that multiple infections occurred mainly in hemocytes and in the adipose, tracheal, salivary gland, and moulting gland tissues.

This study also indicated that the resistance of certain strains of insects to infection by NPV can be terminated by a second superinfecting virus. Such a possibility is certainly valuable and can be exploited advantageously in biologic control of arthropods that are disease vectors. This approach, however, should be considered only after invertebrate viruses are proved to be innocuous to man and animals, as pointed out earlier.[12, 13]

SUMMARY

This study of viral interference shows that single cells of *G. mellonella* may undergo multiple infections by DNA viruses, such as DNV, TIV, and NPV. In such cases, simultaneous replication of the viruses occurs and results in the synthesis of DNV or NPV in the nucleus and TIV in the cytoplasm. These viruses can also simultaneously infect host cells *in vitro*. The type of infection depends on the titer and the time of inoculation of the infecting and superinfecting viruses, inducing interference or synergism of viral pathogenesis. Simultaneous replication of DNV, TIV, and NPV has been revealed by histochemical and electron microscopic techniques in the adipose, hypodermal, silk gland, and moulting gland tissues and in hemocytes of the infected larvae. Similar multiple infections also occur in ovarian cells and hemocytes cultured *in vitro*. In such multiple infections, viral interference may cause an incomplete replication of virions and a considerable decrease in the production of polyhedral proteins. The synergism of viral pathogenesis manifests itself through an earlier and higher host mortality. These observations could be exploited advantageously for the preparation of multicomponent viral insecticides. Such insecticides, however, should first be subjected to strict investigations of the safety of the viruses to other forms of life, namely, man and other animals.

REFERENCES

1. ANDERSON, K. 1942. Amer. J. Pathol. **18:** 577–583.
2. SYVERTON, J. T. & G. P. BERRY. 1947. J. Exp. Med. **86:** 145–152.
3. RABSON, A. S., G. T. O'CONNOR, F. J. PAUL & I. K. BEREZESKI. 1966. Science **15:** 1535, 1536.
4. HSIUNG, G. D., T. ATOYNATAN & L. GLUCK. 1966. Proc. Soc. Exp. Biol. Med. **121:** 562–566.
5. ALSTEIN, A. D., N. N. DODONOVA, G. A. NADTOCHEY & A. F. BYKOWSKI. 1969. Arch. Ges. Virusforsch. **28:** 7–18.
6. KURSTAK, E., S. GARZON & P. A. ONJI. 1972. Arch. Ges. Virusforsch. **36:** 324–334.
7. GARZON, S. & E. KURSTAK. 1972. Compt. Rend. **275:** 507–509.
8. KURSTAK, E. 1972. Advan. Virus. Res. **17:** 207–241.
9. KIMURA, M. & A. H. MCINTOSH. 1975. *In* Invertebrate Tissue Culture. E. Kurstak & K. Maramorosch, Eds. Academic Press, Inc. New York, N.Y.
10. GARZON, S. & E. KURSTAK. 1969. Rev. Can. Biol. **28:** 89–94.
11. GARZON, S. & E. KURSTAK. 1975. In preparation.
12. KURSTAK, E. 1971. Ann. Parasitol. Hum. Comp. **46(3):** 277–288.
13. WORLD HEALTH ORGANIZATION. 1973. Technical report series no. 531. : 1–48. Geneva, Switzerland.

ARBOVIRUS INFECTION OF VERTEBRATE AND INSECT CELL CULTURES, WITH SPECIAL EMPHASIS ON MOKOLA, OBODHIANG, AND KOTONKAN VIRUSES OF THE RABIES SEROGROUP *

Sonja M. Buckley

Yale University School of Medicine
Yale Arbovirus Research Unit
Department of Epidemiology and Public Health
New Haven, Connecticut 06510

A unique contribution of The Rockefeller Foundation to public health over the last 24 years (1950–1974) has been a world-wide program that pertains to the study of arboviruses (abbreviation for "arthropod-borne viruses").[1] As of December 31, 1974, 350 arboviruses are recognized.[2] The burgeoning increase is documented in FIGURE 1. By definition, "arboviruses are viruses which are maintained in nature principally or to an important extent, through biological transmission between susceptible vertebrate hosts by hematophagous arthropods."[3] Natural vectors range from mosquitoes to ticks, phlebotomines, and *Culicoides*.

The heterogeneous arboviruses, incorporated into a general system of virus classification,[4] can be arranged for the most part into groups of related, but distinct, agents. They have been put in order on the basis of serology (sharing of common antigens), morphology, morphogenesis, ribonucleic acid (RNA) or deoxyribonucleic acid (DNA) content, and susceptibility to sodium deoxycholate (which indicates the presence of essential lipid constituents in the viral envelope).[5, 6] Four taxons have already been well characterized, namely, alphaviruses, flaviviruses, orbiviruses, and rhabdoviruses; a fifth subset, the bunyaviruses, has been proposed recently.[7] In addition, there is a sixth taxon: the iridoviruses, which was discussed with some of the other taxons in detail in a recent symposium on comparative virology.[8]

Arboviruses may be related to nonarboviruses.[4] In this association, Baker's comments[9] on the evolution of arboviruses are imaginative and enlightening. He surmises that successive evolutionary steps lead from an originally latent virus of an arthropod to a virus that has a primary arthropod-vertebrate cycle, then to another virus with a side or secondary arthropod-vertebrate cycle, and, finally, to a virus with a vertebrate-vertebrate perpetuation. In the latter circumstance, the virus presumably loses its potential to multiply in arthropod vectors. The timely and notable recognition of the rabies serogroup by Shope *et al.*[10] and Kemp *et al.*[11] presents scientists of this decade with a unique evolutionary model. Rabies-related viruses presently consist of the following agents: Lagos bat,[12] Mokola,[10, 13] Nigerian horse,[14] Duvenhage,[15] Obodhiang,[16] and kotonkan.[11] The neutralization studies with plaque-purified Duvenhage virus confirm the observations of Murphy, Tignor, and Shope, and this presentation is not intended to

* Supported by The Rockefeller Foundation and by United States Public Health Service Grant 1-PO1-AI-11132 from the National Institute of Allergy and Infectious Diseases.

supersede the definitive virus description in preparation. Obodhiang and kotonkan viruses, two presumptive arboviruses, have been isolated from *Mansonia uniformis* and *Culicoides* midges, respectively. The overall objective of this communication is to present *in vitro* studies with members of the rabies serogroup in vertebrate and insect cell cultures. Techniques that pertain to reproducible plaquing, cloning, and cross-plaque neutralization tests in Vero cells are reported.

MATERIALS AND METHODS

Mice

Mice derived from the Charles River CD (R)-1 strain were random bred in a barrier colony maintained at this laboratory. Two-day-old mice were used

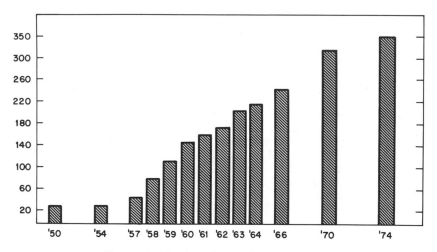

FIGURE 1. Number of recognized arboviruses.

for preparation of virus stocks, and 35–40-day-old mice were used for preparation of immune reagents.

Viruses

Two strains of rabies virus were employed: the CVS strain, 202nd mouse passage, and the TRVL 5843 strain,[1] 3rd mouse passage. An additional strain, used also and known as Nigerian horse virus, prototype, 25th mouse passage, is considered herein a strain of rabies virus, although definitive serologic cross-comparison with standard rabies strains has not been published; it has not yet been established whether Nigerian horse virus is identical or different from rabies virus. The following viruses were also used: Lagos bat, prototype strain, 15th mouse passage; Mokola, strain IbAn 27377, eighth mouse passage; Nigerian horse, prototype strain, 25th mouse passage; Duvenhage, prototype strain, third mouse passage; Obodhiang, strain Sud. Ar.1154–64, third mouse passage, and kotonkan, strain IbAr 23380, ninth mouse passage. Parent virus stocks, which consisted of 10% suspensions of infected newborn mouse brain tissue, were made in 7.5% bovine serum albumin in phosphate-buffered saline (pH 7.2). The suspensions were clarified by centrifugation and were then held in 1-ml amounts in sealed glass ampoules at −65° C in an electrically driven freezer.

Cell Cultures

The Vero cell line was propagated and maintained as follows: stock cultures were carried in Roux bottles with a growth medium that consisted of Eagle's minimal essential medium prepared with Hanks' or Earle's balanced salt solution and 10% fetal bovine serum, supplemented with penicillin (100 units/ml) and streptomycin (100 μg/ml). For viral propagation and plaque assays, 2-oz flint glass prescription bottles were seeded with 10 ml of Vero cell suspension prepared by dispersing cells of one 2-week-old stock culture in 100 or 320 ml of growth medium. These cultures were incubated at 36° C and used 2–5 days after seeding.

The BHK-21 cell line was propagated and maintained as described.[17] Singh's *Aedes aegypti* and *Aedes albopictus* cell lines,[18] propagated in 2-oz flint glass prescription bottles and incubated at 30° C, were grown and maintained with Mitsuhashi-Maramorosch medium[19] supplemented with 20% inactivated (56° C for 30 min) fetal bovine serum. The 2-oz flint glass prescription bottles were seeded with cell suspensions from stock cultures that represented a 1:8 (*A. albopictus*) or 1:4 (*A. aegypti*) split. These cultures were used 3 days after seeding.

Diluent

The diluent consisted of 0.75% bovine serum albumin in phosphate-buffered saline (pH 7.2) and contained 100 μg/ml of diethylaminoethyl-dextran (DEAE-D), from Pharmacia, Uppsala, Sweden.

Titration

For inoculation of virus, the fluid medium was removed from vertebrate and invertebrate cell cultures. Increasing 10-fold dilutions of virus were inoculated in 0.2-ml amounts into two bottles per dilution. Inocula were adsorbed for 1 hr at 36° C, after which time 5 ml of maintenance medium[17] or Mitsuhashi-Maramorosch medium[19] was added; cultures were incubated at 35° C or 30° C, respectively. In addition, Vero cell cultures were also overlaid with 10 ml of a freshly prepared nutrient agar overlay. The nutrient portion of the overlay[20, 21] was composed of 18.0 ml of Earle's balanced salt solution (without $NaHCO_3$ and neutral red) (10×), 3.0 ml of lactalbumin hydrolysate (10%), 1.2 ml of yeast extract (5%), 3.6 ml of fetal bovine serum (inactivated at 56° C for 30 min), 3.0 ml of neutral red (0.1%), 5.4 ml of $NaHCO_3$ (7.5%), 0.9 ml of DEAE-D (2%), 1.8 ml of penicillin-streptomycin solution (10,000 units penicillin and 10,000 μg streptomycin/ml), 1.8 ml of Fungizone® (100×), and sterile, distilled, demineralized water to 90.0 ml.

To complete the agar overlay, the nutrient portion (90.0 ml) was mixed with 90.0 ml of 2% ionagar 2S (Wilson Diagnostics, Inc.). The overlaid Vero cell cultures were incubated in an inverted position at 35° C for 11 days and thereafter at room temperature (20–25° C). Plaque counts were performed at intervals for up to 21 days after inoculation. Plaque assays were terminated 10–21 days after inoculation.

Virus titers are expressed as tissue culture dose (TCD_{50}) or as plaque-forming units (PFU) per milliliter.

Plaque Passaging and Preparation of Cloned Virus Stocks

Cloned viruses were isolated by selecting progenies of single large plaques [22] and plaque passaging them four to seven times. Cloned virus stocks were prepared in Vero cells or in 2-day-old mice and stored as described for parent virus stocks.

Antisera

Mouse hyperimmune antisera for the parent viruses were prepared in mice given five intraperitoneal inoculations [23] of parent stock virus suspended in physiologic saline and bled out 1 week after the last inoculation. Sera were pooled by virus and stored at −20° C. Two pools of normal mouse serum, one collected at the beginning of the experiments and the other after five intraperitoneal inoculations of normal mouse brain suspended in physiologic saline, were processed identically.

Cocultivation

Infected *A. albopictus* or BHK-21 cells were dissociated nonenzymatically with a rubber policeman and a small amount of diluent (1–2 ml/10^6 cells). The resultant cell suspension, after additional dispersal by pipetting, was inoculated into BHK-21 or Vero cell cultures, maintained under fluid medium or under nutrient agar overlay. Cultures were examined for development of cytopathic effect (CPE) or plaque formation.

Plaque Reduction Neutralization Test

Normal and hyperimmune mouse sera were thawed rapidly at 37° C and inactivated for 30 min at 56° C before testing. Serial twofold dilutions of serum, beginning at 1:8, were mixed in equal volumes (0.4 ml) with a virus suspension that contained an estimated 100–200 PFU in 0.1 ml. After incubation at 4° C overnight, the mixtures were inoculated in 0.2-ml amounts into two Vero plaque bottles per mixture. Fifty percent plaque reduction serum titers were determined 10–21 days after inoculation.

RESULTS

Multiplication of Obodhiang and kotonkan, the presumptive arboviruses of the rabies serogroup, was induced in vertebrate cell cultures by using Singh's *A. albopictus* cell cultures as "helper cells," as has been reported in detail.[24] Briefly, neither virus multiplied in cultures of *A. aegypti* incubated at 30° C or in cultures of the Vero and BHK-21 cell lines incubated at 35° C. However, both viruses readily infected *A. albopictus* cell cultures incubated at 30° C. Initially, the presence of virus in the mosquito cells was determined by sub-inoculation of the fluid phase into 2-day-old mice by the intracerebral route. Subsequently, cocultivation of infected *A. albopictus* cells with BHK-21 or Vero cells under fluid medium or nutrient agar overlay induced CPE or plaque formation, respectively. Serial passages of the two viruses were easily estab-

TABLE 1

RESULTS OF TESTING MOUSE BRAIN PREPARATIONS OF RABIES SEROGROUP VIRUSES FOR PLAQUE FORMATION IN VERO CELLS AND ABILITY TO INFECT BHK-21 AND SINGH'S *A. albopictus* AND *A. aegypti* CELLS

Virus	Strain	Mouse Pas-sage Level	Plaques (Vero)	Multiplication *		
				BHK-21	*A. albo-pictus*	*A. aegypti*
Rabies	CVS	202	0 †	+	0	0
Rabies	TRVL 5843	3	+	+	0	0
Lagos bat	prototype	15	+	+	0	0
Mokola	IbAn 27377	8	+	+	+	0
Obodhiang	SudAr 1154–64	3	0	0	+	0
Kotonkan	IbAr 23380	9	0	0	+	0
Nigerian horse	prototype	25	0	+	0	0
Duvenhage	prototype	3	0	+	0	0

* As determined by subinoculation of undiluted fluid phase or combined fluid and cell phases into 2-day-old mice by the intracerebral route.

† +, Plaque formation or multiplication observed; 0, no plaque formation or multiplication observed.

lished in both Vero and BHK-21 cell lines. Infectivity titers varied from 3.5 to 6.5 $\log_{10}$/ml; generally higher TCD_{50} titers were obtained in the BHK-21 cell line. Plaque formation in Vero cell cultures and development of CPE in both Vero and BHK-21 cell cultures under fluid medium were specifically inhibited by immune reagents.

When mouse brain preparations of the other five viruses (six strains), namely, rabies, Lagos bat, Mokola, Nigerian horse, and Duvenhage, were tested for *in vitro* characteristics, only three of them, rabies (TRVL 5843), Lagos bat, and Mokola, contained plaque-producing viral progenies (PPVP) capable of initiating serial plaque passages in Vero cells. Mokola, isolated from shrews (insectivores), multiplied in both BHK-21 and *A. albopictus* cells; the other five strains, all isolated from vertebrates, multiplied only in BHK-21 cells. None of the viruses multiplied in *A. aegypti* cells. TABLE 1 summarizes the *in vitro*

TABLE 2

PLAQUE PASSAGING OF RABIES SEROGROUP VIRUSES IN VERO CELLS

Virus	Passage History	Cocultivation	No. Plaques Examined	No. Plaque Passages	Maximum No. PPVP * from One Plaque	Plaque Appearing on Day	Diameter (mm) Day 21
Rabies, CVS	BHK-21 [†]	+ [‡]	20	5	> 200	6	3
Rabies, TRVL 5843	3 MB [§]	ND [‖]	39	4	> 200	10	3
Lagos bat	15 MB	ND	30	4	> 200	8	7
Mokola	8 MB	ND	8	4	> 10,000	7	10
Obodhiang	3 MB, 1 *A. albopictus*	+	8	4	38	5	4
Kotonkan	9 MB, 1 *A. albopictus*	+	5	4	94	6	2
Nigerian horse	25 MB, 2 BHK-21	+	50+	7	> 200	8	2
Duvenhage	3 MB, 1 BHK-21	+	50+	7	> 200	6	3

* Plaque-producing viral progenies.
† This rabies CVS strain was kindly supplied by Dr. F. A. Murphy as a BHK-21-adapted strain. It was given one additional passage in BHK-21 cells in our laboratory.
‡ Cocultivation performed successfully.
§ Mouse brain.
‖ Not done.

TABLE 3

PLAQUE-FORMING UNIT TITERS OF CLONED VIRUS STOCKS

Cloned Virus Stock	Prepared in	Plaque-Forming Unit Titer per Milliliter	Mouse Pathogenicity *
Rabies, CVS	mice	1.20×10^8	+
Rabies, TRVL 5843	mice	1.50×10^8	+
Lagos bat	Vero	1.00×10^6	+
Mokola	Vero	1.00×10^7	+
Obodhiang	Vero	4.25×10^4	0
Kotonkan	Vero	7.00×10^4	0
Nigerian horse	mice	1.00×10^7	+
Duvenhage	mice	6.00×10^7	+

* +, Test for infectivity in mice positive; 0, no illness observed.

characteristics of viruses of the rabies serogroup with regard to plaque formation in a primate cell line and multiplication in rodent and mosquito cells. Mokola virus is unique: it emerges biologically as the bridging agent.

Plaque formation in Vero cells under a nutrient agar overlay was subsequently obtained with rabies, CVS strain, and with Nigerian horse and Duvenhage viruses, by cocultivation of infected BHK-21 cells with Vero cells. The details have been reported elsewhere.[25] TABLE 2 summarizes facts that pertain to the plaque passaging of rabies serogroup viruses in Vero cells as observed in our laboratory. Plaques began to appear within 5–10 days. They were well defined and readily countable 10–21 days after inoculation. Plaque-derived clones were obtained by selecting progenies of well-separated plaques and plaque passaging them four to seven times. Cloned stocks were prepared in Vero cells or in mice. TABLE 3 lists the PFU titers obtained.

Cross-plaque reduction neutralization tests with cloned viruses that represented the three human pathogens rabies, Duvenhage and Mokola and the two presumptive arboviruses, Obodhiang and kotonkan, were performed next. The results are summarized in TABLES 4 and 5. Especially relevant from TABLE 4

TABLE 4

SHARING OF COMMON ANTIGENS OF CLONED VIRUSES OF THE RABIES SEROGROUP EXPRESSED AS PERCENTAGE OF PLAQUE REDUCTION

Hyperimmune Mouse Serum, Diluted 1:8	Cloned Viruses and Percentage of Plaque Reduction Obtained				
	Rabies, CVS	Duvenhage	Mokola	Obodhiang	Kotonkan
Rabies, CVS	100	100	99	0	0
Duvenhage	100	100	50	0	0
Mokola	*100*	*50*	*100*	68	39
Obodhiang	0	0	0	*100*	50
Kotonkan	0	0	0	55	100

is that Mokola emerges as the serologic bridge between the nonarboviruses and the presumptive arboviruses.

DISCUSSION

In old and well into modern scientific history, rabies virus has been outstanding in that it does not share any antigenic components with other viruses. Rabiesologists, on the one hand, concurred on an international level in this concept of antigenic unity. Their collective, creative consciousness went as far as to recognize strain variations. However, when such a strange bedfellow as Lagos bat[12] was isolated in Nigeria during an intensive search for new rabies strains, this unknown agent disappeared in the deep freezer, labeled simply as a nonrabies strain. Arbovirologists, on the other hand, faced with the explosive increase of recognized arboviruses, knew from experience that to isolate agents

TABLE 5

CROSS-PLAQUE NEUTRALIZATION TESTS WITH CLONED RABIES, DUVENHAGE, MOKOLA, OBODHIANG, AND KOTONKAN VIRUSES AND RESPECTIVE 50% PLAQUE REDUCTION TITERS

Cloned Virus	Titer of Hyperimmune Serum *				
	Rabies, CVS	Duvenhage	Mokola	Obodhiang	Kotonkan
Rabies, CVS	65536	8192	64	<8	<8
Duvenhage	4096	16384	8	<8	<8
Mokola	512	128	8192	<8	<8
Obodhiang	<8	<8	8	8192	8
Kotonkan	<8	<8	<8	8	512

* Titers expressed as reciprocals of serum dilution that give a 50% reduction of plaques.

does not solve the problems. This restless breed of scientists had to cope with hundreds of new arboviruses with regard to identification and classification. Thus, the creative consciousness of an arbovirologist is like that of the "Cosmic Dancer" (Friedrich Wilhelm Nietzsche). When Mokola virus was isolated by Kemp et al.,[13] it was Shope et al.,[10] who by challenging the concept of antigenic unity of rabies, put the rabies serogroup on the scientific globe. Other viruses, such as Obodhiang[16] and kotonkan,[11] which are presumptive arboviruses, have been identified and classified as rabies-related viruses.[26]

In this communication, evidence is presented that Mokola virus,[10, 13] possibly, might be the biologic and serologic bridge between the nonarboviruses, rabies and Duvenhage,[15] and the presumptive arboviruses, Obodhiang[16] and kotonkan.[11] It is of interest that the bridging virus is a human pathogen.[27] Very little is known presently with regard to the epidemiology or disease potential of kotonkan and Obodhiang viruses.[26]

In view of Baker's comments[9] on the evolution of arboviruses from insect viruses to nonarboviruses, the rabies serogroup emerges as a challenging evolutionary virus model.

SUMMARY

Multiplication of rabies serogroup viruses, Obodhiang and kotonkan (two presumptive arboviruses), was induced in vertebrate cell cultures with Singh's *A. albopictus* cell cultures used as "helper cells" in cocultivation experiments. Plaque formation without prior *in vitro* adaptation was induced in Vero cell cultures with eight rabies serogroup viruses: in all five instances by cocultivation of either infected BHK-21 or *A. albopictus* cells with Vero cells under agar overlay and in three of eight instances by direct plaque assay of infected mouse brain suspensions.

In cross-plaque reduction neutralization tests with cloned viruses that represented human pathogens, rabies, Duvenhage, and Mokola, on the one hand, and the presumptive arboviruses Obodhiang and kotonkan, on the other hand, Mokola virus shared common antigenic components with both the nonarboviruses and the arboviruses. Biologically, Mokola virus was different from the other two human pathogens, rabies and Duvenhage, in that it multiplied in both vertebrate and invertebrate cell cultures. Mokola virus thus appears to be the biologic and serologic bridging agent.

ACKNOWLEDGMENTS

The valuable technical assistance of C. Mullen, E. Gilson, and M. Malhoit is greatly appreciated. I am indebted to C. Bierwirth for her competent assistance with the typescript.

REFERENCES

1. THEILER, M. & W. G. DOWNS. 1973. The Arthropod-Borne Viruses of Vertebrates. Yale University Press. New Haven, Conn.
2. BERGE, T. O. 1975. International Catalogue of Arboviruses. U.S. Department of Health, Education and Welfare, DHEW Publication (CDC) 75-8301. : 1–789.
3. WHO SCIENTIFIC GROUP. 1967. W.H.O. Tech. Rep. Ser. No. 369.
4. CASALS, J. 1971. *In* Comparative Virology. K. Maramorosch & E. Kurstak, Eds. : 307–333. Academic Press, Inc. New York, N.Y.
5. ANDREWES, C. H. & D. M. HORSTMANN. 1949. J. Gen. Microbiol. **3:** 290–297.
6. THEILER, M. 1957. Proc. Soc. Exp. Biol. Med. **96:** 380–382.
7. PORTERFIELD, J. S., J. CASALS, M. P. CHUMAKOV, S. Y. GAIDAMOVICH, C. HANNOUN, I. H. HOLMES, M. HORZINEK, M. MUSSGAY & P. K. RUSSELL. 1973–74. Intervirology **2:** 270–272.
8. BROWN, F. & T. W. TINSLEY. 1973. J. Gen. Virol. **20**(Suppl.): 1–130.
9. BAKER, A. C. 1943. Amer. J. Trop. Med. Hyg. **23:** 559–567.
10. SHOPE, R. E., F. A. MURPHY, A. K. HARRISON, O. R. CAUSEY, G. E. KEMP, D. I. H. SIMPSON & D. L. MOORE. 1970. J. Virol. **6:** 690–692.
11. KEMP, G. E., V. H. LEE, D. L. MOORE, R. E. SHOPE, O. R. CAUSEY & F. A. MURPHY. 1973. Amer. J. Epidemiol. **98:** 43–49.

12. BOULGER, L. R. & J. S. PORTERFIELD. 1958. Trans. Roy. Soc. Trop. Med. Hyg. **52:** 421–424.
13. KEMP, G. E., O. R. CAUSEY, D. L. MOORE, A. ODEOLA & A. FABIY. 1972. Amer. J. Trop. Med. Hyg. **21:** 356–359.
14. PORTERFIELD, J. S., D. H. HILL & A. D. MORRIS. 1958. Brit. Vet. J. **114:** 1–9.
15. MEREDITH, C. D. 1971. S. African Med. J. **45:** 767–769.
16. SCHMIDT, J. R., M. C. WILLIAMS, M. LULU, A. MIVULE & E. MUJOMBE. 1965. E. African Virus Res. Inst. Rep. **15:** 24.
17. KARABATSOS, N. & S. M. BUCKLEY. 1967. Proc. Soc. Exp. Biol. Med. **130:** 888–892.
18. SINGH, K. R. P. 1971. Curr. Sci. (India) **36:** 506–508.
19. MITSUHASHI, J. & K. MARAMOROSCH. 1964. Contrib. Boyce Thompson Inst. **22:** 435–460.
20. SIMIZU, B., J. S. RHIM & N. WIEBENGA. 1967. Proc. Soc. Exp. Biol. Med. **125:** 119–123.
21. KARABATSOS, N. 1969. Amer. J. Trop. Med. Hyg. **18:** 803–810.
22. SCHMIDT, N. J. 1964. *In* Diagnostic Procedures for Viral and Rickettsial Diseases. E. H. Lennette & N. J. Schmidt, Eds. 3rd edit. : 78–176. American Public Health Association. New York, N.Y.
23. CLARKE, D. H. & J. CASALS. 1958. Amer. J. Trop. Med. Hyg. **7:** 561–573.
24. BUCKLEY, S. M. 1973. Appl. Microbiol. **25:** 695, 696.
25. BUCKLEY, S. M. & G. H. TIGNOR. 1975. J. Clin. Microbiol. **1:** 241, 242.
26. SHOPE, R. E. 1975. *In* The Natural History of Rabies. G. M. Baer, Ed. Academic Press, Inc. New York, N.Y. In press.
27. FAMILUSI, J. B. & D. J. MOORE. 1972. African J. Med. Sci. **3:** 93–96.

NEUTRALIZATION OF A TOGAVIRUS BY ANTIVECTOR ANTISERA *

Fred M. Feinsod, Andrew Spielman, and Joseph L. Waner

Department of Tropical Public Health
Harvard School of Public Health
Boston, Massachusetts 02115

Because the envelopes of viruses include components derived from the host cell,[1,2] certain surface properties of viral particles may be shared with the host. Indeed, host antigen is present on various enveloped viruses.[3-5] However, it has not been determined whether such host-associated factors may influence infectivity of mosquito-propagated togavirus. Accordingly, we determined whether Sindbis virus may be neutralized by antisera produced against vector tissues and by antisera obtained from animals naturally exposed to the bites of vector mosquitoes. A more complete description of these experiments has been reported elsewhere.[6]

MATERIALS AND METHODS

Two lots of Sindbis virus were prepared: one (designated Sindbis-Vero) was propagated in Vero cells maintained on basal medium Eagles (BME) supplemented with 5% fetal calf serum, and the other (designated Sindbis-*Aedes*) was obtained after two serial passages in adult female *Aedes aegypti*. Sindbis-*Aedes* was harvested 10 days after intraabdominal injection of virus so as to maximize viral propagation in salivary gland tissue.[7,8]

Guinea pigs were inoculated with extracts of whole ground female *A. aegypti* or, alternatively, were exposed to the bites of noninfected *A. aegypti*. Sera were obtained from guinea pigs immediately before initial exposure and after treatment. Known quantities of both Sindbis-*Aedes* and Sindbis-Vero virus were incubated in various dilutions of pretreatment and posttreatment sera and then assayed in Vero cell cultures.

Globulin fractions were prepared [9] from pooled pre- and posttreatment sera obtained from guinea pigs exposed to whole mosquito antigen or to vector bites. The presence of immunoglobulin was established by immunodiffusion with antiserum prepared against guinea pig IgG, and various dilutions of these fractions were tested for neutralizing activity.

RESULTS

Sera from guinea pigs immunized by injection of extracts of ground whole mosquitoes neutralized more mosquito-propagated than Vero-propagated virus. In at least half (7 of 12) of the tests that employed such sera, about twice as many viral particles retained infectivity after incubation with preimmunization

* Supported by Grant AI 10,274 from the National Institutes of Health.

sera (diluted 1:4) as compared to postimmunization sera (diluted 1:8). Thus, neutralization titer for mosquito-propagated virus with this group of sera is expressed as "1:8" (TABLE 1). In only one-fourth (3 of 12) of tests that used more dilute postimmunization sera (1:16) was this level of neutralization observed. The neutralizing activity of sera from two animals exceeded 50% at the 1:32 dilution. In contrast, when Vero-propagated virus was incubated with these sera, similar numbers of viral particles retained infectivity in each serum pair. Sera from guinea pigs naturally immunized via bites by mosquitoes appeared to be less antiviral. Half of the serum pairs tested (5 of 10) indicated the above level of neutralization when diluted 1:4. Vero-propagated virus appeared not to be neutralized by these sera.

To investigate possible nonspecific neutralizing factors that result from the immunization procedure per se, guinea pigs were immunized with Freund's incomplete adjuvant (which contained *Mycoplasma*) following the protocol described for mosquito-injected guinea pigs. Postimmunization sera from three such guinea pigs neutralized neither Sindbis-Vero nor Sindbis-*Aedes* virus.

TABLE 1

NEUTRALIZATION OF SINDBIS VIRUS PROPAGATED IN MOSQUITOES
AND IN VERO CELL CULTURES WITH ANTISERA OBTAINED FROM GUINEA PIGS
INOCULATED WITH EXTRACTS OF MOSQUITOES OR NATURALLY BITTEN BY MOSQUITOES

Virus Propagated in	Neutralization Titer * of Sera from Guinea Pigs Exposed to			
	n	Mosquito Extracts	n	Bites by Mosquitoes
Mosquitoes	12	1:8	10	1:4
Vero cell cultures	12	0	10	0

* Neutralization titer is expressed as the dilution of serum that neutralizes at least half of expected viral plaques in half of sera tested.

Globulin fractions were prepared from pools of sera obtained from guinea pigs before and after injection of mosquito extracts, and such sera were tested for neutralizing activity against Sindbis-*Aedes* and Sindbis-Vero virus. Whereas the immunoglobulin fraction of postinoculation sera did not neutralize Sindbis-Vero virus, 75% of mosquito-propagated virus was neutralized at a 1:4 serum dilution, and 60% was neutralized at a dilution of 1:8. In an additional experiment, an immunoglobulin preparation, diluted 1:8, obtained from sera of guinea pigs repeatedly exposed to bites by mosquitoes, neutralized 35% of Sindbis-*Aedes* virus but did not neutralize Sindbis-Vero virus. The presence of immune globulin was confirmed by gel diffusion.

DISCUSSION

We have shown that guinea pigs exposed to mosquito antigens produce serum that possesses low-titer neutralizing activity against virus propagated in such mosquito hosts. This neutralization of homologous virus by antibody to host tissues may be due to incorporation of host cell membrane into the developing virion.[1, 10]

These results suggest certain epidemiologic interrelationships. Salivary fluid of mosquitoes contains fragments of membrane visible by electron microscopy,[11] which would provide membrane antigen to animals bitten by these insects. Togavirus, which replicates in salivary glands, acquires membrane components while budding through membranous structures. In this manner, salivary secretions of noninfected mosquitoes and virus naturally delivered from those mosquitoes would contain common antigens.

The potency of antiserum produced in this work was less than that generally considered to afford protection against intravenous challenge with a togavirus.[12] However, the more natural intradermal route of inoculation may render togavirus peculiarly vulnerable to antibody. In mammalian hosts sensitive to mosquito bites, local inflammation is evident within 10 min of exposure to salivary antigen of the vector.[13, 14] Numerous polymorphonuclear leukocytes wall off the bite area for as long as 12 hr, and a transudate bathes the site for at least 90 min. This reaction resembles Arthus-like cutaneous anaphylaxis,[15] which involves rapid phagocytosis of antibody-antigen complexes and subsequent degranulation of polymorphonuclear leukocytes.[16] Because, in sensitized hosts, virus is injected into dermis, which rapidly becomes isolated from contiguous skin by cellular infiltrate and which is exposed to antibody-containing transudate, the neutralizing activity of low-titer antibody may be enhanced.

The pattern of host reactivity to bites by mosquitoes depends upon prior exposure to mosquitoes.[17] Immediate cutaneous hypersensitivity follows after about 1 month of exposure, and this activity is lost after several months of intensive vector-bite exposure. The pattern of the delayed response is independent of the immediate response.

SUMMARY

An *A. aegypti*-propagated togavirus (Sindbis) is neutralized by antisera to both whole-body extracts and to salivary fluid of the vector mosquito. Virus propagated in Vero cells is not neutralized by such antisera.

Neutralizing activity resides in the immune globulin fraction of sera.

Sera from animals injected with adjuvant neutralized neither virus propagated in mosquitoes nor virus obtained from Vero cells.

Although neutralizing titers were low, such activity may protect, to some degree, vertebrate hosts normally exposed to vector antigens.

REFERENCES

1. ROTT, R., R. DRZENICK, M. S. SABER & E. REICHERT. 1966. Blood group substances, Forssman and mononucleosis antigens in lipid-containing RNA viruses. Arch. Ges. Virusforch. **19:** 273–288.

2. ACHESON, N. H. & I. TAMM. 1967. Replication of Semliki Forest virus: an electron microscope study. Virology **32:** 128–143.

3. CARTWRIGHT, B. & C. A. PEARCE. 1968. Evidence for a host cell component in vesicular stomatitis virus. J. Gen. Virol. **2:** 207–214.

4. IWASAKI, T. & R. OGURA. 1968. Studies on complement-potentiated neutralizing antibodies induced in rabbits inoculated with Japanese encephalitis virus. Virology **34:** 46–59.

5. KOSYAKOV, P. N., A. I. ROVNOVA & A. P. SCHAVELYOVA. 1966. Neutralization of myxoviruses by anticellular sera. Acta Virol. (Prague) **10:** 218–225.
6. FEINSOD, F. M., A. SPIELMAN & J. L. WANER. 1975. Neutralization of Sindbis virus by antisera to antigens of vector mosquitoes. Amer. J. Trop. Med. Hyg. **24:** 533–536.
7. LAMOTTE, L. C. 1960. Japanese B encephalitis virus in organs of infected mosquitoes. Amer. J. Hyg. **72:** 73–87.
8. WHITFIELD, S. G., F. A. MURPHY & W. D. SUDIA. 1971. St. Louis encephalomyelitis virus: an electron microscopic study of *Aedes triseriatus* salivary gland infection. Virology **43:** 110–122.
9. WILLIAMS, C. A. & M. W. CHASE. 1967. Methods in Immunology and Immunochemistry. Vol. I: 399–401. Academic Press, Inc. New York, N.Y.
10. STRAUSS, J. H., B. W. BURGE & J. E. DARNELL. 1970. Carbohydrate content of the membrane protein of Sindbis virus. J. Mol. Biol. **47:** 437–448.
11. WRIGHT, K. A. 1969. The anatomy of salivary glands of *Anopheles stephensi*. Can. J. Zool. **47:** 579–587.
12. HALSTEAD, S. B. & N. E. PALUMBO. 1973. Studies on the immunization of monkeys against dengue. Amer. J. Trop. Med. Hyg. **22:** 375–381.
13. GOLDMAN, L., E. ROCKWELL & D. F. RICHFIELD. 1952. Histopathological studies on cutaneous reactions to the bites of various arthropods. Amer. J. Trop. Med. Hyg. **1:** 514–525.
14. FRENCH, F. E. 1972. *Aedes aegypti:* histopathology of immediate skin reactions of hypersensitive guinea pigs resulting from bites. Exp. Parasitol. **32:** 175–180.
15. TAICHMAN, N. S. & H. Z. MOVAT. 1966. Do PMN-leucocytes play a role in passive cutaneous anaphylaxis of guinea pigs? Int. Arch. Allergy Appl. Immunol. **30:** 97–102.
16. MULLER, H. K. & D. L. HEALY. 1973. Active cutaneous anaphylaxis in the guinea pig. Immunological and inflammatory reactions. Immunology **24:** 1099–1112.
17. MELLANBY, K. 1946. Man's reaction to mosquito bites. Nature (London) **158:** 554.

VIRAL RECEPTORS AND THEIR ROLE IN HOST AND TISSUE SPECIFICITY

John A. Wise

Department of Pathobiology
School of Public Health and Community Medicine
University of Washington
Seattle, Washington 98195

The broad host range of arboviruses includes invertebrates and vertebrates as diverse as reptiles, mammals, and man. This ability of a single type of arbovirus to infect a variety of animals is quite different from that of most viruses, which have very restricted patterns of infectivity. In the latter case, host specificity was proposed to be due largely to the interaction of viruses with specific viral receptors on the surface of susceptible host tissues.[1] However, this proposal becomes less tenable when one considers the remarkable host range of the arboviruses and prompted a reevaluation of the role of viral receptors in host and tissue specificity.

The major work that described receptors for animal viruses was that of Holland and McLaren [2, 3] with human enteroviruses. These and subsequent *in vitro* experiments by others have led to the concept of viral receptors that incorporates the following points: strong interactions of virus with receptor(s) (only strong interactions are seen due to experimental methods); specificity, for example, with human enteroviruses, adsorption is restricted to certain types of primate tissues; [1] definitive molecular composition, such as protein or carbohydrate, probably in the form of surface glycolipids or glycoproteins.

However, several types of evidence indicate that the *in vitro* studies on which the receptor concept is based may not give an accurate picture of *in vivo* infections. Even with *in vitro* studies, there is frequently a lack of correlation between the presence of receptors and the ability of the cells to yield progeny virus. Buck *et al.*[4] found that mouse picornaviruses adsorbed with equal efficiency to cells from human, mouse, chicken, or bovine origin. In addition, extensive cytopathology was noted in infected cells of all types, but the total virus yield varied as much as 10,000-fold between cell types. Although some early stage of virus infection was noted in all cells, the production of infectious viral RNA and viral protein by any cell type was proportional to the yield of intact virus produced by that cell type. In another example, shown in TABLE 1, we found that the primate enterovirus coxsackie B_3 adsorbed well to mouse 3T3 cells but was unable to initiate even the earliest stages of infection, as evidenced by the absence of any cytopathologic effect. Similar results have been reported by Medrano and Green with coxsackie B_3 and 3T3 cells.[5] However, just the opposite situation was seen when human fetal tonsil cells were exposed to coxsackie B_3 (TABLE 1). No detectable adsorption was observed (less than one virus particle per cell), but there was a significant virus yield (average of 50 virions per cell). Limited replication of coxsackie A_{13} in primary fetal mouse cells was also reported despite the absence of detectable receptors.[6]

The primary isolation of virus from clinical specimens provides an even more interesting example of virus growth in the absence of adsorption. Human fetal tonsil cells are used routinely in our laboratory for the primary isolation of

TABLE 1

EFFECT OF COXSACKIE B₃ ON VARIOUS CELL LINES

Cell Line	Relative Adsorption	CPE	Percentage Virus Yield
HeLa M	1.0	4+	100
Hep 2	1.0	4+	86
Fetal tonsil (human)	< 0.01	2+	0.4
3T3 (mouse)	0.4	0	0

human rhinoviruses and are more efficient than any other cell line we have tried.[7] However, the adsorption of virus to fetal tonsil cells is very poor (TABLE 2). Furthermore, Tyrrell has reported that nasal epithelium organ culture is the most sensitive means of primary isolation of rhinoviruses,[8] but, in our hands, these organ cultures had no measurable receptor activity. It should be noted that the primary isolation of virus from clinical specimens is a very stringent test of cell susceptibility, because only a small number of virus particles may be present. Also, it is more analogous to an *in vivo* infection, where only minimum infectious doses of virus are likely.

Even though virus adsorption is not measurable *in vitro*, viral receptors in some form are probably present on susceptible cells. Certainly, some specificity of virus uptake by cells is indicated by the existence of mutant cells that are resistant to poliovirus due to the absence of receptors[5] and by the infection of naturally insusceptible cells with enterovirus RNA.[9]

The possibility that viral receptors could be present but not readily measurable can be explained if receptors are capable of interacting with virus in a multivalent form, as has been proposed by Lonberg-Holm and Philipson.[10] They hypothesize that a virus particle is bound only weakly (if at all) by a single receptor molecule, while two or three receptors interacting simultaneously with a virion increases the binding affinity, and multiple receptor molecules in close proximity are capable of binding a symmetric virus particle very tightly. This proposal is consistent with several observations on the *in vitro* adsorption of picornaviruses to cells. First, Holland reported that primate cells freshly prepared from a variety of organs failed to adsorb enteroviruses, but these cells

TABLE 2

SUSCEPTIBILITY OF CELL LINES TO RHINOVIRUSES

Cell Line	Type	Primary Isolation	Relative * Adsorption
Fetal tonsil	diploid	+++	0.05
WI–38	diploid	++	0.1
HeLa M	heteroploid	+	1.0
Nasal epithelium	organ	(++++)†	<0.01

* Adsorption of rhinoviruses 1A and 2.
† Isolations not performed in this study; data from Tyrrell.[8]

acquired virus receptors after growth in culture for 24 hr or more.[11] In several cases, freshly dispersed organ cells failed to adsorb coxsackie virus, even though those particular organs commonly serve as foci of infection *in vivo*. Careful experiments ruled out the selection of a subpopulation of receptor-carrying cells due to culturing. The conclusion from this study was that organ cells contain significant numbers of virus receptors that are unmasked by culturing or that culturing promotes the synthesis of viral receptors. However, even such tissue as intestinal epithelium, which will adsorb poliovirus, exhibits an increase in poliovirus receptors after culturing.

Generalizations from these and other experiments are that organ cultures demonstrate little or no receptor activity for picornaviruses, primary cell cultures have an increased capacity to bind virus, and established cell cultures have even greater numbers of receptors and are capable of adsorbing 10^4–10^5 virus particles per cell. Interestingly, the large number of high-affinity receptors in cell culture may be the cause of the large percentage of abortive infections with picornaviruses. It has long been known that adsorbed virus spontaneously elutes from cells, and this eluted virus can represent as much as 80% of the total in the case of poliovirus. Recently, it was shown that eluted picornaviruses have been structurally altered by interaction with cells: they are no longer infectious, and they lack one of four structural proteins.[10] In addition, if virions that contain radioactively labeled RNA are used for infection, as much as 50–80% of the radioactivity is degraded into acid-soluble counts.

These two types of observation could be explained by postulating that the high affinity of the receptors *in vitro* results in abnormal distortion of the virion structure and loss of capsid protein before penetration can occur, in distortion of the protective coat of the virus to expose the RNA to nucleases, in premature uncoating of the viral nucleic acid at unfavorable sites, which causes degradation; virus could also be irreversibly bound at the surface of the cell, which would thus prevent the normal penetration and uncoating process. This hypothesis also offers an explanation for the large number of particles required to initiate a plaque *in vitro*. For most rhinovirus types, for example, the ratio of physical virus particles to plaque-forming units is 2000/10,000. Although it is argued that this ratio represents a normal infectious dose, because 5000–10,000 particles are required to initiate an infection *in vitro*, the two values are not equivalent. Because the virus faces a hostile environment and host defense mechanisms, it would appear that the real efficiency of infection is actually much greater *in vivo*.

The discussion thus far has been restricted to interactions of picornaviruses with cells because these viruses have been intensely studied. Although much less is known about arbovirus-cell interactions, it is tempting to speculate that infectivity by arboviruses also does not require cell receptors with strong affinities. In fact, because of the remarkable lack of tissue specificity exhibited by arboviruses, it seems questionable whether receptors are necessary for infection. Not only do these viruses successfully infect invertebrates and a variety of vertebrate hosts, but they are also capable of replicating in virtually every tissue and organ in these hosts. A common component on the surface of such a variety of cells would appear unlikely, except the lipid membrane itself.

Recently, Mooney *et al.*[12] found that Sindbis virus was capable of binding to liposomes that contain no membrane proteins or glycolipids. However, phospholipids and cholesterol greatly enhanced virus binding. Phospholipids are found universally in biologic membranes and therefore could be involved with surface binding of Sindbis and possibly other arboviruses. Thus, the mechanisms for limitation of arbovirus growth and tissue tropisms are quite likely to involve steps in infection subsequent to the initial nonspecific binding of virus to cells. Possible mechanisms of cellular resistance to arboviruses have already been discussed by Murphy in this monograph.

REFERENCES

1. HOLLAND, J. J. 1964. Bacteriol. Rev. **28:** 3–13.
2. HOLLAND, J. J. & L. C. MCLAREN. 1959. J. Exp. Med. **109:** 487–504.
3. HOLLAND, J. J. & L. C. MCLAREN. 1961. J. Exp. Med. **114:** 161–171.
4. BUCK, C. A., G. A. GRANGER, M. W. TAYLOR & J. J. HOLLAND. 1967. Virology **33:** 36–46.
5. MEDRANO, L. & H. GREEN. 1970. Virology **54:** 515–525.
6. GOLDBERG, R. J., M. GRAVELL & R. L. CROWELL. 1969. Proc. Soc. Exp. Biol. Med. **132:** 743–748.
7. COONEY, X. X. 19xx. Unpublished results.
8. TYRRELL, D. A. J. 1968. Virol. Mon. **2:** 67–124.
9. HOLLAND, J. J., L. C. MCLAREN & J. T. SYVERTON. 1959. J. Exp. Med. **110:** 65–80.
10. LONBERG-HOLM, K. & L. PHILIPSON. 1974. Monographs in Virology. Vol. 9. S. Karger. Basel, Switzerland.
11. HOLLAND, J. J. 1961. Virology **15:** 312–326.
12. MOONEY, J. J., J. M. DALRYMPLE, C. R. ALVING & P. K. RUSSELL. 1975. J. Virol. **15:** 225–231.

PATHOGENIC EFFECTS OF PLANT DISEASE AGENTS ON VECTOR INSECTS: AN INTRODUCTION

Robert F. Whitcomb

Insect Pathology Laboratory
Plant Protection Institute
Agricultural Research Service
United States Department of Agriculture
Beltsville, Maryland 20705

This Conference has so far emphasized an interdisciplinary approach to pathobiology, and this session is no exception. The various authors deal with such diverse pathogens as small RNA viruses of plants, spiroplasmas of plants and insects, walled prokaryotes of plants and insects, and nuclear polyhedrosis viruses (NPV) of insects. In indicating the hosts of these pathogens, I have reflected the current view that the pathogens are indeed confined to "usual" hosts. In retrospect, it seems that one central thread throughout this session is the current degree of uncertainty with respect to the limits of host ranges and specificities of pathogenic organisms. I am reminded of earlier work, in which we discovered, purely by accident, that acholeplasmas (which had been regarded before that time as saprophytes or commensals of vertebrates) multiplied in insects. It had been our intention to use them as control mycoplasmas, which were *not* expected to multiply! They did not, however, in our hands, cause plant disease. A central feature of host relationships is the necessity for pathogenic organisms to be adapted to each of the microenvironments of a biologic cycle. Perhaps what we are learning is that whereas organisms may be adapted to some of these microenvironments, the chance occurrence of the entire series of adaptations that might enable an organism to maintain itself in a reservoir in nature is a rare event. Such adaptations, in fact, apparently occur on an *evolutionary* time scale rather than on a *contemporary* one.

Certainly, the production, licensing, and use of live vaccines depend on the rapid drift away from pathogenicity in different *in vivo* systems. With our spiroplasmas, we also observe such a drift after passage of the corn stunt agent in *Drosophila;* the ability to complete the biologic cycle in leafhoppers and plants is lost. The existence of plant viruses that apparently do not multiply, but that are acquired from and transmitted to plants by the circulative route, should be of considerable importance in studies on host specificity of viruses.

True insect viruses have great potential as cornerstones in integrated insect control programs, so that their host range capabilities are of special interest. Detailed knowledge of the manner in which they infect cells is an a priori requirement for such an assessment. The careful observations of Hirumi *et al.* on one NPV-host cell system further this understanding. But, what is the range of potentially infectable cells? This important question is now being addressed by McIntosh *et al.*, and the progress of this group, as reported here and in forthcoming publications, will have bearing on the speed with which insect viruses are made available for agricultural purposes. Perhaps, the NPV (baculovirus) and granulosis groups, which have no known counterparts as plant or vertebrate pathogens, will prove to be unable to replicate in vertebrate cells. In any event, there is good reason to hold high hope that potentially useful viruses will prove to be as safe as live vaccines for human use.

HELICAL WALL-FREE PROKARYOTES IN INSECTS: MULTIPLICATION AND PATHOGENICITY *

R. F. Whitcomb

Insect Pathology Laboratory
Plant Protection Institute
Agricultural Research Service
United States Department of Agriculture
Beltsville, Maryland 20705

D. L. Williamson

Department of Anatomical Sciences
State University of New York
Stony Brook, New York 11790

INTRODUCTION

Spiroplasmas as Organisms

Spiroplasmas, helical motile wall-free prokaryotes, have only recently been recognized as a distinct new group of microorganisms [1] referrable to the Mollicutes [2, 3] but meriting an assignment to a new family within the class.[4] In the past, spiroplasmas were regarded as spirochetes by workers who observed them in the hemolymph of insects, as viruses by workers who observed the symptoms of plant diseases they induced, or as mycoplasmas by workers who used thin-section electron microscopy for their visualization. Only one spiroplasma (*Spiroplasma citri*) has been assigned [5] a Latin binomial, but techniques derived for its culture [6, 7] have enabled its repeated isolation, and many strains from diverse geographic locations are now available for laboratory study. Some of these strains were shown to multiply in leafhoppers,[8, 9] and eventually these insects were used experimentally to transmit the agent to citrus and other plants.[10, 11] Also, the agent could be cultured from two leafhopper species in the field,[12] one of which, *Circulifer tenellus* (Baker), is already well known for its ability to transmit the destructive beet curly top virus. The other insect, *Scaphytopius nitridus* (DeLong), breeds on citrus and can acquire and transmit the pathogen.[13]

Progress in the culture of two other spiroplasmas has been less rapid. The sex ratio organism (SRO) of *Drosophila* was discovered [14] as a result of its ability to eliminate male progeny from female flies in which it is inherited maternally. Actually, there are several SROs, each of which was isolated from different but closely related neotropical species of *Drosophila* but which can be differentiated by differential susceptibility to lysis by strain specific viruses. At first, the SRO was considered to be a spirochete,[14] but it was later shown [15, 16] to lack an axial filament and an outer envelope or cell wall; both structures are characteristic of spirochetes. The SRO, then, appears, to possess features more similar to the spiroplasmas than to the spirochetes. In addition, antiserum

* Supported in part by United States Public Health Service Grant AI-10950.

against the corn stunt agent severely deformed the SROs.[16] Although this same test in the reciprocal direction did not cause a deformation of the corn stunt organism (CSO), the one-way reaction between CSO antiserum and the SRO may indicate a relationship between them.

A third spiroplasma is associated with the corn stunt disease. This disease [17] was thought to be viral in origin [18] for many years, but in 1968, wall-free prokaryotes were envisioned in association with the disease.[19] These organisms were found in both plant and insect hosts [20] and could be observed in sap stained with phosphotungstic acid.[20] Although the identification of these negatively stained organisms as the etiologic agent was challenged,[21] it is apparently now agreed [22] that the identification was correct. It remained, however, for Davis et al.[23, 24] to show that the CSO occurred in plants and insects [25] in helical form. It is now possible, in light of this subsequent research, to see in the earlier micrographs the vestiges of the helical configurations that are characteristic and diagnostic [26, 27] of spiroplasma cultures whether such cultures are in the insect, the plant, or the test tube.

Although the causal agent of corn stunt was thus pinpointed as a helical wall-free prokaryote, its culture proved far more difficult than that of S. citri. Chen and Granados [28] succeeded in obtaining primary isolation, but sustained culture was not achieved. Brazilian workers [29, 30] may also have achieved a similar but limited success. The early optimism then turned to caution,[23] and, finally, some workers concluded [31-33] that the corn stunt agent provided a special culturing problem.

Within the past year, however, two groups, simultaneouly and independently, who used different approaches and media, achieved cultivation. Chen and Liao,[34] who employed a very slight modification of the initial medium [28] of Chen and Granados, achieved isolation from the plant. The present authors [35] were able to adapt the CSO to grow in the hemolymph of Drosophila pseudoobscura Frolova,[16] from which cultivation could be readily achieved in a medium based on a compromise between media used for Drosophila cell culture and those used for cultivation of S. citri. This compromise medium also permitted culture from infected corn.[35] Both groups agreed that the CSOs were serologically related [36] to S. citri but that a large bloc of antigens, perhaps a majority, were not shared by the two spiroplasmas. McIntosh et al.[61] made a similar claim, but without supporting evidence. Because different geographic isolates of the corn stunt disease agent are known,[37-39] it is clear that a third natural cluster of spiroplasmas exists. The eventual taxonomic resolution awaits the careful characterization required by the set of proposed minimum standards for naming species of mycoplasmas.[40] Regardless of the final taxonomic resolution, however, the discovery of a new family of organisms associated with insects is of considerable importance to the study of pathobiology in invertebrates.

Spiroplasmas as Pathogenic Agents

For many years, it was a nostrum that plant disease agents were harmless to their insect hosts; indeed, there were many instances in which pathogenesis was carefully sought and found absent. In 1958, however, the agent of Western-X disease, considered to be a virus at that time, was shown to be lethal to its leafhopper vector.[11] The agent was later shown to cause histopathologic conditions in the alimentary tract, adipose tissue, endocrine glands, neural tissue, connective tissue, pericardium, and salivary glands of infected insects.[42] The most conspicuous pathologic features were an accumulation of "material" that intensely absorbed Mallory's or Giemsa stains. This material was later found to be an accumulation of wall-free prokaryotes.[43] No helical forms were found in insect or plant. Rather, Nasu et al.[43] proposed that diverse forms of organisms they observed may have a function in the reproductive cycle and that, furthermore, these forms could be maintained for several weeks in a recognizable state in cell-free media.[44]

Spiroplasmas also exert pathogenic effects upon insect hosts that they colonize in large numbers. The effect of CSO on the leafhopper vector Dalbulus elimatus (Ball) was studied by Granados[20] and by Granados and Meehan.[45] The organisms could be envisioned both intra- and extracellularly. As with the Western-X disease agent, cells of the supraesophageal ganglion and salivary glands appeared to be favored sites for accumulation of organisms. In the neural tissue, degeneration of axons was apparently associated with spiroplasma multiplication. In salivary cells, large electron-dense bodies, which often occupied large portions of the infected cells, were associated with or surrounded the spiroplasmas.[45]

MATERIALS AND METHODS

Enumeration of Helices

Enumeration of helical bodies from in vitro cultures or from hemolymph was achieved by placing 5 μl of liquid beneath a cover slip and counting the number of bodies visible in randomly selected fields under dark-field illumination.[46] The concentration of bodies could be calculated from the area of the field. If 5 μl of hemolymph could not be obtained, we calibrated small glass needles to deliver 0.1 μl. This volume is also the approximate amount of fluid we injected into the insects. The small hemolymph droplets could be examined directly under dark-field illumination if they were covered with immersion oil or could be diluted in M1 medium[35] if the numbers of helical bodies were too numerous to count in the sampled droplet.

Colony-Forming Unit (CFU) and Color-Changing Unit (CCU) Assays

Extracts or diluted hemolymph that contained S. citri (Maroc strain, passage levels 150–180) could be plated on conventional solid mycoplasma medium; 10–12 days after inoculation, the umbonate colonies could be counted. Corn stunt organisms (strain B, clone 2, ATCC no. 27953) could also be assayed in this way by using the solid medium developed for that organism.[35] Colony formation by CSOs, however, is irregular, and the CFU assay is therefore not entirely satisfactory. In all cases, serial 10-fold dilutions of CSOs could be made in M1 medium, and the tubes incubated at 30° C. Development of spiroplasma cultures was indicated by a color change of the phenol red indicator from red to yellow. The highest dilution at which this change occurred was defined as containing 1 CCU.

Culture Methods

Spiroplasma cultures were maintained in M1 medium by passage of 0.2 ml of inoculum every 3–4 days to 5 ml of fresh medium. The cultures and all experimental assays were maintained at 30° C for CSO or at 32° C for *S. citri.* The SROs were transferred by injection of hemolymph from their natural host species, *Drosophila willistoni* Sturtevant, into a wild-type strain of *D. pseudoobscura* kept at 20° C and maintained as male-free stocks by mating naturally infected females with males from the uninfected strain.

Leafhoppers and flies were injected abdominally with about 0.1–0.2 μl of spiroplasma inocula. For assessment of the ability to transmit spiroplasma to plants, insects were transferred to healthy corn seedlings about 10–17 days after injection and then weekly as long as they remained alive. Records were kept of survival through the postinjection period. For bioassay of ability to induce sex ratio abnormality in *Drosophila,* injected flies were transferred at 3-day intervals to fresh bottles, and the sex ratio of successive broods that hatched from the bottles was determined.

RESULTS

Morphology of Spiroplasmas in Cell-Free Medium

Observations of Cole *et al.*[47] with *S. citri* were confirmed in our studies with both plant spiroplasmas. The CSOs achieved titers in excess of 10^8 CFU or CCU within 3–4 days after passage; *S. citri* achieved titers as high as 10^9 in 2–3 days. Younger cultures, which corresponded to lag phase or very early log phase, contained many very short or possibly spheroidal bodies; in log phase, the predominant morphologic characteristic was a short helix. Bodies of CSOs appeared to have one end more pointed than the other.[16] In later stages, which probably corresponded to the stationary phase, the length of helical forms increased, sometimes spectacularly, and aggregates of bodies appeared in which longer forms were entangled. These "medusae" were also irregularly observed in some younger cultures. Although these forms probably arise, at least initially, from aggregation, an alternative but less likely explanation for their origin might involve repeated branching of a single helical filament. In older cultures, helicity itself was lost.

Parallel studies by Jones *et al.*[48] have shown that both osmotic and nutritional factors influence spiroplasma morphology in cultures. Organisms growing under suboptimal conditions lose helicity or become more elongate, with a tendency for some turns of the helices to open, which results in twisting and distortion. Spiroplasmas maintained in suboptimal environments may also develop "blebs;" these structures were originally thought to have some significance in the life cycle of the organisms but are perhaps better interpreted[49] as degenerating bodies.

In *Drosophila,* the SROs apparently develop to lengths of about 4–8 μm, but smaller forms are sometimes observed.

These observations of spiroplasma morphology, which are preliminary and not to be regarded as an attempt to construct an interpretation of the mode of spiroplasma reproduction, point to the necessity for caution in the interpretation of helices as significant indicators of the disease process in infected hosts.

Multiplication of Spiroplasmas in Usual Hosts

Spiroplasma citri

The "usual" insect host for *S. citri* is uncertain, but it has been shown experimentally to multiply to high titer in the leafhoppers *Macrosteles fascifrons* (Stål), *Dalbulus elimatus*,[9] and *Euscelis plebejus* (Fallén).[8] Natural multiplication occurs in the leafhoppers *Circulifer tenellus* and *Scaphytopius nitridus*.[12, 13] The spiroplasma also multiplied[9] with some difficulty in *Draeculacephala* spp., members of a subfamily of leafhoppers (Cicadellinae) that feed in the xylem and that are phylogenetically remote from the other insect hosts. In *D. elimatus,* multiplication was better, but in *M. fascifrons, S. citri* reached levels as high as $3–5 \times 10^6$ CFU per insect and reduced the longevity of the insects.[9] The maximum titer of CFU was achieved rapidly (in 2–4 days), even after injection of diluted inocula. In *Macrosteles* and *Dalbulus,* multiplication was imperfectly correlated with production of helical forms in the hemolymph. Cultural tests showed that between 2×10^2 and 3×10^3 CFU or CCU could be demonstrated from droplets of hemolymph (~0.1 μl) collected from insects in which few helical forms were present (0–20 helical forms per hemolymph droplet). Thus, many of the small, not readily identifiable bodies present in such hemolymph preparations must have been viable, but nonhelical, spiroplasma bodies. It should be emphasized that immediately after injection, or at 24–48 hr postinjection, helical forms can be readily detected. In any case, whether the organisms were injected into *Macrosteles* or *Dalbulus,* by the fourth day, their numbers had declined by $2–3 \log_{10}$ units. Instead of helical forms, there arose, in some, but not all insects, an extremely high number of forms, some of which may have been spheroidal but many of which appeared to be very short forms of a half turn at the most. These populations of bodies resemble those seen in early stages in culture, but the bodies were often more numerous, and the identification of individual organisms as spiroplasmas was, of course, uncertain. In a comparative experiment, we found that spiroplasma CCU titer in hemolymph remained high 11, 22, and 29 days after injection, but at no time did large numbers of helical spiroplasmas appear in these insects.

CSO in Natural Leafhopper Hosts

Previous work has indicated that the presence of helical forms in plants[23] and leafhoppers[25] is diagnostic of CSO infection. In the plant, there is a suggestion that large accumulations of these helical forms occur principally in advanced stages of symptomatic expression.[24] We have now studied the relationship of helical CSO filaments to leafhoppers in two ways: by examination of naturally infected insects and by following the course of infection after injection of cultured microorganisms. In all, 10 CSO isolates were injected into *D. elimatus* and examined for the presence of helical forms. Helical forms were found in the hemolymph at all times up to 24 days after injection, by which time the majority of insects had died. When injected with large numbers of helical forms, large numbers of such forms tended to persist until Days 10–12 postinjection, at which time a noticeable decline in number had occurred. Then, 18–24 days after injection, the number of helical forms seemed to rise again to levels that equaled or exceeded the input dose (FIGURE 2). Titers of

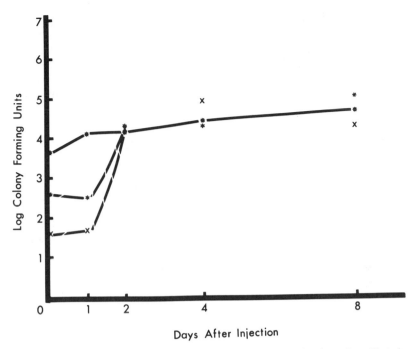

FIGURE 1. Multiplication of *S. citri* in *D. elimatus* after injection of undiluted culture (*) and dilutions of 10^{-1} (*) and 10^{-2} (×) of the cultured organisms.

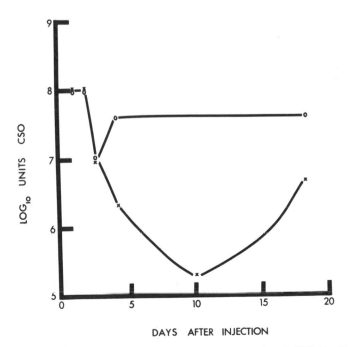

FIGURE 2. Comparison of number of colony forming units of CSOs in *D. elimatus* (○) and count of helical spiroplasma bodies (×) in hemolymph droplets placed under immersion oil and examined by dark-field microscopy.

viable CSOs did not follow this pattern, however (FIGURE 2). The results from several other experiments were similar. However, considerable caution should be used in interpretation of such results. Helical forms are easily deformed, and their absence from hemolymph samples might indicate osmotic or other abnormalities. Also, bacteria may exclude spiroplasmas; the level of bacterial multiplication required for this suppression is unknown.

Insects infected naturally were not titered by either CFU or CCU methods because of the uncertainty of success of primary isolation. Although primary isolations were achieved in 76/111 attempts when droplets of hemolymph that ranged from about 0.1 to 1.0 μl were placed in 1 ml of M1 medium, such cultures grew more slowly than organisms that had been first adapted to grow in the M1 medium and were then injected into leafhoppers. Colonies of CSO also formed irregularly, or failed to form, without a period of prior cultural adaptation. Helical CSOs could be found in insects before completion of the latent period, in some cases as early as 8 days after their first exposure to infected corn. The number of helical forms in the hemolymph of exposed insects varied greatly between individual insects, but in late stages of infection (about 30 days after the first exposure), it was not unusual to find insect hemolymph that contained in excess of 10^8 helical forms per milliliter.

SRO in Drosophila

In the species in which SROs occur naturally and in species to which they have been artificially transferred, infection results in the total, or nearly total, elimination of the males from the progeny. Each of the SROs appears to have a characteristic numerical density in their species of origin. The following numbers were obtained from direct counts of hemolymph samples: *D. equinoxalis* Dobzhansky, $2 \times 10^6/\mu$l; *D. nebulosa* Sturtevant, $2 \times 10^6/\mu$l; *D. willistoni*, $13 \times 10^6/\mu$l.[15] Comparable numbers are obtained when the SROs are transferred by injection to other species of *Drosophila*.

Multiplication of Spiroplasmas in Unusual Hosts

Spiroplasma citri

Introduction of large numbers of *S. citri* into *Drosophila* is followed by an abrupt drop in number of CFU, which may be as great as 3 $\log_{10}$ units.[50] This initial drop is paralleled by a significant drop in the number of helical forms. The course of the infection thereafter was variable from experiment to experiment and between individual insects in the same experiment, but there was a tendency for recovery in CFU to at least the input dose by Days 7–9 post-injection. By the 14th day after injection, large numbers of helical forms could be observed in some, but not all, infected flies.

We also attempted to maintain *S. citri* in the large milkweed bug, *Oncopeltus fasciatus* (Dallas), and the German cockroach, *Blattella germanica* (L.). In each of these hosts, numbers of CFU decayed rapidly 1–3 days postinjection. No CFU were recovered from *Blattella* after that date, but as long as 41 days after injection, a low level of CFU could be demonstrated in extracts of whole *Oncopeltus* adults. Spaar *et al.*[51] also demonstrated long-term persistence of

S. citri in unusual hosts (hemipteran and coleopteran insects). Such persistence is most likely to be achieved through limited multiplication of the organisms.

CSO in Drosophila

The CSO could be established in *D. pseudoobscura* by injection of sap squeezed from infected corn plants.[16] After the first few days, during which time the number of helical forms decreased abruptly, their numbers slowly increased. After five monthly passages, their numbers had increased greatly, and we were able to demonstrate retention of the ability to infect leafhoppers and corn.[16] From these passage experiments, our first *in vitro* isolates of corn stunt were obtained.[16, 35] The initial passage of corn stunt has been maintained at Stony Brook and at the time of this Conference has approached its 16th monthly passage. The adaptation to *Drosophila* has improved during this 12-month period, and the number of helical organisms now exceeds 10^{11}/ml, a number far in excess of our best growth in cell-free media.

The CSO in *D. pseudoobscura* does not cause any distortion of the sex ratio among the progeny of infected females, nor have we observed any instances of transmission of helical forms to progeny flies.

SRO in Macrosteles fascifrons

Injection of SROs into *M. fascifrons* was accomplished by transferring droplets of hemolymph from infected *D. pseudoobscura* into young adult leafhoppers. Although helical bodies were numerous 24 hr after injection, most of them appeared to be deformed, and many exhibited blebs that seemed to be attached to, or derived from, the filament. By the 48th hr after injection, however, all helical forms had disappeared, and the hemolymph of the leafhoppers contained large numbers of spheroidal bodies. Presumably, at least some of the bodies represented deformed SROs.

To evaluate whether viable SROs might be retained in the leafhopper, we used a simple bioassay for SRO infectivity. This assay, which was based in part on earlier work [52] with leafhoppers, measured the ability of extracts to induce the sex ratio abnormality. We first made 10-fold dilutions of SROs from *Drosophila* hemolymph in phosphate-buffered saline (PBS) and then injected the diluted organisms into normal *Drosophila* females. The sex ratios of successive 3-day broods of these females were then noted (TABLE 1). Undiluted SROs, estimated by enumeration to be 4.35×10^{10}, produced an immediate elimination of male progeny, but expression of the sex ratio trait was delayed after injection of diluted preparations. The "latent period" [52] before this expression was an inverse function of SRO concentration, which enabled us to construct a dose-response curve (FIGURE 3) that related dosage of SROs to the length of time before expression of the sex ratio trait.

This bioassay method permitted us to compare the multiplication of SROs in leafhoppers with their multiplication in *D. pseudoobscura*. A dilution of 1/100 of *Drosophila* hemolymph that contained SROs was injected into normal *Drosophila* or young *Macrosteles* adults. Then, at intervals of 1, 2, 3, and 6 days, 0.1 μl of hemolymph was transferred from the injected insects into normal *D. pseudoobscura,* and the brood progenies were recorded (TABLES 2

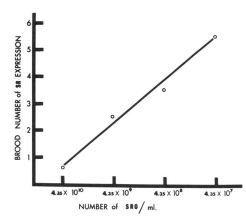

FIGURE 3. Relationship between number of SROs injected into *D. pseudoobscura* and the brood number (3-day intervals) that first exhibits an altered sex ratio.

and 3). From these data, we could interpolate on the dose-response curve (FIGURE 3) and construct growth (or decay) curves for SRO in the two hosts. The SROs multiplied (FIGURE 4) in their natural host, *D. pseudoobscura*, to a level that at 6 days gave an immediate elimination of male progeny in the first brood. In leafhoppers, however, there was no indication (FIGURE 4) of retention of male-killing ability after 24 hr. In this instance, therefore, disappearance of biologic activity paralleled disappearance of the helical forms of the microorganisms.

Pathogenicity of Spiroplasmas for Insects

Pathogenicity of Spiroplasma citri for Macrosteles

S. citri multiplies in and reduces the longevity of *M. fascifrons,* a vector of several wall-free prokaryotes that cause plant diseases of the "yellows" type.[9] We further reported [50] that the enhancement of this pathogenicity by nine serial

TABLE 1

SEXES OF PROGENY FROM *D. pseudoobscura* INJECTED WITH DILUTIONS OF SROs IN PBS

	Dilutions of SROs							
	1/10		1/10		1/100		1/1000	
Broods	♀	♂	♀	♂	♀	♂	♀	♂
1	7	0	11	4	13	12	9	11
2	16	0	11	4	33	44	21	32
3	14	0	22	0	35	21	48	44
4	4	0	28	0	31	1	22	25
5	1	0	6	0	2	0	2	8
6	0	0	25	0	2	0	6	0
7	12	0	14	0	11	0	7	0

TABLE 2

SEXES OF PROGENY FROM *D. pseudoobscura* INJECTED WITH HEMOLYMPH
FROM FLIES INJECTED WITH A 1/100 DILUTION OF SROs IN PBS

	Time Interval (hr) between Injection of First and Second Sets of Flies									
	0		24		48		72		154	
Broods	♀	♂	♀	♂	♀	♂	♀	♂	♀	♂
1	9	21	32	28	9	17	3	4	13	0
2	28	30	27	25	7	12	51	55	5	0
3	43	40	8	5	21	15	35	1	0	0
4	0	0	13	6	15	1	26	0	0	0
5	16	0	9	0	3	0	12	0	0	0
6	11	0	3	0	11	0	6	0	0	0
7	39	0	3	0	9	0	2	0	0	0

passages in *Macrosteles* without increasing the final achieved titer of CFUs indicates that populations of spiroplasmas are capable of adaptation.[50] Although *S. citri* multiplies in *D. elimatus*, the corn stunt vector, it did not reduce the longevity of that insect.[50]

Pathogenicity of SROs for Drosophila

The elimination of male progeny from *Drosophila*, at first thought to be due to a "plasmagene," was shown by Poulson and Sakaguchi[14] to be caused by a helical organism which they regarded as a spirochete. The condition has no known selective advantage for flies in the field and can be regarded as pathologic for male progeny, although females that transmit the SRO have life-spans and fecundities comparable to those of uninfected females. There is some evidence that the male-killing factor can be separated from the micro-organism,[53, 54] but we have no data to indicate its nature or its mode of action.

TABLE 3

SEXES OF PROGENY FROM *D. pseudoobscura* INJECTED WITH HEMOLYMPH
FROM *M. fascifrons* INJECTED WITH A 1/100 DILUTION OF SROs IN PBS

	Time Interval (hr) between Injection of Leafhoppers and Flies									
	0		24		48		72		154	
Broods	♀	♂	♀	♂	♀	♂	♀	♂	♀	♂
1	35	40	32	31	6	9	16	25	19	39
2	54	59	64	67	59	49	53	62	13	22
3	35	34	62	64	53	56	51	53	11	12
4	47	42	41	33	13	9	40	26	39	30
5	15	8	16	9	38	45	10	7	3	5
6	3	0	26	3	13	6	4	9	10	3
7	12	0	17	0	17	28	5	3	8	6

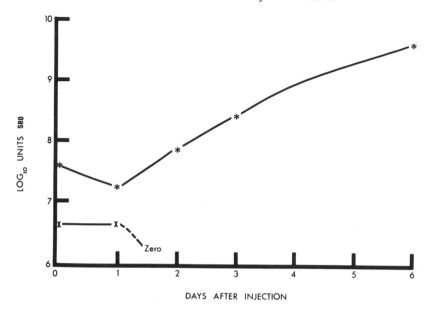

FIGURE 4. SROs multiply after injection into *D. pseudoobscura* Frolova (*) but disappear from *M. fascifrons* Stål (×) after 24 hr.

Pathogenicity of CSO for Dalbulus *Spp.*

Spiroplasmas produce conspicuous symptoms in the plants that they infect. The pathogenicity of *S. citri* to plants has been shown by Daniels and Meddins to result from a toxin, which they partially purified.[55] This toxin was ineffective against insects, however, and the citrus spiroplasma was able to multiply to high titer in *Euscelis* without adversely affecting the insect.[10] Such is not the case with the CSOs in the natural vectors *D. elimatus* and *Dalbulus maidis* DeLong. Granados and Meehan[45] have reported that the corn stunt spiroplasma is pathogenic to both of these natural vectors. We later showed,[35] as did Chen and Liao,[34] that cultured CSOs are also pathogenic to *D. elimatus.* However, our B isolate, obtained after extended passage in *Drosophila,* apparently lost its ability to complete the biologic cycle of multiplication in plants and insects. CSO isolates obtained directly from plants, however, retained this ability. We therefore wished to compare the pathogenicity of various isolates to insects. In one experiment, we injected pelleted organisms of our B (nonpathogenic) isolate and of our E and G isolates (pathogenic). In addition, we injected insects with medium in which CSOs had grown to stationary phase but from which all organisms had been filtered. All three CSO isolates significantly reduced the longevity of leafhoppers into which they had been injected (FIGURE 5), and 22 days after injection, hemolymph from leafhoppers injected with the isolates contained large numbers of helical filaments. Therefore, the B isolate has apparently retained its ability to proliferate in, and induce pathogenicity to, *Dalbulus.*

Discussion

In this paper, we have attempted to summarize the existing knowledge on the pathogenicity of spiroplasmas for insects. The pathobiology of the insect infections is complex, because the variables of host susceptibility and host defense are added to the complexity of the growth cycle of the organisms themselves. Therefore, each infection is unique and appears to follow a different course to a somewhat different end. The plant spiroplasmas have proved to be adaptable to a variety of situations *in vivo* and *in vitro*. In particular, adaptation to a new insect host may require a considerable period of time. There is therefore great danger in concluding that plant spiroplasmas have really disappeared from a host, and such a claim cannot be made, for example, for *S. citri* in *Blattella germanica*.

It would, however, be of considerable interest to observe the fate of the plant spiroplasmas in insects in which host defense mechanisms have been well documented. Steady-state infections of *Drosophila* with enteric bacteria have been reported to confer immunity.[56] It would be interesting to know whether the steady-state spiroplasma infections also confer immunity to other microorganisms. Injection of spiroplasmas from culture or hemolymph into a new insect host invariably results in at least a short-term decrease in number of helices and recoverable infectivity, although the course of disappearance and reappearance of both properties is imperfectly correlated. Is this drop intermediated in part by a host defense reaction, which would be expected[57] to be most intense during the first 24–48 hr of an infection? If such a defense is operating in *Drosophila*, it is imperfect, because the spiroplasmas eventually adapt and are able to multiply to spectacularly high numbers. Our observations on the growth cycle of spiroplasmas in culture are preliminary but suggest that young vigorous cultures in early log phase consist of very short helices or, perhaps, spheroidal bodies. As long ago as 1961, Poulson and Sakaguchi[14] noted that SROs in hemolymph samples maintained under immersion oil exhibited an increasing number of granules; after 1 week, the granules were the principal form observed. These granules appeared to have a small nearly invisible tail and displayed movement distinguishable from Brownian movement.[14] Whether elongated filaments contain more than one genome and whether fragmented filaments are viable, as recently suggested for *S. citri,*[58] is conjectural

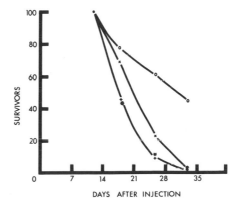

FIGURE 5. Survival of *D. elimatus* leafhoppers that were injected with CSO isolates B (×), G or E (*+), and of control insects that were injected with filtered medium in which CSOs had been grown (○). All isolates were pathogenic to the insect, but other experiments[35] showed that the B isolate had lost its ability to complete the biologic cycle in the plant.

and desperately needs experimental attention. It is unlikely that further progress on the significance of spiroplasma morphology *in vivo* will be made until the growth cycle *in vitro* has been elucidated.

Although pathogenicity of spiroplasmas for insects is associated with multiplication to high titers, it is not an inevitable result of high titer. The data of Granados and Meehan [45] strongly suggest, but do not prove, that plant spiroplasmas can multiply intracellularly in certain insect cells. Similarly, it has been claimed,[41] on the basis of infectivity tests, that SROs are present in the ovary, fat body, and muscle of infected flies. Loss of the ability to multiply intracellularly upon cultural adaptation could account for loss of the ability of the B strain of CSO to complete the biologic cycle; this is at present, of course, mere conjecture. The occurrence of extremely high numbers of spiroplasmas in hemolymph of leafhoppers and *Drosophila* strongly suggests that extracellular multiplication occurs. Definitive proof of multiplication *in situ* could be approached with autoradiography, as was done with the clover phyllody agent by Gouranton and Maillet.[60] An explicit demonstration of the sites of spiroplasma multiplication in their insect hosts would shed interesting light on the cultivation of fastidious pathogens and of their pathogenic interrelationships.

SUMMARY

At least three helical, motile, wall-free prokaryotes (spiroplasmas) are known to be associated with insects. Two of them, the agents of corn stunt disease (CSO) and citrus stubborn disease (*Spiroplasma citri*), are pathogenic to both plants and insects. A third spiroplasma [the sex ratio organism (SRO)] is found in neotropical species of *Drosophila,* is maternally inherited, and eliminates male progeny but is not known to be associated with plants. Recent success in cultivation of *S. citri* and the CSO has facilitated study of their pathogenicity to insects. Measurement of the growth of plant spiroplasmas in insects is possible by enumeration of colony-forming units (CFU) or color-changing units (CCU). Because SROs have not been cultivated, they must be enumerated microscopically or their viability must be bioassayed by injection into normal *Drosophila*. Microscopic enumeration of helical bodies is also possible in hemolymph from leafhoppers infected with *S. citri* or CSO. In some cases, we observed 100- to 1000-fold discrepancies in number of infectious units, as measured by CFU or CCU titrations, and in number of helical forms counted in hemolymph droplets. In optimal cell-free medium, both *S. citri* and CSO have variable morphology. In lag phase or very early log phase, the organisms are short or possibly spheroidal; in log phase, the helical forms are short, and only in late log phase or stationary phase do elongated helical forms appear. When the organisms are growing on suboptimal medium, their morphology may also be distorted, with the appearance of blebs or loss of helicity. Thus, different mechanisms may underlie discrepancies between observed titer and number of helical forms.

Introduction of CSOs or SROs into natural hosts is followed by attainment of high numbers or titers of organisms in the hemolymph, but helicity of organisms is not always preserved. Introduction of spiroplasmas into unusual hosts is followed by disappearance of most helical bodies and abrupt reduction in titer. Loss of helical bodies from the hemolymph of leafhoppers 48 hr after injection of SROs is paralleled by a loss of "infectivity" for *Drosophila* (ability to eliminate male progeny). *S. citri*, when introduced into *Drosophila* or *Oncopeltus*, is apparently maintained for long periods and probably multiplies. The CSO also multiplied in *Drosophila*, retained pathogenicity to plants and insects through at least the fifth monthly passage, and eventually reached levels in the hemolymph in excess of those obtainable in culture media. Spiroplasma populations, therefore, are adaptable, particularly on extended passage. CSOs could be cultured from *Drosophila* after such extended passage or directly from corn or leafhoppers. Two isolates from corn retained their ability to infect and cause disease in both plants and insects. However, the isolate from *Drosophila*, although retaining pathogenicity to insects, apparently lost its ability to be transmitted to and/or infect corn. Pathogenicity of *S. citri* to leafhoppers is associated with multiplication to high titer and can be enhanced by serial passage in the insect. The histopathologic basis for pathogenicity is unknown. Although it is not known with certainty whether spiroplasmas multiply intra- or extracellularly, evidence suggests that both modes may be utilized. Elucidation of this aspect would strengthen our understanding of pathogenic interrelationships and the cultivation of fastidious pathogens.

ACKNOWLEDGMENTS

We thank J. Rosen, M. E. Coan, Sharon Parrish, and A. Friedman for excellent technical assistance.

REFERENCES

1. DAVIS, R. E. & J. F. WORLEY. 1972. Phytopathology **63:** 403–408.
2. BEBEAR, C., J. LATRILLE, J. FLECK, B. ROY & J. M. BOVÉ. 1974. Colloq. Inst. Nat. Sante Rech. Med. **33:** 35–41.
3. SUBCOMMITTEE ON TAXONOMY OF *Mycoplasmatales.* 1974. Int. J. Syst. Bacteriol. **24:** 390–392.
4. SKRIPAL, I. G. 1974. Mikrobiol. Zh. Akad. Nauk Ukr. SSR **36:** 462–467.
5. SAGLIO, P., M. L'HOSPITAL, D. LAFLÈCHE, G. DUPONT, J. M. BOVÉ, J. G. TULLY & E. A. FREUNDT. 1973. Int. J. Syst. Bacteriol. **23:** 191–204.
6. FUDL-ALLAH, A. E.-S. A., E. C. CALAVAN & E. C. K. IGWEGBE. 1972. Phytopathology **62:** 729–731.
7. SAGLIO, P., D. LAFLÈCHE, C. BONISSOL & J. M. BOVÉ. 1971. Physiol. Veg. **9:** 569–582.
8. DANIELS, M. J., P. G. MARKHAM, B. M. MEDDINS, A. K. PLASKITT, R. TOWNSEND & M. BAR-JOSEPH. 1973. Nature (London) **244:** 523, 524.
9. WHITCOMB, R. F., J. G. TULLY, J. M. BOVÉ & P. SAGLIO. 1973. Science **182:** 1251–1253.
10. MARKHAM, P. G. & R. TOWNSEND. 1974. Colloq. Inst. Nat. Sante Rech. Med. **33:** 201–206.
11. MARKHAM, P. G., R. TOWNSEND, M. BAR-JOSEPH, M. J. DANIELS, A. PLASKITT & B. M. MEDDINS. 1974. Ann. Appl. Biol. **78:** 49–57.
12. LEE, I. M., G. CARTIA, E. C. CALAVAN & G. H. KALOOSTIAN. 1973. Calif. Agr. **27:** 14, 15.
13. KALOOSTIAN, G., G. N. OLDFIELD, H. D. PIERCE, E. C. CALAVAN, A. L. GRANETT, G. L. RANA & D. J. GUMPF. 1975. Calif. Agr. **29:** 14, 15.
14. POULSON, D. F. & B. SAKAGUCHI. 1961. Science **133:** 1489, 1490.
15. WILLIAMSON, D. L. 1969. Jap. J. Genetics **44**(Suppl. 1)**:** 36–41.

16. WILLIAMSON, D. L. & R. F. WHITCOMB. 1974. Colloq. Inst. Nat. Sante Rech. Med. **33:** 283–290.
17. ALTSTATT, G. E. 1945. Plant Disease Rep. **29:** 533, 534.
18. GRANADOS, R. R. 1969b. *In* Viruses, Vectors, and Vegetation. K. Maramorosch, Ed. : 327. Interscience Publishers. New York, N.Y.
19. MARAMOROSCH, K., E. SHIKATA & R. R. GRANADOS. 1968. Trans. N.Y. Acad. Sci. Ser. II **30:** 841–855.
20. GRANADOS, R. R. 1969a. Contrib. Boyce Thompson Inst. **24:** 173–187.
21. WOLANSKI, B. & K. MARAMOROSCH. 1970. Virology **42:** 319–327.
22. WOLANSKI, B. S. 1973. Ann. N.Y. Acad. Sci. **225:** 223–235.
23. DAVIS, R. E., R. F. WHITCOMB, T.-A. CHEN & R. R. GRANADOS. 1972. *In* Pathogenic Mycoplasmas. K. Elliott & J. Birch, Eds. : 205. ASP (Elsevier, Excerpta Medica, North-Holland Publishing Co.). Amsterdam, The Netherlands.
24. DAVIS, R. E., J. F. WORLEY, R. F. WHITCOMB, T. ISHIJIMA & R. L. STEERE. 1972. Science **176:** 521–523.
25. DAVIS, R. E. 1974. Plant Disease Rep. **58:** 1109–1112.
26. DAVIS, R. E. 1973. Plant Disease Rep. **57:** 333–337.
27. DAVIS, R. E. 1973. *In* Proceedings of the 3rd International Symposium on Virus Diseases of Ornamental Plants. : 289–302.
28. CHEN, T.-A. & R. R. GRANADOS. 1970. Science **167:** 1633–1636.
29. PEREIRA, A. L. G. & B. S. OLIVEIRA, JR. 1971. Arq. Inst. Biol. Sao Paulo **38:** 191–200.
30. PEREIRA, A. L. G., J. R. JULY & B. S. OLIVEIRA, JR. 1972. Arq. Inst. Biol. Sao Paulo **39:** 59–62.
31. DAVIS, R. E., G. DUPONT, P. SAGLIO, B. ROY, J.-C. VIGNAULT & J. M. BOVÉ. 1974. Colloq. Inst. Nat. Sante Rech. Med. **33:** 187–193.
32. MARAMOROSCH, K. 1974. Annu. Rev. Microbiol. **28:** 301–324.
33. SKOWRONSKI, B. S., A. H. MCINTOSH & K. MARAMOROSCH. 1974. Plant Disease Rep. **58:** 797–801.
34. CHEN, T.-A. & C. H. LIAO. 1975. Science **188:** 1015–1017.
35. WILLIAMSON, D. L. & R. F. WHITCOMB. 1975. Science **188:** 1018–1020.
36. TULLY, J. G., R. F. WHITCOMB, J. M. BOVÉ & P. SAGLIO. 1973. Science **182:** 827–829.
37. BRADFUTE, O. E., D. ROBERTSON & L. R. NAULT. 1975. In preparation.
38. GRANADOS, R. R., K. MARAMOROSCH, T. EVERETT & T. P. PIRONE. 1966. Contrib. Boyce Thompson Inst. **23:** 275–280.
39. MARAMOROSCH, K. 1955. Plant Disease Rep. **39:** 896–898.
40. SUBCOMMITTEE ON TAXONOMY OF *Mycoplasmatales.* 1972. Int. J. Syst. Bacteriol. **22:** 184–188.
41. JENSEN, D. D. 1959. Virology **8:** 164–175.
42. WHITCOMB, R. F., D. D. JENSEN & J. RICHARDSON. 1968. J. Invert. Pathol. **12:** 202–221.
43. NASU, S., D. D. JENSEN & J. RICHARDSON. 1970. Virology **41:** 583–595.
44. NASU, S., D. D. JENSEN & J. RICHARDSON. 1974. Appl. Entomol. Zool. **9:** 115–126.
45. GRANADOS, R. R. & D. J. MEEHAN. 1975. J. Invert. Pathol. **26:** In press.
46. TURNER, T. B. & D. H. HOLLANDER. 1957. World Health Org. Mon. Ser. No. 35.
47. COLE, R. M., J. G. TULLY, T. J. POPKIN & J. M. BOVÉ. 1973. J. Bacteriol. **115:** 367–386.
48. JONES, A., R. WHITCOMB, D. L. WILLIAMSON & M. COAN. 1975. In preparation.
49. RAZIN, S., M. HASIN, Z. NE'EMAN & S. ROTTEM. 1973. J. Bacteriol. **116:** 1421–1435.
50. WHITCOMB, R., D. L. WILLIAMSON, J. ROSEN & M. COAN. 1974. Colloq. Inst. Nat. Sante Rech. Med. **33:** 275–282.

51. SPAAR, D., H. KLEINHEMPEL, H. M. MULLER, A. STANARIUS & D. SCHIMMEL. Colloq. Inst. Nat. Sante Rech. Med. **33:** 207–213.
52. WHITCOMB, R. F. 1972. U.S. Dep. Agr. Tech. Bull. 1438.
53. WILLIAMSON, D. L. 1965. J. Invert. Pathol. **7:** 493–501.
54. WILLIAMSON, D. L. 1966. J. Exp. Zool. **161:** 425–429.
55. DANIELS, M. J. & B. M. MEDDINS. 1974. Colloq. Inst. Nat. Sante Rech. Med. **33:** 195–200.
56. BOMAN, H. G., I. NILSSON & B. RASMUSON. 1972. Nature (London) **237:** 232–235.
57. WHITCOMB, R. F., M. SHAPIRO & R. R. GRANADOS. 1974. *In* The Physiology of Insecta. M. Rockstein, Ed. 2nd edit. Vol. V: 447–536. Academic Press, Inc. New York, N.Y.
58. FUDL-ALLAH, A. E.-S. A. & E. C. CALAVAN. 1974. Phytopathology **64:** 1309–1313.
59. SAKAGUCHI, B. & D. F. POULSON. 1959. Ann. Rep. Nat. Inst. Genetics Jap. **10:** 27, 28.
60. GOURANTON, J. & P. L. MAILLET. 1973. J. Invert. Pathol. **21:** 158–163.
61. MCINTOSH, A. H., B. S. SKOWRONSKI & K. MARAMOROSCH. 1974. Phytopathol. Z. **80:** 153–156.

MOLLICUTES AND *RICKETTSIA*-LIKE PLANT DISEASE AGENTS (ZOOPHYTOMICROBES) IN INSECTS

Karl Maramorosch,* Hiroyuki Hirumi,† Michio Kimura,‡ and Julio Bird §

* Waksman Institute of Microbiology
Rutgers University
New Brunswick, New Jersey 08903
† Boyce Thompson Institute for Plant Research
Yonkers, New York 10701
‡ Wakayama Medical College
Wakayama, Japan
§ University of Puerto Rico
Mayaguez Campus
College of Agricultural Sciences
Agricultural Experiment Station
Rio Piedras, Puerto Rico 00928

INTRODUCTION

In 1967, it became apparent that there exists a large group of prokaryotes that infect plants and insects.[1-3] Earlier, this group of pathogens had been classified as viruses, because they passed through filters that retained bacteria, were transmissible by plant grafting, and multiplied in certain species of insects, mainly leafhoppers and psyllids, some of which were proven vectors of viruses. Proper recognition of the microorganisms was hampered by the failure to isolate and characterize them properly.[4] Numerous reviews have been published during the past 8 years on the newly recognized plant pathogens and their relation to plant and invertebrate hosts.[5-33] At first, there was a tendency to consider all of the microorganisms as mycoplasmas, that is, microorganisms devoid of cell walls and belonging to the class Mollicutes.[34] Recently, in addition to such membrane-bound disease agents, walled bacteria or, perhaps, rickettsia were described.[25]

A new term, zoophytomicrobes, is being proposed here to comprise both the walled and the wall-less agents with alternate plant and invertebrate hosts, associated with yellows-type proliferation diseases of plants. This term is not taxonomic and is used merely for convenience, in the same manner in which the term arboviruses is applied to a heterogeneous group of viruses. Zoophytomicrobes are infectious agents that contain ribonucleic acid, in the form of ribosomes and deoxyribonucleic acid in the nuclear strand material. The natural propagation of most zoophytomicrobes requires alternating plant and invertebrate (insect) hosts. In addition, certain zoophytomicrobes are carried vertically to the progeny of insects (by transovarial passage) or are propagated in plants by vegetative means or by grafting. Most of the zoophytomicrobes have not yet been properly isolated and cultured. Their accurate characterization and taxonomic classification, with only one exception, is not possible at present. The zoophytomicrobes include mycoplasma-like organisms (MLO) and spiroplasmas that are bounded by unit-type membranes and possess no cell wall;

276

they also comprise walled microorganisms that might be confined to either the phloem or the xylem of certain diseased plants and, in many instances, have known insect vectors that carry them from plant to plant and serve as alternate hosts. Herein, we use the term MLO for the members of the class Mollicutes that are bounded by unit membranes 8–10 nm thick with ribosome-like particles that contain RNA and with DNA strands in the nuclear region. Monocotyledenous and dicotyledenous plants have been reported to have diseases associated with, and most likely caused by, MLO.[34] Many MLO have been found to be susceptible to tetracycline antibiotics when such antibiotics were applied to diseased plants via roots, leaves, or stems. Such applications usually result in temporary disease remission, and also in the deterioration and disappearance of MLO, as ascertained by electron microscopy. Known alternate hosts and vectors of MLO include leafhoppers, planthoppers, and psyllids.[13, 25]

Spiroplasmas are a subgroup of MLO that possess all the characteristics of MLO but that are distinguished by a peculiar spiral form that has been observed in certain conditions and that might be one of the morphologic forms of their life cycle. Spiroplasmas are always devoid of cell walls, and the vernacular name [35, 36] applies at present to two plant disease agents and to the agent associated with *Drosophila* sex ratio and known as the "SR spirochete of Drosophila." [37] At present, the causative agent of citrus stubborn disease, *Spiroplasma citri*, is the first and only cultured zoophytomicrobe properly characterized and available to the scientific community through the intermediary of the American Type Culture Collection.[38] Reports of cultivation [39, 40] of the serologically related [62, 79, 80] spiroplasma of corn stunt disease require proper confirmation and evidence that the presumptive isolates differ from *S. citri*. The MLO, including spiroplasmas, belong to the Mollicutes, as defined in the 8th edition of Bergey's manual.[34]

In the past, several reports and reviews have referred to walled plant-pathogenic microorganisms as rickettsiae or rickettsial-like organisms, and the term has been abbreviated and used as RLO. The proper characterization of these walled zoophytomicrobes is inadequate to conclude that they are rickettsiae, and there is no justification for this term, except for obligate parasitism and affinity to insect hosts. The distinction between MLO and RLO can be made morphologically by comparing ultrathin sections. MLO have a unit-type membrane, whereas RLO have a cell wall. The latter differs with respect to the type of RLO, as is discussed below. Penicillin has proven to be a useful tool in distinguishing between the walled and the wall-less zoophytomicrobes. Remission of disease and hampering or interruption of the insect vectors' ability to transmit the disease agents by penicillin administration *in vivo* provided an indication that the respective zoophytomicrobes might be walled microorganisms. Lack of response to penicillin and temporary remission after tetracycline treatment has been interpreted as evidence for MLO etiology. For spiroplasma infections, dark-field and phase microscopy have been used successfully to detect the microorganisms in extracts from diseased plants and insect vectors.[41] The use of antibiotics for diagnostic purposes has its pitfalls,[86] and their improper use has led to embarrassing errors.[42]

Xylem-Restricted RLO

The RLO, or "plant rickettsiae," comprise at least two different groups of microorganisms. One, confined to the zylem of diseased plants, is characterized by a cell wall of three layers, 80–100 nm thick. Intracytoplasmic invaginations of the plasma membrane are sometimes noted, as are ribosome-like particles. Fibrous structures, believed to contain DNA, are sometimes observed, and thin DNA-like strands that form a network of fibrils are also seen. The first report of such xylem-confined RLO in diseased plants referred to microorganisms detected in sugar cane affected by the ratoon stunt disease.[43–49] Subsequently, similar RLO were detected associated with the xylem of plants with phony peach disease [50, 52, 53] and Pierce's disease of grapes.[51, 54, 55] The reports of successful cultivation of RLO associated with Pierce's disease of grapes [56] and ratoon stunt of sugar cane [46] indicate that these microorganisms apparently have the ability to grow in cell-free media in conditions that resemble the mature xylem vessels, free of living protoplasm. The evidence that the cultured microorganisms are the causative agents of the respective diseases requires further tests, but their ability to proliferate in artificial media comes as no surprise.

PHLOEM-RESTRICTED RLO

The RLO associated with the phloem of diseased plants, and with alternate leafhopper vectors, differ morphologically from the xylem-associated RLO with respect to the thickness of the cell wall. The walled phloem-associated zoophytomicrobes have a comparatively thin cell wall, approximately 20 nm thick. Their overall diameter has sometimes been reported to be about one half of the diameter of the xylem-associated RLO, but this difference is not well established. Their affinity to functional phloem cells and phloem parenchyma cells, rich in protoplasm and cell organelles, indicates that they might prove more fastidious than the xylem-confined RLO. The phloem-restricted RLO might represent very small bacteria, rickettsiae, chlamydia, or a new, as yet undescribed, group of microbial disease agents.

During the past 5 years, that is, since 1970, eight different plant diseases caused by phloem-restricted RLO have been reported. The first was detected in a malformation disease of *Cuscuta subinclusa*.[78] In 1972, the precise measurements of microorganisms associated with citrus greening revealed that, instead of a unit-type membrane, the microorganisms possessed a cell wall approximately 20 nm thick.[71] Similar dimensions of cell walls were illustrated in cross sections of willow witches' broom microorganisms.[72] Phloem-restricted RLO have also been described associated with wheat chlorosis [81] for the agent of carrot proliferation transmitted by a psyllid, *Trioza nigricornis*,[82] and a disease temporarily called "rickettsial disease of clover." [83] In most instances, no tests were reported about the effect of penicillin on remission of the respective diseases. Such tests were first performed on plants with clover club leaf disease,[73, 87] which was once considered a classic example of a plant virus disease [67] and has now been demonstrated to be caused by a phloem-restricted zoophytomicrobe. Recently, we discovered a similar microorganism in the phloem of *Sida cordifolia* little leaf disease.[74] Because the findings have been described only in an abstract, a detailed account of the work will be given now, to illustrate the morphologic features of these microorganisms.

MATERIALS AND METHODS

Leaf and petiole samples were obtained from *S. cordifolia* plants growing in a wooded area approximately 40 miles from San Juan, Puerto Rico near the north shore of the island. The plants differed from healthy ones in that they had very small leaves growing densely in a proliferation-type witches' broom fashion. Healthy appearing leaves and petioles were taken a few miles away, from *S. cordifolia* growing near sand dunes. The material was processed in the field by immersing excised leaves in cacodylate-buffered glutaraldehyde, cutting small pieces of petioles and leaves approximately 1 × 2 mm, and placing them in vials that contained the glutaraldehyde fixative. Further processing for electron microscopy was performed according to routine techniques.[75-77]

RESULTS

Microorganisms that resemble small bacteria or rickettsiae were detected in the phloem of samples from little leaf-diseased plants but not in the healthy appearing controls. The microorganisms were rod shaped or elongated, 1–3 μm long, some with rippled cell walls. The cell walls were 20–30 nm thick and thus differed from the MLO of aster yellows disease, which are bounded by unit-type 10-nm thick membranes. The microorganisms were detected in the phloem but not in the xylem of diseased plants.

The abundance of the microorganisms in nine adjoining cells is illustrated in FIGURE 1. Although most microorganisms appeared to be rounded in this electron micrograph, a few happened to be positioned so as to be sectioned longitudinally, revealing their slender, long shape. In some sieve elements, the RLO multiplied to such an extent that the area became completely packed with the pathogens, as shown in FIGURE 2. Depending on the orientation of the RLO within cells at the time of fixation, the electron micrographs revealed either round-shaped forms (FIGURE 2) or predominantly elongated ones (FIGURE 3). In some sieve tube elements, plant organelles were still present, despite the large accumulation of RLO (FIGURE 4). Both the internal structure and the rippled cell wall were clearly observable under higher magnification (FIGURE 5). Some of the RLO were extremely slender (FIGURE 5, *left*) and thus "invisible" by light microscopy, even though their length was approximately 3 μm. Others (FIGURE 5, *right*) were more compact and wider in diameter, revealing the presence of a thin cell wall and a plasma membrane. The passage from cell to cell through the pores of sieve tubes is illustrated in FIGURE 6. This passage is reminiscent of the passage through sieve pores in the sieve plate by MLO, reported earlier by several workers.

One of the most intriguing observations concerned the presence of virus-like particles within the RLO (FIGURE 7). Some of these presumptive viruses contained highly electron-opaque cores, whereas others were apparently empty. The actual nature of these particles remains to be ascertained. Diseased plants, potted and maintained in temperature-controlled chambers at 25° C for 8 weeks, recovered spontaneously, and RLO were no longer detected by electron microscopy. A little leaf-diseased *S. cordifolia* with typical symptoms is illustrated (FIGURE 8).

EFFECT ON INSECT VECTORS

Most of the work on effects of zoophytomicrobes on insect vectors has been performed when these agents were still considered to be viruses. Because the microbial nature of zoophytomicrobes is now well established, a brief summary

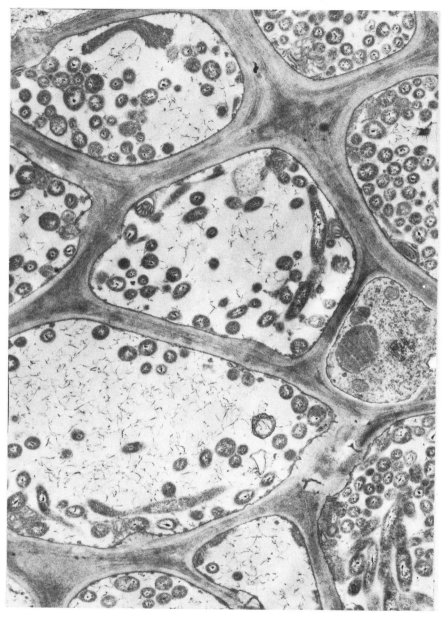

FIGURE 1. Portion of the phloem of little leaf-diseased *S. cordifolia*. Note sieve tube elements that contain several pleomorphic bodies. ×12,900.

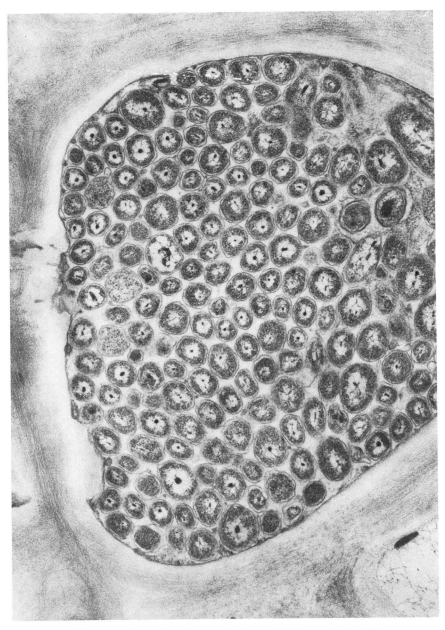

FIGURE 2. Cross section of a sieve tube element fully packed with numerous rickettsia-like organisms. ×30,000.

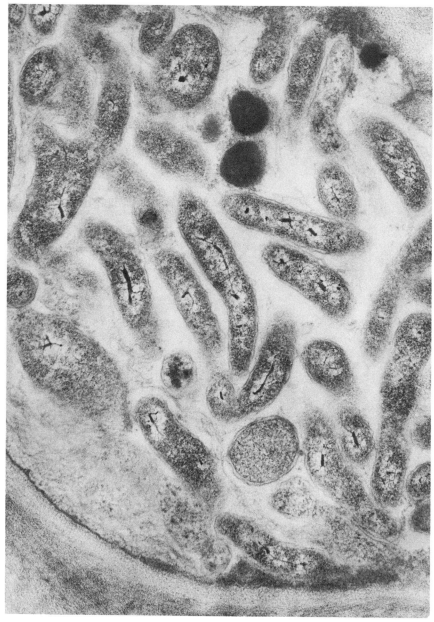

FIGURE 3. Portion of a sieve tube element that contains elongated forms of rickettsia-like organisms. ×42,000.

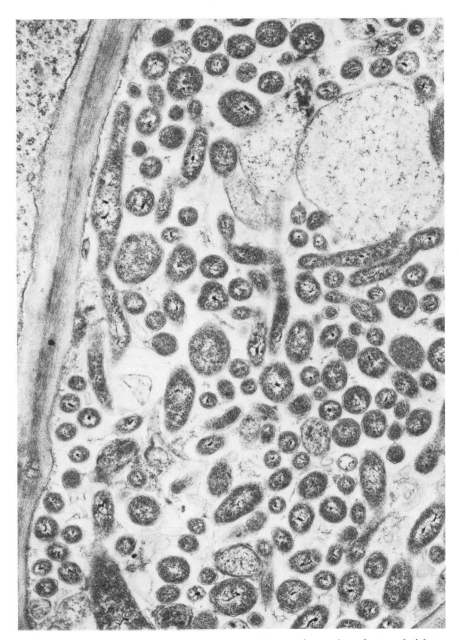

FIGURE 4. Portion of a sieve tube element that contains various forms of rickettsia-like organisms. ×21,900.

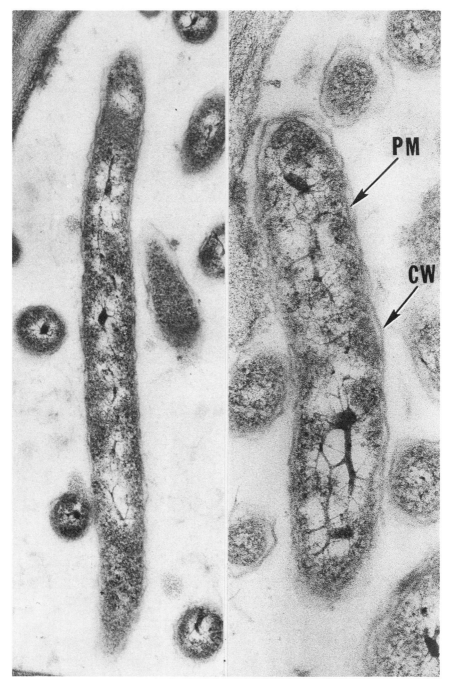

FIGURE 5. Elongated rickettsia-like organisms that contain highly electron-opaque DNA-like strands and peripherally located cytoplasmic matrices. Thin cell wall (CW) and plasma membrane (PM) are clearly seen. *Left,* ×53,000; *right* ×98,100.

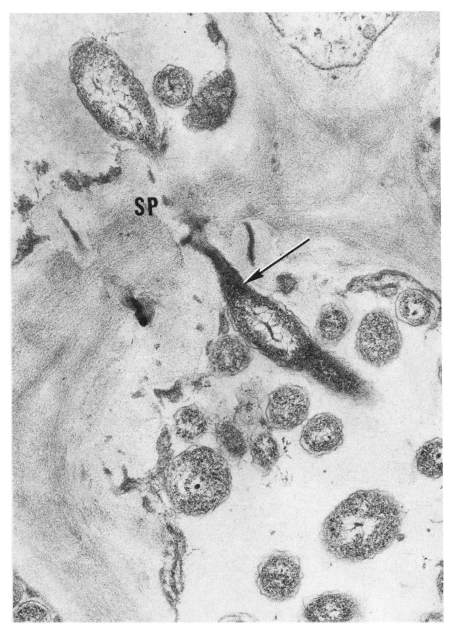

FIGURE 6. Portion of sieve tube elements. Note a rickettsia-like organism (arrow) passing through a sieve pore. SP=sieve plate.

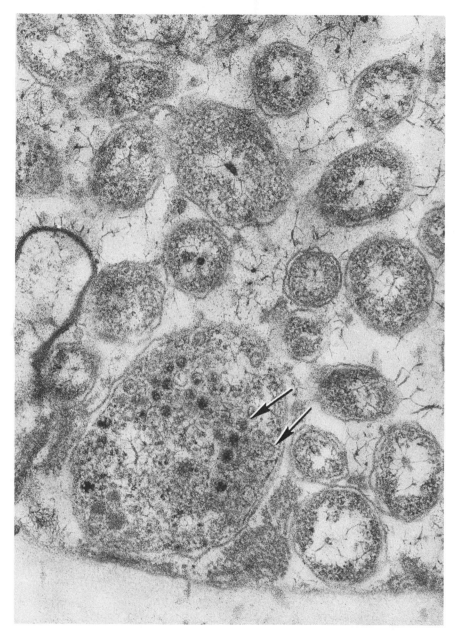

FIGURE 7. Portion of a sieve tube element that contains spherical rickettsia-like organisms. Virus-like particles (arrows) can be seen in a large body. Some particles contain a highly electron-opaque core, whereas others appear to be "empty." ×75,080.

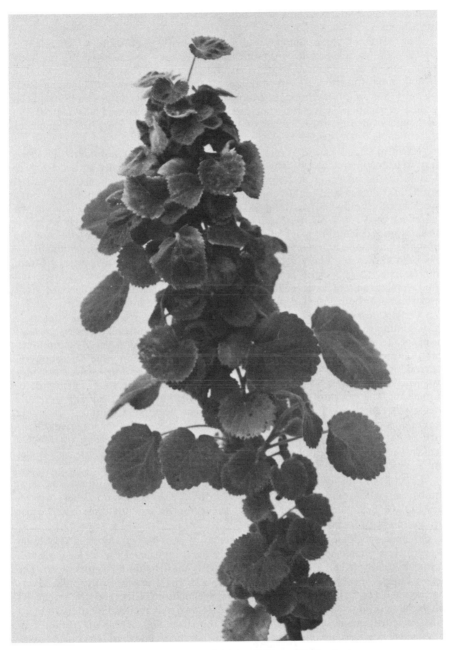

FIGURE 8. Little leaf-diseased *S. cordifolia* plant.

of the earlier findings seems justified, as does a reappraisal of some of the conclusions.

The MLO of aster yellows multiplies in leafhopper vectors, *Macrosteles fascifrons*.[57] A deleterious cytopathic effect has been observed in the fat body tissue cells of male leafhoppers.[58] The oral acquisition, but not the acquisition by abdominal injection, of sap-containing aster yellows MLO affected the feeding of a nonvector leafhopper, *Dalbulus maidis*.[59] This interaction has been termed a beneficial effect on the insect, because it permitted survival of the leafhoppers on numerous species of plants that normally were unpalatable or objectionable to *D. maidis*.

Harmful effects of the Western-X MLO on *Callodonus montanus* has been very well documented.[60, 61] This MLO is carried transovarially to a large proportion of the offspring of female *C. montanus,* and this vertical transmission results in a decrease in viable embryos. Besides, nymphs and adults that carry the MLO live only half as long as noninfected individuals. Observations on the effect of *S. citri* on *M. fascifrons*[62] indicate that plant pathogenic spiroplasmas may deleteriously affect invertebrate animals. The drastic effect of the spiroplasma of *Drosophila*, which causes complete elimination of male offspring, has been known for many years,[37] but its mechanism is still a mystery. Strain interference, termed cross protection by plant pathologists, has been reported for several strains of aster yellows MLO[63-65] and for strains of the corn stunt spiroplasma in both infected plants and in invertebrate hosts.[66]

Vertical transmission of zoophytomicrobes in certain leafhopper vectors is very similar to the vertical transmission of plant pathogenic viruses in leafhoppers. Ironically, one of the best documented experiments on virus multiplication in insect vectors[67] has now been recognized as one in which a zoophytomicrobe is involved. The agent is not only susceptible to tetracycline but also to penicillin and thus is neither a virus nor an MLO but is a walled microorganism. The question is sometimes asked whether there exist any veritable viruses that multiply in both plants and insect vectors. Certainly, there are several, as was exemplified by Fukushi's classic description of rice dwarf virus.[68, 69] This reo-type virus passes transovarially to the progeny of infected female vectors. Its multiplication seems harmless to some *Nephotettix* species but is deleterious to *Inazuma dorsalis*.[69]

In addition to leafhoppers (Cicadellidae), psyllids (Psyllidae) are also known as vectors and alternate hosts of MLO.[23] Although no other invertebrates have been incriminated to date as vectors of zoophytomicrobes, other groups might be found in the future.

Biologic specificity of invertebrate vectors of zoophytomicrobes is very high. Nevertheless, many nonvector species have been reported to be able to sustain the viability of MLO and spiroplasmas, without becoming vectors.[84, 85] The severe effects on plants are in sharp contrast to the comparatively mild effects on invertebrates. These findings led to speculations that zoophytomicrobes might have originated as pathogens of insects and that their adaptation to plant hosts is more recent.[70] Speculation as to the rickettsial nature of certain zoophytomicrobes also involves the symbiont-like interaction of rickettsiae with invertebrates that contrasts with their severe and deleterious effects on vertebrate hosts. The possible existence of rickettsiae that alternate between insects and plants has been considered only very recently, even though alternation between insects, birds, and mammals has been known for a long time.

Discussion

The realization that wall-less mycoplasma type microorganisms are responsible for numerous plant diseases and that such microorganisms constitute a major group of plant disease agents came as a complete surprise to microbiologists. Very few diseases of higher animals caused by mycoplasmas were known in the past, and only one human disease, atypical "virus" pneumonia, has been proven to be caused by a member of this group. Similarly, the finding of filterable walled microorganisms that resemble rickettsiae, or chlamydiae, tentatively classified as rickettsia-like organisms, was unexpected. Morphologic aspects of the fine structure of typical rickettsial cells include some of the features observed in the zoophytomicrobes described as RLO.

The microorganisms are 0.3–0.7 μm in length and 1.5–2.0 μm in diameter. They are bounded by a cell wall 70–100 nm thick, have intracytoplasmic invaginations of the plasma membrane, ribosome-like particles 70–200 nm in diameter in a ground substance of intermediate density, fibers believed to contain DNA, and DNA-like strands. The above characteristics have led to the assumption that these microorganisms, which require alternating plant and insect hosts and are restricted to the xylem of diseased plants, are members of the Rickettsiales.

The phloem-restricted microorganisms of proliferation diseases, such as the described microorganisms visualized in the *S. cordifolia* little leaf disease, differ from xylem-restricted RLO and might belong to a new group of bacteria or, perhaps, to Chlamydia. It is of interest that the original realization that the yellows-type agents are of microbial, rather than viral, nature left their classification open and listed among the possible agents mycoplasmas, chlamydia, or L forms of bacteria. The four diseases originally studied in Japan in 1967, mulberry dwarf, aster yellows, Paulownia witches' broom, and potato witches' broom, have all been associated with phloem-restricted wall-less MLO agents. The same is true for the fifth disease studied in Japan, rice yellow dwarf. The walled, rickettsia- or chlamydia-like agents and their response to penicillin and to tetracycline treatment has been studied in lesser detail than the morphology and antibiotic response of MLO. The possibility that rickettsiae may possess a spheroplast or L-form stage has sometimes been considered, and if such forms should occur in plant-infecting RLO, their morphologic distinction from MLO would be very difficult. Rickettsiae have been found to grow intracellularly in cells of many arthropods, mammals, birds, and reptiles. The nature of obligate parasitism of these microorganisms is not well understood. It seems feasible that, in addition to binary fission, other methods of replication exist that could explain the nature of the obligate parasitism. The availability and use of insect cell cultures from hosts of the zoophytomicrobes might help in the elucidation of the complex relationships and of the diseases caused by these agents.

Whether the virus-like particles within the RLO of *S. cordifolia* little leaf-diseased plants are viruses has not been established, but their morphologic characteristics correspond with those of known viruses. The spontaneous recovery of infected plants is of special interest from theoretic and practical viewpoints. If we assume that the particles represent a virus that infects a rickettsia, the recovery might have been caused by the viral destruction of the RLO. This would indicate a possible means for biologic control of RLO-caused plant diseases.

SUMMARY

The term "zoophytomicrobes" has been coined to describe microorganisms, earlier classified as viruses, that have a biologic affinity to invertebrate animals and plants. Most zoophytomicrobes require alternate plant and insect hosts for their maintenance in nature, and most of them cause severe diseases of plants but no diseases, or comparatively mild ones, in insect vectors. There is no evidence for the existence of different developmental stages in the alternate plant and invertebrate hosts. Electron microscopy permits the morphologic characterization of MLO and spiroplasma agents that are bounded by unit-type membrane and of RLO that possess cell walls. The RLO confined to the xylem of diseased plants have cell walls that are approximately 100 nm thick, whereas the RLO confined to the phloem have cell walls only 20 nm thick. Probably, the two types belong to different groups of bacteria or rickettsiae. RLO are usually susceptible to both tetracyclines and penicillin, whereas MLO are susceptible to tetracyclines and are resistant to penicillin. The susceptibility has been studied *in vivo* in plants and insect vectors and *in vitro* for *S. citri*. A phloem-confined RLO has been discovered in *S. cordifolia* little leaf disease from Puerto Rico. Virus-like particles have been observed intracellularly within the invading RLO. Spontaneous recovery of infected plants with dual, RLO and presumptive virus, infection might be explained by the viral destruction of RLO.

REFERENCES

1. Doi, Y., M. Terenaka, K. Yora & H. Asuyama. 1967. Ann. Phytopathol. Soc. Jap. **33:** 259–266.
2. Ishiie, T., Y. Doi, K. Yora & H. Asuyama. 1967. Ann. Phytopathol. Soc. Jap. **33:** 267–275.
3. Nasu, S., M. Sugiura, T. Wakimoto & T. Iida. 1967. Ann. Phytopathol. Soc. Jap. **33:** 343, 344.
4. Maramorosch, K. 1963. Annu. Rev. Entomol. **8:** 369–414.
5. Amici, A., P. Grancini, R. Osler & E. Refatti. 1972. Riv. Patol. Veg. **8:** 21–50.
6. Anonymous. 1972. Plant Protect. (Japan) **26:** 184–189.
7. Atanasoff, D. 1969. Biol. Zentr. **88:** 571–574.
8. Atanasoff, D. 1972. Phytopathol. Z. **74:** 342–348.
9. Bos, L. 1970. Gewasbescherming **1:** 45–54.
10. Von Casper, R. 1969. Nachr. Pflanzenschutzdienst (Berlin) **21:** 177–182.
11. Cousin, M.-T. 1972. Select. Franc. **15:** 1–27.
12. Darpoux, H. 1971. Phytoma **23:** 16–23.
13. Davis, R. E. & R. F. Whitcomb. 1971. Annu. Rev. Phytopathol. **9:** 119–154.
14. Ghosh, S. K. & S. P. Raychaudhuri. 1972. Current Sci. **41:** 235–241.
15. Hampton, R. O. 1972. Annu. Rev. Plant Physiol. **23:** 389–418.
16. Horne, R. W. 1972. *In* Pathogenic Mycoplasmas. K. Elliott & J. Birch, Eds. : 39–66. Elsevier-Excerpta Medica-North-Holland. Amsterdam, The Netherlands.
17. Horvath, J. 1970. Növenytermeles **19:** 327–337.
18. Hull, R. 1971. Rev. Plant Pathol. **50:** 121–130.
19. Kitajima, E. W. & A. S. Costa. 1970. Ciencia Cult. (Sao Paulo) **22:** 351–363.
20. Kleinhempel, H., H. M. Müller & D. Spaar. 1972. Nachr. Pflanzenschutzdienst (Berlin) **26:** 1–3.

21. MARAMOROSCH, K. 1972. Phytopathology **62:** 1230, 1231.
22. MARAMOROSCH, K., E. SHIKATA & R. R. GRANADOS. 1968. Trans. N.Y. Acad. Sci. **30:** 841–855.
23. MARAMOROSCH, K., R. R. GRANADOS & H. HIRUMI. 1970. Advan. Virus Res. **16:** 135–193.
24. MARAMOROSCH, K., H. HIRUMI, M. KIMURA, J. BIRD & N. G. VAKILI. 1975. FAO Plant Protect. Bull. In press.
25. MARAMOROSCH, K. 1974. Annu. Rev. Microbiol. **28:** 301–324.
26. MARAMOROSCH, K. 1975. *In* Encyclopedia of Plant Physiology. R. Heitefuss & P. H. Williams, Eds. Springer-Verlag. Berlin, Federal Republic of Germany. In press.
27. MARCHOUX, G., F. LECLANT, J. GIANNOTTI & B. CADILHAC. 1972. *In* Troisieme Congres de l'Union Phytopathologique Mediterraneenne, Oeiras-Portugal.
28. MÜLLER, H. M., H. KLEINHEMPEL, D. SPAAR & H. J. MÜLLER. 1973. Advan. Phytopathol. Pflanzenschutz **9:** 95–104.
29. PLOAIE, P. G. 1973. Micoplasma şi Bolile Proliferative la Plante. : 178. Editura Ceres. Bucharest, Rumania.
30. SHIKATA, E., K. MARAMOROSCH & K. C. LING. 1969. FAO Plant Protect. Bull. **17:** 121–128.
31. SPAAR, D., H. KLEINHEMPEL & H. M. MÜLLER. 1972. Arch. Pflanzenschutz **8:** 175–188.
32. VAGO, C. & J. GIANNOTTI. 1972. Physiol. Veg. **10P:** 87–101.
33. WHITCOMB, R. F. & R. E. DAVIS. 1970. Annu. Rev. Entomol. **15:** 405–464.
34. BUCHANAN, R. E. & N. E. GIBBONS. (Eds.) 1974. Bergey's Manual of Determinative Bacteriology. 8th edit. : 929, 955. The Williams & Wilkins Co. Baltimore, Md.
35. DAVIS, R. E. & J. F. WORLEY. 1972. Phytopathology **62:** 752, 753.
36. DAVIS, R. E. & J. F. WORLEY. 1973. Phytopathology **63:** 403–408.
37. POULSON, D. F. & B. SAKAGUCHI. 1961. Science **133:** 1489, 1490.
38. SAGLIO, P., et al. 1973. Int. J. Syst. Bacteriol. **23:** 191–204.
39. CHEN, T.-A. & R. R. GRANADOS. 1970. Science **167:** 1633–1636.
40. McBEATH, J. H. & T. A. CHEN. 1973. Phytopathology **63:** 803.
41. DAVIS, R. E. 1973. Plant Disease Rep. **57:** 333–337.
42. GILLASPIE, A. G., JR. 1970. Phytopathology **60:** 1448–1450.
43. PLAVSIC-BANJAC, B. & K. MARAMOROSCH. 1972. Phytopathology **62:** 498, 499.
44. MARAMOROSCH, K., B. PLAVSIC-BANJAC, J. BIRD & L. J. LIU. 1973. Phytopathol. Z. **77:** 270–273.
45. PLAVSIC-BANJAC, B. & K. MARAMOROSCH. 1973. Mikrobiologija **10:** 43–52.
46. LIU, L. J., A. CORTES MONLLOR, K. MARAMOROSCH, H. RIRUMI, J. G. PEREZ & J. BIRD. 1974. J. Agr. Univ. Puerto Rico **58:** 418–425.
47. WORLEY, J. F. & A. G. GILLASPIE, JR. 1975. Phytopathology **65:** 287–295.
48. TEAKLE, D. S., P. M. SMITH & D. R. L. STEINDL. 1973. Australian J. Agr. Res. **24:** 869–874.
49. GILLASPIE, A. G., JR., R. E. DAVIS & J. F. WORLEY. 1973. Plant Disease Rep. **57:** 987–990.
50. NYLAND, G., A. C. GOHEEN, S. K. LOWE & H. C. KIRKPATRICK. 1973. Phytopathology **63:** 1275–1278.
51. HOPKINS, D. L. & H. H. MOLLENHAUER. 1973. Science **179:** 298–300.
52. FRENCH, W. J. 1974. Phytopathology **64:** 260, 261.
53. HOPKINS, D. L., W. J. FRENCH & H. H. MOLLENHAUER. 1973. Phytopathology **63:** 443.
54. HOPKINS, D. L., H. H. MOLLENHAUER & W. J. FRENCH. 1973. Phytopathology **63:** 1422, 1423.
55. GOHEEN, A. C., G. NYLAND & S. K. LOWE. 1973. Phytopathology **63:** 341–345.
56. AUGER, J. G., T. A. SHALLA & C. I. KADO. 1974. Science **184:** 1375–1377.
57. MARAMOROSCH, K. 1952. Phytopathology **42:** 59–64.
58. LITTAU, V. C. & K. MARAMOROSCH. 1956. Virology **2:** 128–130.

59. MARAMOROSCH, K. 1958. Tijdschr. Plantenziekten **63:** 383–391.
60. JENSEN, D. D. 1959. Virology **8:** 164–175.
61. MARAMOROSCH, K. & D. D. JENSEN. 1963. Annu. Rev. Microbiol. **17:** 495–530.
62. WILLIAMSON, D. L. & R. F. WHITCOMB. 1974. Inserm **33:** 283–290.
63. KUNKEL, L. O. 1955. Advan. Virus Res. **3:** 251–273.
64. KUNKEL, L. O. 1957. Science **126:** 1233.
65. FREITAG, J. H. 1964. Virology **24:** 401–413.
66. MARAMOROSCH, K. 1958. Virology **6:** 448–459.
67. BLACK, L. M. 1950. Nature (London) **166:** 852, 853.
68. FUKUSHI, T. 1940. J. Fac. Agr. Hokkaido Univ. **45:** 83–154.
69. FUKUSHI, T. 1969. *In* Viruses, Vectors and Vegetation. K. Maramorosch, Ed. : 279–301. John Wiley & Sons, Inc. New York, N.Y.
70. MARAMOROSCH, K. 1972. *In* Symposium on Ecosystematics. R. T. Allen & F. C. James, Eds. : 195–213. University of Arkansas Press. Fayetteville, Ark.
71. SAGLIO, P., D. LAFLECHE, M. L'HOSPITAL, G. DUPONT & J.-M. BOVÉ. 1972. *In* Pathogenic Mycoplasmas. K. Elliott & J. Birch, Eds. : 187–203. Elsevier-Excerpta Medica-North-Holland. Amsterdam, The Netherlands.
72. HOLMES, F. O., H. HIRUMI & K. MARAMOROSCH. 1972. Phytopathology **62:** 826–828.
73. WINDSOR, I. M. & L. M. BLACK. 1973. Phytopathology **63:** 44–46.
74. HIRUMI, H., M. KIMURA, K. MARAMOROSCH & J. BIRD. 1974. Phytopathology **64:** 581, 582.
75. HIRUMI, H. & K. MARAMOROSCH. 1972. Phytopathol. Z. **75:** 9–26.
76. HIRUMI, H. & K. MARAMOROSCH. 1973. Phytopathol. Z. **77:** 71–83.
77. HIRUMI, H. & K. MARAMOROSCH. 1973. Ann. N.Y. Acad. Sci. **225:** 201–222.
78. GIANNOTTI, J., C. VAGO, G. MARCHOUX, G. DEVAUCHELLE & J. L. DUTHOIT. 1970. Compt. Rend. **271:** 2118, 2119.
79. McINTOSH, A. H., B. S. SKOWRONSKI & K. MARAMOROSCH. 1974. Phytopathol. Z. **80:** 153–156.
80. TULLY, J. G., R. F. WHITCOMB, J. M. BOVÉ & P. SAGLIO. 1973. Science **182P:** 827–829.
81. PLOAIE, P. G. 1973. Abst. Proc. 2nd Int. Congr. Plant Pathol. : 643.
82. GIANNOTTI, J., L. CLAUDE, F. LECLANT, G. MARCHOUX & C. VAGO. 1974. Compt. Rend. **278:** 469–471.
83. MARKHAM, P. G., R. TOWNSEND & A. PLASKITT. 1975. *In* John Innes Institute Annual Report 1974. In press.
84. MARAMOROSCH, K. 1952. Phytopathology **42:** 663–668.
85. WHITCOMB, R. F., D. L. WILLIAMSON, J. ROSEN & M. COAN. 1974. Inserm **33:** 275–282.
86. KLEIN, M., R. FREDERICK & K. MARAMOROSCH. 1973. Ann. N.Y. Acad. Sci. **225:** 522–530.
87. WINDSOR, I. M. & L. M. BLACK. 1973. Phytopathology **63:** 1139–1148.

A MECHANISM OF VECTOR SPECIFICITY FOR CIRCULATIVE APHID-TRANSMITTED PLANT VIRUSES *

W. F. Rochow, M. J. Foxe,† and Irmgard Muller

Department of Plant Pathology
Cornell University
Ithaca, New York 14850

INTRODUCTION

Despite the importance of aphids as vectors of plant viruses, little is known about pathogenic effects of the viruses in aphids. This dearth of information results mainly from the kinds of virus-vector relationships that occur. Plant viruses are not often associated with aphids in ways that would be expected to produce pathogenic effects.

Aphids transmit plant viruses in at least two distinct ways. Most of the aphid-transmitted viruses are spread by the vectors during brief probes into plant tissue. This virus-vector relationship is called nonpersistent or stylet-borne, because the aphid soon loses the ability to transmit virus, often within seconds or minutes. Since transmissible virus is associated with the vector for such short periods, there is little reason to expect virus to affect the vector in ways detectable by usual physiologic or anatomic studies. Nonpersistent transmission will not be considered here.

In the other kind of relationship, virus circulates through the vector, and transmission occurs during feeding. Because an aphid often retains the ability to transmit such viruses for most of its life, the central question raised by this persistent or circulative type of virus-vector relationship is whether the virus replicates in the vector. Current evidence suggests that several Rhabdoviruses, such as lettuce necrotic yellows virus, sowthistle yellow vein virus, and strawberry crinkle virus, do replicate in the aphid.[1,2] Replication of potato leafroll virus in the vector has been reported, but the work apparently has never been repeated. Other aspects of the virus-vector relationship do not support the idea for replication of potato leafroll virus in *Myzus persicae* (Sulzer).[1] For still other viruses, such as pea enation mosaic virus and barley yellow dwarf virus, there is general agreement that circulation without replication occurs.

Some relatively minor effects of circulative and propagative viruses on aphid vectors are known. Jensen [3] and Ponsen [4] reviewed reports of cytologic and metabolic changes associated with plant viruses in aphids. Such effects have

* Cooperative Investigation, Agricultural Research Service, United States Department of Agriculture, and Cornell University Agricultural Experiment Station. Supported in part by National Science Foundation Grants GB-35242 and BMS-74-19814. Mention of a trademark name, proprietary product, or specific equipment does not constitute a guarantee or warranty by the U. S. Department of Agriculture, and does not imply its approval to the exclusion of other products also available.

† Present address: Department of Plant Pathology, University College, Dublin, Ireland.

been detected for several aphid-virus systems, but the role or importance of the relatively small changes is not clear. Recently, Sylvester and Richardson [5, 6] studied sowthistle yellow vein virus, a propagative virus, in *Hyperomyzus lactucae*. Of several effects noted, decreased longevity of viruliferous aphids was the main evidence for pathogenicity.

This paper focuses on even more subtle relationships between circulative plant viruses and their aphid vectors. Mechanisms for specificity in virus-vector relationships are a basic concern for many investigators. Here, we will discuss the mechanism of vector specificity for two isolates of barley yellow dwarf virus and two aphid species. The discussion will be based on our working hypothesis for a model of vector specificity, first described in 1969.[7] We will summarize evidence that contributes to evaluating the model, and we will discuss some current approaches to test it.

THE VIRUS-VECTOR SYSTEM

Barley yellow dwarf virus (BYDV) is transmitted by aphids in the circulative manner. Failures to maintain virus by serial transfers from aphid to aphid provide some evidence that BYDV does not replicate and accumulate in the vector.[7, 8] BYDV has not been transmitted mechanically to plants; it can, however, be injected into hemolymph of aphids, and bioassays by acquisition feeding of aphids through membranes on virus preparations can be done.[9] The BYDV system is useful in studies of vector specificity because of the range of variation in transmission of different virus isolates by different aphid species.

We use two isolates of BYDV in most studies. One virus isolate (RPV) is transmitted efficiently by *Rhopalosiphum padi* (L.) but only rarely by *Macrosiphum avenae* (F.). The other isolate (MAV) is transmitted by *M. avenae* but not by *R. padi*. Although this specificity is relative, not absolute, it has been consistent in our studies for many years.[10] For example, in more than 100 comparative tests used to maintain the virus isolates by transfer to Coast Black oats (*Avena byzantina* C. Koch), groups of *R. padi* transmitted RPV to 352 of 359 plants, but groups of *M. avenae* transmitted RPV to only three of 310 plants in parallel tests. In the same experiments, *M. avenae* transmitted MAV to 362 of 365 plants; *R. padi* transmitted MAV to six of 310 plants. None of 618 control plants became infected. To make a comparative test, one leaf from each source plant is removed, cut in two, and each half-leaf is infested with one of the aphid species. Acquisition feeding on the detached half-leaves is for 2 days at 15° C. Inoculation test feeding, with about 10 aphids for each of three 6-day-old oat seedlings, is for 5 days at 21° C in a growth chamber.

We make purified preparations of BYDV from frozen infected oats.[11] Crude extracts are clarified with chloroform. Concentrated preparations are then made by differential and sucrose gradient centrifugation. Scanning patterns in the ISCO density gradient fractionator are used to estimate virus concentration. Virus-specific antiserum can be used in several kinds of tests, including a type of neutralization of infectivity based on blocking of virus transmission by aphids fed through membranes on virus-antiserum mixtures.[11, 12]

A limitation in much work with BYDV, and with other aphid-transmitted phloem-limited viruses that are not mechanically transmissible, is the small amount of virus obtained in purified preparations. This low titer of BYDV is a disadvantage for some lines of research. For example, in a recent study,

Harris *et al.*[21] used milligram amounts of pea enation mosaic virus as the inoculum, but we usually are restricted to microgram amounts of BYDV. This difference in virus concentration is probably a major reason why we, with Dr. H. W. Israel, have more difficulty in using electron microscopy to study BYDV in vectors than did Harris and coworkers with pea enation mosaic virus. The dependent transmission systems of BYDV, however, offer advantages over some other virus-vector combinations.[14]

MECHANISM OF SPECIFICITY

Our current working hypothesis for the model of BYDV specificity is based on interactions of virus capsid protein with membranes of the aphid salivary glands. Thus, *R. padi* transmits RPV because the structure of the RPV capsid protein confers a basis for entrance of virions into the salivary glands and movement through the salivary system. However, the protein capsid of MAV does not interact with membranes of *R. padi* in the same way, and thus MAV is excluded from the glands. Within *M. avenae,* the picture is reversed. An obvious and important aspect of this model is that changes in specificity can result from either variations in the virus and/or in the aphid. Specificity might change as a result of variations in protein structure among virus isolates or among virions of one isolate. Similarly, physiologic or morphologic differences in salivary glands of aphids, as illustrated by differences among aphid species or variations among biotypes of one aphid species, could also change the pattern of specificity. Because much of the earlier work that contributed to the development of this hypothesis has been reviewed,[7] we will summarize the evidence for the model, with an emphasis on more recent work.

The apparent contribution of the virus capsid protein to specificity is suggested by two general lines of research. One involves various comparisons between purified preparations of RPV and those of MAV. Both virus isolates are generally similar in size, morphology, and in sedimentation rates in sucrose gradients.[11] Both contain a single component of single-stranded RNA of molecular weight 2.0×10^6, although the RNA of RPV may be slightly more compact than that of MAV.[13] The two virus isolates, however, do differ markedly in serologic properties[11, 12] and, probably, in aromatic amino acid content.[13] Evidence for the role of such differences in specificity derives from a second line of work with mixed infections.

Although *R. padi* does not regularly transmit the MAV isolate of BYDV from oats infected only with MAV, it often transmits MAV, together with RPV, from doubly infected plants. This system of dependent transmission of MAV by *R. padi* provided evidence for the role of virus protein in vector specificity.[11] During simultaneous replication of the two viruses, some nucleic acid of MAV apparently becomes incorporated into virus particles that contain the protein capsid of RPV. Evidence for transcapsidation (genomic masking) as the explanation for the dependent transmission of MAV came from tests of virus purified from doubly infected plants. When such virus preparations were treated with MAV antiserum, and aphids then fed through membranes on the treated preparations, *M. avenae* did not transmit virus; MAV in the preparation was neutralized by the specific antiserum. From the same preparation, however, *R. padi* transmitted both RPV and MAV to test plants.[15] The "mixed" virus particles appear to function in *R. padi* like RPV (because of the RPV protein capsid) and in the plant like MAV (because of the MAV nucleic acid).

Other evidence that supports this conclusion includes failures to duplicate the dependent transmission by using inoculum made by mixing together concentrated preparations of the separate viruses.[16] All attempts to duplicate dependent transmission of MAV by permitting interaction of the two viruses within *R. padi* have also been unsuccessful.[16] Experiments based on neutralizing MAV in preparations made from doubly infected plants have been performed in several ways. Tests have included feeding aphids through membranes on virus-antiserum mixtures, feeding aphids on samples removed from sucrose gradients, injection of treated virus samples into aphids, and injection of virus-specific antiserum into aphids before they feed on doubly infected leaves.[17]

Our choice of salivary glands as the probable selective site in the circulation of BYDV within the aphid results from work that tends to eliminate other sites. The gut wall is often considered the major barrier to virus circulation in insects, largely because of the classic work of Storey[18] on transmission of maize streak virus by the leafhopper, *Cicadulina mbila*. Three lines of evidence suggest that the aphid gut wall is not the selective site for RPV and MAV. First, each virus isolate was detected in hemolymph of "nonvector" aphids that fed on infected plants.[19] For example, *M. avenae* fed on RPV-infected plants did not transmit RPV, but the virus was recovered from hemolymph of some of the aphids. Second, vector specificity of MAV and RPV occurred whether aphids acquired virus by feeding on leaves or whether virus concentrates were injected into hemolymph of aphids before test feedings.[10] Third, our attempts to alter specificity by puncturing the gut wall, as in the experiments of Storey, have been negative.[19] Taken together, these observations are evidence that the gut wall is not the major selective site for circulation of RPV and MAV in the two aphid species.

Specificity could be controlled during circulation of virus in hemolymph. Phagocytic or encapsulation mechanisms in hemolymph offer a range of possibilities for virus inactivation or inhibition.[20] Perhaps, mycetocytes and their symbiotic microorganisms play some role. Our elimination of hemolymph as the major selective site for RPV and MAV is based mainly on the fact that active virus was recovered from hemolymph of "nonvector" aphid species.[19] Because these tests were performed by transferring hemolymph from "nonvectors" to the vector species, it is possible that virus was inhibited in the "nonvector" hemolymph and that this inhibition was merely reversed by injection into vectors. However, other observations support the view that hemolymph, is not the most likely selective site. Ponsen[4] found no circulating hemocytes in *M. persicae*. Specificity of phagocytic reactions is not a pronounced attribute of many systems. For example, in at least two systems where efficient virus transmission occurs,[4, 21] virions were present in a variety of mesodermal cells within aphid vectors, which suggests that phagocytic activity within aphids is not especially selective.

Because there is evidence that the gut wall does not limit circulation of RPV and MAV, and since there is no evidence for selectivity of virus during circulation within hemolymph, we favor salivary glands as the site of selectivity. This choice is influenced by at least two general considerations. Because aphids lack Malpighian tubules, salivary glands function, at least in part, as excretory organs in aphids. Thus, it seems reasonable to expect that in aphids, salivary glands might have more selective functions than in some other insects. A recent anatomic study of *M. persicae* by Ponsen[4] emphasized the complex structure of salivary glands and illustrated their different cell types. The spectrum of specialization underscores the cytologic potential of salivary glands for differential selection.

Recent studies of some other circulative virus systems also point to the importance of aphid salivary glands. Ponsen [4] suggested that the myoepithelioid cell in the distal region of each principal salivary gland regulates transport of potato leafroll virus from hemolymph into the lumen of salivary ducts of *M. persicae*. Harris *et al.*[21] obtained evidence for the selective role of salivary glands in the transmission of pea enation mosaic virus by *Acyrothosiphon pisum* (Harris). Electron microscopy of salivary glands revealed virions of pea enation mosaic in glands of aphids exposed to a transmissible isolate of the virus but not within glands of aphids exposed to a nontransmissible isolate of the virus. Pea enation mosaic virus was especially concentrated in the basal laminae of the accessory gland, and virions were also found in cisternae of the plasma membrane of accessory gland cells.

Little is known about the method by which virus could penetrate membranes of the salivary glands. Pinocytosis (endocytosis) and membrane flow have been suggested. As Forbes [22] pointed out, membrane flow, pinocytosis, vesiculation, and phagocytosis are really all variations of the same dynamic phenomenon. The various stages of the process represent additional steps where selectivity in the penetration could occur. For example, perhaps RPV does not usually adsorb to the salivary membranes of *M. avenae* at sites where entrance could occur.

Although there is no reason to suspect that replication of BYDV in aphid vectors plays a part in specificity, neither is there any basis for ignoring the possibility that limited virus replication could occur in certain cells. Virus synthesis in salivary glands coupled with constant secretion during aphid feeding could not be detected in experiments based on detection of virus accumulation within the vector. This possibility is one of many that needs to be investigated before specificity will be fully understood.

CURRENT TESTS

Some current studies of the hypothesis of vector specificity are based on the concept that variations can result from properties of either the virus or the aphid. One approach is directed at the virus capsid protein. The importance of the protein to circulation of virus through aphids is being tested by attempts to change either the conformation of the coat protein or its amino acid residues. If vector specificity could be modified by altering the capsid protein, it would not only provide direct evidence for the role of the capsid but also would provide a way to study the mechanism in depth.

In a typical experiment, a chemical known to affect proteins was mixed with partially purified virus, usually MAV. After predetermined periods of incubation, the mixture was layered on sucrose gradients and centrifuged. The gradients were scanned and the virus zones collected for use in membrane feeding assays, by means of both aphid species, to permit detection of a change in vector specificity. In such tests, virus concentrations usually were about 20 μg/ml. A range of concentrations of each chemical was usually tested; details will not be given, because none of the treatments altered specificity of the virus.

In some instances, the treatments inactivated MAV; transmission by *M. avenae* was prevented or reduced. Compounds that caused this response were succinic anhydride, diethyl pyrocarbonate, and iodine (TABLE 1, *top*). Size and location of virus zones in sucrose gradients were often, but not always, affected by treatments that inactivated MAV. In more extensive tests with urea, RPV was more sensitive than MAV to inactivation. Only three of 28 plants became infected in tests with *R. padi* and RPV treated with 1 M urea for 30 min. *M. avenae,* however, continued to transmit MAV after treatment with urea at concentrations up to 3 M when incubated for 30 min (TABLE 1, *top*). When treatment with 3 M urea was continued for 60 min, however, MAV was inactivated, although only slight denaturation was evident in the sucrose gradient scanning patterns. None of the treatments resulted in MAV transmission by *R. padi* or in RPV transmission by *M. avenae.*

A second approach to test the hypothesis of vector specificity is directed at the aphid. We attempt to alter specificity by inducing physiologic changes in the vector. Some studies are based on use of chemicals known to affect properties of membranes by enhancing pinocytosis, by causing leakage, or by expediting transfers across them. Chemicals used in these tests include polyamino acids, ionophores, and polyenes. In some experiments, chemicals were

TABLE 1

INFECTIVITY OF THE MAV ISOLATE OF BARLEY YELLOW DWARF VIRUS MIXED WITH VARIOUS CHEMICALS BEFORE USE IN TRANSMISSION TESTS BY MEANS OF *R. padi* AND *M. avenae*

Chemical Treatment *	Transmissions by Aphid Species Shown After Feeding through Membranes on the Treated MAV Preparation Mixed with Sucrose †	
	R. padi	*M. avenae*
1–2 M urea	0/304	243/304
3 M urea (30 min)	0/16	16/16
3 M urea (60 min)	0/16	0/16
Succinic anhydride	0/160	0/160
Diethyl pyrocarbonate	0/208	1/208
O-methylisourea	0/96	2/96
N-ethylmaleimide	0/36	18/36
Iodine	0/12	0/12
Carboxypeptidase	0/60	60/60
Poly-L-ornithine	0/48	48/48
Poly-D-lysine	4/144	136/144
Filipin®	0/108	37/108
Nystatin	0/108	58/108
Amphotericin B	0/108	57/108
Ouabain	0/24	24/24
Gramicidin D	0/24	4/24
Aphid controls	0/220	0/220

 * MAV concentration was about 20 µg/ml; concentrations of chemicals varied with each experiment.
 † Numerator is number of plants that became infected; denominator is number infested each with 10 aphids for a 5-day inoculation test feeding at 21° C. Acquisition feeding through membranes was for about 20 hr at 15° C.

TABLE 2

TRANSMISSION OF THE MAV ISOLATE OF BARLEY YELLOW DWARF VIRUS BY APHIDS
INJECTED WITH VARIOUS CHEMICALS BEFORE OR AFTER ACQUISITION FEEDING
ON VIRUS-INFECTED LEAVES

Chemical Injected	Transmission by Aphid Species Shown *	
	R. padi	M. avenae
Poly-L-ornithine	4/152	40/40
Filipin	1/64	16/16
Nystatin	0/64	16/16
Amphotericin B	0/64	16/16
Ouabain	0/32	8/8
Gramicidin D	0/32	8/8
Aphid controls	0/120	0/120

* Numerator is number of plants that became infected; denominator is number infested with three to five injected aphids for a 5-day inoculation test feeding at 21° C. Acquisition feedings were for 1–2 days on detached leaves at 15° C.

mixed with concentrated MAV and used in membrane-feeding experiments with both vectors and "nonvectors" (TABLE 1, *bottom*). In other experiments, the chemicals were evaluated by injecting them into the hemolymph of aphids before, or sometimes after, aphids were permitted a 1- or 2-day acquisition feeding on virus-infected leaves (TABLE 2). None of the compounds tested to date has consistently altered virus-vector specificity. In one experiment, when poly-L-ornithine, at a concentration of 50 μg/ml, was injected into *R. padi* after acquisition feeding on MAV-infected leaves, four plants became infected (TABLE 2). We have been unable to reproduce this result, however.

In a related series of experiments, we tested the possible effect of NaCl, KCl, $CaCl_2$, $HgCl_2$, $MgCl_2$, and $AlCl_3$ at concentrations of 25–100 mM. The salts were mixed with concentrated MAV and used in membrane-feeding experiments with *R. padi*. None of 336 plants infested with the treated aphids became infected. All 96 control plants also remained healthy.

In a final series of experiments, mixtures of chemicals were injected into hemolymph of "nonvectors" together with concentrated preparations of MAV or RPV. Untreated virus was used as a control in each experiment. Parallel injections of both treated and untreated virus were also performed with vectors. Current emphasis in these tests is on use of various salts, polyamino acids, and mixtures of salts and polyamino acids. Some of the treatments have inactivated MAV or RPV, but none has changed vector specificity.

Despite prevailing failures in our current attempts to alter specificity, this approach seems worthwhile if kept in balance with other lines of investigation. The current failures certainly emphasize the need for a variety of approaches to such a complex problem. We do not consider these current failures to be evidence against the model of specificity, because of the preliminary nature of the tests, because we have no sound basis for selecting the chemicals to test, and because of the many factors that could influence results of such tests, even if we had chosen a potentially useful material. When we know more about the chemical nature of the protein capsid of the virus isolates, we will have a better basis for attempts to alter it.

The relative nature of the BYDV specificity presents some advantages in study of the process. When occasional transmissions by a "nonvector" occur, we have tested the infected plants to determine whether the virus transmitted was different from the isolate in the source plant. In all past tests, during many years, we found that occasional transmissions by "nonvectors" involved the original isolate and not a mutant or some selection from it. Such studies have included occasional transmissions from leaves or whole plants. They have also included occasional transmissions from virus preparations treated by many different procedures, from incubation with enzymes to single drop samples from sucrose gradient tubes. In recent experiments, however, some unexpected evidence for a change was encountered.

In a separate study, BYDV yields in virus preparations made from tissue extracted in liquid nitrogen were compared with virus yields from tissue extracted without liquid nitrogen.[23] Occasional transmissions of RPV and MAV by "nonvectors" occurred from both kinds of highly concentrated preparations. Eleven of 348 plants became infected in tests with *R. padi* of MAV preparations made with liquid nitrogen. In comparative transmission tests from the 11 plants, *M. avenae* transmitted virus, but *R. padi* did not. As in the past, transmission by the "nonvector" had not altered the MAV. In contrast, when we tested nine of 23 plants infected by *M. avenae* in tests of RPV preparations made with liquid nitrogen, the virus transmitted from eight of the nine plants had properties of MAV. At first, we thought that the pattern resulted from contamination or mislabeling, but it has occurred in six separate experiments during about one year. We tested a total of 89 plants infected by *M. avenae* that fed through membranes on RPV preparations. From 83 of the 89 plants, virus was transmitted by *M. avenae* (to 249 of 267 plants) but not by *R. padi* (to two of 267 plants). Thus, 83 of the 89 plants appeared to be infected by MAV. From the same RPV preparations, in each of 30 separate tests, *R. padi* transmitted virus subsequently identified as "ordinary" RPV. None of the aphid control plants became infected.

The apparent alteration of the RPV transmitted by *M. avenae* in these experiments is of interest, because this represents the first such occurrence in many kinds of experiments that tested the possibility of a change in vector specificity.[10, 19] The anomaly occurred only in tests of RPV preparations made by means of liquid nitrogen. We tested relatively few parallel preparations made without liquid nitrogen, but preliminary results suggest that the anomaly might be associated with the use of liquid nitrogen. Further tests of the apparent, unexpected change in RPV seem warranted.

ACKNOWLEDGMENTS

We are grateful to the Squibb Institute for gifts of nystatin and amphotericin B. We thank Dr. G. B. Whitfield, The Upjohn Company, for the gift of Filipin.

REFERENCES

1. PETERS, D. 1973. Persistent aphid-borne viruses. *In* Viruses and Invertebrates. A. J. Gibbs, Ed. Chap. **24:** 463–475. North-Holland Publishing Co. Amsterdam, The Netherlands.
2. SYLVESTER, E. S., J. RICHARDSON & N. W. FRAZIER. 1974. Serial passage of

strawberry crinkle virus in the aphid *Chaetosiphon jacobi*. Virology **59:** 301–306.

3. JENSEN, D. D. 1969. Insect diseases induced by plant-pathogenic viruses. *In* Viruses, Vectors, and Vegetation. K. Maramorosch, Ed. : 505–525. Interscience Publishers. New York, N.Y.

4. PONSEN, M. B. 1972. The site of potato leafroll virus multiplication in its vector, *Myzus persicae*. Mededel. Landbouwhogeschool (Wageningen) 72–16.

5. SYLVESTER, E. S. & J. RICHARDSON. 1971. Decreased survival of *Hyperomyzus lactucae* inoculated with serially passed sowthistle yellow vein virus. Virology **46:** 310–317.

6. SYLVESTER, E. S. 1973. Reduction of excretion, reproduction, and survival in *Hyperomyzus lactucae* fed on plants infected with isolates of sowthistle yellow vein virus. Virology **56:** 632–635.

7. ROCHOW, W. F. 1969. Specificity in aphid transmission of a circulative plant virus. *In* Viruses, Vectors, and Vegetation. K. Maramorosch, Ed. : 175–198. Interscience Publishers. New York, N.Y.

8. PALIWAL, Y. C. & R. C. SINHA. 1970. On the mechanism of persistence and distribution of barley yellow dwarf virus in an aphid vector. Virology **42:** 668–680.

9. ROCHOW, W. F. 1963. Variation within and among aphid vectors of plant viruses. Ann. N.Y. Acad. Sci. **105:** 713–729.

10. ROCHOW, W. F. 1969. Biological properties of four isolates of barley yellow dwarf virus. Phytopathology **59:** 1580–1589.

11. ROCHOW, W. F., A. I. E. AAPOLA, M. K. BRAKKE & L. E. CARMICHAEL. 1971. Purification and antigenicity of three isolates of barley yellow dwarf virus. Virology **46:** 117–126.

12. AAPOLA, A. I. E. & W. F. ROCHOW. 1971. Relationships among three isolates of barley yellow dwarf virus. Virology **46:** 127–141.

13. BRAKKE, M. K. & W. F. ROCHOW. 1974. Ribonucleic acid of barley yellow dwarf virus. Virology **61:** 240–248.

14. ROCHOW, W. F. 1972. The role of mixed infections in the transmission of plant viruses by aphids. Annu. Rev. Phytopathol. **10:** 101–124.

15. ROCHOW, W. F. 1970. Barley yellow dwarf virus: phenotypic mixing and vector specificity. Science **167:** 875–878.

16. ROCHOW, W. F. 1973. Selective virus transmission by *Rhopalosiphum padi* exposed sequentially to two barley yellow dwarf viruses. Phytopathology **63:** 1317–1322.

17. ROCHOW, W. F. & I. MULLER. 1975. Use of aphids injected with virus-specific antiserum for study of plant viruses that circulate in vectors. Virology **63:** 282–286.

18. STOREY, H. H. 1933. Investigations of the mechanism of the transmission of plant viruses by insect vectors. I. Proc. Roy. Soc. London Ser. B **113:** 463–485.

19. ROCHOW, W. F. & E. PANG. 1961. Aphids can acquire strains of barley yellow dwarf virus they do not transmit. Virology **15:** 382–384.

20. LAFFERTY, K. J. & R. CRICHTON. 1973. Immune responses of invertebrates. *In* Viruses and Invertebrates. A. J. Gibbs, Ed. Chap. **16:** 300–320. North-Holland Publishing Co. Amsterdam, The Netherlands.

21. HARRIS, K. F., J. E. BATH, G. THOTTAPPILLY & G. R. HOOPER. 1975. Fate of pea enation mosaic virus in PEMV-injected pea aphids. Virology **65:** 148–162.

22. FORBES, A. R. 1964. The morphology, histology, and fine structure of the gut of the green peach aphid, *Myzus persicae* (Sulzer) (Homoptera: Aphididae). Mem. Entomol. Soc. Can. **36.**

23. FOXE, M. J. & W. F. ROCHOW. 1975. Importance of virus source leaves in vector specificity of barley yellow dwarf virus. Phytopathology **65:** In press.

MORPHOGENESIS OF A NUCLEAR POLYHEDROSIS VIRUS OF THE ALFALFA LOOPER IN A CONTINUOUS CABBAGE LOOPER CELL LINE

Hiroyuki Hirumi and Kazuko Hirumi

Boyce Thompson Institute for Plant Research
Yonkers, New York 10701

Arthur H. McIntosh

Institute of Microbiology
Rutgers University
New Brunswick, New Jersey 08903

INTRODUCTION

Nuclear polyhedrosis viruses (NPVs) are an important group of insect pathogenic viruses placed in the genus *Baculovirus*.[1] Of particular interest are the NPVs that infect members of the order Lepidoptera. Because these viruses have a potential use as biologic control agents of lepidopteran insect pests, they have recently received considerable attention. In general, NPVs are species specific. Certain viruses, however, are known to be cross infective to alternate hosts.[2-5] An NPV isolated from the alfalfa looper, *Autographa californica,*[4] is of special interest, because it is known to be cross infective to six alternate hosts, which belong to four genera.[4, 5]

Continuous cell cultures derived from either original (homologous) or alternate (heterologous) host insects facilitate the study of the morphogenesis, species specificity, pathogenicity, and possible changes that occur during prolonged passages *in vitro* of the NPVs.[6-8] In addition, cell cultures have the advantage of economic production of "clean" virus under highly controlled conditions, in comparison with *in vivo* systems.[6, 9, 10] Complete replication of various NPVs in their homologous [6-8, 11-14] and heterologous [6, 10, 15, 16] host cell lines has been reported. Several NPVs have been successfully propagated *in vitro* through several passages without loss of their infectivity to host insects.[6, 10, 11, 14] However, it was demonstrated recently that long-term serial passages of the cabbage looper, *Trichoplusia ni,* NPV in the homologous host cell cultures greatly diminished the infectivity of polyhedral inclusion bodies (PIBs).[8] Prolonged serial passages of the silkworm, *Bombyx mori,* NPV in larvae of the rice stem borer, *Chilo suppressalis,* also exhibited production of morphologically different PIBs.[17]

Before field applications of NPVs can be made, it is important that their biologic characteristics be fully understood. This is especially true for NPVs that are cross infective to various alternate hosts. An attempt, therefore, was made to elucidate the ultrastructural aspects of *A. californica* NPV replication in an established cell line of its alternate host, *T. ni,* with special emphasis on morphogenesis after prolonged serial passages *in vitro*.

302

MATERIALS AND METHODS

Cell Line

The established cabbage looper, *T. ni,* cell line (TN-368) [18] was obtained from Dr. W. F. Hink, The Ohio State University, in September, 1971. Since receipt, the cell line has been maintained in Hirumi-Maramorosch leafhopper (HML) medium [19, 20] for 23 passages and thereafter in TC199-MK medium [21] with Falcon plastic 25 cm^2 T flasks (T-25) at 27° C.

Virus

The multiple-embedded alfalfa looper, *A. californica,* nuclear polyhedrosis virus (ACNPV) was supplied by Dr. P. V. Vail, Western Cotton Research Laboratory, in powder form in 1973. One gram contained 10^9 PIBs. Cabbage looper larvae were inoculated per os with 10^5 PIBs/0.1 ml on each artificial diet surface. Hemolymph from 150 infected loopers was diluted 1:5 in TC199-MK medium and was sterilized by passage through a 0.45-μm Millipore® filter. TN-368 cells grown in a roller tube were inoculated with 0.2 ml of this material. Cytopathic effects and the production of PIBs were observed for 1 week. Subsequently, the virus was used to inoculate cell cultures by adding 0.5 ml of virus-containing supernatant to fresh TN-368 cells in 4.5 ml of TC199-MK medium. This addition resulted in a 1:10 dilution of virus at each passage. TN-368 cells, at total passages 132, 135 and 200, were inoculated with the ACNPV at virus passages 4, 47, and 99, respectively. Inoculation of these three groups were made as follows.

Low-passage (P4) group. Fluid and cells of ACNPV-infected TN-368 cell cultures in the third passage were frozen and thawed alternately three times in dry ice-acetone and a 37° C water bath. Cell debris was removed by centrifugation at 300g for 10 min. The titer of virus in the supernatant fluid was approximately 10^6 TCID$_{50}$/ml. The TN-368 cell cultures, which contained 1.5 × 10^6 cells/T-25 flask in 4.5 ml of TC199-MK medium, were inoculated by adding 0.5 ml of the virus inoculum. After a 1-hr adsorption period on a rocker platform, the inoculated cultures were incubated at 27° C.

High passage (P47 and P99) groups. Virus-containing culture fluids were removed from 10 dilution bottles at passages 46 and 98 72 hr postinoculation and were concentrated by centrifugation at 52,200g in a Beckman L2–65B ultracentrifuge with an SW27 rotor for 1 hr at 4° C. The pellets were resuspended in 15 ml of TC199-MK medium and were sterilized as described above. The inoculum had a titer of 10^6 TCID$_{50}$/ml. TN-368 cell cultures were inoculated as described above. A total of 58 inoculated and uninoculated cell cultures (48 and 10 cultures, respectively) were examined at various times (from 10 min to 6 days) after inoculation.

Electron Microscopy

Loosely attached TN-368 cells were mechanically suspended in the culture medium and were collected by low-speed centrifugation at 300g for 15 min.

After rinsing with Earle's balanced salt solution, the cells were fixed in 1.5% glutaraldehyde in 0.05 M sodium cacodylate buffer (pH 7.2) for 15 min at room temperature. The cells were rinsed three times with the buffer, which contained 5% sucrose, utilizing low-speed centrifugation, and the final cell pellets were then postfixed in 2% osmium tetroxide in the sucrose-containing buffer. After brief rinsing with the buffer, the postfixed cell pellets were passed through a cold ethanol series and propylene oxide. Subsequently, the pellets were embedded in an Epon® 812-Araldite® 506 mixture.[22] Thin sections were stained with 8% uranyl magnesium acetate in distilled water, followed by 0.4% lead citrate in 0.1 N sodium hydroxide, and were examined with a Siemens Elmiskop-I, modified to IA, at 80 KV.

RESULTS

Phase-Contrast Microscopy

Although no precise counts of PIBs were made, most cells infected with the low-passage virus contained approximately 50–80 PIBs per nucleus, within 48 hr postinoculation. In the high-passage groups, hypertrophy of the nucleus was observed in a few cells as early as 3 hr after inoculation (FIGURE 1). During the next 10–15 hr, most cells became rounded. After 18 hr, PIBs were first observed in a few cells (less than 1%), and 24 hr after inoculation, 8% of the cells contained PIBs (FIGURE 2). At 48 hr postinoculation, approximately 70–80% of cells contained PIBs; however, the number of PIBs per nucleus did not significantly increase (FIGURE 3). After 72 hr, most cells detached from the surface of the culture flasks and contained from 1 to 20 PIBs (FIGURE 4). By that time, degeneration of the cytoplasm had become apparent in some cells. After 6 days, more than 80% of cells had disintegrated. This reduction in PIBs of high-passage virus *in vitro* has also been described in the homologous *T. ni* NPV system.[8]

Ultrastructure of Uninfected Cells

The ultrastructural morphology of uninfected TN-368 cells was similar to that described previously for *B. mori* cells.[7] The majority of TN-368 cells at the interphase contained a large, slightly elliptical nucleus enclosed by a relatively smooth nuclear envelope and typical cytoplasmic organelles, such as ribosomes, mitochondria, agranular and granular endoplasmic reticulum, lysosomes, and small cytoplasmic vacuoles. In general, chromatinic substance was evenly distributed throughout the nucleus. However, some clumps of the substance also occurred at the periphery of the nucleus and near the nucleolus.

Ultrastructure of Infected Cells

Free Virions and Their Aberrant Forms

Virus Entry. Enveloped virions attached to the plasma membrane of the host cells within 10 min postinoculation (FIGURE 5). Virions partially engulfed in

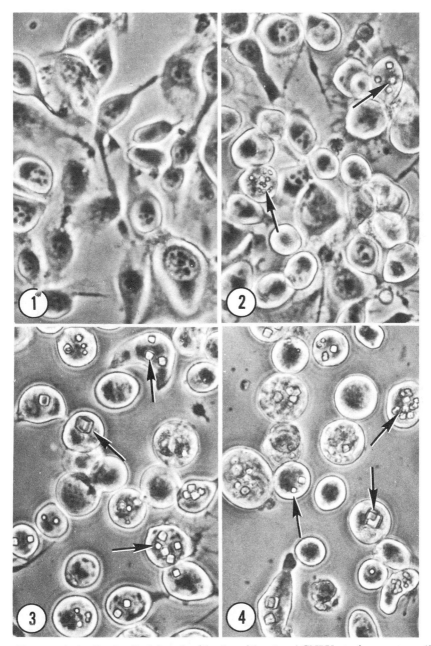

FIGURES 1–4. *T. ni* cells infected with *A. californica* ACNPV at virus passage 47 *in vitro*. Phase-contrast micrographs. FIGURE 1, 3 hr; FIGURE 2, 24 hr; FIGURE 3, 48 hr; FIGURE 4, 72 hr after inoculation. ×500.

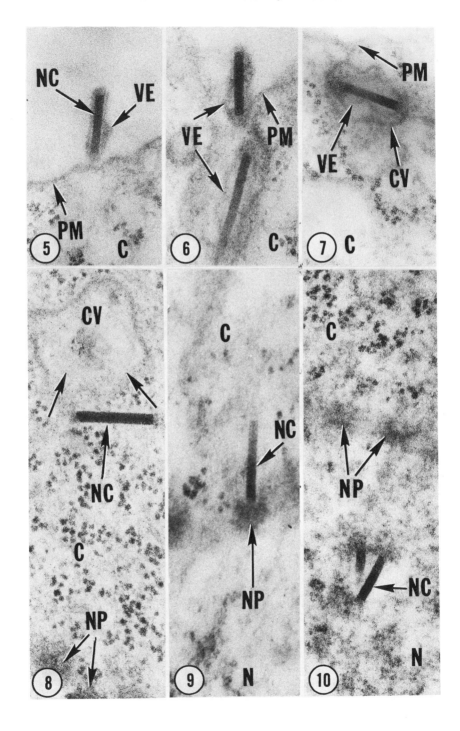

invaginations of the plasma membrane were often seen (FIGURE 6). Subsequently, virions appeared in cytoplasmic vacuoles bounded by a membrane that was presumably acquired from the invaginated plasma membrane (FIGURE 7). Within these vacuoles, the viral rod was still enclosed by a viral envelope. The virus-containing vacuoles appeared only at the periphery of infected cells. No naked virus rods entering the host cell surface were observed. Partially ruptured vacuoles, releasing the virus rods into the cytoplasmic matrix, often appeared in the middle region of the cytoplasm (FIGURE 8). By that time, the viral rods were nonenveloped. At 3 hr postinoculation, naked virus particles were located vertically near the nuclear envelope and were often attached to nuclear pores in an "end-on" orientation (FIGURE 9). Intact virus rods were also seen in the nuclei (FIGURE 10). No enveloped virions were observed either near the nuclear envelopes or inside the nuclei. Empty capsids, described previously as attached to the nuclear pores with an "end-on" association,[23] were not detected.

Formation of Virogenic Stroma. The first morphologic changes of the nucleoplasm were seen in a few infected host cells as early as 3 hr after inoculation. In most cells, the alterations became apparent 6–12 hr postinoculation. Many small aggregates of fine, electron-opaque granules appeared throughout the nucleus (FIGURE 11). These structures are probably the precursors of the virogenic stroma.[7, 24] Subsequently, numerous small particles, approximately 22–24 nm in diameter, were often observed (FIGURE 12). After 18 hr, the aggregates increased in size and density. Nucleoplasmic matrices became considerably electron lucent after 24 hr, whereas the virogenic stroma increased in size and electron opacity and formed a large mass in the central region of the nucleus. No virus rods were detected in the nuclei at this time.

Formation of Viral Progeny. During the period from 24 to 48 hr postinoculation, many naked virus rods, presumably newly formed viral progeny, appeared in the nucleus and were closely associated with the virogenic stroma (FIGURE 13). At this stage, no virus particles were seen in the areas between the virogenic stroma and the nuclear envelope. Shortly thereafter, many membranous profiles, which varied in size and shape, appeared in those nuclei in which numerous naked virus rods were seen around the virogenic stroma (FIGURE 14). Forty-eight hours after inoculation, these intranuclear membranes were closely associated with these naked rods (FIGURE 15). Many bundles of virus particles, in addition to single virus rods, were partially or completely enclosed by the intranuclear membranes (FIGURES 16 & 17). These enveloped virions were scattered throughout the nuclei (FIGURE 17). At this stage, no morphologic alterations of either nuclear envelopes or cytoplasmic organelles were observed.

Virus Release. The majority of the virions were not occluded in PIBs but were released from the nucleus into the cytoplasm and subsequently from the host cell surface to the extracellular space by budding. At 48 hr postinoculation,

---

FIGURES 5–10. *T. ni* cells infected with ACNPV at the early stages of infection, from 10 to 180 min after inoculation, at virus passage 47. C, cytoplasm; CV, cytoplasmic vesicle: N, nucleus; NC, nucleocapsid; NP, nuclear pore; PM, plasma membrane; VE, viral envelope. ×74,000. FIGURE 5, enveloped virus particle closely associated with the plasma membrane of the host cell; FIGURE 6, virions entered the host cell cytoplasm by phagocytosis; FIGURE 7, virus-containing cytoplasmic vesicle; FIGURE 8, cytoplasmic vesicle partially ruptured (arrows) in the cytoplasm, FIGURE 9, nucleocapsid attached to the nuclear pore with an end-on orientation; FIGURE 10, naked nucleocapsids appeared in the nucleus.

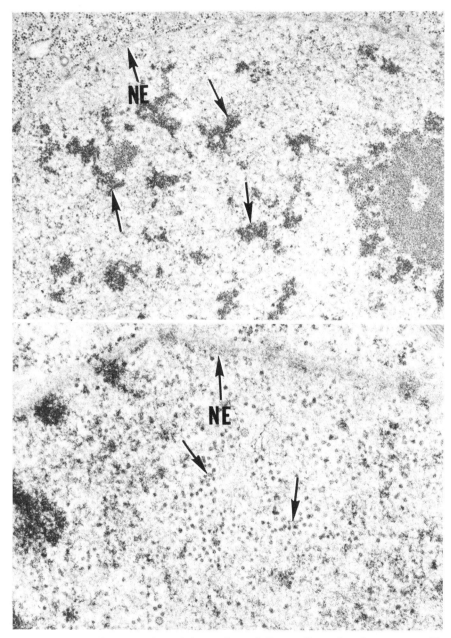

FIGURES 11 and 12. Portion of the nucleus of *T. ni* cells at the virus passage 47. NE, nuclear envelope. FIGURE 11 (*top*), fine electron-opaque granules (arrows) appeared throughout the nucleus, 6 hr after ACNPV inoculation. ×22,050. FIGURE 12 (*bottom*), many small particles (arrows) were seen 12 hr after ACNPV inoculation. ×49,700.

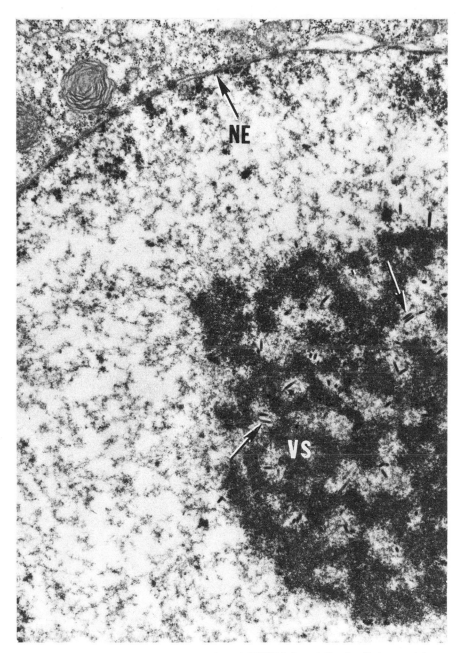

FIGURE 13. Portion of the nucleus of an ACNPV-infected *T. ni* cell that contains a mass of the virogenic stroma (VS). Naked viral progeny (arrows), closely associated with the virogenic stroma, were seen 48 hr after inoculation with virus passage 4. NE, nuclear envelope. ×21,000.

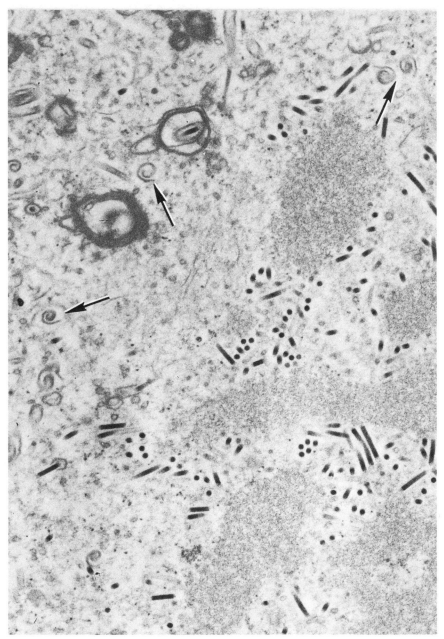

FIGURE 14. Portion of the nucleus of an ACNPV-infected *T. ni* cell 48 hr post-inoculation with virus passage 4. Many membranous profiles (arrows) appeared in the nucleus. ×36,050.

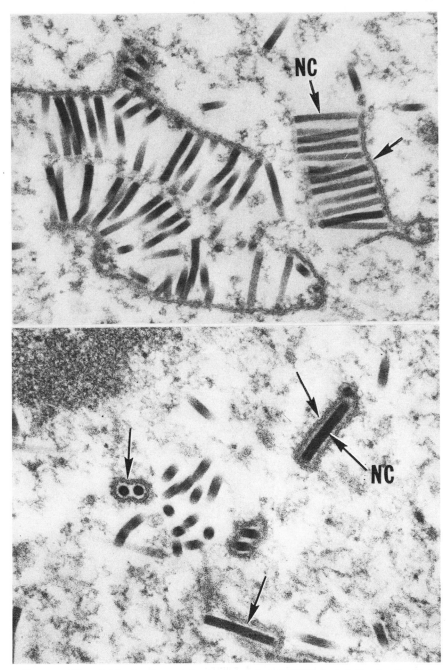

FIGURES 15 and 16. Portion of the nucleus of ACNPV-infected *T. ni* cells 48 hr postinoculation with virus passage 47. Nucleocapsids (NC) were closely associated or completely enclosed with intranuclear membranes (arrows). FIGURE 15 (*top*), ×66,000; FIGURE 16 (*bottom*), ×74,100.

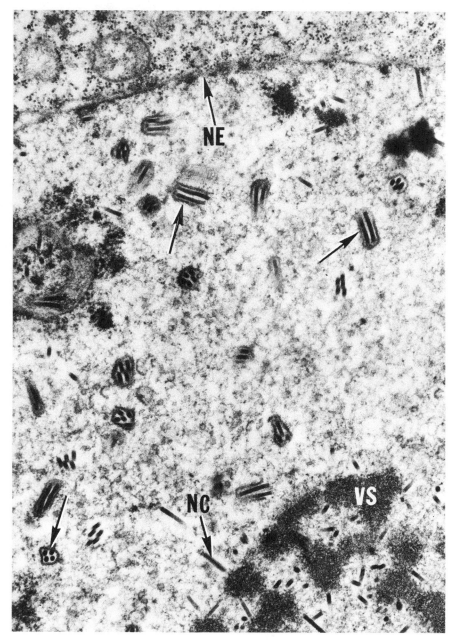

FIGURE 17. Portion of the nucleus of an ACNPV-infected *T. ni* cell 48 hr post-inoculation at the virus passage 47. A number of partially or completely enveloped virus particles (arrows) were scattered throughout the nucleus. NC, nucleocapsid; NE, nuclear envelope; VS, virogenic stroma. ×30,450.

the nuclear envelope partially protruded into the cytoplasm, forming several blebs. The outer and inner membranes of these nuclear protrusions consisted of the outer and inner membranes of the nuclear envelope, respectively (FIGURE 18). In general, the outer membrane protruded more extensively than the inner one, forming a wide, electron-lucent space between the two membranes. Naked virus rods, which varied in number, were released into the inner blebs. No virions enveloped by the intranuclear membranes were observed inside the nuclear blebs. Subsequently, the virus-containing protrusions were separated from the nuclei and became intracytoplasmic vacuoles (FIGURES 19 & 20).

In most infected cells, the outer membranes of virus-containing vacuoles ruptured in the middle region of the cytoplasm. Partially broken inner membranes of the vacuoles were seen at further peripheral regions, releasing naked virus rods into the cytoplasmic matrices of the host cells (FIGURE 20). In these cells, many naked virus rods attached to the plasma membrane were also observed. These virus particles budded from the host cell surface, acquired the plasma membrane, and subsequently were released from the host cell surface (FIGURE 20, *insets*).

No significant differences as to entry, replication, and release of ACNPV in the heterologous host cells were seen between the low (P4) and the high (P47 and P99) passage groups *in vitro*.

Formation of Long Tubular Structures. At 3–6 days postinoculation, many long tubular profiles, which varied in length, appeared in those nuclei in which numerous naked virus rods were seen (FIGURES 21 & 22). They were partially filled with a dense substance that had an electron opacity similar to that of the virus particles (FIGURE 22). Occasionally, they contained bandlike structures (FIGURE 23). These tubular profiles were more abundant in the high-passage groups than in the low-passage group. Similar structures have been reported in several homologous systems, both *in vitro* [8] and *in vivo*,[23, 25] and were suggested to be aberrant forms of the viral capsids.

PIB Formation and Virus Occlusion

Low-Passage Virus. Ultrastructural aspects of PIBs and occluded virions were similar to those reported earlier by Vail *et al.*[26] in the same heterologous *in vitro* system.

High-Passage Virus. A few developing PIBs and accumulations of fine fibrous substances were seen in some infected cells during the early stages of infection (FIGURE 24). Morphologic profiles of these fibrous substances were very similar to those observed by others in the cabbage looper NPV-infected homologous host cell systems, both *in vivo* [27] and *in vitro*.[8] Many naked and enveloped virus particles appeared around the smooth-edged PIBs, which contained no occluded virions (FIGURE 24). Subsequently, partially or completely occluded virus particles were seen in the PIBs (FIGURE 25). Both single virus particles and bundles of virions, which were either naked or enveloped by the intranuclear membranes, were incorporated within PIBs. Viral envelopes of particles that were partially occluded into PIBs were often compressed (FIGURE 25, *inset*). During the late periods of infection, from 3 to 6 days postinoculation, many "empty" spaces were observed in the majority of PIBs (FIGURE 26). Several small vesicles, presumably residuals of viral envelopes, appeared on the surface of rough-edged PIBs (FIGURE 26). The occluded virions did not in-

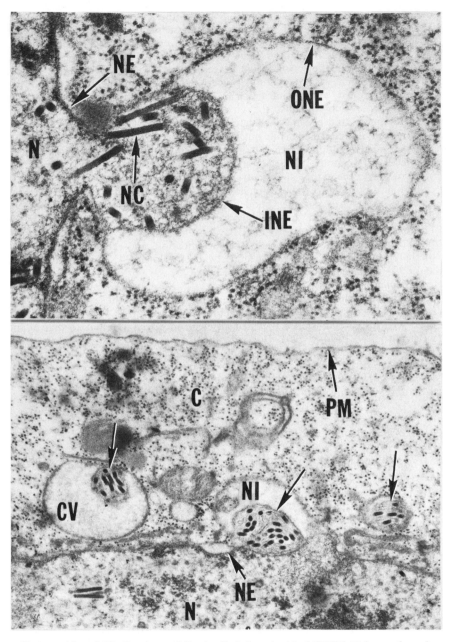

FIGURES 18 and 19. Portions of *T. ni* cells infected with ACNPV 48 hr postinocula-tion with virus passage 47. C, cytoplasm; CV, cytoplasmic vacuole; INE, inner nu-clear envelope; N, nucleus; NC, nucleocapsid; NE, nuclear envelope; NI, nuclear in-vagination; ONE, outer nuclear envelope; PM, plasma membrane. FIGURE 18 (*top*), Naked nucleocapsids were released into the nuclear invagination. ×47,900. FIGURE 19 (*bottom*), nuclear invaginations and cytoplasmic vacuoles contained bundles of naked virus rods (arrows). ×27,000.

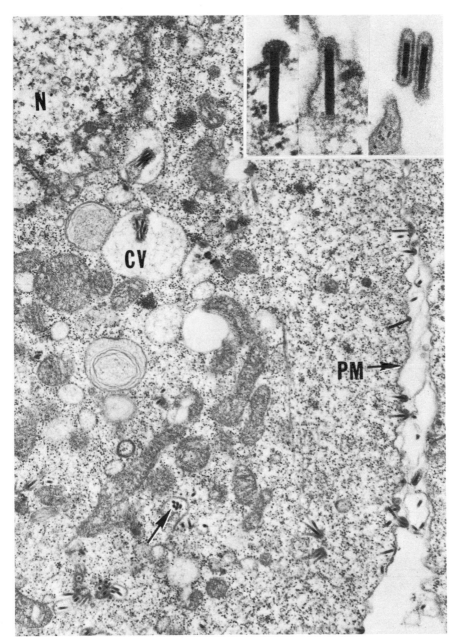

FIGURE 20. Portion of an ACNPV-infected *T. ni* cell 48 hr postinoculation with virus passage 47. Partially ruptured inner membrane of virus-containing cytoplasmic vacuole (arrow) at the middle region of the cytoplasm and many naked virus rods attached to the plasma membrane (PM) at the periphery of the host cell were seen. × 19,300. Insets: virus particles budding from the host cell surface; *left & middle,* ×74,100; *right,* ×49,700. CV, virus-containing cytoplasmic vacuole; N, nucleus.

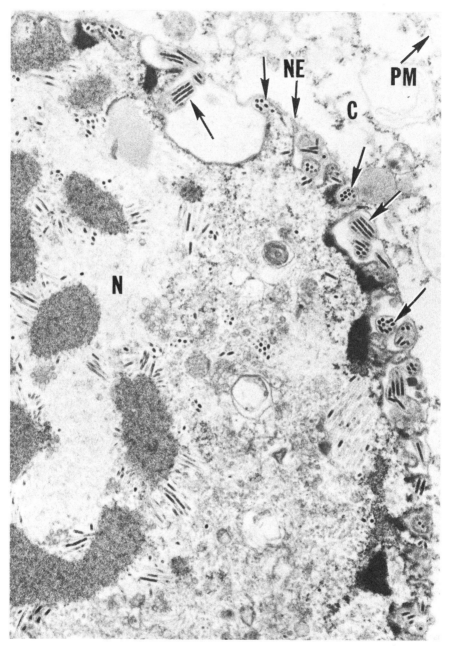

FIGURE 21. Portion of a degenerated *T. ni* cell infected with ACNPV 6 days post-inoculation with virus passage 99. Numerous aberrant forms of virus particles were seen in the nucleus (N). Many bundles of virus rods enclosed at periphery of the nucleus. C, cytoplasm; NE, nuclear envelope; PM, plasma membrane. ×24,000.

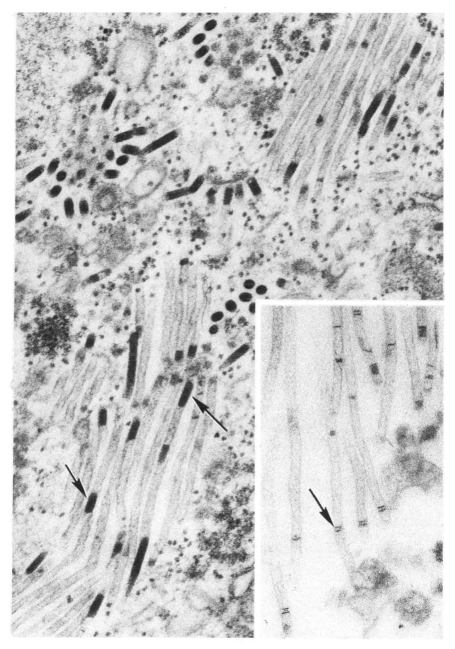

FIGURES 22 and 23. Long tubular profiles appeared in the nuclei of ACNPV-infected *T. ni* cells at virus passage 47. FIGURE 22 (*left*), many tubular structures were partially filled with high electron-opaque substances (arrows) 3 days postinoculation. ×68,200. FIGURE 23 (*inset*), some tubular profiles contained band type structures (arrow) 6 days postinoculation. ×74,400.

crease significantly in number during this period. PIBs, which contained few or no virions, were also often observed (FIGURES 27–29). The number of morphologically normal virions occluded per PIB considerably decreased with the high-passage virus, as compared with those occluded with the low-passage virus.

Degeneration of Host Cells

PIB-Free Infected Cells. During late stages of infection, several PIB-free infected cells were lysed, losing most of their cytoplasmic components. The

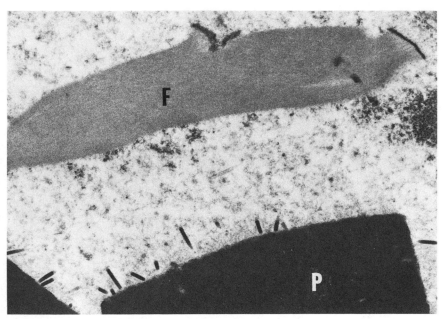

FIGURE 24. Portion of an ACNPV-infected *T. ni* cell that contains a polyhedral inclusion body (P) and fine fibrous substance (F) in the nucleus 48 hr postinoculation with virus passage 47. ×27,000.

nuclei of these cells still contained the nucleoplasm and numerous virus particles (FIGURE 21). In the nuclei, most virus particles were naked, and no intranuclear membranes were seen. At the periphery of the nuclei, bundles of naked virus rods, enclosed by the inner membrane of the nuclear envelope, appeared in the irregularly enlarged perinuclear cisterna.

PIB-Containing Infected Cells. At the developmental stages of PIBs, from 18 to 48 hr postinoculation, the nuclear envelopes of PIB-containing cells became highly irregular, forming many nuclear protrusions (FIGURE 27). At this stage, the cytoplasm of the infected cells was still intact and contained normal cytoplasmic organelles. At later stages, from 3 to 6 days after infection, cell lysis of many PIB-containing infected cells was evident. In the nuclei of these

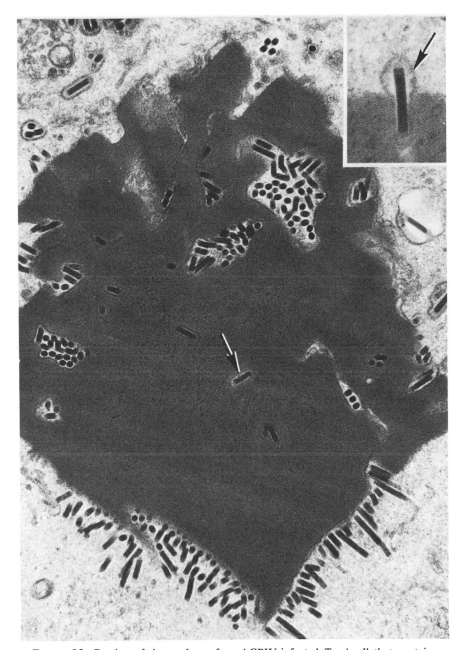

FIGURE 25. Portion of the nucleus of an ACPIV-infected *T. ni* cell that contains a PIB 48 hr postinoculation with virus passage 47. Both naked and enveloped (arrow) virus particles were occluded in the PIB. ×43,600. Inset: virus particle whose envelope was compressed at the edge of the PIB. ×74,400.

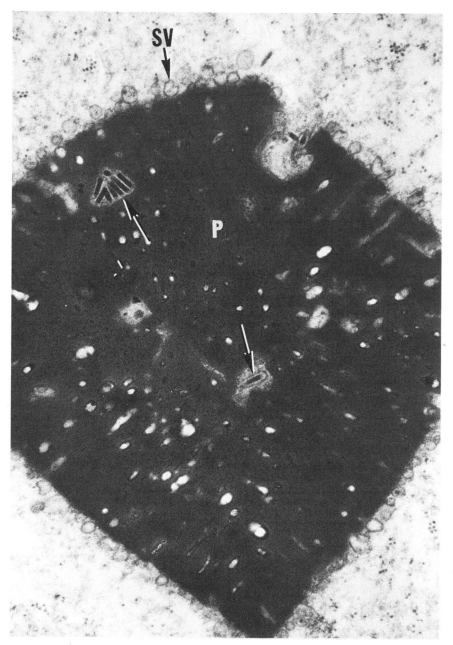

FIGURE 26. PIBs (P) that contained many "empty" spaces and a few intact virus particles (arrows) were seen in the nucleus of an ACNPV-infected *T. ni* cell 3 days postinoculation with virus passage 47. SV, small vesicle. ×34,800.

host cells, numerous naked virus rods, aberrant forms, such as empty capsids and long filamentous structures, and small vesicles were observed, but no complete enveloped virions were present (FIGURES 28 & 29).

DISCUSSION

It was demonstrated earlier that the infectivity of the corn earworm, *Heliothis zea,* NPV represented a dilution of 10^{-8} of the original inoculum after seven consecutive passages in the homologous host cell line *in vitro,* although no free

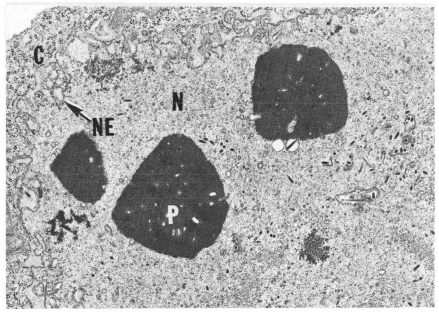

FIGURE 27. Portion of an ACNPV-infected *T. ni* cell that contains a few PIBs (P) 48 hr after inoculation with virus passage 47. The cytoplasm (C) was still intact; however, the nuclear envelope (NE) became highly irregular. N, nucleus. × 17,500.

virions or PIBs were detected in the cell cultures.[14] Faulkner and Henderson,[11] who worked with *T. ni* NPV in the homologous host cell line, suggested that serial propagation of NPVs may be continued for many passages without apparent loss of virulence to the host insect. Vail *et al.*[10] successfully propagated ACNPV in the heterologous host, *T. ni,* cell line through five consecutive serial passages. By use of fluid phases of ACNPV-infected cultures, they demonstrated that ACNPV produced *in vitro* were qualitatively and quantitatively as infective as those produced *in vivo.* It was also reported that NPVs of *T. ni, H. zea,* and the fall armyworm, *Spodoptera frugiperda,* can be propagated in their homologous cell lines without loss of supernatant infectivity obtained from NPV-infected cell cultures through several virus passages *in vitro.*[6] On the other

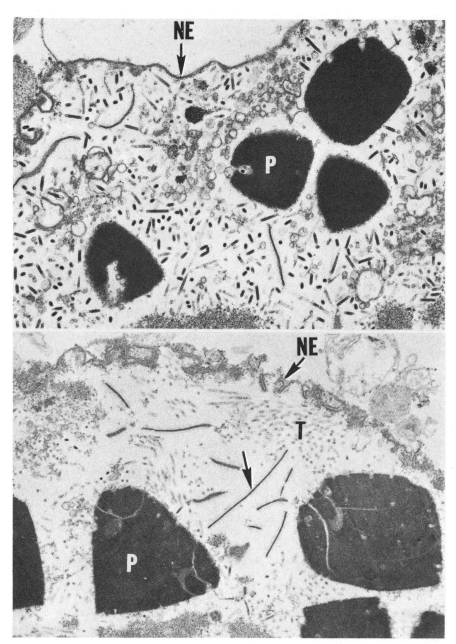

FIGURES 28 and 29. Portion of degenerated *T. ni* cells infected with ACNPV that contain numerous aberrant forms of virus particles and a few PIBs (P). NE, nuclear envelope. FIGURE 28 (*top*), 3 days postinoculation with virus passage 47. ×22,050. FIGURE 29 (*bottom*), 6 days postinoculation with virus passage 99. Numerous empty tubular structures (T) and long filamentous structure (arrow) were seen. ×17,500.

hand, MacKinnon *et al.*[8] reported that prolonged serial passages of *T. ni* NPV in the homologous host cells *in vitro* resulted in a great loss of infectivity of both PIBs and of the supernatants of infected cell cultures. They also observed that long-term passages of the *T. ni* NPV decreased both the total number of PIBs produced *in vitro* and the number of morphologically normal occluded virions.

The present study demonstrated that both the number of PIBs produced per cell and the number of normal virions occluded per PIB decreased considerably after prolonged passages in the heterologous host cells *in vitro*. However, no significant difference was observed in the infectivity of the filtrated cell culture supernatants, as measured by $TCID_{50}$, between the low- and the high-passage levels. These findings are in agreement with the electron microscopic observation that revealed the release of numerous complete, free ACNPV particles in the extracellular space during long-term passages *in vitro*.

With respect to the mode of NPV entry, two concepts have been proposed. One is that the virus particles enter the host cells *in vivo* by fusion of the viral envelope and the plasma membrane of the microvilli of the host insects. Supporting evidence has been reported for the small tortoiseshell butterfly, *Aglais urticae*,[28] and *T. ni*[23] inoculated with their homologous NPVs, and also *T. ni* larvae inoculated with heterologous *Rachiplusia ou* NPV.[29] The other concept is that the virus enters the cell by pinocytosis. This phenomenon has been demonstrated in *T. ni*[30] and *Spodoptera littoralis*[31] host insects infected with their homologous granulosis virus and NPV, respectively. Recently, Raghow and Grace[7] reported the occurrence of *B. mori* NPV entry by phagocytosis into the homologous host cells *in vitro*. The present study supports the latter concept. However, further studies are necessary before any generalization can be made with regard to the mechanism of NPV entry, because there may be certain differences between *in vivo* and *in vitro* systems and between homologous and heterologous systems.

Based on the finding of empty or partially empty capsids that attached to the nuclear pores with "end-on" orientation and the absence of viral rods in the host cell nucleus during the early stages of *T. ni* granulosis virus infection *in vivo*, it has been suggested that the contents of the nucleocapsids enter the nucleus.[23] Raghow and Grace[7] also observed similar attachments of non-enveloped viral rods of *B. mori* NPV to the nuclear pores of the homologous host cells *in vitro*. They pointed out that clear-cut evidence for the entry of the whole nucleocapsid or its contents is lacking, although the mechanism suggested earlier[23] would very likely operate in *B. mori* NPV *in vitro*. On the contrary, Kawanishi *et al.*[29] observed naked viral rods in the *R. ou* NPV-infected homologous host cells *in vivo* as early as 4 hr after inoculation. In the present study, naked viral rods of ACNPV were also seen within 3 hr postinoculation. Because the formation of the virogenic stroma and viral progeny occurred at least 18 hr after inoculation, the naked viral rods observed at the early stage of infection were very likely virions of the original inoculum, which indicates the possible entry of the whole viral rod into the nucleus through the nuclear pore.

The appearance of nonoccluded *A. urticae* NPV particles in the cytoplasm of the homologous host cells *in vivo* was observed earlier and was suggested to be significant in the pathway of the NPV infection.[32] The release of nonoccluded NPV particles from the infected nuclei in the cytoplasm was also reported in *S. littoralis*[31] and *T. ni*[8] host cells infected with their homologous NPVs *in vitro*. The present study has demonstrated further details about the morphogenesis of nonoccluded ACNPV particles in heterologous host cells *in vitro*. These findings suggest that the following sequential events may occur in host cells: entry of complete, free virions into the host cells by phagocytosis; uncoating of the viral envelope in the phagocytotic vesicles; rupture of the vesicles, releasing naked virus rods into the cytoplasmic matrix; entry of naked virions into the nucleus through nuclear pores; formation of the virogenic stroma in the infected nucleus; formation of virus progeny closely associated with the virogenic stroma; coating of virus rods with intranuclear membranes; uncoating of the intranuclear membranes at the periphery of the nucleus; formation of nuclear protrusions that contain naked virus rods; separation of the nuclear protrusions from the nuclear membrane into the cytoplasm, forming virus-containing cytoplasmic vacuoles; rupture of the outer membrane of the vacuoles; rupture of the inner membrane of the vacuoles, releasing the naked rods into the cytoplasmic matrix; and subsequent release of nonoccluded virus particles from the host cell surface to the extracellular space by budding, acquiring a viral envelope derived from the host cell plasma membrane. These sequential events most likely occur in both low- and high-passage virus levels *in vitro*.

SUMMARY

Morphogenesis of the *A. californica* NPV was studied in the cells of an alternate host *T. ni, in vitro* at low (P4) and high (P47 and P99) virus passage levels. PIBs and normal virions occluded in them decreased considerably in number at the high-passage levels, although numerous free virions were propagated in both low- and high-passage groups. Free enveloped virions entered the host cell cytoplasm by phagocytosis. Naked virus rods entered the nucleus through the nuclear pores. Numerous viral progeny closely associated with the virogenic stroma were observed 18–24 hr postinoculation. At 48 hr postinoculation, nuclear envelopes that contained naked virus rods protruded into the cytoplasm, separated from the envelope, and subsequently ruptured into the cytoplasm. Many naked virus rods budded from the cell surface, acquiring an envelope derived from the plasma membrane of the host cell. PIBs in which both enveloped virions and naked virus rods were occluded appeared 24 hr, or later, after inoculation. At later stages (3–6 days postinoculation), only a few complete virions were seen in PIBs produced at high-virus passage levels. Many aberrant forms of the virus particles were frequently observed in the nuclei of degenerating cells at the high-passage levels.

REFERENCES

1. WILDY, P. 1971. Classification and nomenclature of viruses. Mon. Virol. **5:** 81.
2. IGNOFFO, C. M. 1968. Specificity of insect virus. Bull. Entomol. Soc. Amer. **14:** 265–276.
3. TOMPKINS, G. J., J. R. ADAMS & A. M. HEIMPEL. 1969. Cross infection studies with *Heliothis zea* using nuclear-polyhedrosis viruses from *Trichoplusia ni*. J. Invert. Pathol. **14:** 343–357.
4. VAIL, P. V., D. L. JAY & D. K. HUNTER. 1970. Cross infectivity of a nuclear polyhedrosis virus isolated from the alfalfa looper, *Autographa californica*. *In* Proceedings of the IVth International Colloquium on Insect Pathology. : 297–304.

5. VAIL, P. V., D. L. JAY & D. K. HUNTER. 1973. Infectivity of a nuclear poly-hedrosis virus from the alfalfa looper, *Autographa californica,* after passage through alternate hosts. J. Invert. Pathol. **21:** 16–20.
6. GOODWIN, R. H., J. L. VAUGHN, J. R. ADAMS & S. J. LOULOUDES. 1973. The influence of insect cell lines and tissue-culture media on *Baculovirus* polyhedra production. Misc. Publ. Entomol. Soc. Amer. **9:** 66–72.
7. RAGHOW, R. & T. D. C. GRACE. 1974. Studies on a nuclear polyhedrosis virus in *Bombyx mori* cells *in vitro.* 1. Multiplication kinetics and ultrastructural studies. J. Ultrastruct. Res. **47:** 384–399.
8. MACKINNON, E. A., J. F. HENDERSON, D. B. STOLTZ & P. FAULKNER. 1974. Morphogenesis of nuclear polyhedrosis virus under conditions of prolonged passage *in vitro.* J. Ultrastruct. Res. **49:** 419–435.
9. IGNOFFO, C. M. & W. F. HINK. 1971. Propagation of arthropod pathogens in living systems. *In* Microbial Control of Insects and Mites. H. D. Burges & N. W. Hussey, Eds.: 541–580. Academic Press, Inc. New York, N.Y.
10. VAIL, P. V., D. L. JAY & W. F. HINK. 1973. Replication and infectivity of the nuclear polyhedrosis virus of the alfalfa looper, *Autographa californica,* pro-duced in cells grown in vitro. J. Invert. Pathol. **22:** 231–237.
11. FAULKNER, P. & J. F. HENDERSON. 1972. Serial passage of a nuclear polyhedrosis disease virus of the cabbage looper (*Trichoplusia ni*) in a continuous tissue culture cell line. Virology **50:** 920–924.
12. GOODWIN, R. H., J. L. VAUGHN, J. R. ADAMS & S. J. LOULOUDES. 1970. Replica-tion of a nuclear polyhedrosis virus in an established insect cell line. J. Invert. Pathol. **16:** 284–288.
13. VAUGHN, J. L. & P. FAULKNER. 1963. Susceptibility of an insect tissue culture to infection by virus preparations of the nuclear polyhedrosis of the silkworm (*Bombyx mori* L.). Virology **20:** 484–489.
14. IGNOFFO, C. M., M. SHAPIRO & W. F. HINK. 1971. Replication and serial passage of infectious *Heliothis* nucleopolyhedrosis virus in an established line of *Helio-this zea* cells. J. Invert. Pathol. **18:** 131–134.
15. RAMOSKA, W. A. & W. F. HINK. 1974. Electron microscope examination of two plaque variants from a nuclear polyhedrosis virus of the alfalfa looper, *Auto-grapha californica.* J. Invert. Pathol. **23:** 197–201.
16. SOHI, S. S. & J. C. CUNNINGHAM. 1972. Replication of a nuclear polyhedrosis virus in serially transferred insect hemocyte cultures. J. Invert. Pathol. **19:** 51–61.
17. WATANABE, H., Y. ARATAKE & T. KAYAMURA. 1975. Serial passage of a nuclear polyhedrosis virus of the silkworm, *Bombyx mori,* in larvae of rice stem borer, *Chilo suppressalis.* J. Invert. Pathol. **25:** 11–17.
18. HINK, W. F. 1970. Established insect cell line from the cabbage looper, *Tri-choplusia ni.* Nature (London) **226:** 466, 467.
19. HIRUMI, H. & K. MARAMOROSCH. 1964. Insect tissue culture: use of blastokinetic stage of leafhopper embryo. Science **144:** 1465–1467.
20. HIRUMI, H. & K. MARAMOROSCH. 1971. Cell culture of Hemiptera. *In* Inverte-brate Tissue Culture. C. Vago, Ed. Vol. 1: 307–339. Academic Press, Inc. New York, N.Y.
21. MCINTOSH, A. H., K. MARAMOROSCH & C. RECHTORIS. 1973. Adaptation of an insect cell line (*Agallia constricta*) in a mammalian cell culture medium. In Vitro **8:** 375–378.
22. MOLLENHAUER, H. H. 1964. Plastic embedding mixtures for use in electron microscopy. Stain Technol. **39:** 111–114.
23. SUMMERS, M. D. 1971. Electron microscopic observations on granulosis virus entry, uncoating and replication processes during infection of the midgut cells of *Trichoplusia ni.* J. Ultrastruct. Res. **35:** 606–625.
24. XEROS, N. 1956. The virogenic stroma in nuclear and cytoplasmic polyhedroses. Nature (London) **178:** 412, 413.

25. HUGHES, K. M. 1972. Fine structure and development of two polyhedrosis viruses. J. Invert. Pathol. **19:** 198–207.
26. VAIL, P. V., G. SUTTER, D. L. JAY & D. GOUGH. 1971. Reciprocal infectivity of nuclear polyhedrosis viruses of the cabbage looper and alfalfa looper. J. Invert. Pathol. **17:** 383–388.
27. SUMMERS, M. D. & H. J. ARNOTT. 1969. Ultrastructural studies on inclusion formation and virus occlusion in nuclear polyhedrosis and granulosis virus-infected cells of *Trichoplusia ni* (Hübner). J. Ultrastruct. Res. **28:** 462–480.
28. HARRAP, K. A. 1970. Cell infection by a nuclear polyhedrosis virus. Virology **42:** 311–318.
29. KAWANISHI, C. Y., M. D. SUMMERS, D. B. STOLTZ & H. J. ARNOTT. 1972. Entry of an insect virus *in vivo* by fusion of viral envelope and microvillus membrane. J. Invert. Pathol. **20:** 104–108.
30. TANADA, Y. & R. LEUTENEGGER. 1970. Multiplication of a granulosis virus in larval midgut cells of *Trichoplusia ni* and possible pathways of invasion into the hemocoel. J. Ultrastruct. Res. **30:** 589–600.
31. KISLEV, N., I. HARPAZ & A. ZELCER. 1969. Electron-microscopic studies on hemocytes of the Egyptian cottonworm, *Spodoptera littoralis* (Boisduval) infected with a nuclear-polyhedrosis virus, as compared to noninfected hemocytes. II. Virus-infected hemocytes. J. Invert. Pathol. **14:** 245–257.
32. HARRAP, K. A. & J. S. ROBERTSON. 1968. A possible infection pathway in the development of a nuclear polyhedrosis virus. J. Gen. Virol. **3:** 221–225.

EFFECTS OF THE NUCLEAR POLYHEDROSIS VIRUS (NPV) OF *AUTOGRAPHA CALIFORNICA* ON A VERTEBRATE VIPER CELL LINE *

Arthur H. McIntosh and Rebecca Shamy

Waksman Institute of Microbiology
Rutgers University
New Brunswick, New Jersey 08903

Nuclear polyhedrosis viruses (NPVs) are double-stranded DNA viruses that multiply in the nuclei of infected cells. NPVs have been isolated from insects that belong to the orders Lepidoptera, Diptera, Hymenoptera, and, occasionally, Neuroptera. More recently, a virus that morphologically resembles the NPVs has been isolated from shrimp.[1] Infection of the host with a NPV leads to the production of inclusion bodies (polyhedra), in which many virions become occluded. It is this facet of viral morphogenesis that is utilized for the production of viral insecticides, because the polyhedra afford a certain amount of protection to the occluded virions against adverse environmental conditions. After ingestion of the applied polyhedra, the virions are released in the gut of the insect as a result of alkali and enzymatic action on the inclusion body proteins. The free virions then penetrate the gut wall and infect neighboring cells. Death of the host occurs within 1 week, depending on the age of the larvae.

Because NPVs are highly virulent for their invertebrate hosts, it is necessary that potential biologic control agents, such as these viruses, also be tested for their ability to infect higher animal cells. In this regard, there have been relatively few studies [2-5] conducted with NPVs and other insect viruses in vertebrate cell cultures. In the present study, autoradiography and immunofluorescence techniques were employed to determine whether *Autographa californica* NPV produced biologic effects on the vertebrate VSW cell line.

MATERIALS AND METHODS

Cell Lines. A vertebrate cell line established from the spleen of a tumor-bearing viper,[6] and denoted VSW, was grown in Eagle's basal medium (BME) that contained 10% fetal bovine serum. The cells spontaneously produce C-type particles in culture. The insect cell line TN-368 [7] employed in these studies was grown in TC199-MK.[8] Both vertebrate and invertebrate cultures were propagated at 28° C.

Virus. A. californica NPV,[9] which had been passed more than 90 times in TN-368 cells, was used as the inoculum. The virus had a titer of 10^6 $TCID_{50}$/ml in TN-368 cells.

Labeling Studies. A. californica NPV was labeled by growing the virus in TN-368 cells in the presence of 50 μCi/ml of [³H]thymidine (sp act, 6.7 Ci/mM) for 72 hr. Virus was recovered from the supernatant fluids and from cells by freezing and thawing and was concentrated by centrifugation at 60,000g

* Supported in part by National Science Foundation Grant GB-41997.

for 1 hr. The virus pellet was washed three times with excess TC199-MK and was then passed through a 0.45-μm filter (Millipore Corporation). Fluids from the last wash were saved for the determination of possible residual radioactivity. Controls also included the labeling of uninfected TN-368 cells and extraction of cells as described.

VSW cells grown in Leighton tubes that carried coverslips were inoculated with 0.2 ml of labeled virus for various time periods. Coverslips were then prepared for autoradiography, as previously described.[10]

Immunofluorescence. VSW cells in Leighton tubes were challenged with 10^4 $TCID_{50}$/ml of *A. californica* NPV. Coverslips were removed at various time intervals and were prepared for direct staining by the fluorescent antibody technique, as previously reported.[10] The antiserum against *A. californica* NPV was prepared from infectious hemolymph taken from *Trichoplusia ni* (cabbage looper) by injection of New Zealand white rabbits with a footpad technique.[5]

RESULTS AND DISCUSSION

Seventy-two hours after inoculation of VSW cells with labeled *A. californica* NPV, the virus was detected by autoradiography. As shown in FIGURE 1 (*top*), the NPV was associated with the vertebrate cells. Most of the grains were seen over the nuclear area, although they were also observed over the cytoplasm of some cells. The average grain count above background over inoculated cells was 10 compared to an average of two grains over control cells (inoculated with pelleted extract from uninfected but labeled TN-368 cells). A second control that consisted of TN-368 cells inoculated with the last wash from the labeled virus pellet also resulted in few grains over TN-368 cells (FIGURE 1, *bottom*).

To test the possibility that incomplete viral replication might be occurring in VSW cells inoculated with *A. californica* NPV, immunofluorescent studies were performed on inoculated cultures. FIGURE 2 illustrates positive fluorescence of such cultures 72 hr postinoculation. Antigen was detectable as early as 6 hr postinoculation. Controls (uninoculated cultures) and inoculated cultures first treated with postantiserum before the application of the conjugated anti-serum were negative. Electron microscopy performed on 72-hr inoculated cultures revealed the presence of tubular structures (FIGURE 3) that might represent abnormal forms of capsid tubes.[11, 12]

The findings of this study indicate that *A. californica* NPV becomes associated with the vertebrate VSW cell line and that some viral proteins are synthesized by the inoculated cells. These observations rule out the possibility that lack of infection (complete viral replication) is due to failure of the virus to penetrate VSW cells. The techniques described for study of the interactions between insect viruses and vertebrate cells have also been successfully employed to demonstrate the complete replication of the *Chilo* iridescent virus (CIV) in VSW cells.[13]

ACKNOWLEDGMENTS

We thank Dr. Karl Maramorosch for reviewing this manuscript and Dr. Michio Kimura for the electron photomicrograph.

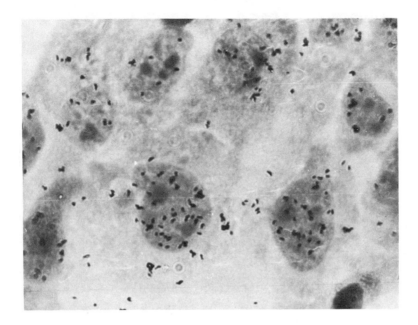

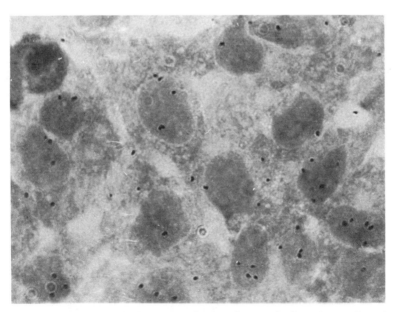

FIGURE 1. *Top:* Autoradiogram of VSW vertebrate cells inoculated with labeled *A. californica* NPV. Note the concentration of grains over the nuclei. ×1344. *Bottom:* Control VSW cells which show the presence of few grains. ×1344.

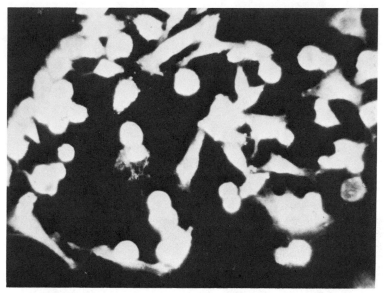

FIGURE 2. Immunofluorescence of VSW cells inoculated with *A. californica* NPV 72 hr postinoculation. ×430.

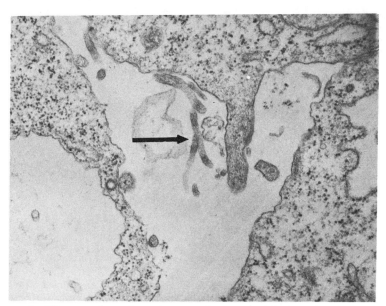

FIGURE 3. Electron photomicrograph of VSW cells inoculated with *A. californica* NPV. Arrow indicates the presence of tubular structures. ×35,772.

REFERENCES

1. COUCH, J. A. 1974. An enzootic nuclear polyhedrosis virus of pink shrimp: ultrastructure, prevalence, and enhancement. J. Invert. Pathol. **24**(3): 311–332.
2. HIMENO, M., F. SAKAI, K. ONODERA, H. NAKAI, T. FUKADA & Y. KAWADE. 1967. Formation of nuclear polyhedral bodies and nuclear polyhedrosis virus of silkworm in mammalian cells infected with viral DNA. Virology **33**: 507–512.
3. KURSTAK, E., S. BELLONCIK & C. BRAILOVSKY. 1969. Transformation de cellules L de souris par un virus d'invertébrés: le virus de la densonucleose (VDN). Compt. Rend. **269**: 1716–1719.
4. IGNOFFO, C. M. & R. R. RAFAJKO. 1972. *In vitro* attempts to infect primate cells with the nucleopolyhedrosis virus of *Heliothis*. J. Invert. Pathol. **20**: 321–325.
5. McINTOSH, A. H. & K. MARAMOROSCH. 1973. Retention of insect virus infectivity in mammalian cell cultures. J. N.Y. Entomol. Soc. **81**: 175–182.
6. ZEIGEL, R. F. & H. F. CLARK. 1969. Electron microscopic observations on a "C"-type virus in cell cultures derived from a tumor-bearing viper. J. Nat. Cancer Inst. **43**: 1097–1102.
7. HINK, W. F. 1970. Established insect cell line from the cabbage looper, *Trichoplusia ni*. Nature (London) **226**: 466, 467.
8. McINTOSH, A. H., K. MARAMOROSCH & C. RECHTORIS. 1973. Adaptation of an insect cell line (*Agallia constricta*) in a mammalian cell culture medium. In Vitro **8**: 375–378.
9. McINTOSH, A. H. & C. RECHTORIS. 1974. Insect cells: colony formation and cloning in agar medium. In Vitro **10**: 1–5.
10. McINTOSH, A. H. & R. S. CHANG. 1971. A comparative study of 4 strains of hartmannellid amoebae. J. Protozool. **18**: 632–636.
11. HUGHES, K. M. 1972. Fine structure and development of two polyhedrosis viruses. J. Invert. Pathol. **19**: 198–207.
12. WATANABE, H., Y. ARATAKE & T. KAYAMURA. 1975. Serial passage of a nuclear polyhedrosis virus of the silkworm, *Bombyx mori*, in larvae of rice stem borer, *Chilo suppressalis*. J. Invert. Pathol. **25**: 11–17.
13. McINTOSH, A. H. & M. KIMURA. 1974. Replication of the insect *Chilo* iridescent virus (CIV) in a poikilothermic vertebrate cell line. Intervirology **4**: 257–267.

PATHOBIOLOGY OF NONINSECT INVERTEBRATES: AN INTRODUCTION

B. J. Bogitsh

Department of Biology
Vanderbilt University
Nashville, Tennessee 37235

The general area of invertebrate pathobiology has been a sorely neglected field, especially the pathobiology of noninsect invertebrates. The diversity of the papers to be presented in this session provides a welcome format in an area in which so much remains to be explored. It is not surprising in such a gathering as this one that a great deal of attention should be directed to the Mollusca; nor is it surprising that the molluscan intermediate host for the human parasite *Schistosoma mansoni* should be a focal point of this particular session. Therefore, it is with considerable interest that we await Dr. Bang's paper, which considers antibody beginnings in an echinoderm and an ascidian, representatives of two groups that precede vertebrates in the phylogenetic tree. Dr. Cheng will then describe a study of phagocytes from three species of mollusks, one of which is *Biomphalaria glabrata.* The studies of Drs. Bang and Cheng, with their divergent emphases, complement each other most effectively. Because a portion of Dr. Bang's discussion will focus upon the activities of amoebocytes, the comparative approach used by Dr. Cheng will be of particular interest in determining whether a thread of uniformity can be discerned among the various invertebrate groups. Continuing with the topic of responses of amoebocytes and similar cells to the presence of parasites, Drs. Carter and Bogitsh will discuss the activities of amoebocytes of *B. glabrata,* including a consideration of these cells not only as encapsulators but also as sources of carbohydrate reserves for the tissues and invading parasites.

The question of susceptibility to parasitic infection in a snail intermediate host is of particular importance to researchers who maintain snail colonies in their laboratories over many snail generations. In this context, the next two papers will be of special interest. Dr. Richards will discuss the genetic implications of *B. glabrata* susceptibility to *S. mansoni.* He will also address himself to the role that hemolymph components play in determining tissue response of various genetic strains of *B. glabrata* to the penetrating parasite. In a related vein, Drs. Michelson and Richards will present a study of neoplasms and tumor-like growths in *B. glabrata* tissues that also demonstrates the influence that microorganisms, genetic patterns, and other factors exert on such growths.

The *in vitro* culturing of various stages of the life cycle of parasitic helminths has special relevance to many in this group. The flexibility that could be achieved with a controlled culture is a dream of all who are involved in the study of various aspects of the physiology, genetics, behavior, and so on, of the organisms being discussed. The report of Dr. Hansen is most appropriate, because it provides a significant addition to our understanding of the transplantation and maintenance of the secondary daughter sporocysts of *S. mansoni.*

Copper salts have been used consistently as a molluscicide for many years throughout the world. With the ever-growing awareness of the potential ecologic hazards from excessive use of chemicals for control of various organisms, the environmental implications in the report of Mr. Sullivan and Dr. Cheng on the pathologic effects of varying concentrations of cupric ions on the tissues of *B. glabrata* afford a timely contribution.

A SEARCH IN ASTERIAS AND ASCIDIA FOR THE BEGINNINGS OF VERTEBRATE IMMUNE RESPONSES

Frederik B. Bang

Department of Pathobiology
The Johns Hopkins University
School of Hygiene and Public Health
Baltimore, Maryland 21205
and Station Biologique
Roscoff 29211, France

INTRODUCTION

"In the study of biological processes, the accumulation of information is often accelerated by a narrow point of view. The fastest way to investigate the body's defenses against injury is to look individually at such isolated questions as how the blood clots or how complement works. We must constantly remind ourselves that such distinctions are man-made. In life, as in the legal cliche, the devices through which the body protects itself form a seamless web, unwrinkled by our artificialities." [1]

Amebocytes * are the circulating cells of the blood of a variety of invertebrates, cells that have a phagocytic function and that, like the macrophage of the vertebrate, are also found in great numbers adherent within the tissues of the animal.[2] Here, they form a mass of phagocytic tissues.[3, 4] This analogy, or perhaps homology, with the vertebrate arrangement of a reticuloendothelial system has been recognized by several investigators.[5, 6] If invertebrates are to be investigated for the evolutionary origin of vertebrate immune responses, at least three points of possible confusion must be avoided.

First, one should study those invertebrates that precede the vertebrates in the evolutionary tree.[7] Insect pathology is of importance in studies of analogous phenomena, but homologous reactions must be looked for in echinoderms and ascidians (protochordates). Unfortunately, studies of the immune responses of mollusks and insects have been more prolific.

Second, the evidence that protochordates are the predecessors of vertebrates, and that echinoderms are the predecessors of ascidians, rests on comparisons of the embryonic forms of both of these invertebrate phyla. The behavior of the amebocytes of the adult animals may therefore have as little relevance to

---

* There is great deal of confusion concerning the terminology of the cells studied in invertebrates, particularly those that are free in the circulating blood or coelomic fluid. We use the term amebocyte in the general sense used by Willmer in his book, *Cytology and Evolution,* as one of the three major types of cells, different from both the mechanocytes (fibroblasts) and epitheliocytes (surface-covering cells). Amebocytes thus are used here in the studies of echinoderms and ascidians to include a variety of granular cells that can phagocytose, that often contain granules, and that are usually not adherent to the tissues. Included in the term would be such specialized cells as the vanadiocytes of the Ascidia.

334

the behavior of amebocytes as the mode of locomotion of a starfish has to human locomotion. Despite the early contributions of Metchnikoff and his students, immune reactions of starfish embryos have not been established. Equally little work has been performed on the pathologic responses of the tadpole-like ascidian embryo, which, through a process of neoteny, may have led to the vertebrate.[8] Many, but not all, ascidian tadpoles lack a circulatory system, so that comparisons of responses must be carefully defined.

Finally, our knowledge of the action of special cells in vertebrate immune responses led to an artificial separation of the phenomena of clotting, inflammation, and immunity. In invertebrates, the same cell is often involved in all three types of responses, and it is not at all clear that they should be separated. The same amebocytes may be involved in the cell clumping that leads to thrombosis of a vessel or to closing of a wound, in an accumulation of granular cells that release various substances (inflammation), or in direct reactions to foreign agents (immune response).

In this paper, I will discuss some recent observations on two species: the beautiful and plentiful sea star, *Asterias rubens,* and the large classic ascidian or tunicate, *Ascidia mentula.* Specimens of both were freshly collected and studied at the Station Biologique in Roscoff. In the context of the central idea of this Conference on economically important invertebrates, I must admit that as far as I can discover, neither of these species is a vector of disease or is eaten by man; among the echinoderms, however, the giant sea cucumber is known as a delicacy, and several ascidians are eaten in Japan as special delicacies. However, animals as dominant in the sea as those that belong to these two phyla are almost by definition economically important, because they are there.

Echinoderms consist of a phylum of diverse animals, such as the holothurians (sea cucumbers), sea urchins, and various sea stars. The remarkable ability of some of the sea cucumbers to completely regenerate after evisceration, and of sea stars to regenerate their limbs, are well known and poorly understood and attest to the ability of these animals to overcome huge bacterial invasions.

We found about 15 years ago that Durham's[9] observations on clumping of cells seen in the tips of starfish papulae after India ink injection could be reproduced by injecting an extract of amebocytes into the coelomic cavity.[10] Direct observation of the papulae allowed one to see the initial loose aggregation of the cells, the later contracted clumping, and the final tight adherence of balls of amebocytes to the inside of the papula. This phenomenon occurred within 2–5 min, lasted only 15–20 min, and then disappeared, leaving the animal susceptible to repeated stimuli of the same kind, without any apparent change in sensitivity. Reinisch and I[11] then showed that injection of sea urchin coelomocytes, about half of which are deeply pigmented, into sea stars was followed by immediate cellular recognition. The pigmented foreign cells were rapidly attached to floccules of the host's circulating amebocytes, and these masses adhered to the inside of the papulae and to the walls of the coelom. The final extrusion of the foreign cells through the papulae could be directly observed. More recently, Reinisch[12] has shown that the clumping induced by the foreign urchin cells causes the release of a clumping factor into the coelomic cavity. Because amebocyte extract acts as a stimulus, it is natural to think of the factor as something released from the amebocytes. However, during the past summer, working with more transparent sea stars, such as *A. rubens* and *Marthasterias* at Roscoff, we found that when the coelomic cavity is injected with 0.1–0.2 cc of heavy bacterial cultures (gram-negative rods, including vibrios), which initiate clumping of the amebocytes in the coelomic cavity,[13] masses of clumped cells also appear in the water vascular system. This finding has significance because the water vascular system is completely separate from the coelomic cavity. This fact is readily demonstrable. When India ink, Evans blue, or even methylene blue are injected into the coelomic cavity, both the feet of the star and several terminal exploratory papulae connected to the water vascular system remain without ink, or dye, during the subsequent hours. Only by the next day are some of the blue-stained cells found in the water vascular system. Yet, the reaction within the feet is just as rapidly (1–2 min) initiated by the bacterial injection, has exactly the same appearance, wanes at about the same time, and occurs after each injection. In one series, six injections of bacteria within 18 hr each produced the same reaction. If the amount of the bacterial suspension injected is increased to 5 cc of a thick suspension, the animal still lives, but cells are slower in reappearing and do so long before the bacteria are removed.

Discarded limbs from traumatized animals that have undergone autotomy remain alive for 1–2 days. A limb of *A. rubens* continued to show clumping in the feet 1 day after coelomic injections, and one remarkable surviving limb of the giant *Marthasterias* still produced clumping 2 days after separation from the main body.

Did this transfer of the stimulus for abnormal clumping from one cavity to another occur by way of the nervous system? All kinds of neurohumoral mechanisms are known in invertebrates. For this reason, the radial nerve was sectioned with a pair of scissors, and the susceptibility of that limb to the production of cellular clumping in the feet was tested and compared with an opposite limb; each limb was injected with 0.1 cc of bacterial suspension, so that the effect would tend to be limited to the injected limb. After the nerve section itself, there was persistent clumping in that limb without injection. In a few days, however, the clumping decreased, and the limbs could be tested for susceptibility to the stimulus. In two animals, sensitivity to clumping remained present on Days 1, 3, 4, and 6 but seemed greatly decreased in the operated limb on Days 11 and 13 and by Day 20 was reapparent. These experiments must be repeated with more accurate determination of the degree of radial nerve damage and regeneration.

ANTISOMES

Ciliates are among the most numerous of the protozoa in the sea sand and may be found on all types of decaying organic material. They are known to cause disease and infection in crabs, lobsters, sea stars, and echinoids.[14] The reaction to them in experimentally infected hosts is readily followed, because they are large enough to be seen in detail, and their immobilization and lysis can be easily observed when the host reacts. Large numbers (~100,000) of *Anophrys* from the blood of naturally infected *Cancer* crabs were introduced into the coelomic cavity of a series of stars. Clearance times were determined by repeated sampling of the coelomic fluid at 30–60-min intervals thereafter. Four healthy *Asterias* were so treated over the next 7 weeks, and the clearance time was determined after each injection. They were scored as cleared when one large drop of the coelomic fluid no longer contained a live ciliate. As shown in FIGURE 1, the first injections were followed by infections that persisted 4–7 hr, but with daily repeated injection of all four, the clearance time was reduced to less than 30 min, and many *Anophrys* exhibited early immobilization and beginning lysis. A 3-day interval before new injections resulted in a return to the original slow clearance of 6 or more hours. With repeated injection, there was again a rapid clearance. Sporadic injections every 4 days were ineffective in maintaining rapid clearance, and finally at the end of the summer, after 7 weeks of injections, repeated daily injections again reduced clearance times to well below 30 min. This series of reactions can hardly be called antibody like, but might it be due to some sort of adaptive enzyme that responds to a variety of foreign agents so long as one of them is present?

Ascidia mentula is a pathobiologist's true dream animal. Grossly, it looks like a rather obscene irregular reddish or white clump of lard. It is covered

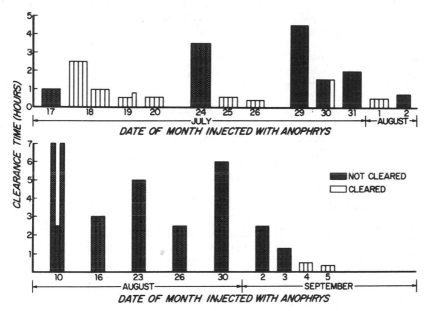

FIGURE 1. Effect of repeated injections of *Anophrys* into the coelomic cavity of sea star on clearance of *Anophrys*.

with debris and is adherent to the substrate. However, it is large (some are as big as a fist), is hardy, and is one of the most beautiful animals I have ever examined under the microscope. In addition, it seems to offer endless opportunities for experimentation. It seems incredible that since the time of Cantacuzène, only two or three scientists have examined ascidians for pathologic responses.[20]

The thick tunic, the origin of the rubric "tunicates," is a very active structure. If the whole animal is immersed for a few minutes in a sea water bath that contains neutral red, one soon finds the entire surface to be covered with a thin continuous layer of neutral red-stained flat cells. The acid tunicin, which comprises the inert structure, is as transparent as the best plastic, so that if one cuts off a slice of the surface, a beautiful complex network of vessels is seen to be embedded in a solid transparent structure. In most places, there are two vessels that run parallel to each other, and as they reach the surface or the tips of the siphons, they merge into capillary loops in which blood cells may be seen moving swiftly through the narrow vessels, from one large vessel to the other. Individual cells leave the main body of the animal and thus are pumped through the big vessels to the capillaries of the tunic and return again in one of the large parallel vessels. The tube-shaped heart reverses its direction of beat at intervals, and with this changeover, the course of the blood may be observed to reverse.[15]

All of these features may not be immediately apparent for several reasons. First, the vast majority of the amebocytes are vanadiocytes (vanadium carrying), which are transparent, while circulating in the vessels. One must therefore train the light on the tips of the siphons in the exact position that allows a direct view of the rapid flow through the capillaries. Second, the great number of orange cells (large granular amebocytes) that are found throughout the animal, which give it a red color, are usually found in the inner wall of the vessel, and the motion of these orange cells is therefore not apparent, except when individual ones break free and are swept away by the current. These large orange cells frequently adhere to the inside of the large parallel vessels, so that the immediate impression is of a line of orange cells in one transparent tube, instead of two vessels. The fact that there are two vessels is clear when, after trauma or intravascular injection of ink, the vessels collapse and can be seen separated from the transparent tunicin that supports them. Whether the vessel walls are cellular is not clear. Immersion of another species of tunicate, *Molgula,* into neutral red solution after the adherent sand grains have been scraped off does lead to intense staining of the vascular network, but this phenomenon did not occur in *Ascidia.*

Animals maintained in the laboratory frequently become infected with fungi that grow all over the surface of the tunic and apparently digest the tunic, leaving empty vascular walls hanging free in the sea water.

When a healthy animal's tunic is cut with a razor blade, there immediately appears a series of tiny volcanic outwellings from the cut vessels all over the transparent surface. The cells within these outwellings soon turn greenish, and a thin clot spreads over the area, which effectively stops further blood loss. Thrombi develop within the tips of the clotted vessels, and retraction of the clot occurs during succeeding hours.

INJECTION METHODS

Cantacuzène[16] studied bacterial infections of *A. mentula* by injecting cultures into the endostylar space but had to sacrifice the infected animals to determine the course of the disease. We have found that material may be injected and fluid sampled at intervals by a relatively simple technique with a small hypodermic syringe with a freely moving barrel and a 27-gauge needle. If a slight pressure is maintained on the barrel as the needle is slowly pushed through the tunic, movement of the barrel will immediately signal the entrance into the subtunic space, here depicted in black (FIGURE 2).[17] About 0.05 cc of fluid may be removed in a similar way by subjecting the syringe to slight suction as the needle moves through the tunic. In this way, we have followed the reaction of individual animals to different agents with as many as 10 samplings for periods up to 1 month. Presumably, they could be studied for much longer.

Injection of India ink, of filtrates of infectious material, and of a crab

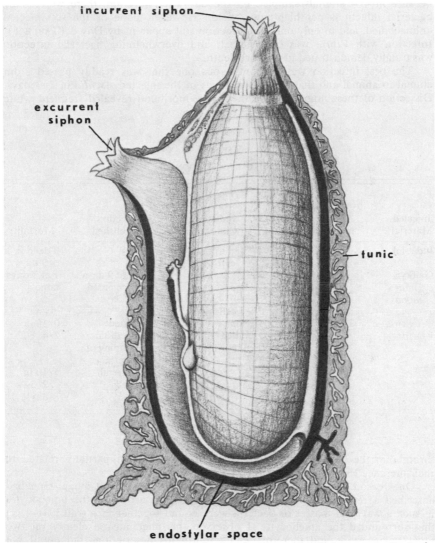

FIGURE 2. Diagram of relationship of subendostylar and pallial spaces to the tunic. Modified from Delage & Herouard.[17]

amebocyte virus produced no significant change in the numbers or kinds of cells found in the subtunic space, nor did they kill the tunicate. India ink was only partially phagocytosed over a period of 1 month. There was frequently a change in the number of both vanadiocytes and of pigmented cells after repeated samplings, presumably related to trauma either to the tunic itself or to the branchial cavity, which comprises the other side of the subtunic space. Active bacterial infections were established by the injection of *Pseudomonas,*† *Vibrio,*† and a natural bacterial infection. The first was clearly able to initiate infection, because in 4/4 animals sampled on the day after injection, there were many bacterial infections per high-power field. However, none of the six injected animals died, and in only one was infection still apparent by Day 3 (TABLE 1). Infection with *Vibrio* was often lethal, and overwhelming bacterial infection was usually demonstrated just before death.

The best infection was a spontaneous one that was readily passed from animal to animal and that killed two thirds of the injected *Ascidia* in 2–3 days. Dissection of these animals when they were moribund revealed frequent white

TABLE 1

EXPERIMENTAL INOCULATION OF *Ascidia*

Injected Material	Animals	Time under Study (Days)	Induced Changes	Infection Established	Mortality
India ink	6	33	slight phago-cytosis	—	3 dead in 9 days
Gaffkya	9	30		? in 1 at 9 days	1 at 7 days
Pseudo-monas	6	27	apparent in 4/4 added cell nos.	only 1 cleared in 3 days	none
CA virus	10	18–25	none	not tested	0/10
Vibrio	10	12	killed at intervals	extracellular clumping of bacteria	2/4
	10			2 days established	5/10 in 2–3 days

thrombi in the larger vessels, and death may have been partially related to their presence (TABLE 2).

One reason for study of infection in ascidians was that Cantacuzène had described a remarkable sticking of bacteria to the surface of the amebocytes in such a way that masses of bacteria were bound together in a transparent gel that surrounded the amebocyte. I observed this phenomenon clearly on two separate occasions and therefore can confirm his descriptions but could not determine its significance in immunity.

We return almost to where we started with infection and thrombosis. This has been summarized in TABLE 3.

† I am indebted to Mlle. Simone Chamroux of the Station Biologique for these cultures.

TABLE 2

ESTABLISHED NATURAL BACTERIAL INFECTION OF *Ascidia*

Injected Material		No. of Animals	Time under Study (Days)	Infection Established	Mortality
Natural infection		6	12	3/6 heavy infection by Day 2	4/6 in 3 days
Passage	1	6	10	heavy infection	4/6 in 3 days
	2	3	9	cells disintegrating	2/3 in 2 days
Filtrate		5	6	no changes	0/6
	3	5	7	heavy infection	4/5 in 3 days

TABLE 3

SUMMARY OF TYPES OF RESPONSES BY ECHINODERMS, ASCIDIANS, AND VERTEBRATES

	Clotting	Immune Response
Echinoderms	bacterial release of extracellular clotpromoting material, spread from one compartment to another	bacterial clearance recognition of foreignness increase of lysis of ciliates Hildeman: increased recognition
Ascidians	amebocyte clumping [18,19] extracellular gel sometimes	subtunic response of amebocytes loss of some bacteria recognition of foreign colonies [6]
Vertebrates	defense reactions that consist of complex interactions involving inflammation, antibody, complement activity, and blood clotting	specialized immunocytes, phagocytic cells, and cells for granular release

REFERENCES

1. RATNOFF, O. D. 1969. Some relationships among hemostasis, fibrinolytic phenomena, immunity, and the inflammatory response. *In* Advances in Immunology. F. Dixon & H. Kunkel, Eds. Vol. **10:** 145–227. Academic Press, Inc. New York, N.Y.
2. WILLMER, E. N. 1970. Cytology and Evolution. 2nd edit. Academic Press, Inc. New York, N.Y.
3. CUÉNOT, L. 1891. Etudes sur le sang et les glandes lymphatiques dans le serie animale. Arch. Zool. Exp. Gen. **19:** 13–90.
4. BAYNE, C. J. 1973. Molluscan internal defense mechanism: the fate of C^{14}-labelled bacteria in the land snail *Helix pomatia* (*L*). J. Comp. Physiol. **86:** 17–25.
5. WIGGLESWORTH, V. B. 1970. The pericardial cell of insects: analogue of the reticuloendothelial system. J. Reticuloendothel. Soc. **7:** 208–216.
6. FREEMAN, G. 1970. The reticuloendothelial system of tunicates. J. Reticuloendothel. Soc. **7:** 183–194.
7. KERKUT, G. A. 1958. The Invertebrate. 3rd edit. revised. Cambridge University Press. Cambridge, England.
8. BERRILL, N. J. 1955. The Origin of Vertebrates. The Clarendon Press. Oxford, England.
9. DURHAM, H. E. 1888. On the emigration of ameboid corpuscles in starfish. Proc. Roy. Soc. London Ser. B **43:** 327–330.
10. BANG, F. B. & A. LEMMA. 1962. Bacterial infection and reaction to injury in some echinoderms. J. Insect Pathol. **4:** 401–414.
11. REINISCH, C. L. & F. B. BANG. 1971. Cell recognition: reactions of the sea star (*Asterias vulgaris*) to the injection of amebocytes of the sea urchin (*Arbacia punctulata*). Cell. Immunol. **2:** 496–503.
12. REINISCH, C. L. 1974. Phylogenetic origin or xenogeneic recognition. Nature (London) **250:** 349, 350.
13. CUÉNOT, L. 1948. Anatomie, ethologie et systematiques des echinodermes. *In* Traite de Zoologie. P. P. Grasse, Ed. Vol. **11:** 1–272. Maison et Cie. Paris, France.
14. BANG, F. B. 1973. Immune reactions among marine and other invertebrates. Bioscience **23:** 584–589.
15. BRIEN, P. 1948. Embranchement des tuniciers, morphologie et reproduction. *In* Traite de Zoologie. P. P. Grasse, Ed. Vol. **11:** 553–894. Maison et Cie. Paris, France.
16. CANTACUZÈNE, J. 1919. Etude d'une infection experimentale chez *Ascidia mentula*. C.R. Soc. Biol. **82:** 1019–1022.
17. DELAGE, Y. & E. HEROUARD. 1898. Les Procordes. *In* Traite de Zoologie Conerete. Schleicher Freres, Ed. Vol. VIII. Maison et Cie. Paris, France.
18. ANDERSON, R. S. 1971. Cellular responses to foreign bodies in the tunicate *Molgula manhattenesis* (DeKay). Biol. Bull. **141:** 91–98.
19. GOODBODY, I. 1974. The physiology of Ascidians. *In* Advances in Marine Biology. : 1–149. Academic Press, Inc. New York, N.Y.
20. WRIGHT, R. K. & E. L. COOPER. 1975. Immunological maturation in the tunicate *Ciona intestinalis*. Amer. Zool. **15:** 21–27.

FUNCTIONAL MORPHOLOGY AND BIOCHEMISTRY OF MOLLUSCAN PHAGOCYTES *

Thomas C. Cheng

Institute for Pathobiology
Center for Health Sciences
Lehigh University
Bethlehem, Pennsylvania 18015

INTRODUCTION

In studies designed to elucidate the mechanisms that may effect or influence the susceptibility and/or nonsusceptibility of mollusks to invading microorganisms, it is essential that consideration be given toward understanding how the internal defense mechanisms of mollusks function when confronted with nonself substances. It should be apparent that such information is essential if rational approaches are to be taken for the development of potential biologic control agents for undesirable mollusks [1] or, on the other hand, if we are to understand and possibly prevent the microbial diseases that weaken or destroy economically important mollusks.

Since Tripp [2-4] demonstrated that microorganisms experimentally introduced into a pelecypod, the American oyster, *Crassostrea virginica,* and a pulmonate gastropod, *Biomphalaria glabrata,* are phagocytized and degraded intracellularly, it has become evident that phagocytosis by molluscan hemolymph cells is the major line of defense in at least these species of mollusks against invading microorganisms.

This information is extremely important for a third practical reason. Specifically, only when we have elucidated the biochemical bases for the recognition of self and nonself, the phagocytosis of nonself materials, and the intracellular degradation of foreign substances can we logically and rationally develop and design methods to depurate edible mollusks that have become biologically polluted. In other words, only when all of the parameters that influence or affect the phagocytosis and degradation of microorganisms that enter mollusks are understood can we devise methods to enhance this innate self-cleansing process and bring about the total and efficient clearing of real and potential pathogens from oysters, clams, and other edible shellfish.

When one considers the various types of reactions of hosts exposed to microorganisms, the development of antibody-mediated immunity naturally comes to mind. This, however, does not appear to be the case in mollusks. The evidence for this is as follows.

Cheng,[5] as a result of a quantitative electrophoretic analysis of the serum of the pulmonate *Helisoma duryi normale,* has concluded that hyperglobulinemia does not occur when this snail is challenged with different species of bacteria and has also concluded that immunoglobulins are not synthesized in mollusks. It is noted, however, that Feng and Canzonier [6] and Gress and Cheng [7] have demonstrated that in *C. virginica* parasitized by larvae of the trematode *Bu-*

* Supported by Grants FD-00416 and AI 12355-01A1 from the United States Public Health Service.

cephalus sp. or the haplosporidian *Minchinia nelsoni* and in *B. glabrata* parasitized by *Schistosoma mansoni* sporocysts, there is an increase in one and three serum protein fractions, respectively. These alterations may represent humoral responses to invasion by the parasites, but it is highly doubtful whether they represent the synthesis of immunoglobulins. In fact, the current consensus among comparative immunobiologists is that none of the invertebrates is capable of true antibody synthesis.

In view of the above considerations, we have concentrated our efforts toward an understanding of what has been commonly designated as "cellular immunity" in mollusks. If immunity is defined as "all those physiologic mechanisms which endow the animal with the capacity to recognize materials as foreign to itself and to neutralize, eliminate or metabolize them with or without injury to its own tissues,"[8] the cellular reactions in mollusks to nonself materials can rightfully be considered as immune reactions.

Because phagocytosis is the main line of defense against invading microorganisms, several individuals at this Institute have been conducting a series of studies aimed at answering the following questions: Are there different types of cells in mollusks? Is one type of cell more important from the standpoint of phagocytosis? Is phagocytic activity in mollusks influenced by ambient factors? How are microorganisms taken into phagocytes? What hydrolytic enzymes occur in phagocytes, and what are the optimal conditions for them to function? What is the fate of bacteria that become degraded intracellularly? Do the intracellular enzymes only function within cells? What are the energy requirements of molluscan phagocytes? These questions, of course, are not the only ones that can be asked, but they appear to be the fundamental questions that need to be answered prior to delving into other studies. Presented below are the answers that we have obtained.

CELL TYPES IN MOLLUSKS

In recent years, the literature pertaining to the types of cells that occur in mollusks has been reviewed by several authors.[9-13] From what is known, it may be concluded that there is no agreement as to the exact number of hemolymph cell types, except that some possess granular cytoplasm, whereas others possess agranular or only slightly granular cytoplasm. Because our studies on phagocytosis were dependent upon knowing how many types of cells occur in molluscan hemolymph and if one type is more important from the standpoint of phagocytosis, we have had to examine the cell types present in each species employed in our studies. Such studies have involved detailed studies of the morphology and *in vitro* behavior of the cells of the American oyster, *Crassostrea virginica*,[14] and of the quahaug clam, *Mercenaria mercenaria*.[20]

Cells of C. virginica

As a result of light microscope studies,[14] it has been concluded that the hemolymph cells of *C. virginica* fall into two size populations. Furthermore, the larger cells are of two classes: granulocytes and fibrocytes. The small cells, designated as hyalinocytes (FIGURE 1), are either agranular or only slightly granular.

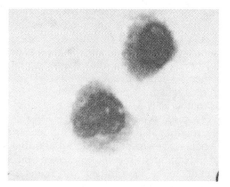

FIGURE 1. Hyalinocytes of *C. virginica* (methanol fixed, Giemsa stain). ×90. (From Foley & Cheng.[14] By permission of *Journal of Invertebrate Pathology*.)

The granulocytes are characterized by the presence of large numbers of cytoplasmic granules, which are primarily restricted to the endoplasm (FIGURE 2). Moreover, when permitted to spread against a solid substrate, these cells produce thin filopodia, each with a supporting riblike structure that originates in the endoplasm (FIGURE 2). Thus, the pseudopods produced by granulocytes are semirigid structures rather than temporary ectoplasmic protrusions.

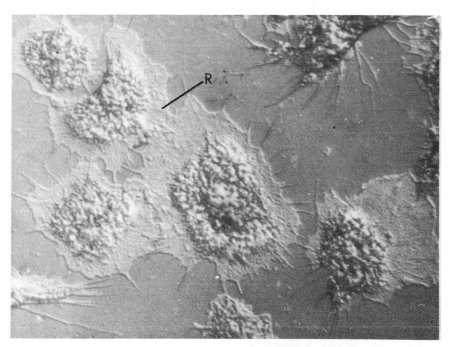

FIGURE 2. Spread granulocytes of *C. virginica*. Note rodlike structure (R) supporting filopodia (glutaraldehyde fixed, Giemsa stain; Nomarski reflected light interference optics). ×40. (From Foley & Cheng.[14] By permission of *Journal of Invertebrate Pathology*.)

It has been reported that when stained with Giemsa's stain, the cytoplasmic granules of *C. virginica* granulocytes may be totally basophilic, totally acidophilic, or a combination of both.[14, 16] Also, Foley and Cheng [14] have demonstrated that granulocytes with primarily acidophilic granules are smaller (19.3 ± 4.0 × 12.1 ± 3.3 μm) than those with primarily basophilic granules (32.7 ± 5.2 × 22.0 ± 4.3 μm). Because a mixture of both types of granules can exist in the same cell, it may be concluded that it is artificial to consider acidophilic and basophilic cells as being of two distinct types. Rather, they are believed to be of the same type; only the pHs of the milieu within their granules fluctuate. The functional reason for this fluctuation remains to be elucidated; however, the occurrence of both acid and alkaline phosphatases in these cells (see below) suggests different metabolic phases that are correlated with pH changes. It also remains to be determined why cells with primarily acidophilic granules are smaller than those with primarily basophilic ones. This difference may reflect a variation in metabolic state, as does the difference in the staining affinities of their granules.

In addition to acidophilic and basophilic granules, a third type, known as refractile granules, may also be present.

According to Foley and Cheng,[14] the fibrocytes of *C. virginica* are less refractile and are essentially devoid of cytoplasmic granules, although vacuoles may be present (FIGURE 3). Based on the morphology of the nuclei, fibrocytes can be recognized as being of the primary and secondary types; each of the former possesses a lobate nucleus, and each of the latter includes a spherical or ovoid nucleus.[14]

Since the earlier report from this Institute,[14] additional studies have caused us to question the validity of recognizing fibrocytes as a distinct category of hemolymph cells in *C. virginica*. The study that leads to this doubt is reported below.

Materials and Methods

Samples, each of which consisted of 0.5 ml of fresh hemolymph, were removed intracardially from *C. virginica* and placed on precleaned glass slides.

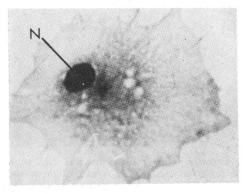

FIGURE 3. Secondary "fibrocyte" of *C. virginica* (glutaraldehyde fixed, May-Grünwald-Giemsa stain). N, nucleus. ×72. (From Foley & Cheng.[14] By permission of *Journal of Invertebrate Pathology*.)

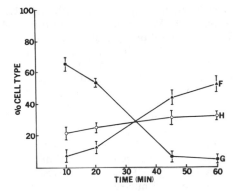

FIGURE 4. Graph that shows the percentage of each cell type in *C. virginica* hemolymph that had been permitted to sit for four predetermined time periods. F, "fibrocytes;" H, hyalinocytes; G, granulocytes.

Ten slides were then permitted to sit in humidified Petri dishes maintained at $21 \pm 1°$ C for each of the following time intervals: 10, 20, 45, and 60 min. The preparations were then fixed by flooding with 2.5% seawater-glutaraldehyde for 5 min. The slides were subsequently rinsed for 2 min in distilled water, dehydrated in 95% ethyl alcohol for 1 min, and air dried. These preparations were stained with May-Grünwald-Giemsa's stain, rinsed with deionized water, and air dried. All of the stained cells were subsequently subjected to differential counts.

Results and Discussion

The results of the differential counts of cells that had been permitted to sit for the four time intervals are presented in FIGURE 4. It is apparent from the results that there is a rapid decline in the number of granulocytes during the initial 45 min of *in vitro* maintenance. Furthermore, concurrent with the decline in the number of granulocytes, there is a corresponding increase in the number of fibrocytes. This information, coupled with the visualization of degranulation of living cells maintained *in vitro* [17] and with biochemical evidence for the release of enzymes from secondary phagosomes (the cytoplasmic granules of light microscopy),[18] has prompted us to conclude that the cells designated earlier as fibrocytes [14] are, in fact, degranulated granulocytes.

It is noted that most, if not all, of the degranulated granulocytes observed in the experiment described were secondary fibrocytes, as originally defined,[14] that is, those with spherical or ovoid nuclei. Consequently, strictly speaking, we believe that secondary fibrocytes are degranulated granulocytes. The function of the primary fibrocytes, if they do, indeed, comprise a distinct cell type, remains unresolved.

Fine Structure

The cytologic features of granulocytes and hyalinocytes of *C. virginica*, as revealed by transmission electron microscopy, have been described by Rifkin *et al.*[19] and by Feng *et al.*[16] Although Rifkin *et al.* recognize only one type of hyalinocyte, Feng *et al.* recognize three. According to the latter authors, there are three types of agranular cells or hyalinocytes. Type-I cells have been reported to be "lymphocyte-like," with a relatively large oval-shaped nucleus and scanty cytoplasm. In addition, there are dilated vesicles of smooth endoplasmic reticulum that are distributed throughout the cytoplasm. Also, the mitochondria present are restricted to certain regions of the cell, and a small amount of glycogen granules are dispersed randomly throughout the cytoplasm.

Type-II agranular cells have been characterized primarily by their considerably greater amount of cytoplasm, which contains clusters of glycogen granules, isolated vesicles of smooth endoplasmic reticulum, long cisternae of rough endoplasmic reticulum, and mitochondria.

According to Feng *et al.*,[16] type-III agranular cells are characterized by a dense spherical nucleus and numerous localized vesicles and tubules of smooth endoplasmic reticulum. Furthermore, the rough endoplasmic reticulum appears to be either contiguous with the nucleus or limited to certain areas of the cytoplasm.

The question that should be raised is whether the morphologic features employed by Feng *et al.*[16] are valid for recognizing three types of agranular hyalinocytes. This is especially true in the case of the so-called type-II agranular cells. As will be reviewed at a later point, it has been demonstrated that during the degradation of bacteria within granulocytes, the carbohydrate constituents of the microorganisms are, via an undetermined pathway, synthesized and stored as clusters of glycogen granules in the cytoplasm.[20] Critical inspection of the electron micrograph of a type-II agranular cell presented by Feng *et al.*[16] gives the impression that this is a granulocyte that has lost its granules, that is, secondary phagosomes,[20] and is at the stage of its metabolic cycle where glycogen granules are clumped in the cytoplasm.

Again, it is our opinion that what Feng *et al.*[16] have designated as types-I and -III agranular cells are of the same type but at different stages of metabolic activity. The reason for this interpretation is that it has been reported that hyalinocytes involved in the encapsulation of the metacestode of *Tylocephalum* differ in certain aspects, depending on their proximity to the parasite.[19] Those closer to the nonself material include larger numbers of vesicles and more conspicuous rough endoplasmic reticulum, whereas those more distant include fewer vesicles and less rough endoplasmic reticulum. These criteria, as stated, are the major ones employed by Feng *et al.*[16] to distinguish between types-I and -III agranular cells.

It is generally agreed that there is only one type of granulocyte in *C. virginica.*[12, 16, 19, 21] When examined with the transmission electron microscope, these cells include both smooth and rough endoplasmic reticulum, lysosomes, mitochondria, free and bound ribosomes, Golgi apparatuses, and occasionally lipid droplets (FIGURE 5). In addition, Feng *et al.*[16] have reported the occurrence of what they have interpreted to be digestive vacuoles and water vacuoles. It is noted that what they have designated as digestive vacuoles are what Cheng and Cali[20] have named primary phagosomes. These structures, from our experience, do not usually occur in resting granulocytes; however, when granulocytes are exposed to bacteria *in vivo* or *in vitro,* the microorganisms, upon being phagocytized, become incorporated in a vesicle lined by a unit membrane (FIGURE 6). Such a vesicle, now known as a primary phagosome, is most probably what Feng *et al.*[16] mean when they describe a "digestive vacuole."

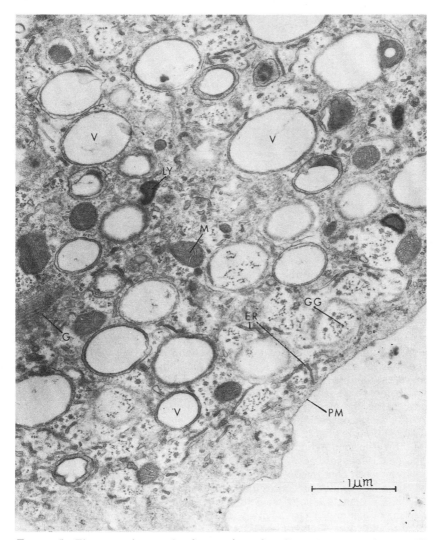

FIGURE 5. Electron micrograph of a portion of a *C. virginica* granulocyte. ER, endoplasmic reticulum; G, Golgi apparatus; GG, glycogen granules; LY, lysosome; M, mitochondrion; PM, plasma membrane; V, vesicle. (From Cheng *et al.*[21] By permission of University of South Carolina Press.)

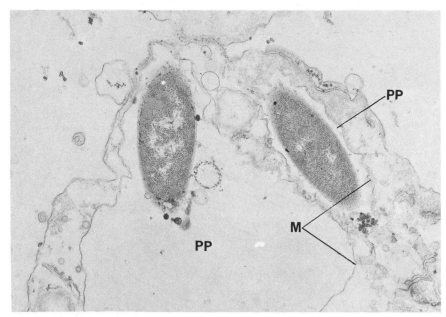

FIGURE 6. Electron micrograph that shows bacteria (*Bacillus megaterium*) within membrane (M)-lined primary phagosomes (PP) of a granulocyte of *C. virginica*.

It is uncertain what Feng *et al.*[16] mean by the term "water vacuole." After examination of one of their electron micrographs that depicts such a vacuole, we believe that their "water vacuole" is a section through a primary phagosome, which, as stated, is lined by a unit membrane. Although their micrograph does not reveal the inclusion of any phagocytized material, the size and structure of the "vacuole" are reminiscent of a profile of a primary phagosome cut at such an angle that the enclosed material is not visible.

The most conspicuous feature of *C. virginica* granulocytes is the presence of large numbers of vesicles, each of which has a complex wall. These structures are the cytoplasmic granules of light microscopy, which have been designated as secondary phagosomes.[20]

It has been confirmed[20, 21] that Feng *et al.*[16] are correct in stating that the cytoplasmic granules of *C. virginica* are walled vesicles (FIGURE 7). Feng *et al.*[16] have designated the outer delimiting membrane as the surface membrane, the zone of medium electron density mediad to it as the cortex, and the vesicular space as the core. Thus, these secondary phagosomes are readily distinguished from primary phagosomes not only by their smaller sizes but also by the more complex nature of their walls.

Feng *et al.*[16] have chosen to recognize three distinct types of secondary phagosomes based on such criteria as dimensional differences of profiles, thickness of the cortex, and the absence or presence of a lucid zone between the surface membrane and the cortex. Furthermore, they have attempted to correlate the three types of vesicles with the acidophilic, basophilic, and refractile granules seen with the light microscope. However, Cheng *et al.*[21] have pointed

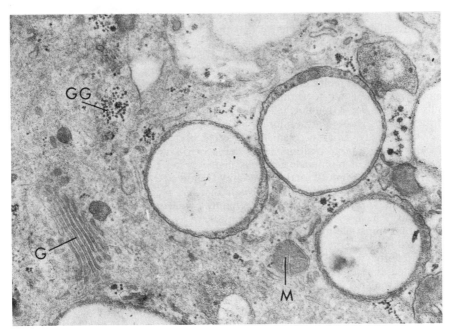

FIGURE 7. Electron micrograph that shows three secondary phagosomes, the cytoplasmic granules of light microscopy, in a granulocyte of *C. virginica*. Notice the complex wall of each secondary phagosome. G, golgi apparatus; GG, glycogen granules; M, mitochondrion. (From Cheng & Cali.[20] By permission of *Contemporary Topics in Immunobiology*.)

out that both their attempt to categorize the vesicles into three types and their suggestion that each fine structural type represents one of the differently stained types observable with the light microscope are questionable. Cheng *et al.*,[21] who based their opinion on a stereomorphologic model of a secondary phagosome, were able to explain why the three types of vesicles described by Feng *et al.*[16] are actually optical sections of the same structure. Subsequently, by employing scanning electron microscopy, it has been demonstrated[22] that the model presented earlier[21] was correct, in that each secondary phagosome is oval shaped.

It is also noted that Feng *et al.*[16] have described a type of granule (vesicle) that is electron dense. According to them, these dense granules lack a delimiting membrane and are comprised of fine dense particles distributed in a homogeneous matrix. The nature and function of these organelles remain to be elucidated. These structures have not been observed in our electron microscope studies of *C. virginica* granulocytes.

Cells of M. mercenaria

The morphology, hematologic parameters, and behavior of the hemolymph cells of the quahaug clam, *M. mercenaria*, have been reported by Foley and

Cheng.[15] As a result of light microscope studies of both stained and living cells, these investigators have concluded that there are three types of cells: granulocytes, fibrocytes, and hyalinocytes.

At the light microscope level, the granulocytes of *M. mercenaria* are similar to those of *C. virginica;* however, some differences are apparent. Specifically, the cytoplasmic granules of *M. mercenaria* granulocytes are not only denser in appearance but elongate vermiform granules are also present in most of the cells (FIGURE 8). Granulocytes are also capable of spreading on a solid substrate, such as glass. Furthermore, they also produce spikelike filopodia.

Occasionally, adjacent granulocytes have been observed to fuse, a process that results in a large multinucleated cell. Sparks and Pauley[23] have reported the occurrence of multinucleated cells in the oyster *Crassostrea gigas* that had been subjected to injury, and Cheng and Galloway[24] have found similar cells in the gastropod *Helisoma duryi normale* that had received allografts and xenografts. The function of such cells remains conjectural; however, Cheng and Galloway[24] have suggested that they may serve as an additional line of defense against incompatible materials, such as allografts and xenografts, which are not lysed and are too large to be phagocytized.

The fibrocytes of *M. mercenaria* (FIGURE 9) are similar to what had been designated as secondary fibrocytes of *C. virginica*[14] and which are now believed to be degranulated granulocytes.

The hyalinocytes of *M. mercenaria* (FIGURE 10) are also similar to those of *C. virginica,* in that they include less cytoplasm than granulocytes, are less

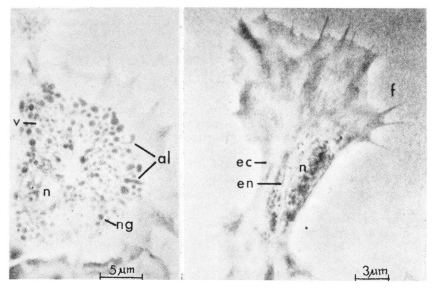

FIGURE 8 (*left*). Living, spread granulocyte of *M. mercenaria* enclosing spherical and elongate granules. al, Elongate granules; n, nucleus; ng, spherical granule; v, vacuole. (From Foley & Cheng.[15] By permission of *The Biological Bulletin.*)

FIGURE 9 (*right*). Living fibrocyte of *M. mercenaria*. ec, Ectoplasm; en, endoplasm; f, filopodia; n, nucleus. (From Foley & Cheng.[15] By permission of *The Biological Bulletin.*)

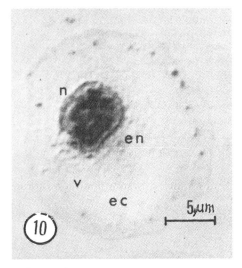

FIGURE 10. Hyalinocyte of *M. mercenaria* that shows ectoplasm with no filopodial projections (Nomarski interference; Giemsa stain). ec, Ectoplasm; en, endoplasm; n, nucleus; v, vacuole. (From Foley & Cheng.[15] By permission of *The Biological Bulletin*.)

motile, and are essentially without cytoplasmic granules. However, vacuoles, vermiform bodies (possibly mitochondria), and a few refractile bodies occur in the cytoplasm.

Fine Structure

The hemolymph cells of *M. mercenaria* have been studied with the transmission electron microscope by Cheng and Foley.[25] As a result, it has been suggested that fibrocytes are actually granulocytes that are at the end of the continuous process of uptake and degradation of nonself materials. This interpretation was based on the finding of large aggregates of glycogen granules in the cytoplasm of fibrocytes and of primary phagosomes enclosing digestive lamellae and partially digested cellular debris (FIGURE 11). It is known from earlier studies on the granulocytes of the American oyster, *C. virginica,* that phagocytized nonself organisms, such as certain bacteria, are eventually digested within secondary phagosomes and that the carbohydrate constituents of the bacteria, via an undetermined pathway, are synthesized into glycogen. Concurrent with the appearance of glycogen granules within secondary phagosomes, there is a breakdown and eventual disappearance of the phagosomal wall. Consequently, large aggregates of glycogen granules are deposited in the cytoplasm. Also, during the degradation process of bacteria in phagosomes, digestive lamellae and cellular debris are present.[20, 21] These features, as stated, have been observed in *M. mercenaria* fibrocytes; therefore, if the assumption that the basic processes involved in the degradation of nonself materials that occur in *C. virginica* granulocytes are also present in *M. mercenaria* granulocytes, the cells of this pelecypod originally defined as fibrocytes [15] may be considered as cells at the end of the physiologic cycle relative to phagocytosis and intracellular degradation.

There are some differences between the cytoplasmic granules of *M. mercenaria* and those of *C. virginica* at the fine structural level. Specifically, those of *C. virginica,* which are now known as secondary phagosomes, are electron-lucid vesicles, each of which possesses a complex wall (FIGURE 7). On the other hand, the granules of *M. mercenaria* are membrane delimited and include a homogeneously electron-dense material (FIGURE 12) and thus are reminiscent of the granules of mammalian granulocytes, especially those of eosinophils and basophils. Furthermore, some of these granules are elongate and vermiform. Until the function(s) of these organelles is known, it cannot be stated whether they are functionally identical to the secondary phagosomes of *C. virginica.* It is noted, however, that Feng *et al.*[16] have reported the occurrence of electron-

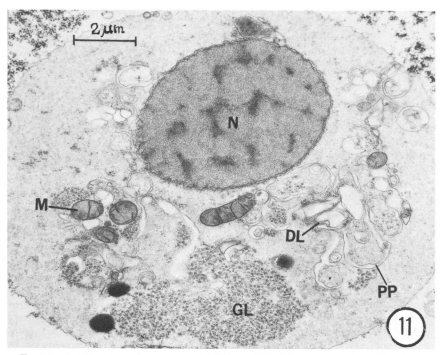

FIGURE 11. Electron micrograph of a "fibrocyte" of *M. mercenaria,* which is now interpreted to be a granulocyte near the terminal of the phagocytosis-degradation physiologic cycle. DL, digestive lamellae; GL, glycogen deposits; M, mitochondrion; N, nucleus; PP, primary phagosome enclosing partially digested material. (From Cheng & Foley.[25] By permission of *Journal of Invertebrate Pathology.*)

dense granules in *C. virginica* granulocytes, although we have yet to observe such organelles.

In addition to the dense granules, *M. mercenaria* granulocytes include mitochondria, membrane-bound electron-lucid vesicles, lysosome-like bodies, glycogen granules, Golgi apparatuses, smooth and rough endoplasmic reticulum, and lipid droplets in their cytoplasm. Some cells include a centrosome.

The hyalinocytes of *M. mercenaria* lack the large electron-dense cytoplasmic granules; however, a few smaller electron-opaque membrane-bound vesicles occur in the cytoplasm (FIGURE 13). In addition, electron-lucid vesicles of

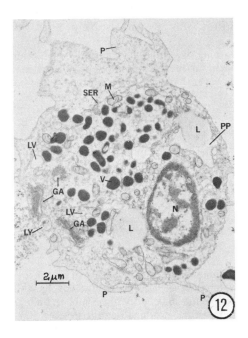

FIGURE 12. Electron micrograph of *M. mercenaria* granulocyte with prominent Golgi structure. GA, Golgi apparatus; L, lipid droplet; LV, lucid vesicle; LY, lysosome; N, nucleus; M, mitochondrion; P, pseudopodium; PP, primary phagosome; SER, smooth endoplasmic reticulum; V, electron-dense vesicle.

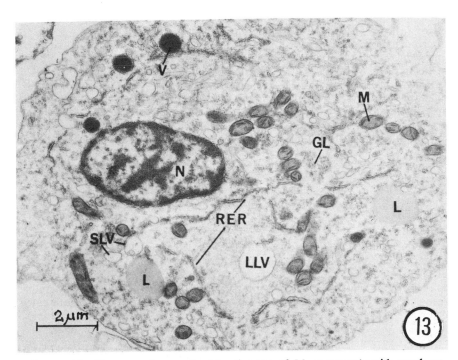

FIGURE 13. Electron micrograph of hyalinocyte of *M. mercenaria* with rough endoplasmic reticulum. GL, glycogen granules; L, lipid droplet, LLV, large lucid vesicle; M, mitochondrion; N, nucleus; RER, rough endoplasmic reticulum; SLV, small lucid vesicles; V, electron-dense vesicle. (From Cheng & Foley.[25] By permission of *Journal of Invertebrate Pathology*.)

varying sizes, lipid droplets, glycogen granules, and rough endoplasmic reticulum occur in the cytoplasm of hyalinocytes. Centrosomes and Golgi apparatuses, however, have not been observed in these cells.

Cells of B. glabrata

The hemolymph cells of *B. glabrata*, one of the intermediate hosts for the human pathogen *S. mansoni*, have been studied at this Institute by Harris and Cheng. With the permission of Dr. K. R. Harris, some of our findings are presented below.

Materials and Methods

Samples of the hemolymph of *B. glabrata* were obtained by inserting a capillary tube into the heart after the overlaying shell had been removed with watchmaker's forceps. Hemolymph, which filled the tube by capillary action, was gently expelled with a rubber bulb onto precleaned glass slides. The cells were either examined immediately after a cover glass was mounted or were permitted to stand on slides for 5–10 min in a humidified chamber. The chamber consisted of a closed glass Petri dish, the bottom of which was covered with damp filter paper, and of a support that allowed the slide to rest off the bottom of the dish.

Nomarski interference microscopy was employed on both fresh and fixed and stained cells. The latter were those allowed to spread for 5 or 10 min prior to being fixed with cold 10% formalin that contained 1% anhydrous $CaCl_2$ (formol-calcium) or with cold 2% glutaraldehyde in 0.1 M Sörensen's phosphate buffer at pH 7.2. Each slide was subsequently rinsed twice in the buffer and once in deionized water. Some slides were air dried, whereas others were postfixed in 95% ethanol before drying. The slides were routinely stained in a 1:40 dilution of stock Giemsa's stain in 0.1 M Sörensen's phosphate buffer (pH 6.5), followed by two rinses with the buffer and an additional rinse with deionized water. In addition, some cells were stained with Harris's hematoxylin, destained in acid alcohol, toned in basic alcohol, and rinsed with tap water.

Observations

When living *B. glabrata* hemolymph cells are first placed on glass slides, their shapes range from spherical to slightly oval. It is extremely difficult to distinguish between the types of cells in fresh preparations. However, as the cells are permitted to stand, in time, two distinct morphologic types can be recognized: granulocytes and hyalinocytes. Descriptions of both are presented below.

Granulocytes. Once contact is made by granulocytes with the slide, they begin producing pseudopodia. These structures first appear as lobopodia or filopodia; however, in time, they become more extensive, spreading in all directions. Fine filopodia eventually extend from the ectoplasmic edge, and like those of *C. virginica* and *M. mercenaria*, they each include a supporting rib (FIGURE 14).

Each granulocyte measures $23.5 \pm 5.4 \times 16.1 \pm 3.7$ μm and includes conspicuous cytoplasmic granules, which are primarily limited to the endoplasm. Its nucleus measures 7.2 ± 0.9 μm in diameter, and these cells comprise $86.6 \pm 12.8\%$ of the total cell population.

In stained preparations, the nucleus is deeply colored with either Giemsa's solution or hematoxylin, whereas the endoplasm is lightly basophilic, and the pseudopods remain clear. In general, formol-calcium fixation results in sharper nuclear definition, whereas glutaraldehyde fixative produces better staining of the cytoplasm and its inclusions.

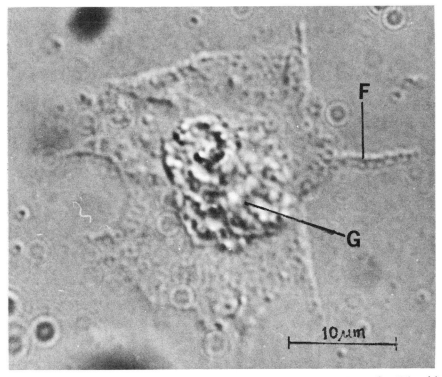

FIGURE 14. Spread, living *B. glabrata* granulocyte that shows filopodia (F) with supporting rodlike structures and cytoplasmic granules (G) limited to the endoplasm (Nomarski optics).

Hyalinocytes. Cells of this category are generally spherical or slightly oval in living preparations. They differ from granulocytes in that although they will adhere to glass slides, they do not flatten and spread against the substrate to any degree. The only pseudopodia formed are lobose and do not include riblike rays (FIGURE 15).

The cytoplasm of hyalinocytes is only sparsely granular and is uniformly basophilic when stained with Giemsa's solution or hematoxylin.

Each hyalinocyte measures $6.9 \pm 1.0 \times 6.6 \pm 0.8$ μm, and its nucleus is

2.6 ± 6.6 μm in diameter. Hyalinocytes comprise 13.4 ± 12.8% of the total cell population.

Conclusions Relative of Molluscan Hemolymph Cells

Although we have only studied the hemolymph cells of three species of mollusks to date, it would appear that although two or more types of cells can be recognized by employing light microscopy on stained and living cells, the essentially morphologic criteria employed in distinguishing between types of cells are deceiving. What have been designated as fibrocytes in *M. mercenaria*, by interpretation of electron micrographic data,[25] appear to be granulocytes that are at or near the terminus of a functional cycle relative to phagocytosis and degradation of nonself materials. Also, from the results presented about *in vitro* degranulation of *C. virginica* granulocytes, it would appear that this phenomenon occurs spontaneously *in vitro* and that the granulocytes assume the morphologic

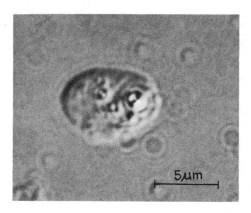

FIGURE 15. Living *B. glabrata* hyalinocyte.

characteristics of fibrocytes, at least of what have been described as secondary fibrocytes.[14] Based on the evidence available for the granulocyte-fibrocyte complex, it would appear that, functionally, there are only two types of cells in the molluscan species studied: granulocytes and hyalinocytes. This, as reported, is the situation in *B. glabrata*.

We reemphasize that the presence of eosinophilic or basophilic granules in granulocytes does not constitute a valid criterion for recognizing different types of cells. The basis for this opinion is the finding that in *C. virginica* granulocytes, mixtures of both types of granules, and of the so-called refractile granules, can occur;[14, 16] the staining affinities of the granules (vesicles of electron microscopy) probably therefore reflect the pH of the intravesicular milieu at different phases of a metabolic cycle.

Based on electron micrographic evidence, it appears that the secondary phagosomes of *C. virginica* granulocytes are different from the electron-dense membrane-bound vesicles of *M. mercenaria* granulocytes. Until the function of the latter is resolved, it remains unknown whether the structural differences reflect functional differences.

Finally, it is relevant to our subsequent discussion to reemphasize that lysosome-like bodies have been observed in granulocytes and hyalinocytes of *C. virginica* and *M. mercenaria*.

COMPARATIVE PHAGOCYTIC ACTIVITIES OF HEMOLYMPH CELLS

Having resolved the cell types present in a few species of mollusks, the question could then be raised as to which type was more important from the standpoint of phagocytosis. Studies designed to obtain an answer have been conducted by Foley and Cheng.[26] An abbreviated account of their results is presented below; however, it should be mentioned that earlier qualitative observations by Bang,[27] Galtsoff,[28] and Cheng and Rifkin [12] have led to the conclusion that the granulocytes of *C. virginica* are the phagocytic cells. On the other hand, Ruddell [29] has inferred that a type of agranular cell is the actively phagocytic cell.

By exposing whole hemolymph of *C. virginica* and *M. mercenaria* to 8.9×10^{6},[3] 1.5×10^{5},[3] and 1.81×10^5 cells/mm^3 of *Bacillus megaterium*, *Escherichia coli*, and *Staphylococcus aureus*, respectively, and by quantifying the association between the various types of hemolymph cells and the bacteria, Foley and Cheng [26] have demonstrated that a significantly greater percentage of granulocytes of both species of mollusks were associated with bacteria. Furthermore, it was found that both hyalinocytes and "fibrocytes" also were associated with bacteria, although to lesser extents.

In view of the fact that the types of hemolymph cells in both *C. virginica* and *M. mercenaria* are dimensionally different,[14, 15] the question was raised as to whether the greater association index between granulocytes and bacteria was due to the greater surface areas of this type of cell. To provide an answer, the following computations were made. The approximate mean surface areas for the different types of cells from both species of mollusks were computed from the dimensions of 10 randomly selected cells of each type. Then, the mean number of bacteria associated with each cell of each type was divided by the ratio of the mean area of each cell type to that of the granulocyte. The resultant values are presented in TABLE 1. From these data, it is evident that the number of bacteria per unit area is greatest in the case of granulocytes in both *C. virginica* and *M. mercenaria*.

As a result of the study referred to above, it is evident that molluscan granulocytes are the most important cells from the standpoint of phagocytosis.

Conclusions Relative to Phagocytosis

Two related points are being raised relative to the phagocytic capability of molluscan hemolymph cells. First, at the time Foley and Cheng [15] performed their study, electron microscopic evidence was not available to permit our present tentative conclusion that the fibrocytes and granulocytes of *M. mercenaria* are of the same type but at different phases of a metabolic cycle. Consequently, fibrocytes were considered a distinct type of cell. This, however, proved to be a fortuitous misinterpretation, because it is now known that even granulocytes near the end of the phagocytosis-degradation cycle still retain some capability to encounter bacteria.

TABLE 1

MEAN NUMBERS OF BACTERIA ASSOCIATED WITH HEMOLYMPH CELLS
OF *M. mercenaria* AND *C. virginica* CORRECTED FOR DIFFERENCES IN APPROXIMATE
MEAN SURFACE AREA OF EACH CELL TYPE * †

	C. virginica (bacteria per unit area)			
Experiment	Granulocytes	Primary Fibrocytes	Secondary Fibrocytes	Hyalinocytes
S. aureus (22° C)	6.44	2.45	1.15	5.69
E. coli (22° C)	22.54	3.12	5.69	19.16

	M. mercenaria (bacteria per unit area)		
Experiment	Granulocytes	Fibrocytes	Hyalinocytes
B. megaterium (4° C)	<1	<1	<1
B. megaterium (22° C)	10.90	1.25	2.68
B. megaterium (37° C)	15.06	2.05	3.54

* At the time these data were collected, evidence was not available to permit the interpretation that fibrocytes are degranulated granulocytes.
† After Foley & Cheng.[28]

Second, as in the case of *M. mercenaria*, there was no evidence available to Foley and Cheng[14] to suggest that the fibrocytes, especially the secondary fibrocytes, of *C. virginica* are degranulated granulocytes. The earlier information, nevertheless, is useful, because it has revealed that granulocytes of *C. virginica* in the "fibrocyte" state are still phagocytic.

INFLUENCE OF AMBIENT FACTORS ON MOLLUSCAN PHAGOCYTES

Stauber[30] had hypothesized that because mollusks are poikilotherms, it would not be surprising if ambient temperature influences the rate of phagocytosis in these invertebrates. This hypothesis has been subjected to testing *in vivo* by Feng,[31] who measured the rate of clearance of suspensions of a *Pseudomonas*-like bacterium, designated as A-3, at three ambient temperatures: 9, 16, and 22–27° C. In brief, he found that at 22–27° C, the number of bacteria, after an initial rise, fell precipitously after the 18th day. At 16 and 9° C, there was a steady decline after 8 days and an immediate steady decline, respectively. It is thus apparent that the ambient temperature influences the clearance rate, although the pattern is not clear.

Feng[32] has tested the same hypothesis by following the fate of bacteriophage 80 injected into *C. virginica* and maintained at 5, 15, and 23.5° C. She found that with an initial inoculum of $9.2 \times 10 \log_{10}$ plaque-forming units (PFU) of bacteriophage 80, it took 43 hr to reduce 1 $\log_{10}$ PFU/ml at 5° C, 3–4 hr to reduce 1 $\log_{10}$ PFU/ml at 15° C, and 1.5 hr to reduce 1 $\log_{10}$ PFU/ml at 23.5° C. These data clearly revealed that the *in vivo* clearing rate of the phage was faster at the higher temperatures. Similarly, Acton and Evans[33] have demonstrated that bacteriophage T2 is cleared *in vivo* by *C. virginica* more rapidly at 32–34° C than at 25° C. Also, Feng and Stauber [34] and Feng and Feng [35] have shown that the flagellate *Hexamita* sp. and chicken erythrocytes, respectively, are cleared faster when injected into *C. virginica* and subsequently maintained at higher ambient temperatures.

Because the reports reviewed above have all been based on *in vivo* studies, the question must be raised as to whether ambient temperatures affect phagocytosis directly. It had been postulated [31, 36] that the influence of temperature on particle clearance *in vivo* may be due to a direct effect of temperature on molluscan heart rate. Specifically, at lower temperatures, the oyster heart rate is depressed, and the decrease in agitation of the hemolymph is associated with a consequent diminution in the number of circulating cells.

Foley and Cheng [26] have performed an *in vitro* study to ascertain the direct effect of temperature on phagocytosis. In this experiment, they exposed samples of fresh whole hemolymph of *M. mercenaria* to *B. megaterium* maintained at 4, 22, and 37° C. After a 15-min exposure, the preparations were fixed, stained, and scored. The mean numbers of *B. megaterium* associated with the different types of cells of *M. mercenaria* at the three temperatures are listed in TABLE 2. It is evident from these data that no association between *M. mercenaria* cells and the bacteria occurred at 4° C, but associations were observed at 22 and 37° C, with the higher rate of association found at 37° C.

Because the cell types of *M. mercenaria* are dimensionally different,[15] corrections were made for differences in mean surface areas by the method presented earlier. These corrections resulted in the association indices listed in TABLE 1. It is evident that even after correction, the frequency of association is highest at 37° C and is essentially nonexistent at 4° C.

Conclusions Relative to Influence of Ambient Factors

At this time, the only ambient factor that has been studied relative to influence on phagocytosis in mollusks is temperature. From the available data, it is now known that phagocytic activity is enhanced by higher temperatures.

TABLE 2

MEAN NUMBERS OF *B. megaterium* ASSOCIATED WITH HEMOLYMPH CELLS OF *M. mercenaria in Vitro* AT THREE DIFFERENT TEMPERATURES ($n=50$) *

		Granulocytes	Fibrocytes	Hyalinocytes
4° C	$x=$	<1	<1	<1
	SD=	—	—	—
22° C	$x=$	10.90	1.92	2.56
	SD=	1.53	0.66	0.96
37° C	$x=$	15.06	2.82	3.08
	SD=	7.54	1.03	1.60
Control (22° C)	x	<1	<1	<1
	SD=	—	—	—

UPTAKE MECHANISMS

Although the ability of molluscan hemolymph cells to phagocytize nonself materials has been known since Haeckel's [37] discovery of the phenomenon, relatively few studies have been made to determine how the foreign material actually enters the cell. With the advent of the electron microscope, Bang [27] was the pioneer in this area of investigation. He reported that when hemolymph cells of *C. virginica* are placed on a glass slide, they spread and produce filamentous pseudopodia, the spaces between which are gradually filled by flowing ectoplasm. In other words, the ectoplasm forms a web between adjacent pseudopods. Bang reported that bacteria that eventually become phagocytized first become adhered to the pseudopodial surfaces and subsequently "glide" into the ectoplasm. Thus, it would appear that the filopodia of molluscan phagocytes play an important role in the phagocytosis of particulate nonself materials.

Bang's [27] report has stimulated us to reexamine the behavior of hemolymph cells of mollusks and the role of the filopodia in the uptake of particles. The

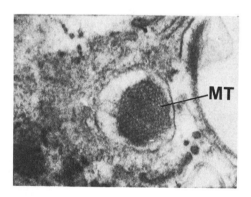

FIGURE 16. Electron micrograph that shows cross section of fascicle of microtubules (MT) that comprise the rodlike rib of a filopodium of *C. virginica* granulocyte. ×40,500.

behavior of cells of *C. virginica* has been described by Foley and Cheng,[14] who have also reported that the production of filopods is characteristic of granulocytes (FIGURE 2). Furthermore, they have demonstrated that each filopod is a semipermanent structure supported by a riblike structure oriented along its length but which extends internally into the endoplasm.

Although earlier efforts to demonstrate the nature of the "rib" by employing electron microscopy were unsuccessful, we have recently succeeded. The particular granulocytes of *C. virginica* studied were fixed at room temperature with 2% glutaraldehyde, sectioned, and positively stained with osmium tetroxide. The rib is now known to be comprised of a fascicle of microtubules that lie in the center of a cytoplasmic sheath (FIGURE 16). Approximately 290 microtubules comprise the bundle. The role of these organelles is assumed to be supportive, that is, to aid in maintaining the rigidity of the filopodia.

Although we have confirmed the phagocytic mechanism described by Bang,[27] additional electron microscopic studies have revealed that bacteria can be taken into *C. virginica* granulocytes via a second mechanism. This information is new and is therefore being reported in detail.

Materials and Methods

The specimens of *C. virginica* used in this study were obtained from a commercial source on the New Jersey coast. After being brought into the laboratory, they were maintained in recirculating seawater tanks with a salinity of 20 o/oo at 20–21° C.

Hemolymph samples were collected by use of sterile hypodermic needles and syringes from the heart, adductor muscle, and mantle cavity of each mollusk after one of the valves had been removed.

Five milliliters of whole hemolymph obtained by the method described were deposited in 15-ml centrifuge tubes, and to each tube was added approximately 10^6 fresh cells of *B. megaterium* harvested from nutrient agar slants. The bacteria had been washed in Seitz-filtered seawater prior to use.

The bacteria were permitted to intermingle with the hemolymph cells with gentle agitation for 30 min, after which time 1 ml of 5% glutaraldehyde in phosphate buffer (pH 7.2) was added to each tube. After 2 hr of fixation, the hemolymph-bacteria mixtures were centrifuged, and the supernatants were discarded. This step was followed by washing with the phosphate buffer, recentrifuging to remove the supernatant, and postfixing with 1% osmium tetroxide in phosphate buffer for 4 hr. After removal of the supernatant by centrifugation, each pellet was embedded in Luft's Epon®, sectioned with a diamond knife on a Sorvall MT-2B ultramicrotome, and the sections, placed on uncoated grids, were stained with a saturated solution of uranyl acetate and lead citrate and examined in a Philips 300 electron microscope operated at 60 kV.

Observations

Numerous oyster granulocytes were observed in the process of engulfing *B. megaterium;* however, the mechanism involved was different from that reported by Bang.[27] Specifically, rather than the bacteria gliding along the filopodia into the ectoplasm, an invagination of the granulocyte's surface occurs, and the bacterium is taken into the endocytotic vesicle (FIGURES 17 & 18). The vesicle that encloses each ingested bacterium is lined with a unit membrane. This vesicle is what has been designated as a primary phagosome.[20]

Each primary phagosome usually includes one bacterium (FIGURE 18), although adjacent phagosomes may fuse, a process that results in a large membrane-lined vesicle that contains several bacteria (FIGURE 19).

Conclusions Relative to Uptake Mechanisms

It is now apparent that there are two ways by which bacteria are engulfed by a granulocyte. The first is via the method originally described by Bang,[27] which involves filopodia, and the second is the one described herein, which involves endocytosis. The existence of the two mechanisms raises the question as to why certain bacteria are phagocytized by one method and others by the second one. A possible answer is provided in a later section.

In addition to phagocytosis of particulate nonself material, the pinocytosis of soluble molecules has been reported.[38] The mechanism(s) involved in pinocytosis by molluscan cells remains uninvestigated.

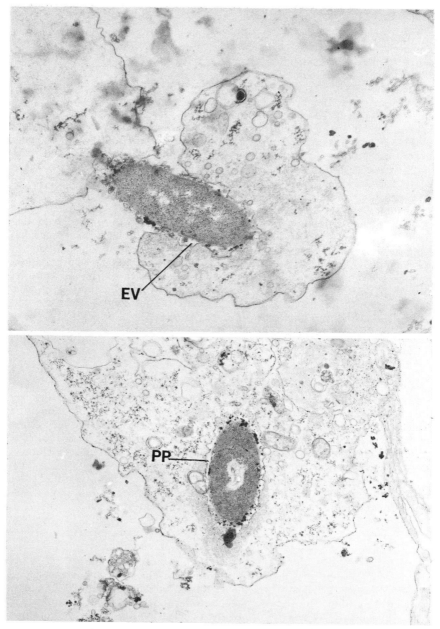

FIGURE 17 (*top*). Electron micrograph that shows uptake of *B. megaterium* by *C. virginica* granulocyte *in vitro* by endocytosis. ×20,000.

FIGURE 18 (*bottom*). Electron micrograph that shows *B. megaterium* in primary phagosome (PP) of *C. virginica* granulocyte. The bacterium had been taken in by endocytosis. ×20,000.

HYDROLYTIC ENZYMES IN MOLLUSCAN HEMOLYMPH

As is reviewed in the following section, there is evidence to suggest that bacteria and other nonself materials are degraded by molluscan phagocytes. Consequently, the logical question to ask is: What hydrolytic enzymes occur in these cells? A search of the literature has revealed several.[17]

We have been studying several lysosomal enzymes in the pelecypods C.

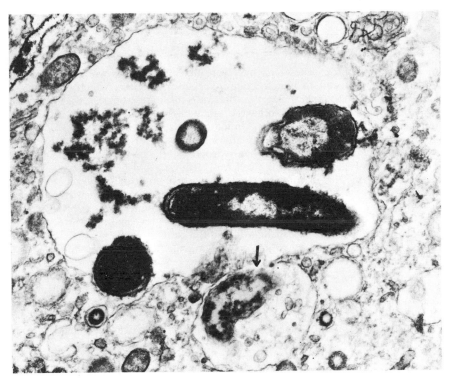

FIGURE 19. Electron micrograph that shows one large primary phagosome that contains several bacteria (B. megaterium) and another one in the process of fusing with it (arrow). ×24,700.

virginica, M. mercenaria, and the soft-shelled clam, Mya arenaria, and in the pulmonate gastropod B. glabrata. Summaries of our findings are presented at this point.

C. virginica

Cheng and Rodrick[39] have examined for the presence and have ascertained the specific activities of lysozyme, acid phosphatase, alkaline phosphatase, β-glucuronidase, amylase, and lipase in the whole hemolymph, serum, and 4000g

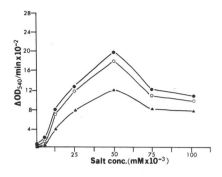

FIGURE 20. Effect of various salt concentrations on the lytic activity of *C. virginica* lysozyme with NaCl (●), KCl (○), and MgCl₂ (▲). Lysozyme activity is expressed as $\triangle OD_{540}$/ min $\times$ 10^{-2} at 25° C and pH 5.5 (From Rodrick & Cheng.[41] By permission of *Journal of Invertebrate Pathology.*)

pellet of *C. virginica.* These enzymes were detected in both whole hemolymph and in the serum and cellular fraction, except for amylase, which only occurs in the whole hemolymph and serum. Because the oyster possesses a crystalline style, the amylase is believed to have originated from this structure. All of the other enzymes studied are lysosomal in nature.[40]

Because lysozyme is known to attack the walls of a variety of bacteria, especially gram-positive species, by hydrolyzing the β-1,4-glucosidic linkages of the mucopolysaccharide in the cell wall, Rodrick and Cheng [41] have studied the kinetic properties of this enzyme in the hemolymph of *C. virginica.* Lysozyme activity, as stated, is associated with both the serum and cell fractions of the American oyster. Examination of the supernatants and pellet fractions produced by centrifugation at 4000 and 10,000*g* has revealed that the enzymatic activity is greater in the supernatant than in the pellet.

The lytic activity of *C. virginica* lysozyme on *Micrococcus lysodeikticus* is salt dependent (FIGURE 20), is relatively heat stable, and is very sensitive to changes in ionic concentration (FIGURE 21). Its optimal pH ranges from 5.0 to 5.5, depending on the buffer employed. When tested against several bacteria, the oyster lysozyme has been found to be active against not only *M. lysodeikticus* but also *Bacillus subtilis, B. megaterium, E. coli, Gaffkya tetragena, Salmonella pullorum,* and *Shigella sonnei,* although it is less active against the last four mentioned. It is not active against *S. aureus.*

It had been postulated that the lysozyme in the serum of *C. virginica* is released from cytoplasmic phagosomes of granulocytes during degranulation.[41] This hypothesis has since been proven.[18]

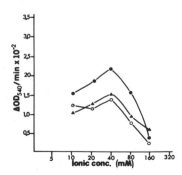

FIGURE 21. Effect of ionic concentration on the lytic activity of *C. virginica* lysozyme at pH 8.0. Lysozyme activity is expressed as $\triangle OD_{540}$/min $\times$ 10^{-2} at 25° C. ●, Ethylene diamine; ○, Mg²⁺ as MgCl₂; ▲, 1,4-diaminobutane. (From Rodrick & Cheng.[41] By permission of *Journal of Invertebrate Pathology.*)

M. mercenaria

Cheng and Rodrick [39] have shown that lysozyme, acid and alkaline phosphatases, β-glucuronidase, and lipase occur in both the serum and cells of *M. mercenaria.*

Mya arenaria

Rodrick [42] has reported the occurrence of β-glucuronidase, acid and alkaline phosphatases, lipase, and lysozyme in both the serum and cell fractions of *M. arenaria* hemolymph.

Because of the known antibacterial activity of lysozyme, some of its properties have been characterized, as has its activity against several species of bacteria.[43] It is now known that lysozyme activity occurs in both the serum and cell pellets produced by centrifugation at 4000 and 10,000g. Furthermore, the enzyme activity is greater in the two supernatants than in the corresponding pellets.

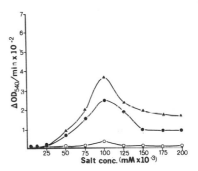

FIGURE 22. Effect of various salt concentrations on the lytic activity of *Mya arenaria* lysozyme with NaCl (▲), KCl (●), and MgCl₂ (○). The lysozyme activity is expressed as $\Delta OD_{540}/min \times 10^{-2}$ at 25° C and pH 5.5. (From Cheng & Rodrick.[43] By permission of *The Biological Bulletin.*)

As is the case with the lysozyme from *C. virginica* hemolymph,[41] hemolymph lysozyme from *M. arenaria* is salt dependent (FIGURE 22), relatively heat stabile, and very sensitive to alterations in ionic concentration. Moreover, the *M. arenaria* lysozyme is very sensitive to heavy metals. It has an optimal pH of 5.0 when 0.1 M glycylglycine, 0.1 M imidazole, or 0.1 M phosphate buffers are employed but has an optimal pH of 4.5 when 0.1 M Tris-HCl buffer is used.

The *M. arenaria* lysozyme is most active against *M. lysodeikicus* and *B. megaterium.* It is less active against *Proteus vulgaris, S. pullorum, S. sonnei, B. subtilis,* and *E. coli.* It is not active against *S. aureus.*

B. glabrata

Rodrick and Cheng [44] have reported activities of lysozyme, alkaline and acid phosphatases, β-glucuronidase, lipase, and amylase in whole hemolymph of *B. glabrata.* None of these enzymes, however, has yet been characterized.

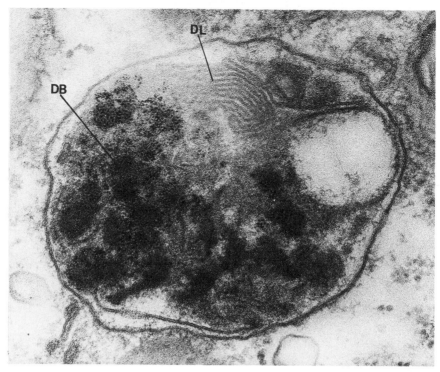

FIGURE 23. Electron micrograph that shows development of digestive lamellae and partially digested bacteria within primary phagosome of *C. virginica* granulocyte. DB, partially digested bacterium; DL, digestive lamellae. ×117,000.

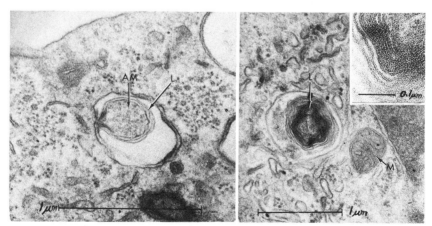

FIGURE 24 (*left*). Electron micrograph that shows transfer of partially digested bacteria from primary to secondary phagosome in *C. virginica* granulocyte. AM, amorphous material (partially digested bacteria); L, digestive lamellae.

FIGURE 25 (*right*). Electron micrograph that shows formation of digestive lamellae

Remarks Relative to Hydrolytic Enzymes of Mollusks

The occurrence of lysozyme in the hemolymph of *C. virginica* was originally discovered by McDade and Tripp;[45] however, for some unknown reason, they were unable to detect activity of this enzyme in the molluscan cells, as Rodrick and Cheng[41] have done. It is possible that during their handling of whole oyster hemolymph, they had caused the complete or near complete release of lysozyme and therefore were unable to detect it in cells.

In a subsequent study, McDade and Tripp,[46] in an attempt to ascertain the source of lysozyme in *C. virginica* hemolymph, assayed extracts of the mantle, adductor muscle, pulp, visceral mass, and gill of this pelecypod. As a result, they reported that the lysozyme activity was greatest in the mantle and postulated that this enzyme is secreted by mantle cells into the mucus. Although this hypothesis is reasonable, in view of the results of Rodrick and Cheng,[41] it is also possible that the lysozyme activity that they detected in the mantle and mucus was due to hemolymph cells incorporated therein, because both the mantle and mucus of oysters are well known to be rich in hemolymph cells.

FATE OF PHAGOCYTIZED BACTERIA

It has been known since the light microscope studies by Tripp[2,3] that bacteria experimentally introduced into the American oyster, *C. virginica,* are phagocytized and intracellular degradation occurs. However, it is noted that this apparently is not the fate of all phagocytized microorganisms. For example, Michelson[47] has reported that in certain planorbid snails, acid-fast bacteria can multiply within phagocytes and presumably can be carried by such cells to uninfected tissues. Also, Pan[48] has shown the apparent inability of *B. glabrata* phagocytes to cope with yeastlike organisms found in the nerve cells and amoebocytes of naturally infected snails. These reports suggest that at least certain microorganisms are resistant to the hydrolytic enzymes in the hemolymph of certain mollusks. The reason for this resistance remains to be examined. Nevertheless, the general rule is that phagocytized bacteria are degraded intracellularly. Consequently, Cheng and Cali[20] performed an electron microscopic study to ascertain the fate of phagocytized bacteria.

By employing *C. virginica* as the molluscan model, these investigators exposed specimens continuously to bacteria in a closed aquarium for 4–6 weeks, after which time hemolymph samples were collected, and the cells were examined with an electron microscope. As a result of this and similar studies, it became known that the bacteria are initially taken into large membrane-lined vesicles, which they have designated as primary phagosomes. The degradation of bacteria is initiated in primary phagosomes, where the development of digestive lamellae occurs (FIGURE 23). Then, the partially degraded bacteria are transferred to secondary phagosomes (FIGURE 24), where constituents of the bacteria are subjected to further degradation. This is indicated by the development of concentric digestive lamellae around the remnants of bacteria (FIGURE 25). Eventually, the digestive lamellae disappear, and the exogenous material, presumably the carbohydrate constituents that had been degraded to a hexose,

---

around degraded bacteria in secondary phagosome of *C. virginica* granulocyte. Inset is a higher-magnification view of digestive lamellae. L, digestive lamellae; M, mitochondrion.

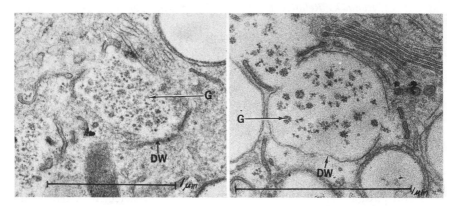

FIGURE 26 (*left*). Electron micrograph that shows glycogen deposits in the core of a secondary phagosome of *C. virginica* granulocyte. Notice disintegrating phagosomal wall. DW, disintegrating wall; G, glycogen.

FIGURE 27 (*right*). Electron micrograph that shows α rosettes of glycogen in the core of a secondary phagosome of *C. virginica* granulocyte. Notice disintegrating phagosomal wall. DW, disintegrating wall; G, glycogen.

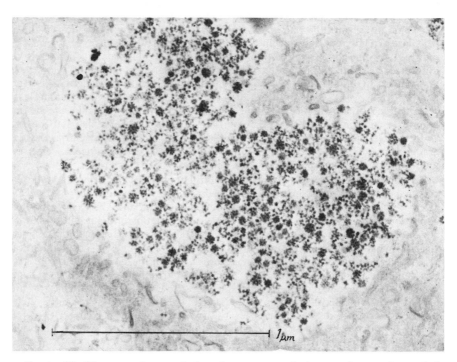

FIGURE 28. Electron micrograph that shows masses of glycogen in cytoplasm of *C. virginica* granulocyte. Notice absence of enveloping phagosomal wall.

probably glucose, is synthesized into glycogen granules (FIGURE 26). Concurrent with the appearance of glycogen granules, primarily as α rosettes, in the core or lumen of the secondary phagosome, the wall of the enclosing phagosome begins to break up (FIGURES 26 & 27), and it eventually disappears. This phenomenon results in the deposition of clumps of glycogen granules free in the cytoplasm (FIGURE 28). These glycogen granules eventually fuse into masses, and from several fortuitous electron micrographs, it is now known that the cytoplasmic glycogen is discharged into the serum enveloped by the plasmalemma of the granulocyte (FIGURE 29).

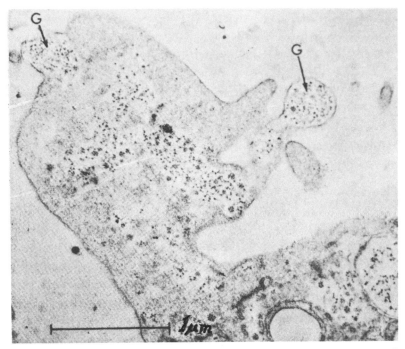

FIGURE 29. Electron micrograph that shows two packets of glycogen granules in consecutive stages of being expelled into the serum. G, glycogen. ×37,00. (From Cheng & Cali.[20] By permission of *Contemporary Topics in Immunobiology*.)

This study,[20] however, left several unanswered questions: What is the source of the enzymes responsible for the degradation of the bacteria within phagosomes? Are there any quantitative data to support the electron microscopic data that glycogen is synthesized in granulocytes? What is the fate of the noncarbohydrate constituents of the phagocytized bacteria? Answers, at least partial ones, to these questions are now available.

It may be recalled that lysosomes have been found in granulocytes of *C. virginica*. An electron micrograph is now available that shows a lysosome attached to a secondary phagosome in a *C. virginica* granulocyte (FIGURE 30). The depicted secondary phagosome includes glycogen granules, which thus indicates that it had been the site of digestion of bacterial remnants. Consequently, it is not surprising to find that the attached lysosome is electron lucid. Its contents most probably had been discharged into the secondary phagosome. Thus, there is now some evidence that lysosomes discharge into secondary phagosomes. The origin of enzymes that mediate digestion within primary phagosomes remains unknown.

There is now also quantitative evidence that the amount of glycogen in hemolymph increases after the phagocytosis of bacteria. Specifically, the glycogen content in 2 ml of whole hemolymph from each of 10 *C. virginica*

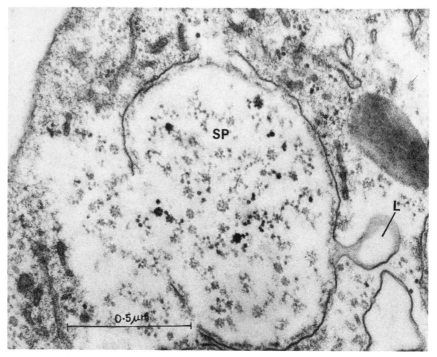

FIGURE 30. Electron micrograph that shows lysosome attached to a secondary phagosome in a *C. virginica* granulocyte. L, lysosome; SP, secondary phagosome.

that had not been exposed to *E. coli* was ascertained. They served as the control group. The experimental group consisted of 10 *C. virginica* evenly matched for size with those of the control group. The valve overlaying the cardiac region of each of them was filed through by a dental drill, and 3×10^3 *E. coli* suspended in 0.5 ml of sterile seawater were injected into the heart. These oysters were returned to seawater after their valves had been sealed with paraffin and left undisturbed for 2 hr. At the termination of this time period, 2 ml of whole hemolymph was removed from the adductor muscle sinus by the method of Feng *et al.*,[16] and the total glycogen content was determined. The method employed for the quantitative determination of glycogen was that of Montgomery.[49]

TABLE 3

AMOUNT OF GLYCOGEN IN 2 ML OF *C. virginica* HEMOLYMPH THAT HAD NOT (CONTROL) AND HAD (EXPERIMENTAL) BEEN EXPOSED TO 3×10^8 *E. coli in Vivo* FOR 2 HR. THE NUMBERS IN BRACKETS REPRESENT THE SAMPLE SIZES

Control	Experimental
65.74 ± 2.69 µg	79.46 ± 2.53 µg
(10)	(10)

Results

The results of the glycogen determinations are presented in TABLE 3. It is evident from these results that there is a significant rise in hemolymph glycogen in the experimental group.

Discussion

Because bacteria are not totally composed of carbohydrates, the question has been raised as to what happens to the noncarbohydrate constituents. There is now electron microscopic evidence that such materials are not passed from primary to secondary phagosomes; rather, they are expelled from primary phagosomes to the exterior of the phagocyte (FIGURE 31). In the accompanying

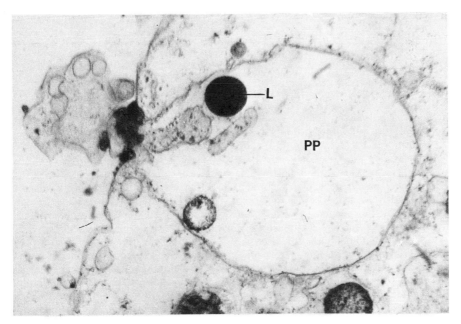

FIGURE 31. Electron micrograph that shows discharge of presumably nondigestible material from a primary phagosome in a *C. virginica* granulocyte into serum. L, lipoidal material; PP, primary phagosome. ×44,300.

micrograph, it appears that lipoidal and proteinaceous material are being discharged. Similarly, Cheng and Foley [25] have found large lipid droplets within a spent phagocyte of *M. mercenaria*.

RELEASE OF LYSOSOMAL ENZYMES FROM HEMOLYMPH CELLS

It has been stated in earlier sections that the lysosomal enzymes that have been studied in *C. virginica, M. mercenaria, M. arenaria,* and *B. glabrata* occur in both the serum and cell fractions of whole hemolymph. This fact led us to the question: What is the source of the serum enzymes? An answer to this question, at least for lysozyme, has been provided.[18] The working hypothesis was that intracellular enzymes were being released into the serum, and to test it, the quantitative shift of lysozyme from hemolymph cells to serum was followed. The hemolymph employed was *M. mercenaria,* and the studies were conducted *in vitro.* As indicated in FIGURE 32, there is a shift of lysozyme activity from cells (pellet) to serum (supernatant) when *B. megaterium* is

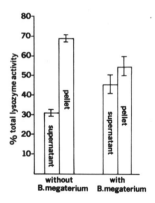

FIGURE 32. Distributions of lysozyme activity in the supernatant (serum) and pellet (cell) fractions of *M. mercenaria* hemolymph that had not or had been incubated with *B. megaterium*. (From Cheng *et al.*[18] By permission of *Journal of Invertebrate Pathology.*)

added to whole hemolymph. This finding indicates that the amount of lysozyme released from cells into serum is enhanced during phagocytosis of the bacteria. Furthermore, the release of lysozyme from cells occurs during phagocytosis and is not a delayed phenomenon.

To be assured that the release of lysozyme is not due to rupture of the cells, the activity of lactate dehydrogenase (LDH), a cytoplasmic enzyme, was also monitored during phagocytosis. No shift of LDH activity from cells to serum occurred during phagocytosis, a finding that thus indicates that the release of lysozyme is not due to cell rupture.

The morphologic basis for enzyme release is the phenomenon of degranulation. During this process, cytoplasmic granules, that is, secondary phagosomes, migrate to the cell surface and rupture. This phenomenon is appreciated as a "popping" of the granules, which is reminiscent of the bursting of a bubble. Degranulation has been observed in granulocytes of both *C. virginica* and *M. mercenaria.*[17] It is not restricted to cells actively phagocytizing but is enhanced during phagocytosis.

The function of lysozyme in molluscan serum remains essentially unexplored, although Tripp[2] has reported that oyster serum is bactericidal. It is possible that the presence of this enzyme in serum serves as an extracellular line of defense against invading microorganisms that are vulnerable. In view of this, it may now be possible that provide an explanation as to why certain bacteria are taken into molluscan phagocytes by the mechanism originally described by Bang,[27] that is, by first becoming attached to the semipermanent filopodia and subsequently being taken into the ectoplasm, whereas others, as reported in an earlier section, are taken in by endocytosis.

It is recalled that the bacterium being endocytosed (FIGURE 17) was *B. megaterium,* which is susceptible to the lysozyme of *C. virginica.* Thus, it is this author's contention that bacteria that are taken into host cells by endocytosis have already been altered by enzymatic action in the serum. In other words, living bacteria are phagocytized by the mechanism first described by Bang,[27] but bacteria whose surfaces have been altered by serum enzymes, such as lysozyme, are endocytosed.

Conclusions Relative to Phagocytosis and Degradation

In FIGURE 33 is depicted what we know about phagocytosis and subsequent intracellular events in mollusks, especially *C. virginica,* at this time.

It is particularly interesting to note that the carbohydrate constituents of phagocytized bacteria are eventually converted into glycogen, which, in turn, is discharged from cells into serum. Future studies will be directed at elucidating the metabolic role of glycogen in serum; however, it appears most likely that this carbohydrate, after hydrolysis to glucose, can be distributed via hemolymph to various tissues of the body and utilized for energy production. Thus, it would appear that phagocytosis in mollusks serves two functions: it eliminates certain nonself materials and provides a nutrient source. In view of the fact that amoeboid engulfment, the most primitive form of phagocytosis in the Animal Kingdom, serves primarily for the uptake of nutrients, it is concluded that during the phylogenetic development of animals, phagocytosis was originally a nutrient-acquiring process, and the second function, that associated with defense, was acquired only later.

It should be pointed out that earlier studies on the specific activities of lysozyme demonstrated that its activity was greater in the serum than in the cells of *C. virginica*[39] and *M. arenaria.*[42] This situation is in contradiction to that in *M. mercenaria.*[18] It is not known at this time whether the lysozyme levels are naturally greater in *C. virginica* and *M. arenaria* serum and naturally lower in *M. mercenaria* serum or whether there is a greater tendency for this enzyme to be released as a result of laboratory manipulations in the case of *C. virginica* and *M. arenaria* hemolymph.

ENERGY REQUIREMENT OF MOLLUSCAN PHAGOCYTOSIS

It is evident from the complex processes involved in phagocytosis and the ultimate deposition of the nonself materials described above that the overall process of phagocytosis in mollusks, especially in *C. virginica,* is a very expensive one from the standpoint of energy utilization. For example, the occurrence of digestion within primary and secondary phagosomes, the deposition of a seg-

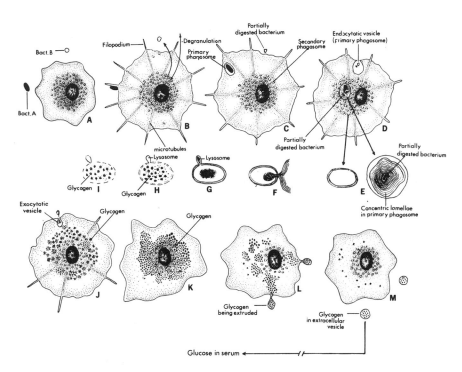

FIGURE 33. Sequence of events now known to occur during the phagocytosis and degradation of bacteria by granulocytes of *C. virginica*. A: Granulocyte in presence of bacteria A and B. B: Bacterium A becomes attached to filopod, while bacterium B is altered by enzyme(s) release from granulocyte during degranulation. C: Bacterium A is within primary phagosome of granulocyte. D: Bacterium B is taken into granulocyte by endocytosis, and digestion of bacterium A has commenced within primary phagosome. E: Formation of digestive lamellae around bacterium in primary phagosome; secondary phagosome in vicinity. F: Transfer of partially digested bacterium from primary to secondary phagosome. G: Lysosome attached and discharging enzymes into secondary phagosome. H: Glycogen synthesized from sugar constituents of degraded bacterium; phagosomal wall disintegrating. I: Phagosomal wall disintegrating. J: Discharge of nondegradable remnants of bacterium via exocytotic vesicle; accumulation of glycogen in cytoplasm of granulocyte. K: Massing of glycogen in cell and disappearance of filopodia. L: Glycogen in process of being discharged into serum in packets. M: Glycogen discharged.

ment of the surface membrane of the granulocyte around the glycogen that is ejected into the serum at the end of the phagocytosis-degradation cycle, and degranulation are all energy-requiring processes. Consequently, some studies have been conducted [50, 51] to ascertain what phagocytes utilize as energy sources during phagocytosis, whether their metabolic rates are altered during phagocytosis, and whether the myeloperoxidase-hydrogen peroxide halide bacteriocidal system, as found in mammalian phagocytes,[52, 53] occurs in molluscan phagocytes.

In brief, it has been ascertained [51] that there is no increase in oxygen consumption by hemolymph cells of *M. mercenaria* during phagocytosis. Furthermore, actively phagocytizing cells utilize glucose and glycogen for energy production, and lactate is produced. These phenomena indicate that glycolysis is the energy-providing pathway. This conclusion is strengthened by the fact that potassium cyanide does not inhibit phagocytosis.

It has also been demonstrated that the myeloperoxidase-hydrogen peroxide-halide antimicrobial system known to occur in mammalian phagocytes does not exist in hemolymph cells of *M. mercenaria*. The same pattern is known to occur in another invertebrate, the roach, *Blaberus craniifer*.

REFERENCES

1. CHENG, T. C. 1975. Use of microorganisms to control aquatic pests other than insects. Environ. Protect. Agency, Ecol. Res. Ser. (EPA-660/3-75-001) : 105–126. Corvallis, Oregon.
2. TRIPP, M. R. 1958. Studies on the defense mechanism of the oyster. J. Parasitol. **44**(2): 35, 36.
3. TRIPP, M. R. 1960. Mechanisms of removal of injected microorganisms from the American oyster, *Crassostrea virginica* (Gmelin). Biol. Bull. **119**: 210–223.
4. TRIPP, M. R. 1961. The fate of foreign materials experimentally introduced into the snail *Australorbis glabratus*. J. Parasitol. **47**: 745–751.
5. CHENG, T. C. 1969. An electrophoretic analysis of hemolymph proteins of *Helisoma duryi normale* experimentally challenged with bacteria. J. Invert. Pathol. **14**: 60–81.
6. FENG, S. Y. & W. J. CANZONIER. 1970. Humoral responses in the American oyster (*Crassostrea virginica*) infected with *Bucephalus sp.* and *Minchinia nelsoni*. *In* A Symposium on Diseases of Fishes and Shellfishes. S. F. Snieszko, Ed. : 497–510. American Fisheries Society. Washington, D.C.
7. GRESS, F. M. & T. C. CHENG. 1973. Alterations in total serum proteins and protein fractions in *Biomphalaria glabrata* parasitized by *Schistosoma mansoni*. J. Invert. Pathol. **22**: 382–390.
8. BELLANTI, J. A. 1971. Immunology. W. B. Saunders Company. Philadelphia, Pa.
9. ANDREW, W. 1965. Comparative Hematology. Grune & Stratton, Inc. New York, N.Y.
10. HILL, R. B. & J. H. WELSH. 1966. Heart, circulation, and blood cells. *In* Physiology of Mollusca. K. M. Wilbur & C. M. Yonge, Eds. Vol. **II**: 125–174. Academic Press, Inc. New York, N.Y.
11. CHENG, T. C., A. S. THAKUR & E. RIFKIN. 1969. Phagocytosis as an internal defense mechanism in the Mollusca: with an experimental study of the role of leucocytes in the removal of ink particles in *Littorina scabra* Linn. *In* Symposium on Mollusca. : 547–566. Marine Biology Association. Bangalore, India.
12. CHENG, T. C. & E. RIFKIN. 1970. Cellular reactions in marine molluscs in response to helminth parasitism. *In* A Symposium on Diseases of Fishes and Shellfishes. S. F. Snieszko, Ed. : 443–496. American Fisheries Society. Washington, D.C.

13. MALEK, E. A. & T. C. CHENG. 1974. Medical and Economic Malacology. Academic Press, Inc. New York, N.Y.

14. FOLEY, D. A. & T. C. CHENG. 1972. Interaction of molluscs and foreign substances: the morphology and behavior of hemolymph cells of the American oyster, *Crassostrea virginica,* in vitro. J. Invert. Pathol. **19:** 383–394.

15. FOLY, D. A. & T. C. CHENG. 1974. Morphology, hematologic parameters, and behavior of hemolymph cells of the quahaug clam: *Mercenaria mercenaria.* Biol. Bull. **146:** 343–356.

16. FENG, S. Y., J. S. FENG, C. N. BURKE & L. H. KHAIRALLAH. 1971. Light and electron microscopy of the leucocytes of *Crassostrea virginica* (Mollusca: Pelecypoda). Z. Zellforsch. **120:** 222–245.

17. FOLEY, D. A. 1974. Studies on hemolymph cells of marine pelecypods. Ph.D. Dissertation. Lehigh University. Bethlehem, Pa.

18. CHENG, T. C., G. E. RODRICK, D. A. FOLEY & S. A. KOEHLER. 1975. Release of lysozyme from hemolymph cells of *Mercenaria mercenaria* during phagocytosis. J. Invert. Pathol. **25:** 261–265.

19. RIFKIN, E., T. C. CHENG & H. R. HOHL. 1969. An electron microscope study of the constituents of encapsulating cysts in *Crassostrea virginica* formed in response to *Tylocephalum* metacestodes. J. Invert. Pathol. **14:** 211–226.

20. CHENG, T. C. & A. CALI. 1974. An electron microscope study of the fate of bacteria phagocytized by granulocytes of *Crassostrea virginica.* Contemp. Topics Immunobiol. **4:** 25–35.

21. CHENG, T. C., A. CALI & D. A. FOLEY. 1974. Cellular reactions in marine pelecypods as a factor influencing endosymbioses. *In* Symbiosis in the Sea. W. B. Vernberg, Ed. : 61–91. University of South Carolina Press. Columbia, S.C.

22. CHENG, T. C. & D. A. FOLEY. 1972. A scanning electron microscope study of the cytoplasmic granules of *Crassostrea virginica* granulocytes. J. Invert. Pathol. **20:** 372–374.

23. SPARKS, A. K. & G. B. PAULEY. 1964. Studies of the normal postmortem changes in the oyster, *Crassostrea gigas* (Thunberg). J. Insect. Pathol. **6:** 78–101.

24. CHENG, T. C. & P. C. GALLOWAY. 1970. Transplantation immunity in mollusks: the histoincompatibility of *Helisoma duryi normale* with allografts and xenografts. J. Invert. Pathol. **15:** 177–192.

25. CHENG, T. C. & D. A. FOLEY. 1975. Hemolymph cells of the bivalve mollusc *Mercenaria mercenaria:* an electron microscopical study. J. Invert. Pathol. In press.

26. FOLEY, D. A. & T. C. CHENG. 1975. A quantitative study of phagocytosis by hemolymph cells of the pelecypods *Crassostrea virginica* and *Mercenaria mercenaria.* J. Invert. Pathol. **25:** 189–197.

27. BANG, F. B. 1961. Reaction to injury in the oyster (*Crassostrea virginica*). Biol. Bull. **121:** 57–68.

28. GALTSOFF, P. S. 1964. The American oyster, *Crassostrea virginica* Gmelin. Fisheries Bull. U.S. Fish Wildlife Serv. **64:** 1–480.

29. RUDDELL, C. L. 1971. The fine structure of oyster agranular amebocytes from regenerating mantle wounds in the Pacific oyster, *Crassostrea gigas.* J. Invert. Pathol. **18:** 260–268.

30. STAUBER, L. A. 1950. The fate of India ink injected intracardially into the oyster, *Ostrea virginica* Gmelin. Biol. Bull. **98:** 227–241.

31. FENG, S. Y. 1966. Experimental bacterial infections in the oyster *Crassostrea virginica.* J. Invert. Pathol. **8:** 505–511.

32. FENG, J. S. 1966. The fate of a virus, *Staphylococcus aureus* phage 80, injected into the oyster, *Crassostrea virginica.* J. Invert. Pathol. **8:** 496–504.

33. ACTON, R. T. & E. E. EVANS. 1968. Bacteriophage clearance in the oyster (*Crassostrea virginica*). J. Bacteriol. **95:** 1260–1266.

34. FENG, S. Y. & L. A. STAUBER. 1968. Experimental hexamitiasis in the oyster *Crassostrea virginica.* J. Invert. Pathol. **10:** 94–110.
35. FENG, S. Y. & J. S. FENG. 1974. The effect of temperature on cellular reactions of *Crassostrea virginica* to the injection of avian erythrocytes. J. Invert. Pathol. **23:** 22–37.
36. FENG, S. Y. 1965. Heart rate and leucocyte circulation in *Crassostrea virginica* (Gmelin). Biol. Bull. **128:** 198–210.
37. HAECKEL, E. 1962. Die Radiolarien. George Reimer. Berlin, Federal Republic of Germany.
38. FENG, S. Y. 1965. Pinocytosis of proteins by oyster leucocytes. Biol. Bull. **128:** 95–105.
39. CHENG, T. C. & G. E. RODRICK. 1975. Lysosomal and other enzymes in the hemolymph of *Crassostrea virginica* and *Mercenaria mercenaria.* Comp. Biochem. Physiol. In press.
40. TAPPEL, A. L. 1969. Lysosomal enzymes and other components. *In* Lysosomes in Biology and Pathology. J. T. Dingle & H. B. Fells, Eds. Vol. **2:** 207–244. North-Holland Publishing Company. Amsterdam, The Netherlands.
41. RODRICK, G. E. & T. C. CHENG. 1974. Kinetic properties of lysozyme from the hemolymph of *Crassostrea virginica.* J. Invert. Pathol. **24:** 41–48.
42. RODRICK, G. E. 1975. Selected enzyme activities in *Mya arenaria* hemolymph. Proc. Oklahoma Acad. Sci. In press.
43. CHENG, T. C. & G. E. RODRICK. 1974. Identification and characterization of lysozyme from the hemolymph of the soft-shelled clam, *Mya arenaria.* Biol. Bull. **147:** 311–320.
44. RODRICK, G. E. & T. C. CHENG. 1974. Activities of selected hemolymph enzymes in *Biomphalaria glabrata* (Mollusca). J. Invert. Pathol. **24:** 374, 375.
45. McDADE, J. E. & M. R. TRIPP. 1967. Lysozyme in the hemolymph of the oyster, *Crassostrea virginica.* J. Invert. Pathol. **9:** 531–35.
46. McDADE, J. E. & M. R. TRIPP. 1967. Lysozyme in oyster mantle mucus. J. Invert. Pathol. **9:** 581, 582.
47. MICHELSON, E. H. 1961. An acid-fast pathogen of fresh water snails. Amer. J. Trop. Med. Hyg. **10:** 423–427.
48. PAN, C. T. 1956. Studies on the biological control of schistosome-bearing snails: a preliminary report on pathogenic microorganisms found in *Australorbis glabratus.* J. Parasitol. **42**(2): 33.
49. MONTGOMERY, R. 1957. Determination of glycogen. Arch. Biochem. Biophys. **67:** 378–386.
50. RODRICK, G. E. & T. C. CHENG. 1974. Biochemistry of molluscan phagocytosis. Amer. Zool. **14:** 1263.
51. CHENG, T. C. 1975. Aspects of substrate utilization and energy requirement during molluscan phagocytosis. Comp. Biochem. Physiol. In press.
52. KLEBANOFF, S. J. 1968. Myeloperoxidase-halide-hydrogen peroxide antimicrobial system. J. Bacteriol. **95:** 2131–2138.
53. KLEBANOFF, S. J. 1971. Intraleukocytic microbicidal defects. Annu. Rev. Med. **22:** 39–62.

HISTOLOGIC AND CYTOCHEMICAL OBSERVATIONS OF THE EFFECTS OF *SCHISTOSOMA MANSONI* ON *BIOMPHALARIA GLABRATA* *

O. S. Carter and B. J. Bogitsh

Department of Biology
Vanderbilt University
Nashville, Tennessee 37235

INTRODUCTION

Studies on pathologic effects of digenetic trematode larvae within their molluscan hosts have dealt primarily with altered histology of the lobular digestive gland cells and with mechanical effects of the presence of sporocysts or rediae within the digestive gland and/or ovotestis,[1-5] the usual sites of daughter sporocyst development and proliferation. Considerable early information on the histology of *Biomphalaria glabrata*, a snail host of *Schistosoma mansoni*, has come from the work of Faust and Hoffman,[1] who utilized both naturally and experimentally infected snails to study intramolluscan development of *S. mansoni*. Their study involved mother sporocysts 8 days and older and daughter sporocysts within the interlobular spaces of the digestive gland (i.e., hepatopancreas).

The role of snail connective tissue in the host-parasite association at the time that massive proliferation of the cercariae-containing daughter sporocysts occurs has received scant attention. Some reports that parasites within mollusks stimulate proliferation and mobilization of so-called amoebocytes may be found in the literature,[6, 7] but these reports are generally associated with destruction of snail tissue by the parasite after the cercariae begin emerging from their sporocysts. Postulations for the role of amoebocytes as a snail defense mechanism have been investigated with the use of introduced exogenous (i.e., foreign) materials, such as India ink, carmine, and polystyrene particles.[8, 9] In addition, amoebocytic infiltration has been studied in invasions of susceptible and non-susceptible snails by miracidia of *S. mansoni*[6, 10-13] and in progressive development of trematodes and associated amoebocytic infiltration.[7] Tissue reactions have also been reported in nematode invasions of snails.[14] Pan[7] has reported an apparent infiltration of amoebocytes into the tissues or spaces that surround developing daughter sporocysts, and his study suggests that a primary function of amoebocytes is of a "house-keeping" nature. He has shown large aggregates of amoebocytes in "old" infections that fill spaces formerly occupied by developing sporocysts. The sporocysts, apparently exhausted of their cercaria-producing ability and, presumably, filled with metabolic waste products and in a state of degeneration, elicit a tissue reaction that results in invasion by these phagocytic cells, which summarily engulf and destroy cellular debris and toxic wastes.

There is a dearth of information about the role of yet another molluscan connective tissue cell type that probably plays an essential role in the carbohydrate-oriented nutrition of the snail, namely, the vesicular connective tissue

* Supported by National Institutes of Health Grant AI 08058 (B.J.B).

380

cell (VCTC), which is variously referred to as glycogen storage cell, cell of Leydig, and so on. Some authors have given limited information on the VCTC's function as a glycogen storage cell.[9, 15, 16] This cell type, we feel, probably plays an essential role in maintaining and nourishing developing daughter sporocysts and cercariae of *S. mansoni* within *B. glabrata*.

Pathologic changes that occur in *B. glabrata* parasitized by *S. mansoni* have been variously compared to the effects of starvation in the snail,[17, 18] in light of findings that implicate the infection as a causative factor in glycogen depletion from the digestive gland.

It is the purpose of the work herein reported, then, to further clarify the pathologic effects of *S. mansoni* on *B. glabrata* with respect to glycogen localization in digestive gland lobular cells, fate of vascular connective tissue cells, amoebocyte activity, and developing parasite tissue, by means of fixation and cytochemical techniques designed to best reveal localization of carbohydrate storage products.

MATERIALS AND METHODS

The digestive glands were removed from Puerto Rican strains of *B. glabrata* maintained in this laboratory for several years. The snails were previously divided into three groups. Members of one group were infected with *S. mansoni,* members of the second group were starved for 1 week, and members of the third group were considered normal controls. Upon excision of the digestive glands, they were divided into three parts. Therefore, the observations reported herein are based on examinations of representative areas of these parts and represent a composite picture.

For light microscopy, the tissue was freeze dried, fixed in formalin vapor, and embedded in paraffin. Resultant sections were stained with the periodic acid-Schiff (PAS) technique for glycogen and mucosubstances or by the colloidal iron technique for acid mucopolysaccharides. For electron microscopy, the tissue was fixed in glutaraldehyde, postfixed in osmium tetroxide, and embedded in Epon®. Sections were subjected to the periodic acid-thiocarbohydrazide-silver proteinate procedure for glycogen localization. Some tissue was exposed to the diaminobenzidine-hydrogen peroxide procedure for peroxidase localization. In addition, one group of snails infected 5 weeks previously was exposed to a solution of [³H]glucose for 3 hr and processed as usual to detect utilization of glucose.

The usual controls were employed in all instances.

RESULTS

With radioactively labeled glucose used to determine the sites of incorporation of this monosaccharide, it is observed that large amounts of the label are associated with the daughter sporocyst wall and in young (i.e., nonmature) cercariae. Older mature cercariae and vesicular connective tissue cells do not incorporate appreciable amounts of glucose (FIGURE 1).

In freeze-dried, paraffin-embedded sections stained with the PAS technique, with diastase-treated controls, the lobular cells of uninfected digestive glands contain variable amounts of glycogen (i.e., diastase-labile, PAS-positive gran-

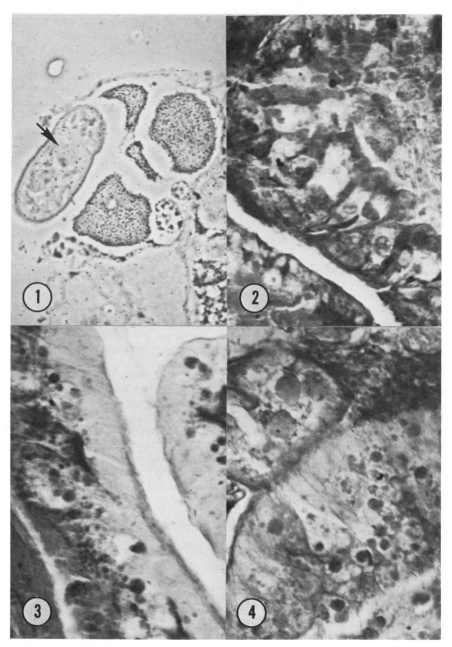

FIGURE 1. [³H]glucose-labeled intrasporocyst cercariae of *S. mansoni* within the digestive gland of *B. glabrata* (14-week infection). Note large amount of glucose incorporation by immature cercariae, in contrast to older, almost mature cercariae (arrow). × 680.

ular material) (FIGURE 2). Interspersed among the glycogen deposits are diastase-fast mucus materials and digestive vacuoles filled with similarly stained material and occasional PAS-positive, diastase-fast mucus cells (FIGURES 2 & 3). At the ultrastructural level, lobular cells from uninfected snails range from those that contain small amounts of glycogen to those richly laden with glycogen. Digestive glands removed from snails infected 5 and 14 weeks previously display little or no glycogen within their lobular cells (FIGURES 4 & 5). Starvation produces the same effects on the digestive gland as does infection with the parasites (FIGURE 6). However, 1-week starvation produces approximately the same effects as a 3-week parasitic infection under the conditions utilized herein.

Effects of parasite development and starvation were further compared by the colloidal iron technique for acid mucopolysaccharides. A reduction in the number and size of digestive vacuoles is observed when one compares normal digestive gland lobular cells (FIGURE 7) with those of 5-week (FIGURE 8) and 14-week (FIGURE 9) infected snails. Again, a similar pattern is observed, although not to the extent of the parasitized condition, in digestive gland lobular cells after a short period (1 week) of starvation (FIGURE 10).

Concomitant with alterations within the lobular cells described above, an increase in extent of intercellular spaces between digestive lobular cells occurs, both in parasitized and starved snails (FIGURE 11), whereas in normal tissue, the intercellular spaces are narrow and few in number. The width and extent of the intercellular spaces appear directly related to pathologic features either induced by starvation or parasitism by *S. mansoni* and probably represent fluid-filled spaces between the adjacent cell membranes. Close apposition of adjacent membranes is not wholly lost, however, because the expansions narrow periodically, forming closely apposed cell junctions (FIGURE 12).

Vesicular connective tissue cells from starved snails were compared to those of uninfected and parasitized snails. The VCTC ranges in size from 30 to 120 μm in the normal well-fed snail and is almost completely filled with glycogen (FIGURE 13). Each cell possesses a thin periphery of cytoplasm with occasional peroxidase-containing lysosomes (FIGURE 14) and a centrally to peripherally situated nucleus. The ratio of glycogen to cytoplasm is extreme. These cells are widely distributed within interlobular areas of normal *B. glabrata* digestive glands.

A major portion of the interlobular area, which is normally occupied by glycogen-packed VCTCs, is replaced by cercariae-filled daughter sporocysts in 5-week and 14-week infections (FIGURE 15). A few moderately well-developed VCTCs are still apparent, and, occasionally, a solitary cell of this type may be found between sporocyst tissue and digestive gland lobules. In general, the VCTCs that are present in infected digestive glands are smaller than normal and are displaced to the periphery of the interlobular areas. The initiation of diminution of the VCTCs, whether in infected or in starved snails, is char-

FIGURE 2. Uninfected digestive gland lobular cells of *B. glabrata* that shows glycogen distribution (PAS). ×680.

FIGURE 3. Uninfected digestive gland lobular cells of *B. glabrata* after diastase digestion. Reaction product is due to diastase-fast mucus droplets (PAS/diastase). ×680.

FIGURE 4. Digestive gland lobular cells in *B. glabrata* at 5 weeks postinfection with *S. mansoni*. Note marked absence of glycogen within cells (compare with previous Figure). ×680.

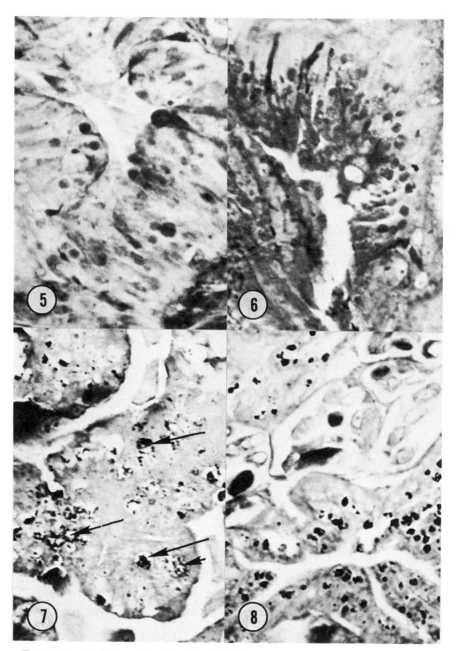

FIGURE 5. *B. glabrata* digestive gland lobular cells, 14 weeks postinfection with *S. mansoni*. Note depletion of glycogen, few digestive vacuoles, and fewer mucus depositions (PAS). ×680.

FIGURE 6. *B. glabrata* digestive gland lobular cells from snail starved for 1 week.

acterized by a stippled appearance of the contents (FIGURE 16). When viewed with the electron microscope, the stippled areas are found to be cytoplasmic "islands" surrounded by glycogen (FIGURES 17 and 18). Glycogen depositions in these cells are less dense than in normal VCTCs, the glycogen to cytoplasm ratio gradually is reduced, and at the same time the cell becomes smaller and more amoeboid in appearance (FIGURE 19). The circular to ovoid inner cytoplasmic areas ("islands") appear to be cross-sectional views of inward invaginations of the peripheral cytoplasm (FIGURE 18). Peroxidase-positive lysosomes appear in greater number in these cells (FIGURE 19).

Amoebocytes may be seen surrounding daughter sporocysts within the host digestive gland (FIGURE 20). These cells are characterized by extensive cytoplasmic extensions and contain well-developed Golgi apparatuses, from which arise primary lysosomal vesicles (FIGURES 21 & 22). They contain large lysosomes that show peroxidatic activity (FIGURE 23).

DISCUSSION

Both mollusks and digenetic trematodes are known to metabolize and store carbohydrates as their major energy source.[19, 20] The precise mechanism by which larval trematodes utilize host carbohydrates is not known. Previous histochemical studies have shown an apparent utilization of host carbohydrates by these parasites;[2, 4, 5, 21-23] there is also evidence that larval trematode infections deplete the glycogen content of their molluscan hosts, but there is some controversy over the degree to which this depletion occurs. Cheng[2, 24] has noted that sporocysts of *Glypthelmins pennsylvaniensis* in *Helisoma trivolvis* removed more glycogen from intact digestive gland cells than do rediae of *Echinoparyphium*. Reader[25] has confirmed the former observation about sporocysts but has also reported severe glycogen depletion in digestive gland cells of snails infected with rediae.

Glucose has been shown to be present in developing larval digeneans associated with either a consequent decrement in host tissue[21] or with no apparent diminution.[25] Cheng and Lee,[26] who used biochemical assays, also have shown depletion of hemolymph glucose in *B. glabrata* infected with *S. mansoni* beyond the third week postinfection and have postulated that the depletion is due to the developing parasite. Studies have shown that infected snails exposed to radioactive glucose solutions incorporated much of the isotope. Subsequent observations revealed an appreciable amount of labeled material incorporated into the tissue of emerged cercariae.[27, 28] Recent quantitative studies of glycogen fluctuation in normal versus parasitized *B. glabrata* have shown a decrease in glycogen in the digestive gland, and in other tissues of the snail, by Day 25 of infection.[17] Glycogen levels remained low for the duration of infection, after having approached zero. In another study, Christie *et al.*[18] investigated

---

Note reduction in glycogen and reduced size and number of digestive vacuoles. Compare with preceding Figure (PAS). ×680.

FIGURE 7. Uninfected *B. glabrata* digestive gland lobular cells stained for acid mucopolysaccharides, which shows large digestive vacuoles that contain positive materials (arrows) (colloidal iron, acid fuchsin). ×200.

FIGURE 8. *B. glabrata* digestive gland lobular cells, 5 weeks postinfection with *S. mansoni*. Note reduction in size and number of digestive vacuoles within cells. Much of the reaction product is due to mucus droplets (colloidal iron, acid fuchsin). ×200.

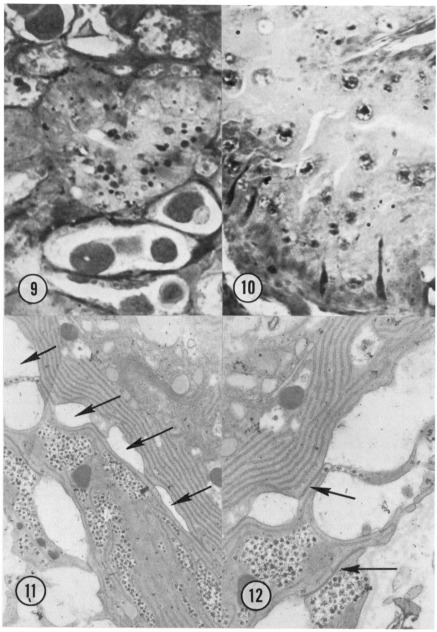

FIGURE 9. *B. glabrata* digestive gland lobular cells, 14 weeks postinfection with *S. mansoni*. Note the almost complete absence of digestive vacuoles in lobular cells and reduced mucus droplets. Compare with previous Figure (colloidal iron, acid fuchsin). ×200.

[14C]glucose uptake by parasitized and normal snail digestive gland-gonad complex and found evidence that nutrient utilization by developing schistosomes may be responsible for the glycogen depletion noted in infected *B. glabrata;* thus, the effect of parasitism is similar to starvation.

It is therefore generally agreed that reduction in carbohydrate levels reflects utilization of these carbohydrates by the parasite. Further, it is reasonable to assume, in light of these and other investigations, that the primary source of glucose utilized by the developing parasite is from glycogen stores in the digestive gland, with the VCTC being the main storage depot. The disappearance of glycogen in the lobular cells probably reflects both the depressed levels of glucose in the hemolymph and possible depressed feeding habits of the mollusk.

Digestive gland function is apparently impaired with progress of infection, as evinced by the reduction in size and number of lobular cell digestive vacuoles, results that thus simulate the effects of starvation, as shown by comparative examination of starved tissues. Infection of *B. glabrata* by *S. mansoni,* then, is twofold in its effects within the digestive gland; it in some manner impairs the digestive function of its snail host and at the same time utilizes the host's glucose for its own nutrient needs and thereby diminishes storage carbohydrates. The storage carbohydrates are converted to glucose and emptied into the circulation, where the parasite takes it up in apparently copious amounts.

The vesicular connective tissue cells are situated anatomically in a position that appears to maximize their proposed function as storage cells. Found immediately beneath the digestive gland lobular cells, digested nutrient in the form of simple carbohydrates could be readily taken up and converted into glycogen by these cells. From these cells, which are constantly bathed by hemolymph (because they are contained in the hemal sinuses of the digestive gland), rapid conversion of glycogen and dumping of the resultant glucose into circulation would be readily accomplished when hemolymph glucose levels fall, whether due to food deprivation or to the presence of developing sporocysts. Thus, triggering the host's own physiologic compensatory mechanisms for reduced levels of blood sugars, the host's enzyme systems act on its storage cells to provide more nutrient (in the form of sugars) than would normally be available. This supports Cheng's [3] hypothesis that the host's enzymes are probably involved in providing glycogenolytic products for maintenance of the parasite.

Amoebocytes that envelope daughter sporocysts have no apparent effects on the integrity of the sporocyst wall or on the developing cercariae within. The presence of active lysosomes within the amoebocytes indicates that utilization of some material was occurring; however, the microvillar surface of daughter sporocysts was intact and apparently in a healthy state. It is possible that the amoebocytes ingest toxic waste products that emanate from the parasite and thus extend the life of the parasitized snail. Obviously, this function of the amoebocyte would also be beneficial to the parasite, especially until the cercariae are mature and infective to the vertebrate.

FIGURE 10. *B. glabrata* digestive gland lobular cells from snail starved for 1 week. Note fewer, smaller digestive vacuoles; the effects, however, are not as dramatic as those observed in 5- or 14-week infections. Compare with previous two Figures. ×200.

FIGURE 11. Portion of digestive gland lobular cells 14 weeks postinfection with *S. mansoni,* which shows intercellular spaces (arrow). ×14,400.

FIGURE 12. Same as preceding Figure and shows persistence of junctions between cells (arrows). ×20,400.

FIGURE 13. Uninfected *B. glabrata* digestive gland that shows glycogen-packed vesicular connective tissue cells (arrows), situated in interlobular areas between acini of digestive gland lobules (d) (freeze dried, PAS). ×250.

FIGURE 14. Vesicular connective tissue cell that shows distribution of glycogen throughout and peroxidase-positive lysosomes (arrow). Note thin cytoplasmic periphery. ×4800.

FIGURE 15. *B. glabrata* digestive gland at 5 weeks postinfection with *S. mansoni* sporocysts that contain cercariae located in areas formerly occupied by vesicular connective tissue cells. Note lack of PAS-positive material in lobular cells (d). Compare with FIGURE 13 (PAS). ×200.

FIGURE 16. Phase-contrast micrograph of vesicular connective tissue cell (arrow) from 1-week starved *B. glabrata* digestive gland. Note stippled appearance of cell and laterally placed nucleus. ×680.

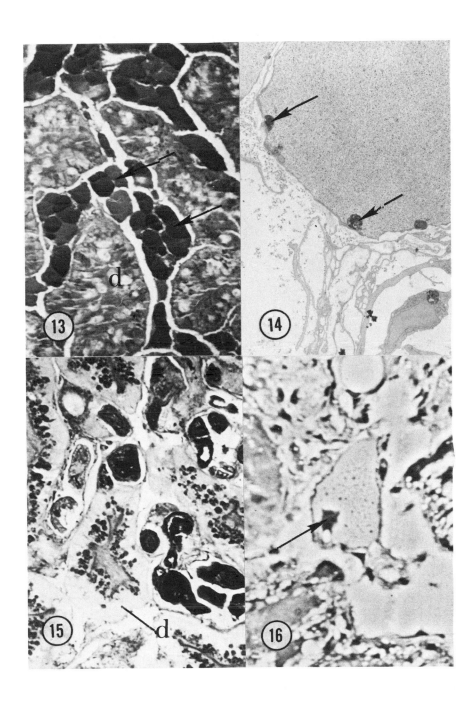

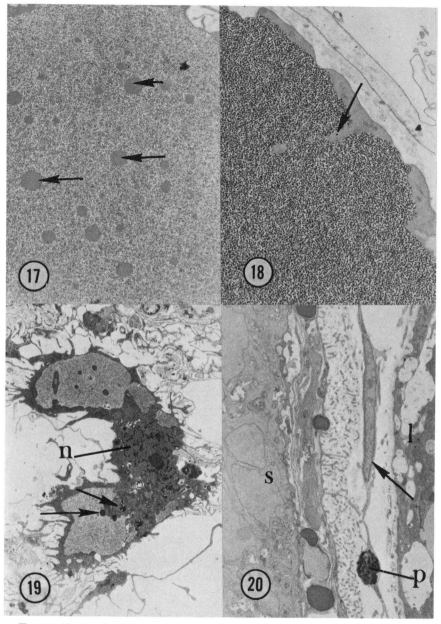

FIGURE 17. Portion of a vesicular connective tissue cell from infected *B. glabrata* that shows cytoplasmic islands (arrows point to several) (PA-TCH-SP). ×4800.

FIGURE 18. Same as previous Figure and shows the intrusion of cytoplasm (arrow) into glycogen mass (PA-TCH-SP). ×7200.

FIGURE 19. Vesicular connective tissue cell shows the spread of cytoplasm with a concomitant decrease in glycogen. Note nucleus (n) surrounded by several lysosomes that display peroxidase activity (arrows) (PA-TCH-SP, DAB-H$_2$O$_2$). ×2400.

FIGURE 20. Amoebocyte (arrow) "walling off" daughter sporocyst (s) from lobule (l). Note peroxidase-containing secondary lysosome (p) (DAB-H$_2$O$_2$). ×4800.

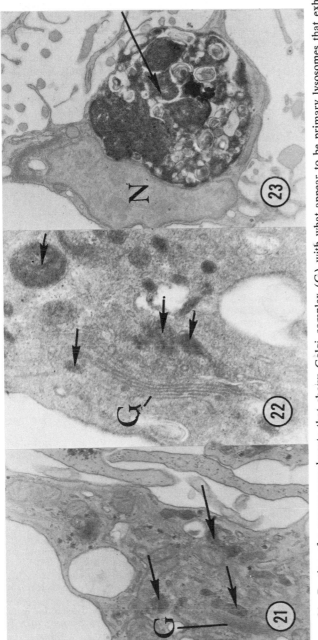

FIGURE 21. Portion of a young amoebocyte that shows Golgi complex (G) with what appear to be primary lysosomes that exhibit peroxidase activity (arrows) (DAB-H₂O₂). ×22,800.

FIGURE 22. Portion of another young amoebocyte as above but at higher magnification. Note Golgi complex (G) and primary lysosomes (arrows) (DAB-H₂O₂). ×44,400.

FIGURE 23. Portion of an older amoebocyte with large secondary lysosome with peroxidase activity (arrow). Note nucleus (N) pushed to one side (DAB-H₂O₂). ×14,400.

Another possibility exists with regard to the surrounding amoebocytes. The presence of cell types intermediate between VCTCs and amoebocytes suggests that the two cell types may be interconvertible or that they might be derived from the same stem cells. It is possible that the cells that overlie and closely abut the secondary sporocysts are remnants of VCTCs, especially if these cells are not capable of movement. We have never observed a cell membrane of a VCTC that appeared to be damaged; therefore, they probably would be squeezed to the periphery as the secondary sporocysts rapidly proliferate into the area in which they are found. A third possibility exists that would be beneficial to the parasite, namely, that these depleted cells might serve as a buffering zone around the parasite, an action that would thus "mask" it from recognition by the snail host until it produces its progeny cercariae, thus further ensuring its survival and dissemination. It has been pointed out that massive amoebocytic proliferation and infiltration into sporocyst tissues does not occur until late in infection, after cercariae begin emerging from the sporocyst and damaging host tissue as they migrate out of the host snail.

REFERENCES

1. FAUST, E. C. & W. A. HOFFMAN. 1934. Studies on schistosomiasis mansoni in Puerto Rico. III. Biological studies. 1. The extra-mammalian phases of the life cycle. Puerto Rico J. Publ. Health Trop. Med. **10:** 1–47.
2. CHENG, T. C. & R. W. SNYDER, JR. 1962. Studies on host-parasite relationships between larval trematodes and their hosts. I. A review. II. The utilization of the host's glycogen by the intramolluscan larvae of *Glypthelmins pennsylvaniensis* Cheng, and associated phenomena. Trans. Amer. Microsc. Soc. **81:** 209–228.
3. CHENG, T. C. 1963. Biochemical requirements of larval trematodes. Ann. N.Y. Acad. Sci. **113:** 289–321.
4. JAMES, B. L. 1965. The effects of parasitism by larvae Digenea on the digestive gland of the intertidal prosobranch, *Littorina saxatilis* (Olivi) subsp. *tenebrosa* (Montagu). Parasitology **55:** 93–115.
5. WRIGHT, C. A. 1966. The pathogenesis of helminths in the Mollusca. Helminthol. Abst. **35:** 207–224.
6. PAN, C. T. 1963. Generalized and focal tissue responses in the snail, *Australorbis glabratus,* infected with *Schistosoma mansoni*. Ann. N.Y. Acad. Sci. **113:** 475–485.
7. PAN, C. T. 1965. Studies on the host-parasite relationship between *Schistosoma mansoni* and the snail *Australorbis glabratus*. Amer. J. Trop. Med. Hyg. **14:** 931–976.
8. TRIPP, M. R. 1961. The fate of foreign materials experimentally introduced into the snail *Australorbis glabratus*. J. Parasitol. **47:** 745–775.
9. SMINIA, T. 1972. Structure and function of blood and connective tissue cells of the freshwater pulmonate *Lymnaea stagnalis* studied by electron microscopy and enzyme histochemistry. Z. Zellforsch. Mikrosk. Anat. **130:** 497–526.
10. NEWTON, W. H. 1952. The comparative tissue reaction of two strains of *Australorbis glabratus* to infection with *Schistosoma mansoni*. J. Parasitol. **38:** 362–366.
11. NEWTON, W. H. 1954. Tissue response to *Schistosoma mansoni* in second generation snails from a cross between two strains of *Australorbis glabratus*. J. Parasitol. **40:** 352–355.
12. COELHO, M. V. 1954. Acao das formas larvarias de *Schistosoma mansoni* sobre a reproducao de *Australorbis glabratus*. Publ. Avulsas Inst. Aggeu Magalhaes Recife, Brazil **3:** 39–53.

13. BROOKS, C. P. 1953. A comparative study of *Schistosoma mansoni* in *Tropicorbis havanensis* and *Australorbis glabratus*. J. Parasitol. **39:** 159–165.

14. CHERNIN, E., E. H. MICHELSON & D. L. AUGUSTINE. 1960. *Daubaylia potomaca*, a nematode parasite of *Helisoma trivolvis*, transmissible to *Australorbis glabratus*. J. Parasitol. **46:** 599–607.

15. PAN, C. T. 1958. The general histology and topographic microanatomy of *Australorbis glabratus*. Bull. Museum Comp. Zool. Harvard Coll. **119:** 237–299.

16. MEULEMAN, E. A. 1972. Host-parasite interrelationships between the freshwater pulmonate *Biomphalaria pfeifferi* and the trematode *Schistosoma mansoni*. Neth. J. Zool. **22:** 355–427.

17. CHRISTIE, J. D., W. B. FOSTER & L. A. STAUBER. 1974. The effect of parasitism and starvation on carbohydrate reserves of *Biomphalaria glabrata*. J. Invert. Pathol. **23:** 55–62.

18. CHRISTIE, J. D., W. B. FOSTER & L. A. STAUBER. 1974. ¹⁴C uptake by *Schistosoma mansoni* from *Biomphalaria glabrata* exposed to ¹⁴C-glucose. J. Invert. Pathol. **23:** 297–302.

19. SMYTH, J. D. 1966. The Physiology of Trematodes. W. H. Freeman and Co. Publishers. San Francisco, Calif.

20. VON BRAND, T. 1973. Biochemistry of Parasites. 2nd edit. Academic Press, Inc. New York, N.Y.

21. CHENG, T. C. & R. W. SNYDER, JR. 1963. Studies on host-parasite relationships between larval trematodes and their hosts. IV. A histochemical determination of glucose and its role in the metabolism of mollusc and parasite. Trans. Amer. Microsc. Soc. **82:** 343–346.

22. CHENG, T. C. 1963. The effects of *Echinoparyphium* larvae on the structure of and glycogen deposition in the hepatopancreas of *Helisoma trivolvis* and glycogenesis in the parasite larvae. Malacologia **1:** 291–303.

23. DENNIS, E. A., M. SHARP & R. DOUGLASS. 1974. Carbohydrate reserves and phosphatase activity in the mollusc-trematode relationship of *Mytilus edulis* L. and *Proctoeces maculatus* (Looss, 1901) Odhner, 1911. J. Helminthol. **48:** 1–14.

24. CHENG, T. C. 1962. The effects of parasitism by the larvae of *Echinoparyphuim* Dietz (Trematoda: Echinostomatidae) on the structure of and glycogen deposition in the hepatopancreas of *Helisoma trivolvis* (Say). Amer. Zool. **2:** 513.

25. READER, T. A. J. 1971. Histochemical observations on carbohydrates, lipids and enzymes in digenean parasites and host tissues of *Bithynia tentaculata*. Parasitology **63:** 125–136.

26. CHENG, T. C. & F. O. LEE. 1971. Glucose levels in the mollusc *Biomphalaria glabrata* infected with *Schistosoma mansoni*. J. Invert. Pathol. **18:** 395–399.

27. LEWERT, R. M. & J. B. PARA. 1966. The physiological incorporation of carbon-14 in *Schistosoma mansoni* cercariae. J. Infect. Diseases **116:** 171–182.

28. BRUCE, J. I., E. WEISS, M. A. STIREWALT & D. R. LINCICOME. 1969. *Schistosoma mansoni:* glycogen content and utilization of glucose, pyruvate, glutamate, and citric acid cycle intermediates by cercariae and schistosomules. Exp. Parasitol. **26:** 29–40.

GENETIC STUDIES OF PATHOLOGIC CONDITIONS
AND SUSCEPTIBILITY TO INFECTION IN
BIOMPHALARIA GLABRATA

Charles S. Richards

Laboratory of Parasitic Diseases
National Institute of Allergy and Infectious Diseases
National Institutes of Health
Bethesda, Maryland 20014

The relationship between a trematode parasite, such as *Schistosoma mansoni,* and a molluscan intermediate host, such as *Biomphalaria glabrata,* includes several stages, from location of snail by miracidia to departure of cercariae. Possibly, the most critical stage is the host-parasite interaction in the first few hours after miracidial penetration (FIGURE 1). Analysis of this interaction will involve genetic studies on variation in snail susceptibility and parasite infectivity, chemical and ultramicroscopic studies to determine how the successful miracidium masks from the snail host the fact it is a foreign object while the unsuccessful miracidium is encapsulated by a tissue reaction, and histopathologic studies of this host reaction and mobilization of amoebocytes.

We have conducted studies on genetics of susceptibility of *B. glabrata* to infection with *S. mansoni* and on genetics of infectivity in *S. mansoni.* Observations on numerous serial generations have provided the opportunity to follow serial transmission of a variety of abnormal conditions in the snails. Some involve genetics, some infectious agents, and some a combination of these factors. Several abnormal conditions currently under investigation in *B. glabrata* involve the amoebocytes and hemopoietic areas and are thus pertinent to studies of host defense mechanisms.

Results of most of our studies on snail susceptibility have been published.[1-4] Newton[5] demonstrated a genetic basis for susceptibility. Our investigations on susceptibility in *B. glabrata* have involved several snail populations and two strains of *S. mansoni,* from Puerto Rico (PR) and St. Lucia (L). Results indicated several different susceptibility combinations, including stocks that showed adult variability in susceptibility, in one of which some individuals refractory as young adults revert to susceptibility in old age. In *B. glabrata,* juvenile susceptibility to the PR strain of *S. mansoni* was found to be regulated by a combination of several genetic factors, probably four or more.[4] In juvenile susceptible snails, adult susceptibility is determined by a single gene, which exhibits simple Mendelian inheritance, with insusceptibility dominant.[2] In adult variable stocks, adult susceptibility is apparently modified by additional genetic factors. In PR susceptible snails, juvenile susceptibility to the L strain of *S. mansoni* appears to be determined by a single gene, with insusceptibility dominant.[3]

The fact that some clonal stocks of *B. glabrata* test susceptible to PR but refractory to L *S. mansoni* indicates a difference in parasite infectivity. To study this difference, snails susceptible to both parasite strains served as controls to demonstrate potential infectivity of the miracidia, while snails PR susceptible but L refractory served as test snails.[3, 6] In these studies, individual snails were exposed to single miracidia, and penetration was observed. This procedure provided single sex infections in snails, so that crosses between the PR and L strains could be established in mice. F_1 hybrid miracidia from the male PR $\times$ female L crosses infected 19% test snails; F_1 hybrid miracidia from female PR $\times$ male L crosses infected 1.7%. The difference in results between the reciprocal crosses suggested sex linkage. Results also agreed with the cyto-genetic results of Short and Menzel [7] that the female schistosome is heterogametic (XY), the male XX. Our clonal "test" stocks of *B. glabrata* are not com-pletely refractory to the L strain of *S. mansoni;* about 4% of the miracidia are infective. Studies in progress, which select for two substrains that differ in infectivity from the L strain, have demonstrated that the parent L strain is heterogenic for infectivity.

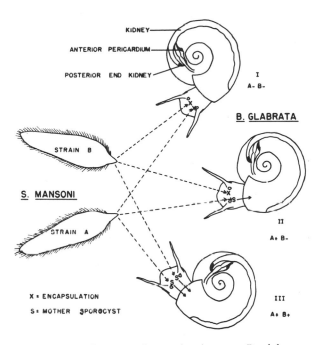

FIGURE 1. Diagram that illustrates interaction between *B. glabrata* snails of three genetic susceptibility types and *S. mansoni* miracidia of two genetic infectivity strains. Type-I snails are refractory to *S. mansoni* strains A and B, type III are susceptible to both, and type II are susceptible to A but refractory to B. Hemopoietic areas of *B. glabrata* in the anterior pericardium and saccular kidney are indicated.

It is understandable why snails and parasites from different geographic areas may differ in susceptibility and infectivity. Interbreeding snail populations and interbreeding trematode populations may vary qualitatively in the genetic alleles present or absent and quantitatively in gene frequencies. Host-parasite relations that result in potential infection frequencies anywhere between 0 and 100% may be expected. The great variability between and within both snail stocks and parasite strains obviously constitutes a factor that should be considered in any experimental studies.

When a miracidium of *S. mansoni* penetrates *B. glabrata,* usually either

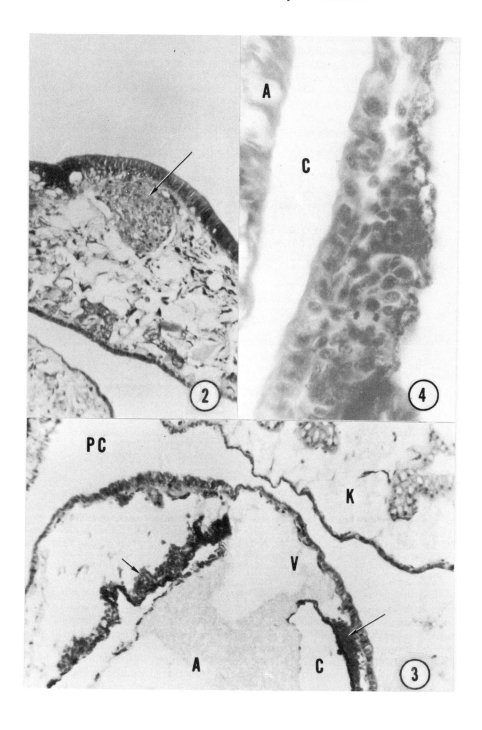

development is normal, with no evidence of host reaction, or the miracidium dies in the first few hours after penetration, accompanied by a host tissue encapsulating reaction.[8, 9] As shown by Tripp,[10] the tissue response by *B. glabrata* is not specific; it is evoked even by inert materials. Wright[11] suggested that the ability of successful miracidia to evade the snail host's cellular responses may be either due to adsorption of host substances, to production by the miracidia of some covering, or to continual synthesis of inhibiting substances. Probably the most interesting host-parasite interaction occurs when a susceptible snail is penetrated by an excess of infective miracidia. Refractory snails exposed to 25 miracidia per snail were fixed after 24 hr and serially sectioned. About half the miracidia were found, which indicates at least 50% penetration. All were encapsulated by the host tissues. In susceptible snails exposed to 25 miracidia and similarly treated, about half the miracidia were again found, of which a few (four or five) appeared normal, with no evident host reaction, whereas the rest were encapsulated and appeared dead. When 25 susceptible snails were exposed to one miracidium each, developing mother sporocysts were evident in 16 (64%) after 10 days. This finding suggests that the failure of many of the miracidia that penetrated a single susceptible snail exposed to 25 miracidia was related to the successful development of the few observed without host reaction. Because some of the encapsulated miracidia were located at an appreciable distance in the snail from the successful miracidia, the circulating hemolymph and hemocytes appear to be involved.

Implication of the hemolymph in the capacity of a miracidium to evade recognition as a foreign object by the snail and the cellular response when the snail does recognize a miracidium as foreign lead to our interest in abnormal conditions that involve the circulating hemocytes and the hemopoietic tissues (FIGURE 1). There is still little known about hemopoiesis in *B. glabrata*. Pan[12] suggested that possible sites of normal production of amoebocytes in *B. glabrata* are the blood sinuses and the wall of the saccular part of the kidney that borders the pericardial cavity. In normal *B. glabrata*, the anterior pericardial wall, which separates the heart from the pulmonary cavity, appears *in vivo* as a thin transparent membrane. We have noted that in some living *B. glabrata* with a variety of pathologic conditions, with or without demonstrated involvement of infectious agents, the anterior pericardial wall appears thick and cloudy. Sections of the pericardium reveal groups of undifferentiated cells, some of which show mitotic figures.[13] Some mitotic figures also occur in the posterior portion of the kidney, as described by Pan.[12]

In one stock of *B. glabrata* under study, lesions occur on the body and mantle collar. The host cellular reaction results in nodules (FIGURE 2) that eventually open to the outside, with destruction of the epithelium and formation of an exudate. Although the cause is unknown, an infectious agent is suspected. These lesions occur at some distance from the heart region. The pericardial wall, however, contains extensive nests of undifferentiated cells, some in mitosis (FIGURES 3 & 4).

FIGURE 2. Photomicrograph that shows lesion (arrow) in mantle of *B. glabrata;* hematoxylin-azure eosin. × 100.

FIGURE 3. Photomicrograph of same snail as in FIGURE 2; pericardium with nests of undifferentiated cells (arrows), atrium (A), vein (V), pericardial cavity (C), pulmonary cavity (PC), kidney (K); hematoxylin-azure eosin. × 100.

FIGURE 4. Photomicrograph of same snail as in FIGURE 2; pericardium with mitotic figure, pericardial cavity (C), atrium (A); Gomori's trichrome. × 400.

METHODS

Studies on the genetics of susceptibility to infection with *S. mansoni* have afforded a unique opportunity to observe abnormal conditions, such as those to be described, and to investigate their causes and transmission. Frequencies of the pathologic conditions suggest serial transmission in clonal stocks, which involves genetics, infectious agents, or a combination of both. Attempts to determine the causal factors involve the following procedures. Offspring produced by self-fertilization of snails that show the condition are isolated as juveniles after a period of association with the parent. This selection procedure is performed for several generations to see if frequencies are maintained or increased. Eggs from an affected snail are removed before hatching to a clean container and are reared to test for transovarial transmission or inheritance. In crossing experiments, precross progeny by selfing are obtained from an affected snail and a normal snail. After reciprocal cross fertilization, hybrid F_1s from each parent are followed through several generations, and when the parent snails resume self-fertilization, postcross progenies by selfing are also observed.

In addition to studies on serial transmission, affected snails are being maintained in containers in association with their own juveniles as controls and with juvenile offspring from normal stock snails of different pigment type to determine whether transmission occurs. We plan to perform transplants of the abnormal cellular accumulations to snails of normal stocks.

Snails fixed in Bouin's have been serially sectioned and stained with either hematoxylin and azure eosin or Gomori's trichrome. Portions of the cellular accumulations from live snails have been mounted in hemolymph in sealed double cover slip preparations and observed.

RESULTS

We have observed several internal pathologic conditions in *B. glabrata,* at least four of which involve the amoebocytes and the pericardium. Pending further histologic studies, these conditions will be referred to, in general, as proliferative amoebocytic accumulations. The first condition to be described consists of hemocyte aggregations in the atrium, observed in a clonal albino stock of *B. glabrata* (FIGURE 5). Nodules that appear to be suspended in the cavity of the atrium move back and forth with the pulse of the hemolymph but maintain a fixed relative position, anchored by association with muscle fibers or the wall of the atrium. Formation of these aggregations is transitory, and frequencies appeared sporadic until it was ascertained that they begin forming soon after onset of egg laying, increase for a few weeks, then decrease and usually disappear. Observed frequencies thus depend on timing of observations. In sections, the aggregations appear to consist of amoebocytes (FIGURE 6). Some contain rod-shaped inclusions that stain bright red with Gomori's trichrome but are unstained by hematoxylin-azure eosin. The pericardium contains groups of undifferentiated cells, and mitotic figures occur here, in the nodules, and in the atrial epicardium (FIGURES 7 & 8). In older snails, when nodules may no longer be evident in the atrial cavity, sections have revealed accumulations in the kidney and in the hemolymph sinuses around the stomach and intestine (FIGURE 9). When an atrial nodule was mounted in hemolymph in a

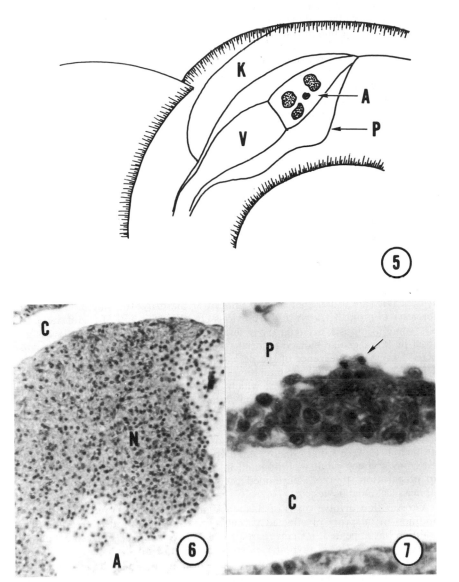

FIGURE 5. Diagram that indicates location of atrial nodules: atrium (A), kidney (K), ventricle (V), pericardium (P).

FIGURE 6. Photomicrograph of *B. glabrata:* atrium (A), atrial nodule (N), pericardial cavity (C), pericardium; Gomori's trichrome. ✕100.

FIGURE 7. Photomicrograph of same snail as in FIGURE 6: pericardium (P), nests of undifferentiated cells with mitotic figure (arrow), pericardial cavity (C), atrium; Gomori's trichrome. ✕ 400.

sealed double cover slip preparation, the cells developed pseudopodia and migrated out from the cell mass as amoebocytes (FIGURE 10).

FIGURE 11 is a diagram that illustrates results of selfing and crossing snails of this stock. Initially, observations on atrial nodules were incidental to other studies. Only the third and fourth filial generations of snail 3 by selfing were observed on a regular schedule, and about half of them developed atrial nodules. Atrial nodule stock snail 3 was mated three times in series, alternating normal stock blackeye and wild-type mates. Hybrid F_1s from all three crosses, and their progenies through three generations of selfing, have been observed with no positive results for atrial nodules. Another snail from the atrial nodule stock (no. 7) was mated with a normal stock blackeye snail. Hybrid F_1s from both parents appeared normal. Following the routine procedure of isolating juveniles for rearing that have been associated with their parent, no F_2s but 5/8 F_3s have formed atrial nodules. Eggs from one of the F_1s were transferred to a fresh container before hatching. From these juveniles, 1/9 F_2s and 3/7 F_3s have developed atrial nodules. The atrial nodule stock is a type-II stock, juvenile susceptible/adult refractory to S. mansoni. All four of the normal stock snails used in the above crosses were type-III S. mansoni-susceptible snails.

The second condition involves proliferative cellular accumulations in the pericardial cavity and has been observed in one clonal albino stock of B. glabrata. In some juvenile snails, hemocyte aggregations occur in the hemocoel by the intestine and in the hepatopancreas. The cellular accumulations in the pericardial cavity are usually not evident until after maturity; they increase in extent thereafter (FIGURE 12). As in the previous condition, groups of undifferentiated cells, some in mitosis, occur in the anterior pericardium, and mitotic figures are found in the saccular kidney (FIGURES 13–15). Sectioned old juveniles, suspected from the appearance of the pericardium and their parentage to be in the initial stage of pericardial accumulation formation, had nests of undifferentiated cells in the pericardium, some of which contained mitotic figures. Adults had massive cellular accumulations intimately associated with the pericardium and the epicardium of the ventricle. Cells in mitosis occurred in the ventricular epicardium and in the pericardium. Cellular accumulations also were observed in the kidney (FIGURE 16) and in areas around the stomach and intestine, and mitotic figures were seen in the intestinal epithelium. When a cellular accumulation from a young adult was mounted in hemolymph in a sealed double cover slip preparation, the cells developed pseudopodia and migrated out from the cell mass as amoebocytes.

Crosses that involve snails of this stock are in progress. Frequencies of the condition in offspring of affected parents by selfing averaged over 50%. The condition has appeared in snails reared from eggs transferred to fresh containers before hatching. This is a type-I S. mansoni-refractory stock.

In a third clonal stock of blackeye B. glabrata, amoebocytic accumulations sometimes form around the aorta (FIGURE 17). These accumulations are usually not evident until after maturity; they increase thereafter. After several months, cellular accumulations may also appear around the junction of the ventricle and atrium. In sectioned snails with nodules around the aorta (FIGURES 18 & 19), cellular accumulations also occurred around parts of the digestive system, and mitotic figures were seen in the kidney and intestinal epithelium. The pericardium contained nests of undifferentiated cells, some in mitosis, and strands of cells connected these areas with the accumulations around the aorta. When periaortic cellular accumulations were mounted in hemolymph in a sealed double

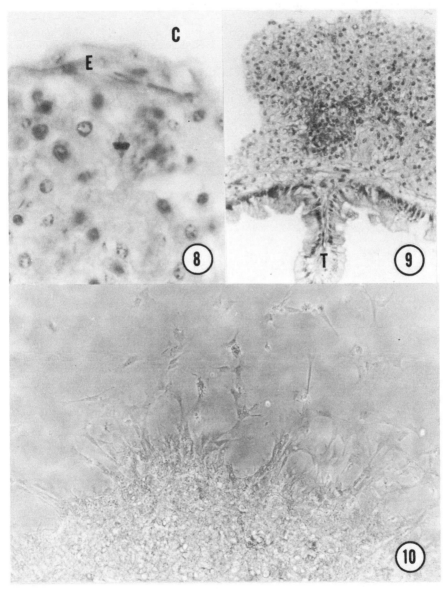

FIGURE 8. Photomicrograph of *B. glabrata:* atrial nodule with mitotic figure, epicardium (E), pericardial cavity (C); Gomori's trichrome. ×400.

FIGURE 9. Photomicrograph of same snail as in FIGURE 8. amoebocytic accumulation by prointestine; typhlosole (T); Gomori's trichrome. ×100.

FIGURE 10. Photomicrograph of *B. glabrata:* atrial nodule in hemolymph, sealed double cover slip preparation, 2 hr, phase-contrast microscopy. ×100.

cover slip preparation, the cells developed pseudopodia and migrated out as amoebocytes. Crosses with this stock are in progress. This is a type-I *S. mansoni*-refractory stock.

The fourth pathologic condition was observed in a clonal stock of *B. glabrata,* including both albino and wild-type snails. Nodules are first evident in juvenile snails about 5 mm in diameter, in the hemocoel near the intestine (FIGURE 20). Nodules and cellular accumulations may then be seen forming around parts of the intestine and in the hepatopancreas. In snails fixed and sectioned, the anterior pericardium contains groups of undifferentiated cells (FIGURE 21), some in mitosis. Mitotic figures also occur in the saccular kidney. Cellular accumulations are found in the hemocoel near the digestive tract, and in older snails,

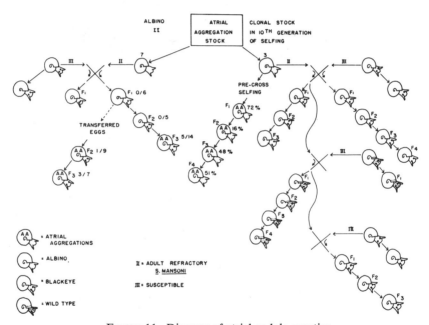

FIGURE 11. Diagram of atrial nodule genetics.

cellular accumulations are seen around the intestine and in sinuses of the hepatopancreas (FIGURES 22 & 23). As in the atrial nodule stock, some cells contain needle-like inclusions that stain bright red with Gomori's trichrome. When one of the nodules from a young snail was mounted in hemolymph in a sealed double cover slip preparation, amoebocytes moved out from the cell mass, with typical pseudopodia (FIGURE 24).

A simplified diagram of crossing experiments is illustrated in FIGURE 25. An albino from the hemocoel accumulation stock, of unknown *S. mansoni* susceptibility, was mated with a homozygous blackeye snail from a normal type-II *S. mansoni* adult refractory stock. The albino parent produced hybrid F_1s, 87% of which developed hemocoel nodules. Two blackeye F_1s were mated, each with an albino from a type-I *S. mansoni*-refractory stock. Both albinos produced

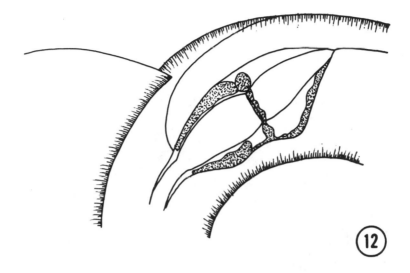

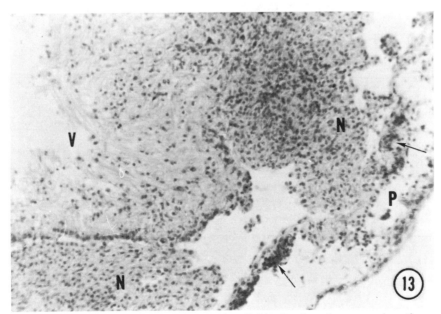

FIGURE 12. Diagram of *B. glabrata* pericardial cavity that shows amoebocytic accumulations.

FIGURE 13. Photomicrograph of *B. glabrata:* ventricle (V), pericardial cavity accumulations (N), pericardium (P) with nests of undifferentiated cells (arrows); hematoxylin-azure eosin. ×100.

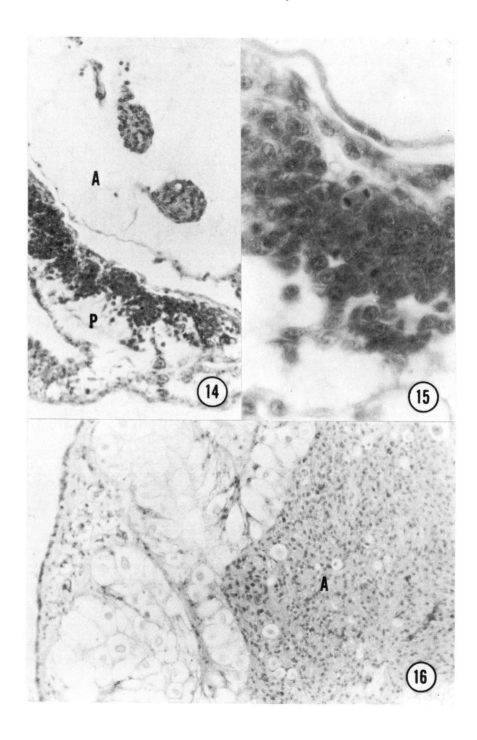

hybrid offspring, 6/26 (23%) with hemocoel nodules. Two homozygous black-eye F_2 snails, which were derived from the original cross and averaged 42% (total 8/19) hemocoel nodule offspring by selfing, were mated to two albinos from two different normal type-III *S. mansoni*-susceptible stock snails. All postcross progeny examined were normal. When eggs from a hemocoel growth snail by selfing were transferred to a separate container before hatching, 50% of the resultant snails reared and examined developed hemocoel nodules.

DISCUSSION

The four proliferative amoebocytic accumulation conditions described in *B. glabrata* display similarities and differences. Hemocoel nodules are usually apparent in young juveniles, whereas the other accumulations are usually first evident in adults. In the stock that develops pericardial cavity accumulations, however, juveniles sometimes show nodules in the hemocoel and hepatopancreas similar to those of the hemocoel nodule stock. Observations on young nodules mounted in hemolymph suggest that all the accumulations originate as aggregations of amoebocytes. Atrial nodules are transitory, regressing after a few weeks, whereas the other accumulations persist. Infiltration of other areas occurs persistently in all four conditions. Nests of undifferentiated cells, some in mitosis, occur in the pericardial wall in snails with all four conditions. These cells may contribute to the accumulations or may be a protective response that attempts to control them.

If the proliferative amoebocytic accumulations are caused by infectious agents, such as viruses, transovarial transmission probably occurs. Four different agents could be involved or the same agent could cause different conditions due to genetic differences in the snail stocks. Preliminary crossing experiments suggest that genetics is involved, either directly or by variation in susceptibility to an infectious agent. Descendents of an atrial nodule stock snail by precross selfing, followed through four generations, showed a frequency of atrial nodule formation of about 50%. When the same parent snail was mated three times in series with normal stock snails, and hybrid offspring were followed through three generations, none was observed to form atrial nodules. When another atrial nodule stock snail was mated with a normal snail, the hybrid F_1s were all normal, but one F_2 and several F_3s developed atrial nodules. In three crosses between hemocoel nodule snails and normal stock snails, hemocoel nodules were observed in a relatively high percentage of the F_1s, whereas in two other crosses, all F_1s appeared normal. If the various amoebocytic accumulations are regulated primarily by genetics, there may be four different genetic factors or complexes involved, or they may be determined by genetic complexes that contain several major genes and modifying genes; the four snail stocks might share some of the same genes but differ in others.

FIGURE 14. Photomicrograph of *B. glabrata* with pericardial cavity accumulations; pericardium (P) with nests of undifferentiated cells, atrium (A); Gomori's trichrome. ×100.

FIGURE 15. Photomicrograph of same snail as in FIGURE 14: pericardium with mitotic figures; Gomori's trichrome. ×400.

FIGURE 16. Photomicrograph of *B. glabrata* with pericardial cavity accumulations; proliferative accumulation (A) in kidney; hematoxylin-azure eosin. ×100.

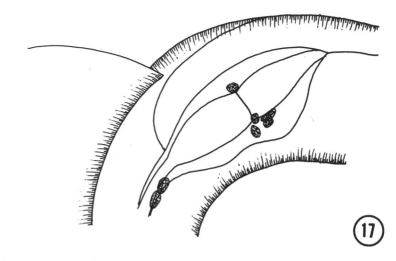

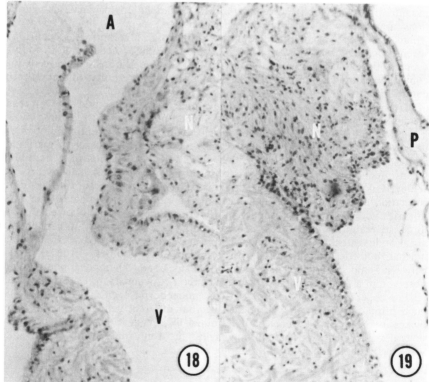

FIGURE 17. Diagram of *B. glabrata* with periaortic amoebocytic accumulations (and accumulation around atrial-ventricular junction).

FIGURE 18. Photomicrograph of *B. glabrata* with periaortic accumulation (N), ventricle (V), aorta (A); hematoxylin-azure eosin. ×100.

FIGURE 19. Photomicrograph of same snail as in FIGURE 18: ventricle (V), periaortic accumulation (N), pericardium (P); hematoxylin-azure eosin. ×100.

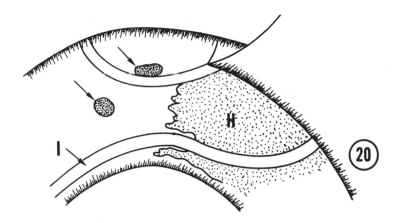

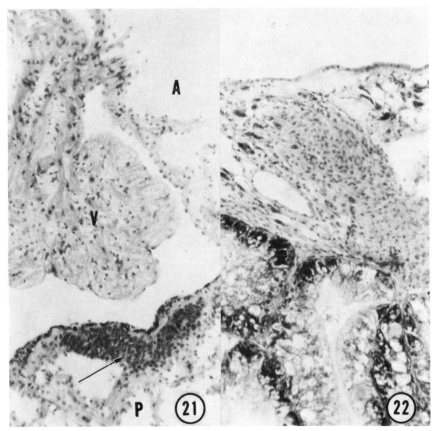

FIGURE 20. Diagram of *B. glabrata* with hemocoel nodules (arrows): hepatopancreas (H), intestine (I).

FIGURE 21. Photomicrograph of adult hemocoel nodule *B. glabrata;* atrium (A), ventricle (V), pericardium (P) with nest of undifferentiated cells (arrow); hematoxylin-azure eosin. ×100.

FIGURE 22. Photomicrograph of same snail as in FIGURE 21: proliferative amoebocytic accumulation by hepatopancreas. ×100.

407

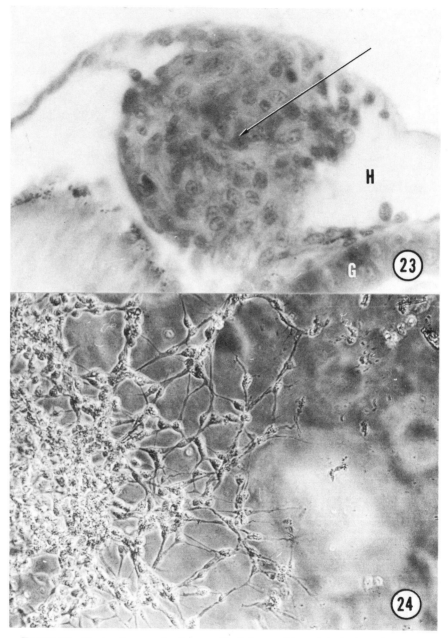

FIGURE 23. Photomicrograph of young *B. glabrata* with nodule by intestine: nodule (arrow), intestine (G), hemocoel (H); hematoxylin-azure eosin. ×400.

FIGURE 24. Photomicrograph of hemocoel nodule from *B. glabrata* in hemolymph in sealed double cover slip preparation, 20 hr, phase-contrast microscopy. ×100.

The apparent association between the occurrence of the accumulations and genetic insusceptibility to infection with *S. mansoni,* suggested by the preliminary crossing data, may merely be coincidental. Crosses in progress that involve combinations of the various amoebocytic accumulation conditions, and between these and normal stock snails of various *S. mansoni* susceptibility types, with miracidial exposures of precross and postcross juveniles and adults, should demonstrate whether there is a relationship between the tendency for amoebocytic accumulations and *S. mansoni* insusceptibility.

The ability to follow the development of the various amoebocytic accumulations through time in individual snails *in vivo,* through successive generations

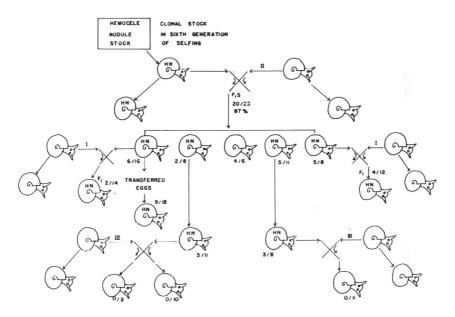

FIGURE 25. Diagram of hemocoel nodule (HN) genetics: snail pigment phenotypes as in FIGURE 11; *S. mansoni* susceptibility types: I, refractory; II, adult refractory; III, susceptible.

of selfing, and through serial crosses, in addition to such procedures as transplants, tissue culture, and electron microscopy, presents an opportunity that should provide additional valuable information.

SUMMARY

During studies on the genetics of variation in susceptibility of *B. glabrata* to infection with *S. mansoni,* four types of proliferative amoebocytic accumulations have been observed. They occur in four different clonal stocks of *B. glabrata,* beginning as amoebocytic aggregations, namely, in the atrial cavity, pericardial cavity, periaortic space, and hemocoel between the stomach and intestine. Persistent amoebocytic accumulations involve the sinuses around the stomach, intestine, and hepatopancreas. In these snails, nests of undifferentiated cells occur in the anterior pericardial wall, which is considered to be a hemopoietic area. Crossing experiments indicate the involvement of genetic factors, possibly in combination with infectious agents.

ACKNOWLEDGMENTS

The technical assistance of Mr. Paul Shade, Mr. Thomas Hallack, and Mr. Rodney Duvall is greatly appreciated.

REFERENCES

1. RICHARDS, C. S. 1970. Genetics of a molluscan vector of schistosomiasis. Nature (London) **227:** 806–810.
2. RICHARDS, C. S. 1973. Susceptibility of adult *Biomphalaria glabrata* to *Schistosoma mansoni* infection. Amer. J. Trop. Med. Hyg. **22:** 748–756.
3. RICHARDS, C. S. 1975. Genetic factors in susceptibility of *Biomphalaria glabrata* for different strains of *Schistosoma mansoni*. Parasitology **70:** 231–241.
4. RICHARDS, C. S. & J. W. MERRITT, JR. 1972. Genetic factors in the susceptibility of juvenile *Biomphalaria glabrata* to *Schistosoma mansoni* infection. Amer. J. Trop. Med. Hyg. **21:** 425–434.
5. NEWTON, W. L. 1953. The inheritance of susceptibility to infection with *Schistosoma mansoni* in *Australorbis glabratus*. Exp. Parasitol. **2:** 242–257.
6. RICHARDS, C. S. 1975. Genetic studies on variation in infectivity of *Schistosoma mansoni*. J. Parasitol. **61:** 233–236.
7. SHORT, R. B. & M. Y. MENZEL. 1960. Chromosomes of nine species of schistosomes. J. Parasitol. **46:** 273–287.
8. NEWTON, W. L. 1952. The comparative tissue reaction of two strains of *Australorbis glabratus* to infection with *Schistosoma mansoni*. J. Parasitol. **38:** 362–366.
9. PAN, C. T. 1965. Studies on the host-parasite relationship between *Schistosoma mansoni* and the snail *Australorbis glabratus*. Amer. J. Trop. Med. Hyg. **14:** 931–976.
10. TRIPP, M. R. 1961. The fate of foreign materials experimentally introduced into the snail *Australorbis glabratus*. J. Parasitol. **47:** 745–751.
11. WRIGHT, C. A. 1974. Snail susceptibility or trematode infectivity? J. Nat. Hist. **8:** 545–548.
12. PAN, C. T. 1958. The general histology and topographic microanatomy of *Australorbis glabratus*. Bull. Museum Comp. Zool. Harvard Coll. **119:** 237–299.
13. LIE, K. J., D. HEYNEMAN & P. YAU. 1975. The origin of amebocytes in *Biomphalaria glabrata*. J. Parasitol. **61:** 574–576.

NEOPLASMS AND TUMOR-LIKE GROWTHS IN THE AQUATIC PULMONATE SNAIL *BIOMPHALARIA GLABRATA*

E. H. Michelson and Charles S. Richards

Department of Tropical Public Health
Harvard University School of Public Health
Boston, Massachusetts 02115
and Laboratory of Parasitic Diseases
National Institutes of Health
Bethesda, Maryland 20014

Tumors or tumor-like growths have been observed or induced in species that represent three of the six classes of living mollusks: most frequently in the Pelecypoda, occasionally in the Gastropoda, and rarely in the Cephalopoda.[1-3] Most reports, with respect to gastropod species, have been concerned with lesions in terrestrial slugs and snails.[4-8] Tumor-like lesions were reported also in a species of marine snail,[9] and Krieg [10-13] successfully induced tumors in an aquatic prosobranch. To date, observations on tumors and tumor-like growths in species of aquatic pulmonate snails have been oriented toward elucidating the genetics of such growths, and their histopathology has been studied only superficially.[14-18]

This paper describes, for the first time, the gross and microscopic features of a series of tumors or tumor-like growths observed in the aquatic pulmonate snail *Biomphalaria glabrata*. Some of these growths arose spontaneously in stock snail colonies and were probably initiated by a variety of factors, including microorganisms. Others appear to be hereditary in nature and were possibly genetically induced.

MATERIALS AND METHODS

All snails employed in this study were derived either directly or from clonal stocks of a Puerto Rican strain (NIH-BPR-M) of *B. glabrata* that has been maintained routinely at the National Institutes of Health.[19]

After removal from the shell, the snails were fixed in Newcomer's solution for 18 hr at 5° C, embedded in Paraplast®, serially sectioned at 7 μm, and the sections stained routinely with hemalum and azure II-eosin, hemalum and eosin, or Gomori's trichrome stain. Selected sections were stained with Wolbach's Geimsa stain for protozoans, Fite's carbolfuchsin and Janus green for acid-fast organisms, Lillie's tissue Gram stain for bacteria, and Gridley's periodic acid-Schiff stain for fungi.

OBSERVATIONS AND RESULTS

Pseudobranchial Growths

One of us (C.S.R.) has observed that pseudobranchial growths occur with high frequency in some clonal stocks of *B. glabrata*. Preliminary breeding experiments suggest that such growths may have a hereditary basis and may possibly be genetically induced. A series of 10 snails, each of which had a similar type growth on the pseudobranch, were studied. The snails ranged in size from 10 to 14 mm in shell diameter and were sexually mature.

In all instances, the growths were found on the ventral surface of the pseudobranch and appeared as either a single or bifurcate finger-like projection (FIGURE 1). The growths showed slight contraction on touch but were not completely retractible. Histologic sections of the growths revealed that their outer surface was a continuation of the epithelium of pseudobranch and consisted of moderately tall, ciliated, columnar epithelial cells. The nuclei of these cells were situated between the middle and basal third of the cells and stained intensely with hemalum. The inner core of the growth consisted of the normal tissue elements found in the pseudobranch and was composed of muscle fibers, connective tissue cells, and gland cells (FIGURE 3). The nature of the connective tissue varied with the specimen; in some, it was dense, and in others, it was loose and vascular. Likewise, the number of pigment cells varied from specimen to specimen. All the growths, however, contained numerous hemolymph sinusoids. Except for one specimen, mitotic figures were not noted in either the tissues of the growth or in the adjacent tissues. Although no microorganisms were detected in any of the growths, several of the snails were infected with a yeast- or microsporidian-like organism. These organisms were found most frequently in the digestive gland and the ovo-testis (FIGURE 4). Many, but not all, of the snails appeared to contain an abnormal amount of pigment in their tissues. This finding may be of some importance, because toxemia and infectious processes frequently induce heavy pigmentation in *B. glabrata* and other freshwater snails.

Foot Polyp

A small (0.77–0.88 mm in height) polyp-like growth was detected on the caudodorsal surface of the foot of a black-eyed, partially pigmented specimen of *B. glabrata* (FIGURE 2). The origin and genetics of this particular phenotype have been described by Richards.[20] There is, however, no evidence that the growth is in anyway genetically induced.

Viewed from above, the growth was oval in shape, with the anterior and posterior surfaces slightly flattened. The growth was not retractible and had a fine line of pigment running down the center of each of its lateral surfaces. On histologic examination, the polyp appeared to be an extension of normal foot tissues and probably represents an example of hyperplasia rather than neoplasia. Except for a decrease in gland cells and a slight increase in muscle fibers near its origin, the tissues of the growth resembled those of the foot (FIGURE 5). No mitotic figures were observed, nor was there any evidence of microorganisms or parasites in or near the growth.

Fungiform Foot Polyp

A fungiform growth, approximately 3 mm in diameter and 1.5 mm in height, was noted on the ventral surface of the foot of a specimen 17 months old. Both the parents of this snail and two surviving offspring were normal, and there

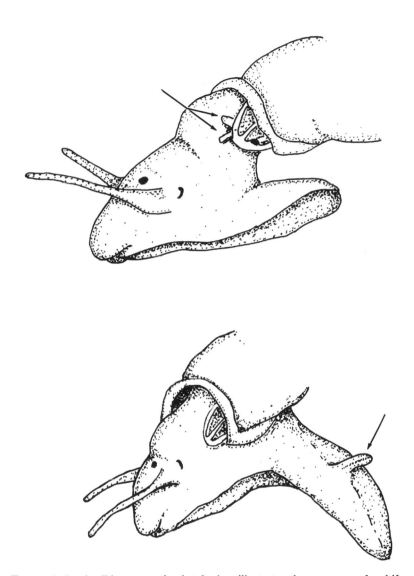

FIGURE 1 (*top*). Diagrammatic sketch that illustrates the presence of a bifurcate pseudobranchial growth in a specimen of *B. glabrata*. Arrows indicate the growth.

FIGURE 2 (*bottom*). Diagrammatic sketch that illustrates the presence of a polyp-like growth on the caudodorsal surface of the foot of a specimen of *B. glabrata*. Arrow indicates growth.

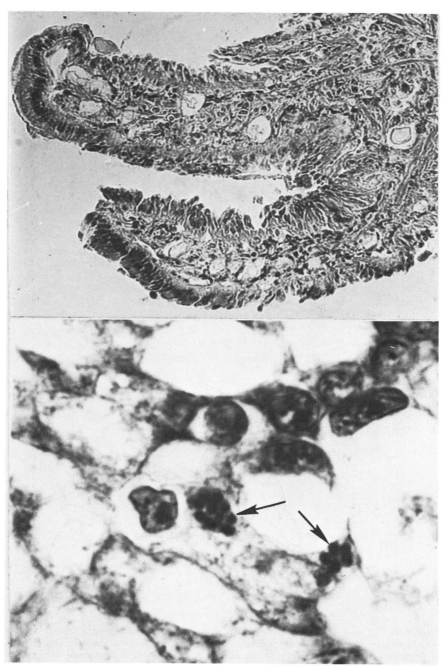

FIGURE 3 (*top*). Section through a bifurcate pseudobranchial growth in the snail *B. glabrata*. Gomori's trichrome; ×670.

FIGURE 4 (*bottom*). Section through the digestive gland of a snail with a pseudobranchial growth that shows the presence of yeast- or microsporidian-like organisms. Hemalum azure II-eosin; ×3445.

was no evidence of similar growths in other members of the stock colony. In the living snail, a discrete pedicle could not be detected, and the growth appeared as a spongy, convoluted, deeply furrowed mass attached directly to the sole of the foot. The growth was unpigmented and contrasted sharply with the dark pigmentation of the snail's body.

On microscopic examination, a cystlike invagination that contained spore-bearing bacilli was found at the base of the growth (FIGURE 6). It is possible that the growth was initiated as a response to the bacteria. This "cyst" appeared to have been formed by the infolding of the epithelium that covers the surface of the foot and the main portion of the tumor. Due to pressure, however, the normally tall columnar epithelial cells were greatly compressed and had lost their cilia. The center of the cyst was filled with necrotic debris, cell fragments, bacteria, and an amorphous material that appeared light pink in hemalum and eosin-stained sections and light purple in Gomori's trichrome-stained sections (FIGURE 7). It is of interest to note that the bacteria (bacilli with terminal spores) resemble those described by Cruz and Dias [21] as *Bacillus pinottii,* a bacillus previously considered to be a potential agent for the biologic control of schistosome-bearing snails.

The polyp appeared, in tissue sections, as a convoluted mass composed of numerous deep, cryptlike depressions (FIGURE 8). Bacteria were found in the lumina of many of the crypts and in the tissues of the tumor. The epithelium covering the surface of the polyp was composed of tall columnar cells, as in the normal tissue of the foot mass; however, there were areas in which the epithelium was depressed and squamous. The core of the polyp consisted of a loose connective tissue in which there were numerous vacuoles and areas of aplasia. Gland cells were present in considerable numbers, but there was a noticeable lack of pigment cells. In addition, muscle fibers were markedly reduced. Mitotic activity was not observed.

Buccal Gland Tumor

This specimen was characterized by the presence of a protruding cyst-like mass that occupied most of the anterior position of the snail's head region (FIGURE 9). The mass appeared to be filled with a whitish material, was firm to touch, and did not pulsate. One margin of the mass anastomosed to the inner lateral surface of the right tentacle, and the posterior edge of the growth encroached upon the right eye. In addition, the right tentacle was bifurcate. Although similar looking growths have been noted on occasion in the stock colony, there is no evidence to suggest that they might be hereditary.

Histologic examination revealed that the tumor probably originated in the region of the buccal gland and subsequently expanded upward and outward. As a consequence of pressure atrophy, the cells comprising the outer epithelium were markedly compressed, had lost their cilia, and contained grossly distorted nuclei (FIGURE 11). A layer of muscle fibers was situated beneath the epithelium. This layer was not uniform but varied in thickness around the circumference of the tumor. Beneath the muscle layer was a region of gland cells that enveloped the innermost core of the tumor. The gland cells were filled densely with secretion granules, and it was difficult to identify nuclei. In some areas, the gland cells were compressed, fragmented, and only granules remained. The central core of the tumor was composed of a dense, collagen-like reticulum

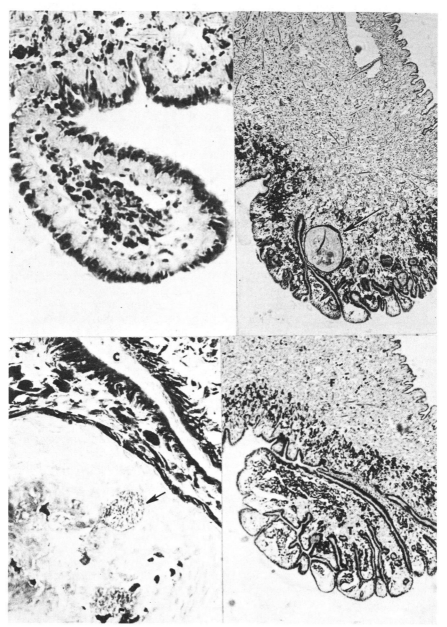

FIGURE 5 (*top left.*) Longitudinal section through a polyp-like growth on the caudodorsal surface of the foot. Note heavy concentration of pigment in the mid-region of the growth. Azure II-eosin; ×455.

FIGURE 6 (*top right*). Longitudinal section through a fungiform growth observed on the ventral surface of the foot. A discrete bacterial lesion (arrow) can be seen that stained bright red with azure II-eosin and greenish purple with Gomori's trichrome stain (FIGURE 12). Scattered among the fibers of the reticulum were secretion granules, gland cells, and cell fragments. Numerous mitotic figures were detected in the epithelium of the growth and in surrounding connective tissue, a finding which suggested that active neoplastic growth was occurring. The tissues of the bifurcate right tentacle appeared normal in all histologic aspects. No microorganisms or parasites were observed in or near the tumor or in other portions of the snail.

Mantle Collar Tumor

The specimen was an albino variant of *B. glabrata,* 12.9 mm in shell diameter, and approximately 5 months old at the time it was studied. A small (0.9–1.0 mm) tubular growth with a terminal opening was observed on the right parietal margin of the mantle collar. Snails of the colony from which this specimen was derived are characterized by preputiums that are continually everted; however, there is no evidence to suggest that this genetic anomaly and the growth are related.

Microscopically, the surface of the growth was covered with tall, ciliated epithelial cells similar to those found covering the mantle collar. At the tip of the tumor, the epithelium was inverted and continued downward to the base. Thus, the structure resembled a tube with a blind end. The epithelium lining the internal channel was extremely active and contained numerous mitotic figures. The stroma of the tumor consisted mainly of muscle fibers and dense connective tissue and, in general, resembled the tissues of the mantle collar (FIGURE 13). Gland cells were found in the distal tip of the tumor and less frequently in other areas. The proximal end of the channel of the tumor appeared to be filled with an amorphous material, possibly mucus. No microorganisms or parasites were found in the tissues of the growth or in other portions of the snail.

Abnormal Tentacle Growths

The snail, approximately 1 year old and 16.4 mm in shell diameter, was unusual in that both tentacles were grossly deformed. The left tentacle was hypertrophic and foreshortened, whereas the right one was hooked and had a subterminal swelling (FIGURE 10). An opaque area was noted in the center of the swelling. The abnormality observed in the left tentacle has been demonstrated by one of us (C.S.R.) to be a hereditary trait in certain clonal stocks and appears to be controlled by a single recessive gene. It is frequently asso-

---

at base of growth. Note the absence of gland cells in region of the foot near the lesion. G, gland cells. Hemalum and eosin; ×57.6.

FIGURE 7 (*bottom left*). Longitudinal section through portion of a bacterial lesion seen in FIGURE 6. Arrow designates clump of bacteria. C, crypt. Azure II-eosin; ×576.

FIGURE 8 (*bottom right*). Longitudinal section through fungiform growth observed on the ventral surface of the foot. Section does not show bacterial lesion. Note numerous cryptlike folds that comprise the growth. F, foot; T, tumor-like growth. Azure II-eosin; ×57.6.

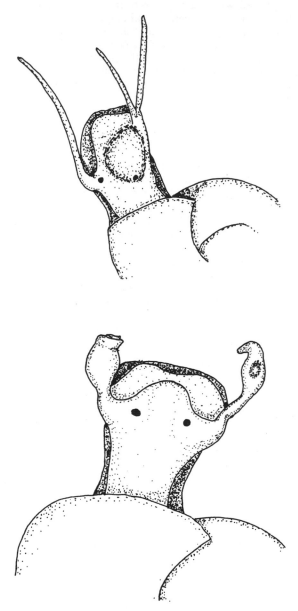

FIGURE 9 (*top*). Diagrammatic sketch that shows a specimen with a buccal gland tumor. Note also that this snail has a bifurcate right tentacle.

FIGURE 10 (*bottom*). Diagrammatic sketch that shows a specimen with abnormal tentacles. The abnormality of the left tentacle is thought to be hereditary; that of the right one arose spontaneously.

ciated with another genetic anomaly, an everted preputium; however, in this specimen, the preputium was normal.

Microscopically, the left tentacle was found covered with short, ciliated, columnar epithelial cells. The inner core of the tentacle was characterized by dense connective tissue and a noticeable lack of loose connective fibers radiating to the epithelium (FIGURE 14). A slight increase in muscle fibers was also apparent. The nuclei of a small proportion of connective tissue cells were hypertrophic, and some of the connective tissue cells had nuclei with questionable mitotic figures. The tentacular nerve and artery were present and appeared normal.

The microscopic structure of the right tentacle was quite different from that of the left one. The proximal portion of the tentacle was covered with an epithelium that resembled that found in a normal snail: tall to moderate, ciliated, columnar cells; however, as one progressed toward the tip of the tentacle, the epithelium became more and more compressed. The nuclei of these compressed cells were distorted, and the cilia were greatly reduced.

Identification of the opaque region could not be made with certainty; however, a portion of the central artery, in what was judged to be the region of opacity, was composed of hypertrophic endothelial cells filled with large amounts of pigment.

The tentacular artery and nerve were clearly seen in the proximal portion of the tentacle, but all traces of discrete structure were lost near the tip of the tentacle. In the proximal portion of the tentacle, the core consisted of dense connective tissue, longitudinal and circular muscle fibers, and scattered pigment cells (FIGURE 15). A decrease in the amount of dense connective tissue and an increase in loose vacuolated tissue were noted as one progressed toward the distal end of the tentacle. The subterminal region consisted of a reduced core of dense connective tissue, from which radiated hypertrophic bands of fibroblasts. Near the tip, large areas of aplasia occurred, and the distalmost portion of the tentacle was composed of completely disorganized tissue elements (FIGURE 16). No microorganisms or parasites were found in the tentacle, and factors that induced this abnormal growth remain unknown.

An unusual feature of this snail was the presence of a large bacterial lesion. This lesion was situated in an area bound by the hindgut, the terminal portion of the salivary glands, and the esophagus. The lesion resembled the type-2 lesions described by Pan [22] and was characterized by hyperactivity of the connective tissue elements. In this lesion, there were numerous hypertrophic amoebocytes filled with bacteria interspersed among hypertrophic fibroblasts. Mitotic activity was noted in the nuclei of the fibroblasts, and dividing forms were observed. The lesion appeared to be invasive and actually destroyed a portion of the hindgut. Although bacteria were common in the lesion per se, it should be noted that there was no evidence of bacteria in either of the tentacles or in other tissues.

DISCUSSION AND SUMMARY

Considerable uncertainty exists in our attempt and those of others to identify and characterize tumors in gastropods and other invertebrates. As a formal discipline, invertebrate oncology is still in its infancy and has progressed little beyond the stage of simple description. The lack of a sufficiently large number

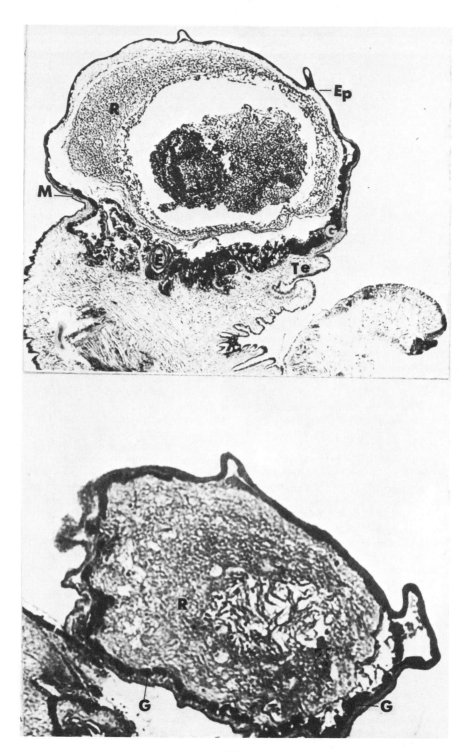

of observations and case histories has impeded efforts to establish firm criteria for evaluating neoplastic growth in these animals. Criteria established for vertebrates are not truly applicable, as noted by Scharrer and Lochhead[1] and by Sparks,[3, 23] because these organisms differ from vertebrates and among themselves with respect to cellular organization and physiology. Moreover, as indicated by Scharrer and Lochhead[1] and by Sparks,[3] it is frequently difficult, if not at times impossible, to differentiate in invertebrate tissues (as in vertebrates) between neoplasia, hyperplasia, and hypertrophy. Thus, in the absence of firm criteria, judgments of what constitutes neoplastic growth are frequently subjective. In mollusks, as in other groups of invertebrates, the pathologist and oncologist are frequently hampered by a lack of information about the normal histology of the species under study. Fortunately, this is not the case with *B. glabrata,* because there exist several excellent studies by Pan[22, 24, 25] and by others[26-31] on the normal histology and the histopathologic responses of this snail to various insults.

Our evaluations, therefore, of the series of growths observed in *B. glabrata* must be judged in the context of the limitations previously noted. The pseudobranchial growths appear, to us at least, to be examples of hyperplasia rather than neoplasia. The tissues of these growths appeared in all cases to resemble that of the pseudobranch, mitotic activity was minimal, and no indication of new or abnormal tissue elements were observed. To be sure, the frequency of occurrence and the regularity of the growths at particular sites suggest that some clonal strains of *B. glabrata* may have a tendency to produce hyperplastic growths in response to various stresses. Fifty percent of the snails with this type of growth were found infected with microorganisms, and several others exhibited abnormal pigmentation indicative of stress. The frequency with which we have found yeast or microsporidian-like organisms in laboratory and field colonies of *B. glabrata* suggests that a true picture of hyperplasia and neoplasia may only be possible in specially cultured "pathogen-free" snails. One such strain has already been developed.[22]

Neither the simple foot polyp nor the fungiform growth observed on the sole of the foot appears to be a true example of neoplasia. In the first case, the polyp seems to be an extension of normal tissues, with no evidence of increased mitotic activity or the presence of new or abnormal tissue elements. Although the causative factors that initiate the growth are unknown, it could well be a simple hyperplastic response to a previous injury. The fungiform growth, on the other hand, appears to be a response to a bacterial infection and probably represents an example of rapid hyperplastic growth rather than neoplasia.

The growth on the mantle collar appears to have characteristics of both a true tumor and of a hyperplastic response and is difficult to categorize. The structure is entirely foreign to the mantle, and the presence of numerous mitotic figures suggests active and rapid growth, yet the tissue elements do not differ from those found in normal mantle tissue.

Of the series of specimens studied, the buccal gland growth and the hooked tentacle both appear to be examples of true neoplastic growth. The buccal

---

FIGURE 11 (*top*). Longitudinal section through anterior region of snail that shows the presence of a buccal gland tumor. E, eye; Tc, tentacle; M, muscle layer; Ep, compacted epithelium; R, collagen-like reticulum. Azure II-eosin; ×84.5.

FIGURE 12 (*bottom*). Section through buccal gland tumor to show collagen-like reticulum that fills the core. R, reticulum; G, gland cells. Azure II-eosin; ×166.

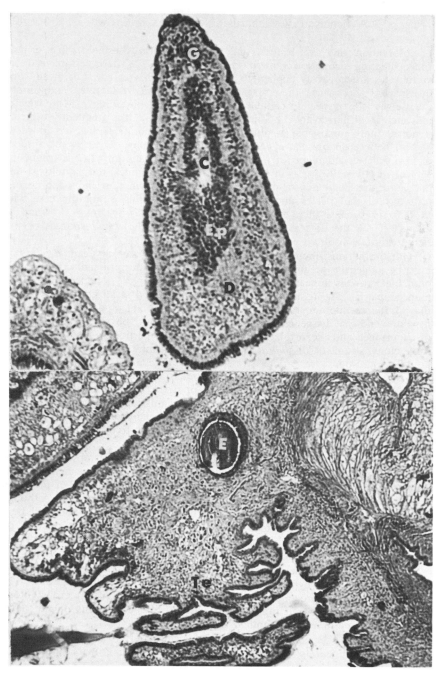

FIGURE 13 (*top*). Longitudinal section through mantle collar growth. Although only a portion of the internal channel is observed in this section, it runs from the tip to the base of the growth. Ep, epithelium lining inner channel; D, dense connective tissue; G, gland cells; C, inner channel. Azure II-eosin; ×166.

FIGURE 14 (*bottom*). Oblique section through a foreshortened tentacle. This growth appears to be hereditary in certain clones of *B. glabrata*. The growth is characterized by the lack of loose connective tissue fibers radiating from a central core to the external epithelium. E, eye; Te, tentacle. Azure II-eosin; ×166.

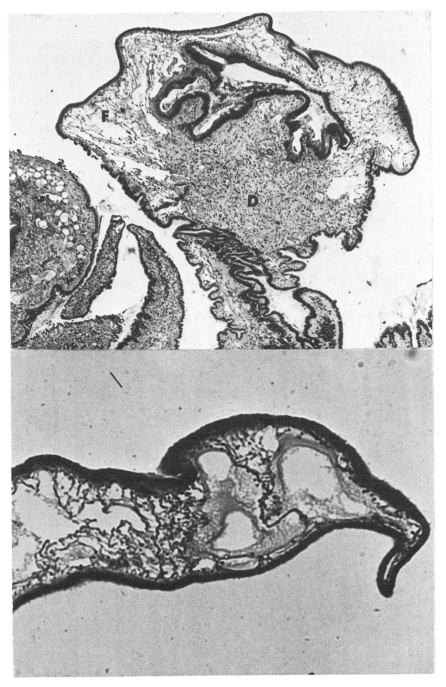

FIGURE 15 (*top*). Semioblique section through left hooked tentacle shown in FIG-URE 13. Section represents portion near swollen midregion of tentacle. D, dense connective tissue core; F, radiating loose connective tissue elements, including fibroblasts. Azure II-eosin; ×84.5.

FIGURE 16 (*bottom*). Longitudinal section through tip portion of hooked tentacle. Note complete disorganization of tissue elements and large regions of aplasia. Azure II-eosin; ×166.

gland growth exhibited invasiveness, abnormal tissue elements, and considerable mitotic activity. On the other hand, mitotic activity was absent in the tissues of the hooked tentacle; however, tissue disorganization and an alteration of normal tissue structure were present.

As noted previously, the classification of these growths is subjective and is fraught with uncertainty. The need to continue to accumulate additional examples of abnormal growth in mollusks is an obvious requisite for the development of any scheme for the eventual classification of tumor-like growths.

ACKNOWLEDGMENTS

We thank Miss Lorin DuBois and Mrs. Lucija Kaulins for their technical assistance and Dr. Steve Pan for his aid in preparing the photographs.

REFERENCES

1. SCHARRER, B. & M. S. LOCHHEAD. 1950. Tumors in the invertebrates: a review. Cancer Res. **10**: 403–419.
2. PAULEY, G. B. 1969. A critical review of neoplasia and tumor-like lesions in mollusks. Nat. Cancer Inst. Mon. **31**: 509–539.
3. SPARKS, A. K. 1972. Invertebrate Pathology. Academic Press, Inc. New York, N.Y.
4. SZABÓ, I. & M. SZABÓ. 1934. Epitheliale Geschwulstbildung bei einem wirbellosen Tier *Limax flavus* L. Z. Krebsforsch. **40**: 540–545.
5. GERSCH, M. 1950. Über Zellwucherungen und Geschwulstbildung in der Lunge von *Helix*. II. Beitrag zur Frage der Zellentartung bei Wirbellosen. Biol. Zentr. **69**: 500–507.
6. FRÖMMING, E., H. PETER & W. REICHMUTH. 1961. Beitrag zur Frage der pathologischen Gestaltsveränderung und der Geschwulste bei unseren Nacktschnecken. Zool. Anz. **166**: 139–147.
7. NOLTE, A. 1962. Eine Geschwulstbildung bei, *Helix pomatia* L. Z. Zellforsch. Mikroskop. Anat. **56**: 149–156.
8. MICHELSON, E. H. 1972. A neoplasm in the giant African snail *Achatina fulica*. J. Invert. Pathol. **20**: 264–267.
9. FISCHER, P. H. 1954. Tumeur fibreuse chez un Pleurobranche. J. Conchyl. **94**: 99–101.
10. KRIEG, K. 1968. Experimentelle Kanzerogenese bei Mollusken. 1. Mitteilung: Chemisch induzierte epitheliale Tumoren bei der La-Plata-Apfelschnecke *Ampullarius australis* d'Orbigny (Gastropoda, Prosobranchia). Arch. Geschwulstforsch. **32**: 20–34.
11. KRIEG, K. 1969. Experimentelle Kanzerogenese bei Mollusken. 2. Mitteilung: Transplantationsversuche mit einem bei der La-Plata-Apfelschnecke *Ampullarius australis* d'Orbigny (Gastropoda, Prosobranchia) chemisch induzierten adenopapillom. Arch. Geschwulstforsch. **33**: 18–30.
12. KRIEG, K. 1969. Experimentelle Kanzerogenese bei Mollusken. 3. Mitteilung: Weitere Untersuchungen zur Geschwulstbildung bei der La-Plata-Apfelschnecke *Ampullarius australis* d'Orbigny (Gastropoda, Prosobranchia) unter besonderer Berücksichtingung des Methylcholanthrens. Arch. Geschwulstforsch. **33**: 255–267.
13. KRIEG, K. 1970. Experimentelle Kanzerogenese bei Mollusken. 4. Mitteilung: Verleichende Untersuchungen zur Geschwulstbildung bei Land-und-Wasserschnecken. Arch. Geschwulstforsch. **35**: 109–113.
14. RICHARDS, C. S. 1973. Genetics of *Biomphalaria glabrata* (Gastropoda: Planorbidae). Malacolog. Rev. **6**: 199–202.

15. RICHARDS, C. S. 1973. Bulbous head growths of *Biomphalaria glabrata:* genetic studies. J. Invert. Pathol. **22:** 278–282.
16. RICHARDS, C. S. 1973. Tumors in the pulmonary cavity of *Biomphalaria glabrata:* genetic studies. J. Invert. Pathol. **22:** 283–289.
17. RICHARDS, C. S. 1974. Antler tentacles of *Biomphalaria glabrata:* genetic studies. J. Invert. Pathol. **24:** 49–54.
18. RICHARDS, C. S. 1974. Everted preputium and swollen tentacles in *Biomphalaria glabrata:* genetic studies. J. Invert. Pathol. **24:** 159–164.
19. RICHARDS, C. S. & J. W. MERRITT, JR. 1972. Genetic factors in the susceptibility of juvenile *Biomphalaria glabrata* to *Schistosoma mansoni* infection. Amer. J. Trop. Med. Hyg. **21:** 425–434.
20. RICHARDS, C. S. 1967. Genetic studies on *Biomphalaria glabrata* (Basommatophora: Planorbidae), a third pigmentation allele. Malacologia **5:** 335–340.
21. CRUZ, O. & E. DIAS. 1953. *Bacillus pinottii* sp. n. Trans. Roy. Soc. Trop. Med. Hyg. **47:** 581, 582.
22. PAN, C.-T. 1965. Studies on the host-parasite relationship between *Schistosoma mansoni* and the snail *Australorbis glabratus.* Amer. J. Trop. Med. Hyg. **14:** 931–976.
23. SPARKS, A. K. 1969. Review of tumors and tumor-like conditions in Protozoa, Coelenterata, Platyhelminthes, Annelida, Sipunculida, and Arthropods, excluding insects. Nat. Cancer Inst. Mon. **31:** 671–682.
24. PAN, C.-T. 1958. The general histology and topographic microanatomy of *Australorbis glabratus.* Bull. Museum Comp. Zool. Harvard Coll. **119:** 237–299.
25. PAN, C.-T. 1963. Generalized and focal tissue responses in the snail, *Australorbis glabratus* infected with *Schistosoma mansoni.* Ann. N.Y. Acad. Sci. **113:** 475–485.
26. BARTH, R. & G. JANSEN. 1959. Contribuicões ao estudo da gametogênese dos planorbideos. I. parto. Célula nutridora e sua funcão. An. Acad. Brasil. Cienc. **31:** 429–445.
27. BARTH, R. & G. JANSEN. 1960. Ueber der begriff "Kinoplasma" in der spermiogenese von *Australorbis glabratus olivaceus* (Mollusca, Pulmonata, Planorbidae). Mem. Inst. Oswaldo Cruz **58:** 209–228.
28. DE JONG-BRINK, M. 1969. Histochemical and electron microscope observations on the reproductive tract of *Biomphalaria glabrata* (*Australorbis glabratus*), intermediate host of *Schistosoma mansoni.* Z. Zellforsch. **102:** 507–542.
29. MICHELSON, E. H. 1961. An acid-fast pathogen of fresh-water snails. Amer. J. Trop. Med. Hyg. **10:** 423–433.
30. TRIPP, M. R. 1961. The fate of foreign materials experimentally introduced into the snail *Australorbis glabratus.* J. Parasitol. **47:** 745–751.
31. SMINIA, T., H. H. BOER & A. NIEMANTSVERDRIET. 1972. Haemoglobin producing cells in freshwater snails. Z. Zellforsch. **135:** 563–568.

SECONDARY DAUGHTER SPOROCYSTS OF *SCHISTOSOMA MANSONI*: THEIR OCCURRENCE AND CULTIVATION *

Eder L. Hansen

561 Santa Barbara Road
Berkeley, California 94707

INTRODUCTION

The interest in secondary daughter sporocysts of *Schistosoma mansoni* arose initially out of our experience with cultivation of primary daughter sporocysts. When cultured, they gave rise to secondary daughter sporocysts that emerged into the medium.[1, 2] When implanted into the snail, they multiplied before producing cercariae.[3] There had been only a few previous reports suggesting that *S. mansoni* can depart from the generally recognized development pattern, in which a single generation of daughter sporocysts precedes cercarial production, the secondary daughter sporocysts being found only rarely and then only as a regenerative phase in old infections.[4, 5] Further studies on secondary daughter sporocysts in infected snails and their *in vitro* cultivation have now been made.

MATERIALS AND METHODS

These studies were conducted with albino [6] *Biomphalaria glabrata* infected with a Puerto Rican strain of *S. mansoni*. Procedures for infecting the snails have been described by Lim and Heyneman.[7] After an initial period of 6 days at 26–27° C, infected snails were placed at 17 or 20° C in the dark. They are referred to below as "low-temperature" snails. They served as a source of secondary sporocysts from Days 42 to 103.

The implantation technique was simplified from those of Chernin [8] and Dönges.[9] Sporocysts were placed in the digestive gland or pericardial region, after selecting the exact location through the semitransparent shell. A finely tapered glass capillary pipette operated by mouth pressure was used for delivery of the sporocysts. The shell could usually be punctured by the pipette tip. Delivery of individual sporocysts could be observed directly under a dissecting microscope and could be checked by rinsing the tip in a drop of culture medium. Aseptic techniques were employed throughout. The snails were handled gently, so that they were not retracted. Consequently, the use of relaxants was abandoned after preliminary trials. There was very little loss of hemolymph through the tiny hole, and it was found better to leave the puncture uncovered than to apply sealing materials. Recipient snails were placed on a moist towel for about 15 min, then transferred to autoclaved aquarium water and kept overnight. The

* Supported by National Institute of Allergy and Infectious Diseases Grant A1-07359 and by Contract NO1-A1-22525 for work at the former Clinical Pharmacology Research Institute, Berkeley, Calif.

next day, they were maintained on lettuce in individual beakers at 26–27° C with a photo period from 9 AM to 4 PM. After 15 days, the water was checked daily for cercariae.

Secondary daughter sporocysts were axenized from parasitized tissues by the following procedures. Low-temperature snails were washed in 70% alcohol, soaked in antibiotics for about 2 hr, then placed in sterile aquarium water, and kept overnight at 27° C. The next day, they were again soaked in antibiotics. The shell was removed, and the snail was placed in saline that contained antibiotics. The digestive gland and rectal ridge were rapidly dissected and cut into small pieces. These pieces were placed in dishes of trypsin [0.05% in calcium and magnesium-free saline with 0.2 mM ethylenediaminetetraacetate (EDTA)] for 1–2 hr at 37° C and then moved to medium that contained antibiotics. Small motile daughter sporocysts were found free in the medium. Larger sporocysts were gently teased out. Cercarial embryos were liberated by disrupting distended sporocysts. The parasites were collected and passed through washes of medium. They were then implanted into recipient snails or inoculated into *in vitro* cultures. The preparative procedures were conveniently performed in covered Bureau of Plant Industry watch glasses. The composition of the antibiotic and trypsin solutions and the salines used to adjust the osmolality to 125–170 mOsm has been described previously.[10]

Procedures for *in vitro* cultivation and study of sporocyst development in culture were adapted from those used in the cultivation of primary daughter sporocysts.[1, 11] Each culture was inoculated with five to 10 small secondary daughters, three to 23 larger sporocysts, or 10 cercarial embryos. The medium described by Buecher et al.[11] was used at one-half fold, and one-half-fold Chernin's salts,[12] nucleic acid precursors at 0.5 μM, and MEM vitamins were added. It was conveniently prepared by mixing equal parts of media M260 and S301.[10] HEPES buffer was added at 3 mM, and dithiothreitol (DTT) at 0.1 mM. The gas phase contained 9% O_2, 0.04% or 0.3% CO_2, and the remainder was N_2. Control cultures without DTT were incubated in humidified air. Inactivated fetal calf serum was included in the medium at 10%. In one experiment, serum was decreased to 0.5%, and 4.5% snail hemolymph was added. The hemolymph had been collected from infected snails, diluted with an equal volume of saline that contained 0.1 mM DTT, filtered for sterility through a Millipore membrane of 0.3 μm porosity, and stored in frozen aliquots.

Synxenic cultures with cells of the Bge cell line[13] were overlaid with the same medium but without addition of DTT or control of the gas phase. Sporocysts were placed directly on the cell layer in 3-cm plastic petri dishes or were placed in Nuclepore chambers.[1]

Sporocyst morphology was examined in both fresh and stained specimens after cultivation or after teasing from snail tissue. Chromosomes were examined in preparations fixed in acetic acid-alcohol and squashed in aceto-orcein.

RESULTS

In snails held at 26–27° C, motile daughter sporocysts were first seen under the tunica propria of the digestive gland on the eighth day after miracidial infection. They were numerous by Day 12. Secondary daughter sporocysts were first found on Day 14. They were contained within sporocysts embedded in the interfollicular connective tissue. They were found also later in the infection;

a dissection made 75 days postinfection is shown in FIGURE 1. The secondary daughter sporocysts occurred in groups of two to eight within thin-walled sporocysts that lay in the more normal appearing tissue of the digestive gland and rectal ridge. From Day 21 on, most of the sporocysts were distended with tailed cercariae and cercarial embryos. Shedding began on Day 25.

Mother sporocysts were found in the digestive gland in only one snail. They were noted on Day 11; one lay under the tunica propria, the other was deep in the distal portion of the gland. Both were large and convoluted and contained

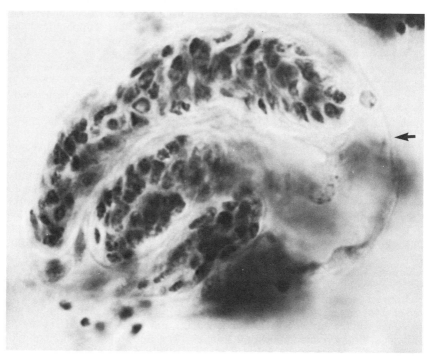

FIGURE 1. Three secondary daughter sporocysts, approximately 90 μm long, contained within a daughter sporocyst wall (arrow). Teased from the digestive gland of *B. glabrata* 76 days after infection with *S. mansoni* incubated at 27.5 ± 0.5° C. Feulgen-fast green stain.

22 and 25 motile daughters, rspectively, and many embryos. All other mother sporocysts were found in their normal location in the head and foot regions.

With low-temperature snails, a few cercariae were shed from those kept at 20° C but none from those at 17° C. On dissection, the 17° C snails were found to contain only sporocysts. The digestive gland and rectal ridge were heavily parasitized with short motile forms, 120–260 μm long, and with long entwined sporocysts more than 500 μm long that were embedded in the connective tissue. The motile forms contained germinal cells; the embedded sporocysts contained embryos and six to eight motile secondary daughters. In the 20° C snails, some of the sporocysts were distended with partially developed cercariae.

In Vitro *Cultivation*

Small secondary daughter sporocysts introduced into axenic culture retained good motility for 3 days. They gradually became more sluggish but remained alive for up to 11 days and grew to 350 μm. There was no development of embryos within them nor appearance of tegumental processes. In media without gas phase adjustment, the sporocysts survived for less than 5 days.

In synxenic cultures, with Bge tissue culture, secondary daughter sporocysts survived for 16 days, reaching a length of 480 μm. Development was best in the culture in which hemolymph from an infected snail had been added to replace part of the fetal calf serum. The sporocysts became covered with the Bge cells by 8 days. This experiment was terminated at 12 days to permit detailed examination. Sporocysts had grown to 370 × 60 μm and contained active flame cells. They were densely packed with clear large germinal cells, and clusters of five to six cells could be discerned in the posterior region of the lumen.

Large sporocysts, 700–1500 μm long and 90–155 μm wide, remained viable in culture as long as 38 days. Motility of the sporocyst apical cone was observed, as were spasmodic contractions in response to light. Tegumental processes, present on sporocysts from both the rectal ridge and digestive gland, persisted for 20 days. The processes were sticky and held the sporocysts together as they became entwined during cultivation. The best culture was a group of 23 sporocysts from the rectal ridge. The largest sporocyst was observed for the first 17 days before it became too entangled with the others to be observed individually. It grew from 900 × 60 μm to 2000 × 100 μm. Twenty-seven secondary daughters and two cercariae emerged from the 23 parental sporocysts over a period of 35 days. The secondary daughters were transferred to other cultures and were maintained up to 8 days, growing from 90 to 300 μm.

Other large sporocysts from the 20° C snails, and showing well-developed cercariae, shed during the first 5 days in culture, averaging four cercariae per sporocyst.

Cercarial embryos developed in only two sporocysts. Two cercariae were shed on Day 13 and one on Day 21. Embryos did, however, develop rapidly if they were first freed from the sporocysts. Most of the larger elongate embryos and those that had tail buds developed cercarial tails. Small round embryos, 30–40 μm in diameter (stage III in the description by Cheng and Bier [14]) also developed. Of 30 such embryos, nine developed tails, and 11 more showed short tails, reaching this stage in 4–7 days. They exhibited swimming and contractile motility for a further 5 days. This development occurred in synxenic cultures. Under axenic conditions, there was only partial tail growth in 10 of 60 embryos.

Cercarial embryos of still smaller size could not be cultured. They disintegrated into balls of cells, a finding that is consistent with the sequence of changes that have been observed in the early cercarial wall.[15, 16]

Implantation

Individual secondary daughter sporocysts were implanted into 37 snails. Only one implant was successful, a lower "take" than the 10% experienced with implants of primary daughter sporocysts. Five cercariae were shed on

Day 63, followed by yields of four to 86 per day until, 9 days later, the rate suddenly increased to more than 150 per day. This rate was maintained for the next 8 days, at which time the snail was sacrificed for examination. It was heavily parasitized in both the digestive gland and rectal ridge. In addition to the sporocysts that produced cercariae, there were numerous motile sporocysts 225 × 30 μm, as well as embedded sporocysts about 600 × 35 μm that contained three to six motile sporocysts, which thus constituted at least a fourth generation of daughter sporocysts.

The long prepatent period seen in this snail occurred also in implants of individual primary daughters. For example, in one snail implanted with a primary daughter sporocyst, the first cercaria was shed on Day 34, followed by a second one on Day 53. Shedding then continued at a rate of three to 60 per day, until the snail died 105 days after implantation. On dissection, the digestive gland and rectal ridge were found to be heavily parasitized. Some of the sporocysts were very large; they contained more than 100 active tailed cercariae at the time of autopsy.

Embryo Morphology

Embryos from mother sporocysts were compared with those from sporocysts producing cercariae. In live preparations, cercarial embryos were more refractile than were the sporocyst embryos. In Feulgen-stained preparations, nuclei in sporocyst embryos were large, vesicular, and lightly stained, and wall cells could be distinguished. In cercarial embryos, the nuclei were smaller and more densely stained, and wall cells could not be seen. In small embryos, cells were twice as numerous in cercarial as in sporocyst embryos. For example, in an 18-μm diameter embryo from a mother sporocyst, there were 24 cells, whereas in a cercaria-type embryo of the same diameter, there were 42 cells.

A further characteristic of cercarial embryos was a bluish appearance with Feulgen stain when examined under phase-contrast microscopy. The distinctive embryo cells can still be distinguished in the black and white reproduction (FIGURE 2).

Well-developed cercariae or elongate cercarial embryos were not found in sporocysts that also contained developing secondary daughters. However, small embryos with a characteristic cercarial appearance were found in the anterior region of sporocysts in which developing secondary daughters lay in the posterior lumen.

Meiosis-type metaphases that showed eight pairs of chromosomes, including one heteromorphic pair, that had been noted in developing sporocyst embryos were also seen in cells of early cercarial embryos. They therefore were not a distinguishing characteristic.

DISCUSSION

The life cycle of the digenetic trematode *S. mansoni* in the snail *B. glabrata* consists of a series of morphologic changes. The snail is first invaded by a miracidium that remains near the site of penetration and transforms to a mother sporocyst. The mother gives rise to many daughter sporocysts that migrate and are carried by the hemolymph to be entrapped in the connective tissue of the interfollicular areas of the digestive gland, between the acini of the gonad, and within the folds of the rectal ridge. The daughters enlarge and produce many cercariae. The latter break through the sporocyst wall, which rapidly heals. They migrate and are carried by the hemolymph to emerge from the snail at moist vascularized surfaces, particularly the mantle edge and pseudobranch. The two phases of multiplication have been well documented. However, a few authors considered the possibility of a second generation of daughter sporocysts. Lim and Heyneman [7] reviewed the early work that first proposed and then discounted the occurrence of this additional sporocyst generation. Pearson [17]

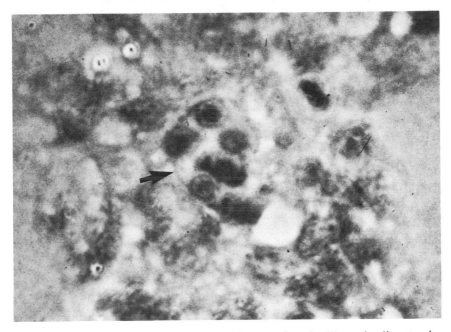

FIGURE 2. Early cercarial embryo (arrow) approximately 10 μm in diameter in *S. mansoni* teased from the digestive gland of *B. glabrata* incubated at 20° C for 60 days. Feulgen-fast green stain, viewed with a Leitz phase-contrast microscope under oil immersion.

noted that to be restricted to a single daughter generation puts an inexplicable difference between daughter sporocysts and rediae.

By implanting secondary daughter sporocysts where their progeny could be traced, we were able to show that at least four generations of daughter sporocysts occurred. It is therefore quite possible that a series of infections of *S. mansoni* could be maintained by sporocyst multiplication after implantation, as Dönges [18] has shown occurs with rediae of echinostomes. This technique could be used to provide a continually available source of sporocysts for experimental work.

Several observations made by other authors can best be accounted for by occurrence of secondary daughter sporocysts as part of the normal cycle in the snail. For example, the number of cercariae shed was not related to the number of miracidia that initiated the infection.[19] The number of sporocysts in infected tissue can exceed the estimated potential [1] of 200 daughters from one mother sporocyst. Small motile daughters have been reported in heavily parasitized tissue from old infections [20] and were noted by Chernin [12] in culture of infected digestive gland fragments. These small sporocysts could be inhibited forms or could have been late arrivals from a mother sporocyst. However, we have not been able to find active daughter sporocysts in mothers older than 27 days. When old mother sporocysts could be detected in the tissue, they contained no embryos and only a few residual daughters, which were sluggish, large, and granular.

By implantation, we were able to demonstrate sporocyst multiplication and had hoped to provide a reasonable answer to the question of the reproductive potential of a miracidium. The long prepatent period after implantation of individual sporocysts and the ensuing stepwise cercarial output suggest that several generations of daughter sporocysts formed. The distribution of sporocysts was discernible through the snail shell, but the organs were partly obscured, and exact observation of increased distribution of sporocysts was not possible. On dissection, they were found to be too tightly entwined to be counted. The large numbers of cercariae retained in some of the sporocysts made it unreliable to attempt to relate number of sporocysts to cercarial shedding. Faust and Hoffman [21] had estimated a yield of several thousand cercariae per sporocyst. In the two implantations that remained as single sporocysts, about 400 cercariae were counted from each, either shed or remaining in the sporocyst.[22] From these two snails, cercariae were first shed on Days 22 and 24 postimplantation.

In view of the possibility that secondary daughters were part of the normal development cycle, we searched for this stage in early infections and found them on Day 14 postinfection. Among the numerous sporocysts that contained cercarial embryos, there were many that contained secondary daughter sporocysts. These sporocysts were easily distinguishable from the two mother sporocysts that were found on a single occasion in the digestive gland. Mother sporocysts have been only rarely reported from the deeper organs.[20, 23]

Additional confirmation was obtained by examination of field-infected snails collected in Puerto Rico.[1] On careful examination, and aided by an exact knowledge of what we were looking for, sporocysts that contained well-developed secondary daughters were found. They were difficult to find because they were small compared to the large swollen sporocysts that contained cercariae. They were transparent and were located deep in the interlobular areas of the digestive gland. It is easy to see how they could have been overlooked by earlier investigators. Except under special circumstances, such as implantation of single daughters, their presence is obscured by the rapid development of all phases in the snail and by the resultant large number of sporocysts that produce cercariae. This finding in field-infected snails ensures that secondary daughters were not merely an artefact of laboratory conditions or a peculiarity of the albino snail that we were using.

The question of what factors determine the direction of development either to cercariae or secondary daughters could not be solved. Clearly, temperature is important, and cercarial production is decreased or arrested at low temperatures.[24, 25] Our finding that reduction in cercarial production is accompanied by an increased production of secondary daughter sporocysts is parallel to the development of daughter rediae reported [26] in *Fasciola gigantica* in response to low temperatures. In contrast to the morphologic differences that aided in distinguishing the successive generations of rediae, none could be detected to separate the secondary sporocyst generations.

The exact location of sporocysts in the digestive gland and rectal ridge does not appear to be a determining factor. Secondary daughters occurred immediately adjacent to sporocysts that contained large cercarial embryos.[22] Nor was the key a response to crowding, because secondary daughter sporocysts were found both in early infections and in densely parasitized tissue. It was noted, however, that in the latter, the secondary daughters were deep in the interlobular areas, embedded in tissue that had retained its normal appearance. Meuleman [27] had noted the persistence in heavily infected *B. pfeifferi* of areas that had retained functional morphology.

The question of the succession of generations could not be answered. Lie [4] had found a mature cercariae and a mature sporocyst within the same regenerated sporocyst. Embryos of the two forms have usually been considered to be indistinguishable,[28] but Maldonado and Acosta [20] did note that cercarial embryos were less granular. We, however, noted several distinguishing characteristics between the two types of embryos. Several sporocysts that contained secondary daughters and embryos with cercarial characteristics were observed. This finding suggests that secondary daughters mature first, followed by development of cercariae.

The overall objective of our study was the cultivation of larval stages of *S. mansoni in vitro*. Information from these cultures was used continually to further our understanding of the infection in the snail. For the present series of cultures of sporocysts isolated from the internal organs, the methods described for cultivation of primary daughters [1, 11] were modified to allow for the more extensive sterilization treatments that were required.

The initial finding that only secondary daughter sporocysts were produced *in vitro* raised the possibility that the culture conditions could not support the new cell formation and the differentiation that occurs in cercarial development. We had hoped to test this directly by promoting cercarial development in secondary daughter sporocysts. However, contrary to our expectations, these sporocysts proved difficult to culture. It is possible that the preparative treatment with antibiotics and trypsin had an inhibitory influence. Damaged cells from the host digestive gland may also have contributed to the inhibiting effects, because we found that sporocysts recovered from the rectal ridge responded better in culture than did those from the digestive gland.

The suitability of the medium for cercarial development was later shown by their development from small embryos that had been liberated from the parent sporocyst. This raises the possibility that under the conditions of *in vitro* culture, the sporocyst wall impedes the availability of nutrients. Furthermore, these cercariae maintained motility for 4–5 days and may provide a means for study of axenic cercariae. Those that had developed from free embryos exhibited a considerable degree of extensibility.

The vertebrate serum component of the medium introduced a continuing problem. The source of the variable toxicity could not be identified. Diconza and Basch [29] found it necessary to use a selected donor. Our work was performed with selected lots of commercial fetal calf serum. In the experiment with filtered hemolymph from infected snails, there was improved sporocyst morphology.

Media of widely differing composition have been used for cultivation of sporocysts.[1, 2, 29] In the current series, the medium was adjusted to include components that had been favorable in snail tissue culture.[10] However, in all cultures to date, sporocyst development *in vitro* is much below that *in vivo*. The balance of components can undoubtedly be improved, and, just as has been shown with defined media for vertebrate tissue culture,[30] improved parasite growth will result.

A further improvement can be expected from adjustment of the gas phase and redox potential. Decrease in oxygen and addition of sulfhydryl compounds[11] improved culture conditions for primary sporocysts, but further adjustment may still be required to initiate development of cercariae from germinal cells. Though some guidance is given by measurements on hemolymph,[31] the extracted hemolymph may be different from that which bathes the cells.

The role of tissue culture in synxenic cultures was reviewed by Chao.[32] In our cultures with Bge cells, there was striking improvement in the sporocyst morphology. These cells were of embryonic origin. Explants of digestive gland have so far shown persistent outgrowths for 2–3 months but were insufficient for association with sporocysts. However, if such cultures can be improved, and if the cells do retain their cellular function for production of specialized compounds, the role of "snail hormone"[33] could be investigated. A culture system as complex as this one might be needed to obtain the full cycle of larval multiplication from the converted miracidium[34, 35] through successive sporocyst generations to the production of cercariae.

CONCLUSIONS

The findings of numerous secondary daughter sporocysts and four generations of daughters under laboratory conditions, their detection in routine laboratory infections and in field-infected snails, together with inferences from the observed prolonged shedding of cercariae, suggest that secondary daughters occur normally and are an important part of the life cycle in the snail. Their role is probably to ensure that there will be heavy infections, even when the miracidial infection is light, and also that the infection and cercarial production will continue for the life of the snail. Their production in culture offers the possibility of eventual study of the controlling factors for sporocyst or cercarial development.

ACKNOWLEDGMENTS

I thank Dr. D. Heyneman, with whom I had many valuable discussions, for his generous cooperation in providing infected snails and Drs. E. J. Buecher, E. A. Yarwood, and K. Hussey for their participation in portions of this investigation.

References

1. HANSEN, E. L., G. PEREZ-MENDEZ, S. LONG & E. YARWOOD. 1973. Emergence of progeny-daughter sporocysts in monoxenic culture. Exp. Parasitol. **33:** 486–494.

2. HANSEN, E. L., G. PEREZ-MENDEZ, E. YARWOOD & E. J. BUECHER. 1974. Second-generation daughter sporocysts of *Schistosoma mansoni* in axenic culture. J. Parasitol. **60:** 371, 372.

3. DICONZA, J. J. & E. L. HANSEN. 1972. Multiplication of transplanted *Schistosoma mansoni* daughter sporocysts. J. Parasitol. **58:** 181, 182.

4. LIE, K. J. 1969. Role of immature rediae in antagonism of *Paryphostomum segregatum* to *Schistosoma mansoni* and larval development in degenerated sporocysts. Z. Parasitenk. **32:** 316–323.

5. PAN, C. 1965. Studies on the host-parasite relationship between *Schistosoma mansoni* and the snail *Australorbis glabratus*. Amer. J. Trop. Med. Hyg. **14:** 931–976.

6. NEWTON, W. L. 1955. The establishment of a strain of *Australorbis glabratus* which embodies albinism and high susceptibility to infection with *Schistosoma mansoni*. J. Parasitol. **41:** 526–528.

7. LIM, H. K. & D. HEYNEMAN. 1972. Intramolluscan inter-trematode antagonism: a review of factors influencing the host-parasite system and its possible role in biological control. *In* Advances in Parasitology. B. Dawes, Ed. Vol. **10:** 192–253. Academic Press, Inc. New York, N.Y.

8. CHERNIN, E. 1966. Transplantation of larval *Schistosoma mansoni* from infected to uninfected snails. J. Parasitol. **52:** 473–482.

9. DÖNGES, J. 1968. Der beweis potentiell unbeschränkter generationsfolge bei redien von *Isthmiophora melis* (Trematoda, Echinostomatidae) durch das transplantationsexperiment. Zool. Anz. Suppl. **32:** 550–558.

10. HANSEN, E. L. 1975. A cell line from embryos of *Biomphalaria glabrata* (Pulmonata): establishment and characteristics. *In* Invertebrate Tissue Culture: Research Applications. K. Maramorosch, Ed. Academic Press, Inc. New York, N.Y. In press.

11. BUECHER, E. J., G. PEREZ-MENDEZ, E. L. HANSEN & E. YARWOOD. 1974. Sulfhydryl compounds under controlled gas in culture of *Schistosoma mansoni* sporocysts. Proc. Soc. Exp. Biol. Med. **146:** 1101–1105.

12. CHERNIN, E. 1964. Maintenance in vitro of larval *Schistosoma mansoni* in tissues from the snail, *Australorbis glabratus*. J. Parasitol. **50:** 531–545.

13. HANSEN, E. L. 1974. A cell line from the fresh water snail *Biomphalaria glabrata*. IRCS, Med. Sci. **2:** 1703.

14. CHENG, T. C. & J. W. BIER. 1972. Studies on molluscan schistosomiasis: an analysis of the development of the cercaria of *Schistosoma mansoni*. Parasitology **66:** 129–141.

15. MEULEMAN, E. A. & P. J. HOLZMANN. 1975. The development of the primitive epithelium and true tegument in the cercaria of *Schistosoma mansoni*. Z. Parasitenk. **45:** 307 318.

16. LEE, D. H. 1972. The structure of the helminth cuticle. *In* Advances in Parasitology. B. Dawes, Ed. Vol. **10:** 347–370. Academic Press, Inc. New York, N.Y.

17. PEARSON, J. C. 1972. A phylogeny of life-cycle patterns of the Digenea. *In* Advances in Parasitology. B. Dawes, Ed. Vol. **10:** 153–181. Academic Press, Inc. New York, N.Y.

18. DÖNGES, J. 1971. The potential number of redial generations in echinostomatids (Trematoda). Int. J. Parasitol. **1:** 51–59.

19. STURROCK, B. M. & R. F. STURROCK. 1970. Laboratory studies of the host-parasite relationship of *Schistosoma mansoni* and *Biomphalaria glabrata* from St. Lucia, West Indies. Ann. Trop. Med. Parasitol. **64:** 357–363.

20. MALDONADO, J. F. & J. M. ACOSTA. 1947. The development of *Schistosoma mansoni* in the snail intermediate host, *Australorbis glabratus*. Puerto Rico J. Publ. Health Trop. Med. **22:** 331–373.

21. FAUST, E. C. & W. A. HOFFMAN. 1934. Studies on Schistosomiasis mansoni in Puerto Rico. III. Biological studies. I. The extra-mammalian phases of the life cycle. Puerto Rico J. Publ. Health Trop. Med. **10:** 1–47.

22. HANSEN, E. L. 1973. Progeny daughter sporocysts of *Schistosoma mansoni*. Int. J. Parasitol. **3:** 267, 268.

23. OLIVIER, L. & C. P. MAO. 1949. The early larval stages of *Schistosoma mansoni* Sambon, 1907 in the snail host *Australorbis glabratus* (Say, 1818). J. Parasitol. **35:** 267–275.

24. FOSTER, R. 1964. The effect of temperature on the development of *Schistosoma mansoni* Sambon 1907 in the intermediate host. J. Trop. Med. Hyg. **66:** 289–291.

25. STIREWALT, M. A. 1954. Effect of snail maintenance temperature on development of *Schistosoma mansoni*. Exp. Parasitol. **3:** 504–516.

26. DINNIK, J. A. & N. N. DINNIK. 1964. The influence of temperature on the succession of redial and cecarial generations of *Fasciola gigantica* in a snail host. Parasitology **54:** 59–65.

27. MEULEMAN, E. 1972. Host-parasite interrelationships between the freshwater pulmonate *Biomphalaria pfeifferi* and the trematode *Schistosoma mansoni*. Neth. J. Zool. **22:** 355–427.

28. CORT, W. W., D. J. AMEEL & A. VAN DER WOUDE. 1954. Review: germinal development in the sporocysts and rediae of the digenetic trematodes. Exp. Parasitol. **3:** 185–225.

29. DICONZA, J. J. & P. F. BASCH. 1974. Axenic cultivation of *Schistosoma mansoni* daughter sporocysts. J. Parasitol. **60:** 757–763.

30. RICHTER, A., K. K. SANFORD & V. J. EVANS. 1972. Influence of oxygen and culture media on plating efficiency of some mammalian tissue cells. J. Nat. Cancer Inst. **49:** 1705–1712.

31. LEE, F. O. & T. C. CHENG. 1971. *Schistosoma mansoni:* respirometric and partial pressure studies in infected *Biomphalaria glabrata*. Exp. Parasitol. **30:** 393–399.

32. CHAO, J. 1973. The application of invertebrate tissue culture to the *in vitro* study of animal parasites. *In* Current Topics in Comparative Pathobiology. T. C. Cheng, Ed. Vol. **2:** 107–144. Academic Press, Inc. New York, N.Y.

33. COLES, G. C. 1970. Snail "metabolite hormone" and snail parasite metabolism. Comp. Biochem. Physiol. **34:** 213–219.

34. BASCH, P. F. & J. J. DICONZA. 1974. The miracidium-sporocyst transition in *Schistosoma mansoni:* surface changes in vitro with ultrastructural correlation. J. Parasitol. **60:** 935–941.

35. VOGE, M. & J. S. SEIDEL. 1972. Transformation in vitro of miracidia of *Schistosoma mansoni* and *S. japonicum* into young sporocysts. J. Parasitol. **58:** 699–704.

HEAVY METAL TOXICITY TO *BIOMPHALARIA GLABRATA* (MOLLUSCA: PULMONATA) *

John T. Sullivan and Thomas C. Cheng

Institute for Pathobiology
Center for Health Sciences
Lehigh University
Bethlehem, Pennsylvania 18015

INTRODUCTION

The sophistication of the invertebrate pathologist working in the field of chemical injury has not kept pace with that of the invertebrate toxicologist involved in pesticide development.[1] Except in the case of insecticides, little information exists on the toxic mechanisms of most agents used to control invertebrate vectors of disease. For example, copper as copper sulfate has been used for the preceding 50 years in attempts to control species of *Biomphalaria,* the intermediate host of *Schistosoma mansoni.* Of course, it is known that even minute concentrations of copper are lethal to snails, particularly in waters of low alkalinity, turbidity, and organic content.[2] As little as 0.07 ppm of copper as $CuSO_4$ in deionized water effects 100% mortality of *B. glabrata* within 72 hr under specific conditions of exposure.[3] However, there is little information on precisely how this mollusk is killed by copper.

Exposure to toxic concentrations of the cupric ion causes a lowering of the oxygen consumption rate in *B. glabrata.*[4] It is possible, however, that this decline is due to the rapid retraction of the snail into its shell upon exposure to copper and, consequently, to a decrease in surface area available for uptake of oxygen rather than to a direct effect of the copper on the oxygen consumption of the snail.

A characteristic behavior of *B. glabrata* in response to toxic concentrations of copper is the so-called distress syndrome, during which the snail displays the same intoxicated behavior as when exposed to narcotizing agents, such as Nembutal® or menthol.[5] It is inferred from this observation that the toxic mechanism involves a neuromuscular phenomenon, because the autonomous ciliary beat of the ciliary epithelium is not altered.

Measurement of the uptake of ^{64}Cu by distressed *B. glabrata,* that is, those exposed to toxic levels of copper, and nondistressed *B. glabrata,* that is, those exposed to nontoxic levels of copper, demonstrates that nondistressed snails accumulate ^{64}Cu in the digestive gland, whereas distressed snails do not.[6] From these data, it is concluded that the permeability of the surface epithelial membranes is disrupted, which thus accounts for less uptake of ^{64}Cu by the digestive glands of distressed snails. Furthermore, it is hypothesized that toxicity is due to this disruption of membrane permeability rather than to the inhibition of some metabolic process.[6]

* Supported by Grant INCRA-193 fom the International Copper Research Association, Inc. Materials used in this study were provided by the U.S.-Japan Cooperative Medical Science Program—National Institute of Allergy and Infectious Diseases.

Copper sulfate inhibits the oxidation of exogenous succinate, glutamate, and reduced tetramethyl-*p*-phenylenediamine (TMPD) by tissue homogenates of *B. alexandrina*.[7] The ability of copper and other heavy metals to interfere with enzyme-mediated pathways is attributed to complex formation between the metal and ligands on the enzyme, substrate, activators, or cofactors that contain sulfur, nitrogen, or oxygen atoms that serve as electron donors.[8] However, there is no evidence at this time that copper exerts its cidal effect on gastropods by direct inhibition of intracellular enzymatic reactions.

Toxic concentrations of copper as copper sulfate have a measurable inhibitory effect on the heart rate of *B. glabrata*.[9] It is speculated, however, that this effect is due to the retraction of the snail into its shell rather than to a direct inhibition of the heart beat by copper. Furthermore, it is known from a study on the effects of two copper compounds, copper (II)-ethylenediamine-*N,N,N′*, *N′*-tetraacetic acid (CuEDTA) and copper (II)-bis-*N,N*-dihydroxyethylglycine [Cu(DEG)$_2$], on the oxygen consumption and survival of *B. glabrata* that the toxicity is inversely correlated with the steric hindrance of the copper.[10] In other words, copper must be exposed in the stereochemical sense to be molluscidal.

Several investigators have employed radioisotopic heavy metals in autoradiographic studies. The deposition of ^{64}Cu in the ovotestis of *B. glabrata* and in the albumin gland of *B. pfeifferi* has been reported.[11] In this study, snails exposed to copper for up to 18 hr were fixed for autoradiography postmortem. In another study,[12] the accumulation of ^{115}Cd in the kidney, oviduct, digestive gland, and parts of the intestine of *B. glabrata* exposed to this radioisotope for 48 hr has been demonstrated. Finally, it has been shown that ^{67}Cu accumulates in four areas of *B. glabrata:* on the surface of the head-foot epithelium, embedded in a layer of mucus; on the epithelium of the rectal ridge; in cells of the oviduct; and in leukocytes along the epithelial border of the postintestine.[2] In these studies, the snails had been exposed to ^{67}Cu for periods of ½, 2, 4, 6, 8, and 10 hr in a solution "spiked" with 1 ppm of nonradioactive copper.

Based on the relatively few studies of mechanisms of copper toxicity to gastropods, one of two conclusions may be drawn. First, it is possible that copper acts on a yet unidentified internal organ or system and causes snail mortality by interfering with the normal function of that organ. It is noted, however, that to reach the internal milieu of a snail, copper must first be taken up across epithelial borders and transported in the hemolymph. Such borders on *B. glabrata* are those that cover the head-foot, mantle, and lining of the digestive tract.

Alternative to the above "target organ" hypothesis, it can be speculated that copper acts primarily on the epithelium of the snail. The epithelial surfaces of gastropods function not only for protection but also in oxygen uptake, osmoregulation, locomotion, perception, and shell formation and regeneration.[13, 14] Presumably, a disruption of the oxygen uptake or osmoregulatory function of epithelia as a result of exposure to copper could result in the death of the organism.

We have chosen to study a specific epithelium of *B. glabrata*, that which covers the rectal ridge, because earlier autoradiographic studies[2] have revealed a heavy accumulation of ^{67}Cu at this site. Furthermore, both the histologic composition of the rectal ridge, over which water is circulated in the mantle cavity,[15] and the fine structure of its epithelium,[16] which characterizes it as a transporting epithelium, suggest that this portion of the body surface is particularly susceptible to copper toxicity. The fine structural histopathology effected in the rectal ridge by exposure to copper is presented in this report.

MATERIALS AND METHODS

Adult specimens of the albino strain of *B. glabrata* [17] that measured from 12 to 15 mm in shell diameter were placed in individual 2.5-in. culture dishes to which 25 ml of 60 ppm of copper as $CuSO_4$ were added. After 12 hr of exposure to this concentration of copper, the rectal ridge was dissected from the mantle of each snail and fixed in a 0.5% solution of 0.075 M cacodylate-buffered acrolein at pH 7.85 for 4 hr. The tissues were postfixed in 1% OsO_4 for 1 hr, dehydrated, and embedded in Luft's Epon®. Sections were cut on an MT-2B Porter-Blum ultramicrotome, stained with lead citrate and uranyl acetate, and examined with a Philips 300 electron microscope operated at 60 kV.

A second group of *B. glabrata* were exposed to 0.06 ppm of copper as $CuSO_4$ for 60 hr. Subsequent to this exposure, during which 50% mortality occurred, the surviving specimens were prepared for transmission electron microscopy, as described above.

Sections of the rectal ridge from snails that had not been exposed to copper served as the controls.

It is noted that both high concentration-short exposure time and low concentration-long exposure time protocols were employed. The rationale for this approach is that molluscicides are usually applied in the field in one of two fashions: either as a "slug dose," where a high initial concentration of molluscicide is attained, or by a controlled-release system, where a low-level application is maintained over an extended period of time.

OBSERVATIONS

In control specimens, a single layer of microvilli-bearing epithelial cells covers the rectal ridge surface in an alternating series of projections and furrows (FIGURE 1). The apical cytoplasm of these microvillar cells is packed with mitochondria. Mucus-secreting goblet cells and ciliated cells also are distributed throughout this epithelium. The digitiform bases of the epithelial cells interdigitate with constrictions of the underlying basal lamina.

Mediad to the basal lamina are bands of myofibers, which are not organized as a continuous sheet. Finally, below the myofibers occurs the matrix of the rectal ridge, which is composed of loose vascular connective tissue. Embedded in this matrix are pigment cells, amoebocyte-like and fibrocyte-like cells, scattered myofibers, and calcium spherites. Membrane-bound vesicles, some containing glycogen, and cytoplasmic strands also occur in this zone. The pigment cells (FIGURE 2) deserve special mention, because unusual microtubule-like structures often are found within cisternae of the granular endoplasmic reticulum of these cells.

The morphology of the rectal ridge of snails that have been exposed to 60 ppm of copper as $CuSO_4$ for 12 hr is markedly different from that of the controls (FIGURE 3). Specifically, the corrugated appearance of the surface is

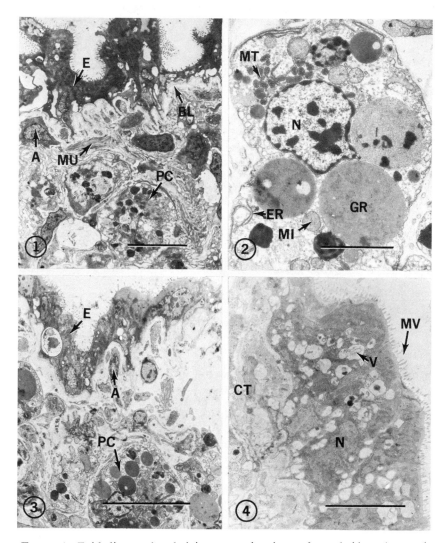

FIGURE 1. Epithelium and underlying connective tissue of rectal ridge. A, amoebo-cyte-like cell; BL, basal lamina; E, epithelial cell; MU, muscle; PC, pigment cell. Bar = 10 μm. (From Sullivan et al.[16] By permission of Cell and Tissue Research.)

FIGURE 2. Pigment cell from loose vascular connective tissue. ER, granular endo-plasmic reticulum; GR, pigment granule; MI, mitochondrion; MT, microtubule-like structures; N, nucleus. Bar = 5 μm.

FIGURE 3. Epithelium of rectal ridge and underlying connective tissue from B. glabrata exposed to 60 ppm of copper as CuSO₄ for 12 hr. A, amoebocyte-like cell; E, epithelial cell; PC, pigment cell. Bar = 20 μm.

FIGURE 4. Vacuolated epithelial cells of rectal ridge from B. glabrata exposed to 0.06 ppm of copper as CuSO₄ for 60 hr. CT, connective tissue; MV, microvilli; N, nucleus; V, vacuole. Bar = 5 μm.

not as prominent, although cilia are present, and the cytoplasmic organelles appear normal. In addition, the number of digitiform projections at the bases of the epithelial cells is greatly reduced; they are entirely absent in some cells. The basal lamina is not present, although fibrous remnants are evident. Finally, the loose vascular connective tissue appears "empty," that is, with large spaces occurring in the matrix. This area is tightly packed with cells in control specimens. It is noted, however, that cells embedded in the connective tissue, for example, pigment cells and amoebocytes, appear normal.

The rectal ridge from snails that had been exposed to 0.06 ppm of copper as $CuSO_4$ for 60 hr also exhibits distinct pathologic features. In addition to those already described, certain cells of the epithelium appear highly vacuolated (FIGURE 4). Also, other epithelial cells have an unusually smooth surface and are devoid of microvilli and cilia (FIGURE 5).

Numerous vesicles occur in the matrix of the rectal ridge of these specimens (FIGURE 6). Certain of these vesicles resemble cisternae of granular endoplasmic reticulum normally found in pigment cells (FIGURE 7). Some of these vesicles contain a crystalline substance (FIGURE 8), which most probably represent fragments of the microtubule-like structures that occur in pigment cells. Other vesicles contain an electron-dense substance and bear a close resemblance to the pigment granules of pigment cells (FIGURE 9). Finally, degenerating mitochondria are free in the matrix (FIGURE 10). The inner and outer membranes of these mitochondria are separated by a wider space than is normally observed. Furthermore, many of the mitochondria, such as the one depicted in FIGURE 10, appear to be abnormally distended. It is noted that normal-appearing pigment cells and amoebocytes also occur in the connective tissue of these specimens.

DISCUSSION

The epithelial cells of the rectal ridge of *B. glabrata* that had been exposed to lethal doses of copper appear to have been greatly distended. Specifically, the loss of the corrugated appearance of the epithelium, the loss of digitiform projections from the bases of the epithelial cells, and the disintegration of the underlying basal lamina imply that a swelling of the tissues mediad to the epithelium has occurred, which thus exerts a stretching force on that epithelium and the basal lamina. Furthermore, the distended, empty appearance of the loose vascular connective tissue of the rectal ridge from these specimens suggests an influx of water into this tissue. This condition implies a failure in the osmoregulatory physiology of the organism, which thus allows water to accumulate in the tissues, resulting in the distention.

A secondary effect of the accumulation of water in the tissues is apparently the lysis of the pigment cells, the vesicular remnants of which are then found free in the intercellular spaces of the matrix. Although, in our opinion, the function of the pigment cells remains uncertain, a hemoglobin-producing role has been attributed to them.[18] If these cells, indeed, are the sites of hemoglobin synthesis, the destruction of pigment cells consequent to exposure to copper should have a measurable effect on hemoglobin levels in the hemolymph of the snail. A study is currently underway to further investigate this hypothesis.

There appears to be a greater amount of tissue damage in snails that had been exposed to 0.06 ppm of copper as $CuSO_4$ for 60 hr than in those that had

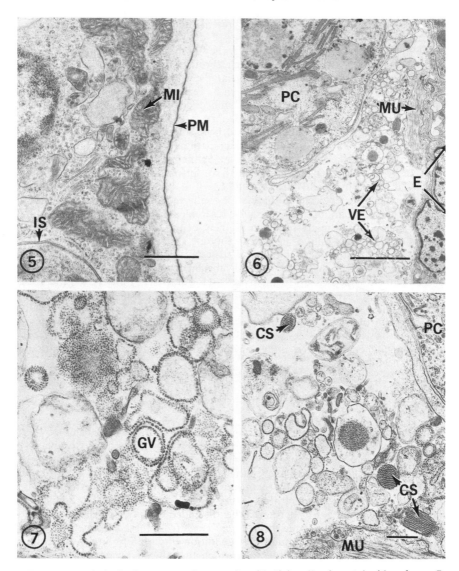

FIGURE 5. Apical plasma membrane of epithelial cell of rectal ridge from *B. glabrata* exposed to 0.06 ppm of copper as CuSO₄ for 60 hr.. IS, intercellular space; MI, mitochondrion; PM, plasma membrane. Bar = 1 μm.

FIGURE 6. Loose vascular connective tissue of rectal ridge from *B. glabrata* exposed to 0.06 ppm of copper as CuSO₄ for 60 hr. Note presence of vesicles. E, epithelial cell; MU, muscle; PC, pigment cell; VE, vesicles. Bar = 5 μm.

FIGURE 7. Granular vesicles in intercellular spaces of loose vascular connective tissue of rectal ridge from *B. glabrata* exposed to 0.06 ppm of copper as CuSO₄ for 60 hr. GV, granular vesicles. Bar = 1 μm.

FIGURE 8. Extracellular vesicles in loose vascular connective tissue of rectal ridge from *B. glabrata* exposed to 0.06 ppm of copper as CuSO₄ for 60 hr. Note occurrence of crystal-like substance in three vesicles. CS, crystal-like substance; MU, muscle; PC, pigment cell. Bar = 1 μm.

been exposed to 60 ppm of copper for 12 hr. This difference may be a result of the dissimilar behavioral reactions of the two categories of snails. When specimens of *B. glabrata* were placed in contact with 60 ppm of copper, they immediately retracted fully into their shells and remained in this retracted state throughout the exposure. Furthermore, a thick layer of mucus was secreted over the basal surface of the head-foot, which further separated each snail from its toxic surroundings. However, snails in contact with 0.06 ppm of copper did not immediately retract but exhibited distress throughout the greater part of the exposure. Thus, the rectal ridges of these specimens were in full contact with the toxic solution for approximately 60 hr and therefore probably sustained more damage as a result of the longer exposure.

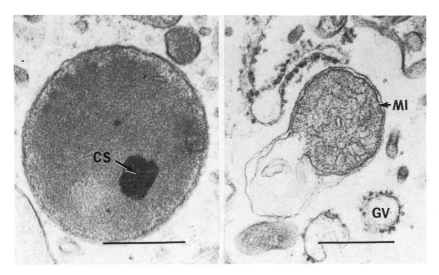

FIGURE 9 (*left*). Extracellular electron-dense vesicle in loose vascular connective tissue of rectal ridge from *B. glabrata* exposed to 0.06 ppm of copper as CuSO₄ for 60 hr. Note occurrence of crystal-like substance in this vesicle. CS, crystal-like substance. Bar=0.5 μm.

FIGURE 10 (*right*). Extracellular mitochondrion in loose vascular connective tissue of rectal ridge from *B. glabrata* exposed to 0.06 ppm of copper as CuSO₄ for 60 hr. GV, granular vesicle; MI, mitochondrion. Bar=0.5 μm.

Relative to the precise toxic effect of copper on the rectal ridge epithelium, which, in turn, brings about the pathologic alterations described above, at least three possibilities exist. 1. Copper elicits the secretion of mucus by goblet cells embedded in the epithelial surface. This mucus may produce a suffocating effect by preventing an exchange of ions and gases across the epithelium. 2. Copper may become bound to hydrophilic regions on the external plasma membrane of the epithelial cells and, as a result, disrupt the permeability of the membrane by altering its biochemical and biophysical properties. 3. Finally, copper may somehow enter the cytoplasm of the epithelial cells and disrupt their normal functions.

REFERENCES

1. SPARKS, A. K. 1972. Invertebrate Pathology. Academic Press, Inc. New York, N.Y.
2. CHENG, T. C. & J. T. SULLIVAN. 1974. Mode of entry, action, and toxicity of copper molluscicides. *In* Molluscicides in Schistosomiasis Control. T. C. Cheng, Ed. : 89–153. Academic Press, Inc. New York, N.Y.
3. MALEK, E. A. & T. C. CHENG. 1974. Medical and Economic Malacology. Academic Press, Inc. New York, N.Y.
4. VON BRAND, T., B. MEHLMAN & M. O. NOLAN. 1949. Influence of some potential molluscicides on the oxygen consumption of *Australorbis glabratus*. J. Parasitol. **35:** 475–481.
5. HARRY, H. W. & D. V. ALDRICH. 1963. The distress syndrome in *Taphius glabratus* (Say) as a reaction to toxic concentrations of inorganic ions. Malacologia **1:** 283–289.
6. YAGER, C. M. & H. W. HARRY. 1964. The uptake of radioactive zinc, cadmium, and copper by the freshwater snail, *Taphius glabratus*. Malacologia **1:** 339–353.
7. ISHAK, M. M., A. A. SHARAF, A. M. MOHAMED & A. H. MOUSA. 1970. Studies on the mode of action of some molluscicides on the snail, *Biomphalaria alexandrina:* I. Effect of Bayluscide, sodium pentachlorophenate, and copper sulphate on succinate, glutamate, and reduced TMPD (tetramethylparaphenylenediamine) oxidation. Comp. Gen. Pharmacol. **1:** 201–208.
8. PASSOW, H., A. ROTHSTEIN & T. W. CLARKSON. 1961. The general pharmacology of the heavy metals. Pharmacol. Rev. **13 :**185–202.
9. CHENG, T. C. & J. T. SULLIVAN. 1973. The effect of copper on the heart rate of *Biomphalaria glabrata* (Mollusca: Pulmonata). Comp. Gen. Pharmacol. **4:** 37–42.
10. CHENG, T. C. & J. T. SULLIVAN. 1973. Comparative study of the effects of two copper compounds on the respiration and survival of *Biomphalaria glabrata* (Mollusca: Pulmonata). Comp. Gen. Pharmacol. **4:** 315–320.
11. DE AZEVEDO, J. F., F. C. GOMES, A. M. BAPTISTA & F. B. GIL. 1957. Studies on the molluscocide action of copper sulphate using [64]Cu. Z. Tropenmed. Parasitol. **8:** 457–464.
12. YAGER, C. M. & H. W. HARRY. 1966. Uptake of heavy metal ions by *Taphius glabratus*, a snail host of *Schistosoma mansoni*. Exp. Parasitol. **19:** 174–182.
13. HESS, O. 1964. Die Haut der Mollusken. Studium gen. **17:** 161–176.
14. ZYLSTRA, U. 1972. Uptake of particulate matter by the epidermis of the freshwater snail *Lymnaea stagnalis*. Neth. J. Zool. **22:** 299–306.
15. SULLIVAN, J. T. & T. C. CHENG. 1974. Structure and function of the mantle cavity of *Biomphalaria glabrata* (Mollusca: Pulmonata). Trans. Amer. Microsc. Soc. **93:** 416–420.
16. SULLIVAN, J. T., G. E. RODRICK & T. C. CHENG. 1974. A transmission and scanning electron microscopical study of the rectal ridge of *Biomphalaria glabrata* (Mollusca: Pulmonata). Cell Tissue Res. **154:** 29–38.
17. NEWTON, W. L. 1955. The establishment of a strain of *Australorbis glabratus* which combines albinism and a high susceptibility to infection with *Schistosoma mansoni*. J. Parasitol. **41:** 526–528.
18. SMINIA, T., H. H. BOER & A. NIEMANTSVERDREIT. 1972. Hemoglobin producing cells in freshwater snails. Z. Zellforsch. **135:** 563–568.

MOLLUSK-PARASITE INTERACTIONS: AN INTRODUCTION

Thomas C. Cheng

Institute for Pathobiology
Center for Health Sciences
Lehigh University
Bethlehem, Pennsylvania 18015

Among the groups of invertebrates that are known to serve as vectors of disease-causing parasites, the mollusks are overshadowed only by the insects. Even then, it cannot be denied that the species of gastropods that act as the intermediate hosts for the human-infecting species of schistosomes must be ranked among the most important invertebrate vectors of disease.

In recent years, we have witnessed an increased interest in the development of methods alternative to chemical control directed toward the control of schistosome-transmitting and other undesirable species of snails. This, of course, requires considerable additional basic information relative to the mollusk-parasite relationship not available at this time. This is not to say that no work is being performed in this area. In fact, several distinguished investigators throughout the world have focused their attention on problems of this nature. The contributions of several of these individuals are included in this section.

Dr. K. R. Harris, one of the more distinguished of my former students, has contributed an excellent account of the encapsulation process in *Biomphalaria glabrata* directed toward the nematode *Angiostrongylus cantonensis,* as revealed by electron microscopy. This study, in my opinion, will serve as a prototype for many others to come.

Dr. P. L. Krupa and his colleagues, L. M. Lewis and P. Del Vecchio, have contributed a significant report that helps to elucidate the surface transport system in schistosome sporocysts. Similarly, Drs. F. J. Etges, O. S. Carter, and G. Webbe have contributed an interesting account of the behavior of schistosome miracidia related to host finding and to the effect of parasitization on the fecundity of the molluscan host.

It is always a pleasure to introduce the work of a former student, in this case Dr. G. P. Hoskin. This enthusiastic investigator has employed the *Nassarius-Himasthla* model to elucidate some salient features of the mollusk-trematode interface and how the parasites affect the snail at the cellular level.

One group of potential candidates for the biologic control of schistosome-transmitting snails is the microsporidians. Therefore, the contribution by Dr. C. J. Bayne and his colleagues, A. Owczarzak and W. E. Noonan, on the cultivation of a microsporidan in *B. glabrata* cells will undoubtedly be read with great interest.

Finally, although not directed toward the understanding of a mollusk-parasite relationship, the contribution by Drs. J. A. Couch, M. D. Summers, and L. Courtney is, in my opinion, a very significant one. These investigators have posed some interesting questions as to the environmental significance of the occurrence of a *Baculovirus* enzootic in penaeid shrimp.

In conclusion, I wish to thank all of the participants in this session. It has been my pleasure to chair such an interesting series of contributions.

445

THE FINE STRUCTURE OF ENCAPSULATION
IN *BIOMPHALARIA GLABRATA* *

Kevin R. Harris

Department of Biology
Adelphi University
Garden City, New York 11530

Most reviews of molluscan immunobiology and pathobiology have concluded that the primary internal defense mechanism, elaborated by gastropod mollusks against metazoan endoparasites, involves the encapsulation of the invasive organism by host cells.[1-6] The destruction of larval helminths, especially digenetic trematodes that have penetrated refractory strains or species of snails, often accompanies the formation of such host tissue responses.[7-11] Similar reactions have also been implicated in the destruction of sporocysts and of cercariae lodged within the tissues of normally susceptible snails.[11-14] It has been pointed out, however, that some other helminths, particularly nematodes, may not be destroyed, even when surrounded by extensive host cellular reactions.[1, 15]

Richards and Merritt [16] have reported that larvae of the metastrongylid nematode *Angiostrongylus cantonensis,* used to experimentally infect *Biomphalaria glabrata,* provoke extensive host tissue reactions. The nematodes are not destroyed by this host response, and viable third-stage larvae can be recovered from infections of long duration.[16] Harris and Cheng [15] have suggested that this might be a particularly useful parasite-host system for examining certain aspects of the encapsulation process in mollusks and, as the result of a light microscope study, have reported that encapsulation of *A. cantonensis* within *B. glabrata* occurs as a biphasic process. The initial response involves the infiltration and aggregation of basophilic hemolymph cells around the parasite. Subsequently, such cellular aggregations become transformed into more fibrous-appearing nodules. Enzyme histochemistry has been employed to demonstrate a marked localization of acid phosphatase, nonspecific esterase, alkaline phosphatase, and β-glucuronidase activities within these capsules.[17]

To more clearly elucidate the cellular defense mechanisms of *B. glabrata,* electron microscope observations, reported herein, have been made on the formation of host encapsulation reactions provoked in this mollusk by infection with larvae of *A. cantonensis.* Because cells of the hemolymph have been suggested to participate in the formation of these capsules,[15] the fine structure of hemocytes of *B. glabrata* has also been studied.

MATERIALS AND METHODS

All specimens of *B. glabrata* used in this study were of the National Institutes of Health albino strain [18] and were maintained as described previously.[15]

* Supported in part by Grant FD-00416 from the United States Public Health Service to Dr. Thomas C. Cheng.

446

Before collection of hemolymph samples to be prepared for transmission electron microscopy, the shells of snails, each of which measured 10–16 mm in diameter, were carefully cleaned with 70% ethanol and wiped dry. Hemolymph collected intracardially with microcapillary tubes were expelled directly into centrifuge tubes that contained fixative. Hemolymph cells were fixed for 1–3 hr in cold 2% glutaraldehyde in Sörenson's 0.1 M phosphate buffer (pH 7.2). They were washed for 12 hr in cold buffer and postfixed in 2% phosphate-buffered osmium tetroxide for 1 hr, prior to being dehydrated and embedded in Luft's Epon®.

Snails were infected with first-stage larvae of *A. cantonensis* as described earlier.[15] Mantle collar tissue of *B. glabrata* was prepared for transmission electron microscopy at 3, 8, 28, and 63 days postinfection. Tissues were fixed for 1½ hr, in 2% acrolein in 0.1 M Sörenson's phosphate buffer at pH 7.2. Subsequent processing of mantle collar tissues was as described for snail hemolymph cells, except that postfixation with osmium tetroxide was performed for 3 hr.

Sections of hemolymph cells and mantle collar tissue were made with a diamond knife (DuPont) on a Sorvall MT-2B ultramicrotome. Sections were collected on uncoated copper grids and stained with a saturated solution of uranyl acetate and Reynolds'[19] lead citrate. Stained sections were examined with an RCA EMU-3G electron microscope operated at 50 kV or with a Philips 300 electron microscope operataed at 40 kV.

RESULTS

Transmission electron microscopy reveals the presence of two distinct morphologic types of cells in the hemolymph of *B. glabrata*. By far the more numerous are cells that possess a moderately electron-opaque cytoplasm and exhibit numerous cytoplasmic extensions from the main cell body (FIGURES 1 & 2). The cytoplasm includes considerable amounts of glycogen and of mitochondria and rough endoplasmic reticulum (FIGURE 3). Large numbers of mitochondria are frequently found aggregated in the main portion of the cell body near the nucleus (FIGURE 3). Also present, often in aggregations, are numerous lysosome-like bodies. They may contain only a few central membraneous figures (FIGURE 4) or varying amounts of concentrically whorled lamellae (FIGURES 5 & 6).

The second type of cell is present in fewer numbers and is roughly oval in sections. Such cells do not possess cytoplasmic extensions and exhibit a relatively less electron-opaque cytoplasm (FIGURES 7 & 8). Considerable amounts of mitochondria, Golgi apparatuses, smooth endoplasmic reticulum, and membrane-bound vesicles are distributed throughout the cytoplasm (FIGURES 7–9).

Electron microscope observations on mantle collar tissues from infected snails reveal the presence of numerous cells of moderate electron opacity that have aggregated around *A. cantonensis* larvae by 3 days postinfection (FIGURE 10). One of the most striking features of this early cellular response, as visualized in electron micrographs, is the formation by these cells of numerous pseudopodium-like extensions of the peripheral cytoplasm directed toward the surface of the parasite (FIGURES 10–12). Large amounts of glycogen, mitochondria, and endoplasmic reticulum are present within the cytoplasm of these reaction cells. For the most part, however, such organelles are restricted to

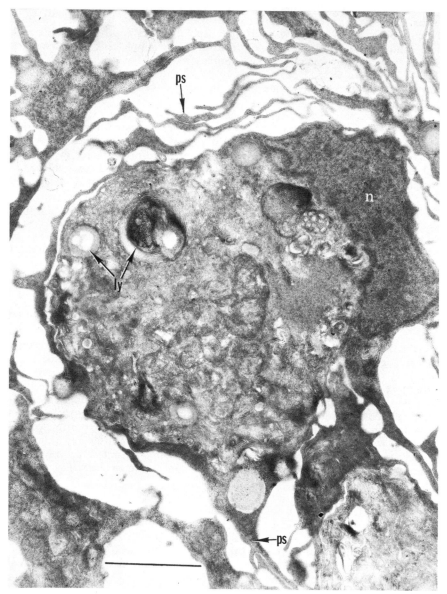

FIGURE 1. Electron micrograph of a granulocyte of *B. glabrata*. Note the formation of pseudopodium-like extensions of the peripheral cytoplasm. Large numbers of lysosome-like inclusions, some of which contain concentric whorls of lamellae, are found within the endoplasm. Bar=2 μm. ly, Lysosome-like inclusion; n, nucleus; ps, pseudopodium.

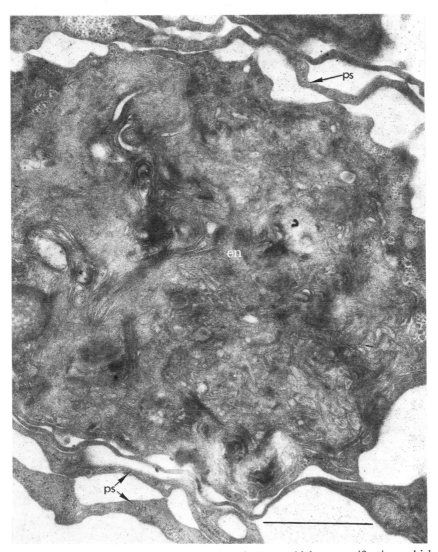

FIGURE 2. Electron micrograph of a granulocyte at higher magnification, which shows the many whorls of membranes characteristically segregated within the endoplasm. Thinly drawn pseudopodium-like projections of the ectoplasm are also evident. Bar—1 μm. cn, Endoplasm; ps, pseudopodium

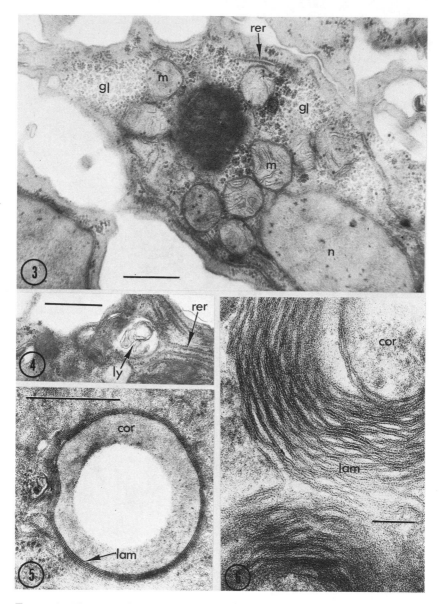

FIGURE 3. Electron micrograph of localized aggregation of mitochondria and glycogen rosettes within the endoplasm of a granulocyte. Rough endoplasmic reticulum is also present within such cells. Bar=0.5 μm.

FIGURE 4. Lysosome-like body near the periphery of a granulocyte. Centrally located membraneous figures may be noted within this inclusion. Bar=0.5 μm.

FIGURE 5. Electron micrograph of a granulocyte, which shows a lysosome-like body with several peripheral membraneous lamellae and a homogeneous cortex. Bar=0.5 μm.

FIGURE 6. Electron micrograph of granulocyte, which shows a lysosome-like body that consists almost entirely of concentric membraneous whorls. The cortex is much reduced. Bar=0.1 μm. cor, Cortex of lysosome-like body; gl, glycogen; lam, concentric membraneous lamellae; ly, lysosome-like body; m, mitochondrion; n, nucleus; rer, rough endoplasmic reticulum.

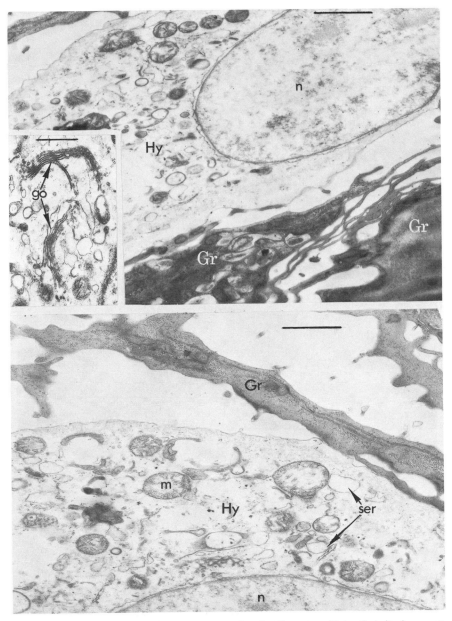

FIGURE 7 (*top*). Electron micrograph of a hyalinocyte. Note that it does not possess pseudopodium-like extensions, as do the surrounding granulocytes. The cytoplasmic matrix in hyalinocytes is also considerably less electron dense than that of granulocytes. Bar—1 μm.

FIGURE 8 (*top* inset). Prominent Golgi apparatuses within the cytoplasm of a hyalinocyte. Bar=0.5 μm.

FIGURE 9 (*bottom*). Hyalinocyte that contains characteristic mitochondria, smooth endoplasmic reticulum, and membrane bound vesicles within the cytoplasm. At the periphery of the hyalinocyte is a cytoplasmic extension from a granulocyte. Bar= 0.5 μm. go, Golgi apparatus; Gr, granulocyte; Hy, hyalinocyte; m, mitochondrion; n, nucleus; ser, smooth endoplasmic reticulum.

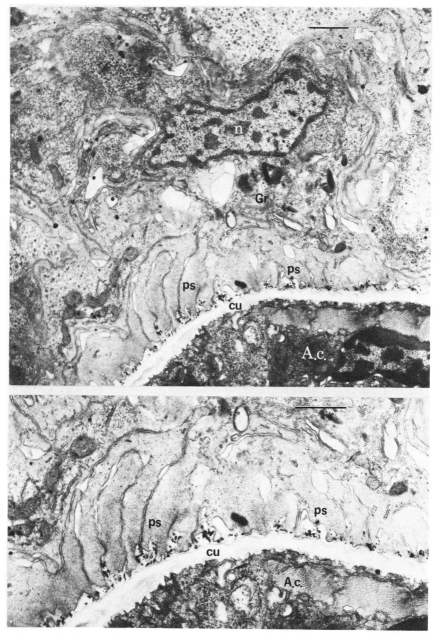

FIGURE 10 (*top*). Electron micrograph that shows the early phase of capsule formation, as granulocytes aggregate around an *A. cantonensis* larva at 3 days postinfection. Pseudopodial processes formed by granulocytes are directed roughly perpendicular to the nematode's cuticle. The major cell organelles are for the most part the major body of the cell (FIGURES 10 & 13); they are seldom found in the finely granular homogeneous cytoplasm of the pseudopodial extensions (FIGURES 10–12). Also present within the central body of the cell are inclusions that resemble lysosomes and that contain numerous concentric whorled lamellae (FIGURES 13 & 14). A certain amount of flattening of the host reaction cells, in addition to elongation and flattening of their nuclei, can occasionally be seen toward the periphery of these cellular aggregations (FIGURE 13). At this time, however, most of the pseudopodial extensions appear as finely granular lamellae of considerable thickness and lie roughly parallel to each other and perpendicular to the parasite's cuticle (FIGURES 10–12 & 14). Accumulations of two types of material are regularly observed between the surfaces of nematode larvae and the surrounding host cells. One type appears granular and extremely opaque, whereas the second one is in the form of membrane-bound vesicles (FIGURES 15 & 16).

As the encapsulation reaction progresses, the lamelliform pseudopodial extensions of the surrounding host cells become thinner and gradually come to lie more nearly parallel to the nematode's cuticle (FIGURES 17 & 18).

By 8 days postinfection, the cytoplasmic extensions of the reaction cells occur in different stages of conversion to concentric cytoplasmic layers surrounding the parasite (FIGURES 19 & 20). Such cytoplasmic extensions, which are arranged in parallel stacks around the nematode, are expanded in regions that contain nuclei or organelles, such as mitochondria (FIGURE 19). In other regions, they are stretched to extreme thinness and form layer upon layer of finely drawn processes (FIGURES 20–22). The thinnest processes of this type (FIGURES 21 & 22) contain few organelles and include a finely granular cytoplasm of moderate electron opacity. Darkly stained granules, which superficially resemble those found between the inner cell layer and the nematode's cuticle, are also present in many of these processes (FIGURES 21 & 22). Although muscle cells may lie close to encapsulated nematodes (FIGURES 20 & 21), at no time do they appear to play a role in the actual cellular reaction.

Large capsules in long-standing infections consist of layer upon layer of thinly drawn cells and processes of the general type described above (FIGURES 23 & 24). In locally expanded regions of these cells are found both the nuclei and concentrations of glycogen and mitochondria (FIGURES 24 & 27). In addition, similar expansions may contain localized aggregations of lysosome-like bodies that frequently contain numerous whorled lamellae (FIGRES 25 & 26). Nematodes become so completely ensheathed by capsules formed by the host that even where the molted cuticle is contorted and two regions closely abut, it is enveloped by multiple layers of cellular processes (FIGURE 28). Even in capsules observed 9 weeks postinfection, neither extracellular elements nor myofibers appear to play a part in the encapsulation process.

---

restricted to the endoplasm near the nucleus of granulocytes and are seldom found within the pseudopodial extensions. Bar = 1 μm.

FIGURE 11 (bottom). Electron micrograph that shows detail of pseudopodial processes that initially extend perpendicularly to the parasite's surface. Such processes contain a finely granular homogeneous cytoplasm. Bar = 1 μm. A.c., A. cantonensis larva; cu, cuticle of nematode; Gr, granulocyte; n, nucleus; ps, pseudopodial extension of granulocyte.

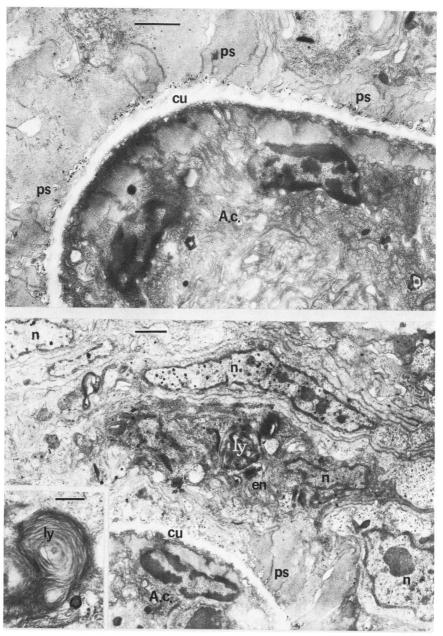

FIGURE 12 (*top*). Pseudopodial extensions from granulocytes, which extend perpendicularly to and completely surround the surface of an *A. cantonensis* larva at 3 days postinfection. Bar=1 μm.

FIGURE 13 (*bottom*). Granulocytes surrounding nematode larva at 3 days postinfection. Lysosome-like inclusions and other cellular organelles characteristic of granulocytes are restricted to the major cell body and are not seen in pseudopodial

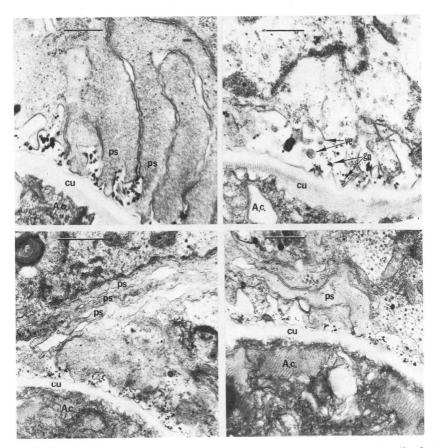

FIGURE 15 (*top left*). Electron micrograph that shows detail of pseudopodia that extend perpendicularly to the surface of an *A. cantonensis* larva; 3 days postinfection. Bar = 0.5 μm.

FIGURE 16 (*top right*). Electron micrograph that illustrates the nature of material found at the nematode-granulocyte interface. One type is granular and extremely electron dense, whereas the other is in the form of membrane-bound vesicles; 3 days postinfection. Bar = 0.5 μm.

FIGURE 17 (*bottom left*). Granulocyte pseudopodia that have begun to flatten and lie more nearly parallel to the surface of the nematode; 3 days postinfection. Bar = 1 μm.

FIGURE 18 (*bottom right*). Granulocyte pseudopodia that have flattened to form thin cytoplasmic processes that lie parallel to the cuticle of the nematode; 3 days postinfection. Bar = 1 μm. A.c., *A. cantonensis* larva; cu, cuticle of nematode; gn, granular electron-dense material at host-parasite interface; ps, pseudopodial process of granulocyte; ve, membrane-bound vesicle found at the host-parasite interface.

extensions. Some flattening of host cells and their nuclei can be noted toward the periphery of this leukocytic aggregation. Bar = 1 μm.

FIGURE 14 (*bottom* inset). Lysosome-like inclusion within the cytoplasm of granulocyte that surrounds an *A. cantonensis* larva. Bar = 0.25 μm. A.c., *A. cantonensis* larva; cu, cuticle of nematode; ly, lysosome-like inclusion within granulocyte; ps, pseudopodial extension of granulocyte.

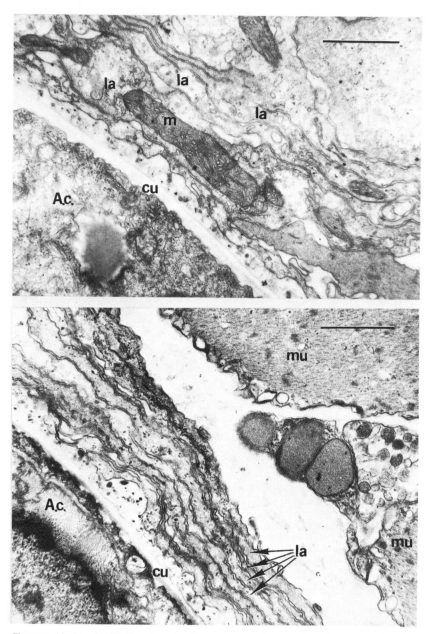

FIGURE 19 (*top*). Flattened extensions of granulocytes that form cytoplasmic lamellae that surround an *A. cantonensis* larva at 8 days postinfection. Note the large mitochondrion within the granulocyte cytoplasm in close proximity to the nematode surface. Bar = 1 μm.

FIGURE 20 (*bottom*). Thinly drawn granulocytes that form concentric lamellae around nematode larva at 8 days postinfection. Although muscle cells lie in close proximity, they play no role in the encapsulation response. Bar = 1 μm. A.c., *A. cantonensis* larva; cu, cuticle of nematode; la, lamellae formed by cytoplasmic extensions of flattened granulocytes; m, mitochondrion within cytoplasm of granulocyte; mu, host muscle cell.

DISCUSSION

Transmission electron microscopy of *B. glabrata* hemolymph cells fixed immediately upon withdrawal from snails has indicated the occurrence of two types of leukocytes based on morphologic criteria. By far the more numerous are cells of moderate electron opacity, which possess considerable numbers of mitochondria and lysosome-like bodies that frequently enclose concentric whorls of lamellae. An electron micrograph of a similar cell from the hemolymph of

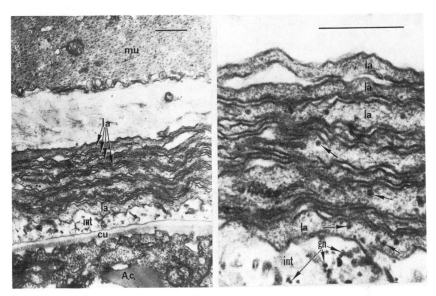

FIGURE 21 (*left*). Thinly drawn cytoplasmic processes of granulocytes that form concentric lamellae that lie parallel to and surround an *A. cantonensis* larva at 8 days postinfection. Bar = 0.5 μm.

FIGURE 22 (*right*). Electron micrograph that shows greater detail of cytoplasmic lamellae that surround the parasite. Found within such lamellae are darkly stained granules (arrows), which superficially resemble those observed at the host-parasite interface. Bar = 0.5 μm. A.c., *A. cantonensis* larva; cu, cuticle of nematode; gn, granular material found at host-parasite interface; int, interface between nematode and host reaction; la, cytoplasmic lamellae formed by granulocytes; mu, host muscle cell.

B. glabrata has been published by Faulk *et al.*[20] Even in cells of this type fixed directly upon removal from snails, the tendency to form fine cytoplasmic processes has been noted. It is believed that these cells correspond to the large amoeboid leukocytes observed with light microscopy [20, 21] and scanning electron microscopy.[21] The numerous mitochondria and large lysosomes in the main cell body, observed with transmission electron microscopy, presumably represent the granular inclusions observed with the light microscope and that characterize this type of cell, which Harris [21] has termed the granulocyte.

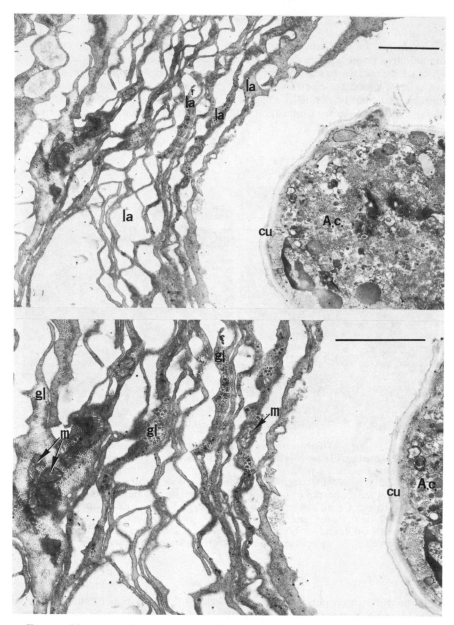

FIGURE 23 (*top*). Large encapsulation reaction that surrounds *A. cantonensis* larva at 63 days postinfection. Numerous concentric lamellae of cytoplasmic processes surround the parasite. Bar=2 μm.

FIGURE 24 (*bottom*). Electron micrograph that shows greater detail of capsules that surround nematode larva at 63 days postinfection. Aggregations of glycogen and mitochondria are noted within local expansions of the cytoplasmic lamellae. Bar=2 μm. A.c., *A. cantonensis* larva; cu, cuticle of nematode; gl, glycogen; la, cytoplasmic lamellae formed by flattened granulocytes; m, mitochondrion.

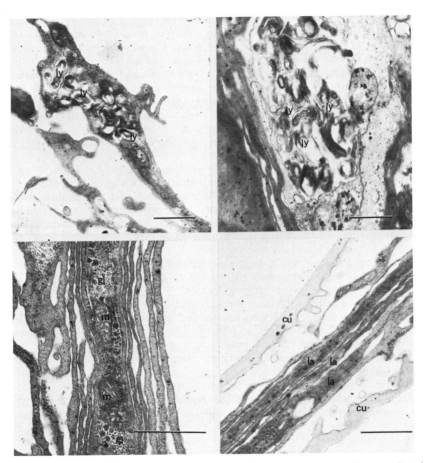

FIGURE 25 (*top left*). Numerous lysosome-like inclusions within cytoplasmic lamellae formed by granulocytes around *A. cantonensis* larva; 63 days postinfection. Bar = 1 μm.

FIGURE 26 (*top right*). Lysosome-like inclusions within a cytoplasmic lamella that surrounds an *A. cantonensis* larva; 28 days postinfection. Bar = 1 μm.

FIGURE 27 (*bottom left*). Glycogen rosettes and mitochondria within expansion of cytoplasmic lamella that surrounds a nematode larva; 63 days postinfection. Bar = 1 μm.

FIGURE 28 (*bottom right*). Electron micrograph of region in which molted cuticle of *A. cantonensis* is contorted so that two regions closely abut. Note that even in this situation, layers of cytoplasmic lamellae completely envelop the parasite; 28 days post-infection. Bar = 1 μm. cu, Cuticle of nematode larva; gl, glycogen; la, cytoplasmic lamella; ly, lysosome-like inclusion; m, mitochondrion.

At the electron microscope level, organelles that morphologically resemble lysosomes occur in aggregates that frequently appear segregated from those of mitochondria. This finding complements the earlier light microscope observation that large numbers of acid phosphatase-positive granules, presumably lysosomal in nature, are often sequestered in one region of the granular endoplasm in *B. glabrata* granulocytes.[16] The accumulations of various amounts of membraneous lamellae, noted within the lysosomes of these cells, are morphologically similar to those that Hohl[22] has reported to be formed within food vacuoles of cellular slime molds after phagocytosis and digestion of bacteria. An identical process may occur in the granulocytes of *B. glabrata*, because Tripp[23] has demonstrated that wandering hemocytes of this gastropod are capable of phagocytosis and intracellular degradation of bacteria and certain other small particulate materials *in vivo*. Similarly, Faulk *et al.*[20] employed electron microscopy to demonstrate the presence of phagocytized erythrocytes within such cells after *in vitro* experiments.

The fine structure of the *B. glabrata* granulocyte closely resembles that reported for hemolymph cells from several other species of gastropods.[24-27] It should also be noted that Sminia[25] has demonstrated acid phosphatase activity localized within lysosomes of such cells from the hemolymph of *Lymnaea stagnalis*. Membrane-bound inclusions that contained concentric membraneous lamellae, similar to those observed within granulocytes of *B. glabrata*, were demonstrated to be secondary lysosomes.[25]

The second type of cell in the hemolymph of *B. glabrata* is both less numerous and less electron dense than the granulocyte. It generally appears oval in section and bears no cytoplasmic processes. It is presumed that these cells correspond to small basophilic leukocytes that have been described with light microscopy and scanning electron microscopy and that have been termed hyalinocytes by Harris.[21] The most numerous inclusions, smooth endoplasmic reticulum and membrane-bound vesicles, are distributed throughout the cytoplasm and probably account for its finely granular appearance when examined with the light microscope.

It should be pointed out that the ultrastructure of the granulocytes of *B. glabrata* does not resemble that of the granular leukocytes of the pelecypod *Crassostrea virginica*, because the cytoplasm of the latter includes numerous large granules that are bounded exteriorly by a limiting membrane and that contain a thin inner ring of cortex.[6, 28-30] However, the hyalinocytes of *B. glabrata* do have certain morphologic affinities to *C. virginica* hyalinocytes,[6, 28] especially to the type of cell designated as a type I agranular cell by Feng *et al.*[28] Such pelecypod hyalinocytes possess oval nuclei surrounded by a relatively scanty cytoplasm that contains large amounts of smooth endoplasmic reticulum and membrane-bound vesicles, in addition to some mitochondria.

An earlier light microscope study by Harris and Cheng[15] indicated that larvae of *A. cantonensis* are encapsulated within *B. glabrata* by the formation of apparently fibrous nodules after an initial leukocytic infiltration of tissues that surround the parasite. Gastropod tissue responses that previous investigators have characterized as encapsulation by amoebocytes, and frequently were reported to involve "fibroblasts," "fibrous elements," or "fibers," have been observed to surround injected pollen grains or polystyrene spheres,[23] transplants of heterologous or formalin-fixed homologous snail tissues,[23] amoebocytes that contained a species of *Mycobacterium*,[31] trematode miracidia or sporocysts,[7-11, 13, 14, 32] or moribund cercariae lodged within snail tissues.[13, 14]

My observations, which represent the first electron microscope study of encapsulation by a gastropod, have provided information on the nature of tissue reactions and the cells forming them, which would not be apparent with light microscopy.

The initial basophilic infiltration phase, recognized with the light microscope, corresponds to the aggregation of one type of snail leukocyte, the granulocyte. Pseudopodial processes directed against the cuticle of *A. cantonensis* by these cells appear finely granular and contain few organelles. Undoubtedly, these cytoplasmic projections correspond to the extensive hyaline pseudopodia that granulocytes form *in vitro* and that have been observed by use of both light [20, 21] and scanning electron microscopy.[21] During early phases of encapsulation, pseudopodia initially extend perpendicularly to the cuticle of the nematode, but they subsequently come to lie more nearly parallel to its surface as surrounding granulocytes flatten in concentric layers around the parasite. The conversion from a loose amoebocytic aggregate to what appears with the light microscope to be a fibrous nodule can now be stated to reflect the stretching and flattening of granulocytes around the nematode.

As the reaction progresses, electron micrographs indicate the addition of layer upon layer of thinly stretched granulocytes. Lamellae of fine cytoplasmic processes, which may be as thin as 40–80 nm, undoubtedly are responsible for the fibrous appearance of such nodules when viewed with the light microscope. No extracellular elements contribute to the formation of the encapsulation reaction. The appearance of expanded cells interspersed within fibrous-appearing nodules observed in an earlier study [15] can be correlated with localized expansion of encapsulating cells that contain nuclei or aggregations of mitochondria and lysosomes. It is also important to note that concentrations of acid phosphatase-positive granules have been observed in the endoplasm of granulocytes in hemolymph samples removed from *B. glabrata*.[21] Lysosome-like bodies observed with the electron microscope probably represent sections through these inclusions. Furthermore, the localized activity of several hydrolytic enzymes, including acid phosphatase, has also been demonstrated within capsules.[17]

Other fibrous or fibroblastic encapsulation reactions observed in *B. glabrata* [7, 9, 13, 14, 23, 31, 32] may very well also involve one type of cell, the granulocyte. Similarly, the so-called fibrous elements or fibers, too fine to be more adequately characterized by light microscopy, may actually be thinly drawn cytoplasmic processes that extend from these cells, as is the case in capsules that surround *A. cantonensis* in *B. glabrata*. Relative to this speculation, some detailed and highly relevant light microscope observations on encapsulation in *B. glabrata* have been published by Tripp [23] and Pan.[13, 14] Tripp [23] has noted that amoebocytes tend to stretch around injected polystyrene spheres and pollen grains prior to the occurrence of a process described as encapsulation by fibroblasts. Pan [13, 14] has suggested that a conversion of amoebocytes into fibroblasts occurs during the encapsulation of cercariae lodged in the tissues of *B. glabrata*. In the *B. glabrata-A. cantonensis* system described herein, the cells that appear to be fibroblast-like with light microscopy are actually flattened granular leukocytes.

In the only other published electron microscope studies on mulluscan encapsulation, Rifkin *et al.*[33] and Cheng and Rifkin [6] have noted that a capsule that includes true extracellular fibers is formed around metacestodes of *Tylocephalum* sp. by the lamellibranch *C. virginica*. Unlike capsules elicited in *B. glabrata* against *A. cantonensis* larvae, the *C. virginica* encapsulation reactions consist of three major cell types, leukocytes, fibroblast-like cells, and brown cells. Not only are intracellular fibers observed, but cells are also embedded in an amorphous matrix that contains two types of intercellular fibers. It is also pertinent that Cheng and Rifkin [6] have pointed out that although leukocytes and fibroblasts are distinguishable by differences in the occurrence of rough endoplasmic reticulum and lysosomes, the two cell types exhibit remarkable morphologic similarities at the fine structural level. It has further been proposed that the two cell types might have differentiated from an immediate common precursor cell or, more likely, that leukocytes have transformed into fibroblast-like cells during encapsulation.[6] Results from my study of encapsulation in *B. glabrata* would tend to support this second hypothesis.

Also germane to my finding that encapsulation reactions in *B. glabrata* are formed by differentiated granular leukocytes is an electron microscope study by Sminia *et al.*[34] of wound healing in *L. stagnalis*. Normal amoebocytes that aggregate at the sites of experimentally produced wounds subsequently differentiate into flattened cells. These cells superficially resemble the flattened leukocytes involved in capsule formation by *B. glabrata*. However, intracellular microfilaments not observed in *B. glabrata* have been observed in *L. stagnalis* leukocytes. Sminia *et al.*[34] have suggested that such filaments probably play a role in the transformation of normal amoebocytes into flattened ones. In addition, intercellular fibers that morphologically resemble collagen are formed between such cells in *L. stagnalis*.

In summary, it has been shown that capsules formed around *A. cantonensis* larvae in *B. glabrata* are not simply static fibrous nodules, merely responsible for sequestration of large foreign materials. Rather, they consist of layer upon layer of finely drawn cells. These observations therefore support the earlier proposition, made as the result of enzyme studies,[17] that the molluscan encapsulation reaction may prove to be a highly dynamic structure of extreme importance in maintaining the internal integrity of the mollusk.

ACKNOWLEDGMENT

Grateful thanks are given to Dr. Thomas C. Cheng, Director of the Institute for Pathobiology and Center for Health Sciences, Lehigh University, for making the facilities of his laboratory available to me and for his helpful suggestions and criticisms relative to the conception and development of these studies.

REFERENCES

1. CHENG, T. C. 1967. Marine molluscs as hosts for symbiosis: with a review of known parasites of commercially important species. *In* Advances in Marine Biology. F. S. Russell, Ed. Vol. **5**: 1–424. Academic Press, Inc. New York, N.Y.
2. BROOKS, W. M. 1969. Molluscan immunity to metazoan parasites. *In* Immunity to Parasitic Animals. G. J. Jackson, R. Herman & I. Singer, Eds. Vol. **1**: 149–171. Appleton-Century-Crofts. New York, N.Y.
3. TRIPP, M. R. 1969. General mechanisms and principles of invertebrate immunity. *In* Immunity to Parasitic Animals. G. J. Jackson, R. Herman & I. Singer, Eds. Vol. **1**: 111–128. Appleton-Century-Crofts. New York, N.Y.
4. TRIPP, M. R. 1970. Defense mechanisms of molluscs. J. Reticuloendothel. Soc. **7**: 173–182.

5. TRIPP, M. R. 1974. Molluscan immunity. Ann. N.Y. Acad. Sci. **234**: 23–27.
6. CHENG, T. C. & E. RIFKIN. 1970. ·Cellular reactions in marine molluscs in response to helminth parasitism. *In* A Symposium on Diseases of Fishes and Shellfishes. F. S. Snieszko, Ed. Vol. **5**: 443–496. American Fisheries Society. Washington, D.C.
7. NEWTON, W. L. 1952. The comparative tissue reaction of two strains of *Australorbis glabratus* to infection with *Schistosoma mansoni*. J. Parasitol. **38**: 362–366.
8. BROOKS, C. P. 1953. A comparative study of *Schistosoma mansoni* in *Tropicorbis havanensis* and *Australorbis glabratus*. J. Parasitol. **39**: 159–165.
9. BARBOSA, F. S. & A. C. BARRETO. 1960. Differences in susceptibility of Brazilian strains of *Australorbis glabratus* to *Schistosoma mansoni*. Exp. Parasitol. **9**: 137–140.
10. SUDDS, R. H., JR. 1960. Observations of schistosome miracidial behavior in the presence of normal and abnormal snail hosts and subsequent tissue studies of these hosts. J. Elisha Mitchell Sci. Soc. **76**: 121–133.
11. KINOTI, G. K. 1971. Observations on the infection of bulinid snails with *Schistosoma mattheei*. The mechanism of resistance to infection. Parasitology **62**: 161–170.
12. DUKE, B. O. L. 1952. On the route of emergence of the cercariae of *Schistosoma mansoni* from *Australorbis glabratus*. J. Helminthol. **26**: 133–146.
13. PAN, C. T. 1963. Generalized and focal tissue responses in the snail *Australorbis glabratus* infected with *Schistosoma mansoni*. Ann. N.Y. Acad. Sci. **113**: 475–485.
14. PAN, C. T. 1965. Studies on the host-parasite relationship between *Schistosoma mansoni* and the snail *Australorbis glabratus*. Amer. J. Trop. Med. Hyg. **14**: 931–976.
15. HARRIS, K. R. & T. C. CHENG. 1975. The encapsulation process in *Biomphalaria glabrata* experimentally infected with the metastrongylid *Angiostrongylus cantonensis:* light microscopy. Int. J. Parasitol. In press.
16. RICHARDS, C. S. & J. W. MERRITT. 1967. Studies on *Angiostrongylus cantonensis* in molluscan intermediate hosts. J. Parasitol. **53**: 382–388.
17. HARRIS, K. R. & T. C. CHENG. 1975. The encapsulation process in *Biomphalaria glabrata* experimentally infected with the metastrongylid *Angiostrongylus cantonensis:* enzyme histochemistry. J. Invert. Pathol. In press.
18. NEWTON, W. L. 1955. The establishment of a strain of *Australorbis glabratus* which combines albinism and high susceptibility to infection with *Schistosoma mansoni*. J. Parasitol. **41**: 526–528.
19. REYNOLDS, E. S. 1963. The use of lead citrate at high pH as an electron opaque stain in electron microscopy. J. Cell Biol. **17**: 208–212.
20. FAULK, W. P., H. K. LIM, K. H. JEONG, D. HEYNEMAN & D. PRICE. 1973. An approach to the study of immunity in invertebrates. *In* Non-Specific Factors Influencing Host Resistance. W. Braun & J. Ungar, Eds. : 24–32. S. Karger. Basel, Switzerland.
21. HARRIS, K. R. 1974. Studies on encapsulation in *Biomphalaria glabrata*. Ph.D. Dissertation. Lehigh University. Bethlehem, Pa.
22. HOHL, H. R. 1965. Nature and development of membrane systems in food vacuoles of cellular slime molds predatory upon bacteria. J. Bacteriol. **90**: 755–765.
23. TRIPP, M. R. 1961. The fate of foreign materials experimentally introduced into the snail *Australorbis glabratus*. J. Parasitol. **47**: 745–751.
24. STANG-VOSS, C. 1970. Zur Ultrastruktur der Blutzellen wirbelloser Tiere. III. Über die Haemocyten der Schnecke *Lymnaea stagnalis* L. (Pulmonata). Z. Zellforsch. **107**: 141–156.
25. SMINIA, T. 1972. Structure and function of blood and connective tissue cells of the fresh water pulmonate *Lymnaea stagnalis* studied by electron microscopy and enzyme histochemistry. Z. Zellforsch. **130**: 497–526.

26. ABOLINŠ-KROGIS, A. 1972. The tubular endoplasmic reticulum in the amoebocytes of the shell regenerating snail, *Helix pomatia* L. Z. Zellforsch. **128:** 58–68.

27. WOLBURG-BUCHOLZ, K. & A. NOLTE. 1973. Vergleichende Untersuchungen an Amoebozyten und Blasenzellen von *Cepea nemoralis* L. (Gastropoda, Stylommatophora) Unterschiedliche Endozytosefähigkeit der Zellen. Z. Zellforsch. **137:** 281–292.

28. FENG, S. Y., J. S. FENG, C. N. BURKE & L. H. KHAIRALLAH. 1971. Light and electron microscopy of the leukocytes of *Crassostrea virginica* (Mollusca: Pelecypoda). Z. Zellforsch. **120:** 222–245.

29. CHENG, T. C. & A. CALI. 1974. An electron microscope study of the fate of bacteria phagocytized by granulocytes of *Crassostrea virginica*. *In* Contemporary Topics in Immunobiology. E. L. Cooper, Ed. Vol. **4:** 25–35. Plenum Publishing Corporation. New York, N.Y.

30. CHENG, T. C., A. CALI & D. A. FOLEY. 1974. Cellular reactions in marine pelecypods as a factor influencing endosymbiosis. *In* Symbiosis in the Sea. W. Vernberg, Ed. University of South Carolina Press. Columbia, S.C.

31. MICHELSON, E. H. 1961. An acid fast pathogen of fresh water snails. Amer. J. Trop. Med. Hyg. **10:** 423–433.

32. NEWTON, W. L. 1954. Tissue response to *Schistosoma mansoni* in second generation snails from a cross between two strains of *Australorbis glabratus*. J. Parasitol. **40:** 352–355.

33. RIFKIN, E., T. C. CHENG & H. R. HOHL. 1969. An electron microscope study of the constituents of encapsulating cysts in *Crassostrea virginica* formed in response to *Tylocephalum* metacestodes. J. Invert. Pathol. **14:** 211–226.

34. SMINIA, T., K. PIETERSMA & J. E. M. SCHEERBOOM. 1973. Histological and ultrastructural observations on wound healing in the freshwater pulmonate *Lymnaea stagnalis*. Z. Zellforsch. **141:** 561–573.

ELECTRON MICROSCOPY OF OUABAIN-INHIBITED, POTASSIUM-DEPENDENT TRANSPORT ADENOSINE TRIPHOSPHATASE ACTIVITY IN SCHISTOSOME SPOROCYSTS *

Paul L. Krupa, Larry M. Lewis, and Peter Del Vecchio

Department of Biology
The City College of the City University of New York
New York, New York 10031

INTRODUCTION

The properties and behavior of the surface plasma membrane of sporocysts greatly affect the nature of mollusk-parasite interactions, because these trematode larvae must procure all their nutrients at the host-parasite interface. If enzyme activities associated with transport systems for passage of biologically important substances across plasma membranes of well-studied nonparasitologic cell types are also found on or in surfaces of these sporocysts, a more adequate assessment may be obtained of what the parasites can or cannot do.

One of the most widely distributed active transport systems in vertebrates and invertebrates uses Na^+-K^+-activated adenosine triphosphatase (Na-K-ATPase), which is dependent on Mg^{2+} and is inhibited by ouabain (see recent reviews [1-3]). For many years, the histochemical procedure of Wachstein and Meisel [4] has been widely used to demonstate adenosine triphosphatase (ATPase) activity with adenosine triphosphate (ATP) as the substrate and lead as the capture ion of inorganic phosphate released by the enzyme. Nevertheless, the method has been inconsistent for detecting ouabain-sensitive Na-K-ATPase [9] and has been criticized and defended by many workers for other reasons (see reviews [5-8]). To partially bypass the problems of the Wachstein-Meisel medium, Ernst [5, 6] introduced an alternate approach for the cytochemical localization of Na-K-ATPase by using *p*-nitrophenylphosphate (NPP) instead of ATP as the substrate and strontium (Sr) instead of lead (Pb) as the capture ion to demonstrate ouabain-inhibited, potassium-dependent phosphatase (K-NPPase), which is the second step of the two-stage Na-K-ATPase enzyme system.[1, 3, 5] More recently, Leuenberger and Novikoff [9] and Firth [8] found Ernst's method reliable for detecting Na-K-ATPase when appropriate controls are employed.

This paper is an inquiry into the electron microscopy of Na-K-ATPase activity in *Schistosoma haematobium* and *S. mansoni* daughter sporocysts as revealed by the Ernst method.

MATERIALS AND METHODS

Snails of *Bulinus truncatus*, infected with *S. haematobium* (Egyptian strain), and of *Biomphalaria glabrata* (Puerto Rican strain), infected with *S. mansoni* larvae, were obtained from Dr. Harvey D. Blankespoor at the Museum of

* Supported by National Institutes of Health Grant AI 102070 and by grants from the City University of New York Faculty Research Program (P.L.K.).

Zoology, University of Michigan, under the auspices of the U.S.-Japan Cooperative Medical Science Program (NIAID). The snails were used within 1 week after delivery, during which time they were fed lettuce and kept in finger bowls filled with spring water.

Cytochemistry

Shells of infected snails were carefully crushed in a dish filled with spring water. Digestive glands infected with sporocysts and cercariae were cut with a razor into two or three pieces and placed in ice-cold 3% formaldehyde freshly prepared from paraformaldehyde[10] in 0.1 M cacodylate buffer (pH 7.2). After 10 min in the fixative, the infected material was cut on a TC-2 tissue chopper[11] at 100 μm and returned to fresh cold fixative for a total 20-min fixation time. The tissues were rinsed in cacodylate buffer three times (5 min each) and then rinsed similarly with 0.092 M Tris buffer (pH 7.2). This second rinse was performed because cacodylate reversibly inhibits Na-K-ATPase activity.[12]

Tissues chopped at 100 μm were incubated in the standard p-nitrophenyl-phosphate-strontium medium of Ernst[6] that contained (final concentrations) 5 mM NPP (disodium salt, Sigma), 100 mM Tris-HCl buffer (pH 9.0), 10 mM MgCl$_2$, 10 mM KCl, and 20 mM SrCl$_2$ as the heavy metal capture ion. The sections were incubated at room temperature (26° C) for 45 min in a mechanical agitator.

As controls to help interpret staining reactions, 10 mM ouabain was added to the standard medium to test for inhibition of K-NPPase activity, equimolar concentrations of choline chloride were substituted for KCl, Mg^{2+} was deleted from the standard medium, equimolar concentrations of β-glycerophosphate (GP) were substituted for NPP in the standard medium, and specimens were incubated in the standard medium without NPP.

Electron Microscopy

After incubation, all sections were rinsed in three changes of 0.1 M Tris-HCl buffer (pH 9.0). To convert precipitated strontium phosphate (SrP) to lead phosphate (PbP) for visualization in the electron microscope,[6] sections were washed twice (5 min each) in 2% lead nitrate. To remove free Pb, the sections were then washed in two 5-min rinses with 5% sucrose and were postfixed at 26° C in 1% OsO$_4$-0.1 M cacodylate buffer (pH 7.5) with 5% sucrose added. Finally, the sections were rinsed briefly in distilled water, dehydrated with acetone, embedded in an Araldite®-Epon® mixture, sectioned with an ultramicrotome, and examined in a Philips 300 electron microscope. The sections were not stained to avoid masking small amounts of reaction product deposits with counterstains.

RESULTS

Although parasite tissues fixed in formaldehyde retained only fair to good morphology, with cercariae tending to fix better than sporocysts, inadequate preservation was more than offset by precise localization of enzyme activities in distinct regions of sporocysts and their intrasporocyst cercariae.

In formaldehyde-fixed parasites incubated with NPP as the substrate, the reaction product is found only on the cytoplasmic side of the apical plasma membrane that covers the microvilli and tegument of sporocysts of *S. haematobium* (FIGURES 1 & 2) and *S. mansoni* (FIGURE 4). In *S. haematobium*, the deposits are small ($\sim$80 Å), numerous, and form dense clumps in the microvilli and tegument (FIGURE 2), often filling the entire length of microvilli so as to clearly demark their single or branched profiles (FIGURES 1 & 2). In *S. mansoni* sporocysts, the deposits are large ($\sim$800 Å) discrete granules, mostly located in microvilli (FIGURE 4). No reaction product is found in deeper subtegumental regions of the sporocyst body wall of either species (FIGURES 1, 2 & 4) or in cercariae (FIGURE 3). No deposits are found in mitochondria, even those of the sporocyst tegument located close to reaction particles (FIGURE 4). No reaction product is found in nuclei or on the extracellular side of plasma membranes of sporocysts and intrasporocyst cercariae incubated with NPP.

As controls, *S. haematobium* larvae were incubated with NPP and ouabain, NPP and no K$^+$, NPP and no Mg^{2+}, or with GP. In the presence of ouabain, little or no K-NPPase activity is found in sporocyst microvilli and tegument (FIGURE 5). Elsewhere in ouabain-incubated specimens, deposits are encountered in the subtegumental portion of the sporocyst body wall (FIGURE 5) and in cercariae on the outer surface of the tegument, in the basal lamina, and on the extracellular side of plasma membranes of penetration gland cells (FIGURE 6). With NPP and no K$^+$ in the incubation medium, little or no reaction product is found in the microvilli or tegument of sporocysts or in the tegument of cercariae (FIGURE 7), but some nonspecific precipitate is seen in the basal lamina of cercariae. Specimens incubated with NPP but without Mg^{2+} have reduced precipitate or none at all in sporocyst (FIGURE 8) or cercarial surfaces. In specimens incubated with GP, much precipitate is found on the outer surface of the cercarial tegument (not illustrated) and within the subtegumental region of the sporocyst body wall (FIGURE 9), but few or no deposits are seen in the sporocyst microvilli and tegument (FIGURE 9).

In the absence of NPP as the substrate, no reaction product is present on either side of the apical plasma membrane of sporocysts of *S. mansoni* (FIGURE 10) and *S. haematobium* or of their intrasporocyst cercariae. *S. haematobium* sporocysts fixed poorly in substrate blanks. In other well-preserved specimens incubated without substrate, mitochondria of *S. haematobium* cercariae contain some dense deposits (FIGURE 11), but mitochondria of *S. mansoni* sporocysts and cercariae do not.

DISCUSSION

In light of previous work by others [6, 8, 9] who found NPP a reliable substrate to localize transport ATPase when used with appropriate controls, our results indicate that a ouabain-sensitive, potassium-activated Na-K-ATPase system occurs in the surface of *S. haematobium* and *S. mansoni* sporocysts. With NPP as the substrate in the incubation medium, reaction product was found on the cytoplasmic side of the apical plasma membrane that covers the microvilli and tegument of daughter sporocysts of *S. haematobium* (FIGURES 1 & 2) and of *S. mansoni* (FIGURE 4). We do not know why reaction particles appeared so different in size in *S. haematobium* (FIGURE 2) and *S. mansoni* (FIGURE 4) sporocysts incubated with NPP. The occlusion of microvilli by precipitate in

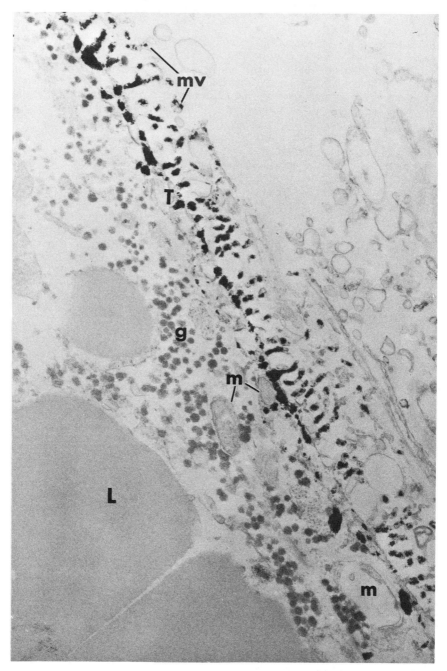

FIGURE 1. An electron micrograph of the apical surface of the body wall of a *Schistosoma haematobium* daughter sporocyst incubated 45 min. for K-NPPase activity. Reaction product is found in microvilli (mv) and in the tegument (T) but not in mitochondria (m) or in deeper regions of the body wall. L, lipid; g, glycogen. ×25,000.

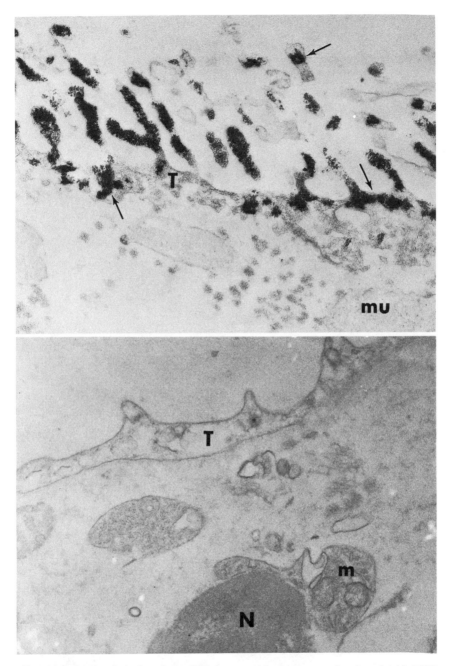

FIGURE 2 (*top*). Apical surface of *S. haematobium* sporocyst incubated with NPP. Arrows show sites where K-NPPase reaction product is seen restricted to the cytoplasmic side of the apical plasma membrane that covers the microvilli and to the cytoplasmic side of the apical and basal plasma membranes of the tegument (T). Note branched microvillous profile. mu, Muscle. ×50,000.

FIGURE 3 (*bottom*). Apical surface of *S. haematobium* cercaria in brood chamber of sporocyst illustrated in FIGURES 1 and 2. No precipitate is found in or on tegument (T) or elsewhere. N, nucleus; m, mitochondrion. ×25,000.

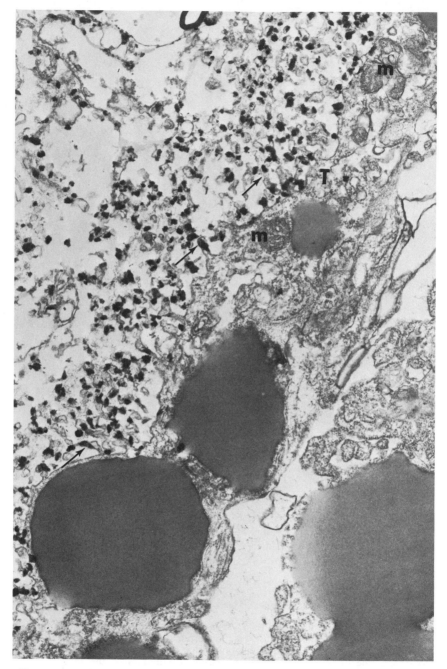

FIGURE 4. Apical surface of *S. mansoni* sporocyst incubated with NPP. Most reaction product deposits are restricted to the cytoplasm of microvilli (arrows). A few granules are seen in the tegument (T), but mitochondria (m) have none. ×25,000.

S. haematobium (FIGURES 1 & 2), however, is probably due to the relatively lengthy incubation period (45 min). As precipitation continues, Ernst[6] found densities of deposits increased with increasing incubation periods. K-NPPase activity was virtually or completely abolished in the presence of ouabain (FIGURE 5) and in the absence of K^+ (FIGURE 7) and Mg^{2+} (FIGURE 8). No K-NPPase activity was found in the tegument of intrasporocyst cercariae (FIGURE 3) of either species. With GP as the substrate, little or no reaction product was found in sporocyst microvilli and tegument (FIGURE 9), and no deposits were found here in specimens incubated without substrate (FIGURE 10).

At this writing, only a few electron cytochemical studies of K-NPPase activity are available for comparison with our results. In vertebrate tissues incubated with NPP, reaction product was restricted to the intracellular side of the plasma membranes of certain cells of avian salt glands[6] and of mammalian renal tubules[9] but to the extracellular side of the plasma membranes of certain cells of the rat cornea.[8] In the cornea study, Leuenberger and Novikoff[9] suggested that "sidedness" of K-NPPase reaction deposits of plasma membranes may reflect differences in enzyme sites among different cell types. In observations with electron microscopy of adult trematodes reported in brief to date, alkaline NPPase activity was found in the tegument of *S. mansoni*[13] but not in the tegument of *Megalodiscus temperatus,*[27] which in previous studies was found to possess little ability to transport molecules through its tegument. In addition, Bogitsh[27] has found Na^+-dependent, K^+-independent, ouabain-sensitive NPPase activity on the cytoplasmic side of the apical plasma membrane of the cecum of *M. temperatus.*

The ultrastructural localization of ATPase activity in schistosome sporocysts with the Ernst method in the present study differs from that reported by Krupa and Bogitsh[7] for ATPase activity localized in *S. mansoni* larvae with the Wachstein-Meisel method. With the latter procedure used to incubate formaldehyde-fixed sporocysts and intrasporocyst cercariae with ATP, they found reaction product on the outer surface of the apical plasma membrane that covers sporocyst microvilli and tegument, on the outer surface of the tegumental plasmalemma of cercariae, and in some mitochondria of cercariae. In addition, mitochondria were unreactive for ATPase in formaldehyde-fixed sporocysts but not when sporocysts were incubated prior to fixation. In the present study of schistosomes incubated with NPP in the Ernst medium, reaction product was consistently found only on the intracytoplasmic side of the surface plasma membrane of *S. haematobium* and *S. mansoni* sporocysts. No reaction product was found extracellularly, in mitochondria, or elsewhere in parasites incubated with NPP. Although some workers[14-16] raised serious questions about the validity of the Wachstein-Meisel method for cytochemical localization of phosphohydrolases, others[17-19] have shown that real enzyme activities are found in tissues incubated with different nucleoside phosphates, inhibitors, and activators. Because the results of Krupa and Bogitsh[7] and ours in this study both appear to reveal real ATPase activities associated with plasma membranes, as supported by appropriate controls, it is possible that each method has demonstrated in the surface of schistosome sporocysts and cercariae either different activities of a single ATPase enzyme system or two different ATPase enzyme activities. In well-studied vertebrate and invertebrate cells, Mg^{2+}-activated adenosine triphosphatase (Mg-ATPase) hydrolyzes only ATP present outside, and Na-K-ATPase hydrolyzes only ATP present inside of plasma membranes.[2] In view of numerous additional biochemical dissimilarities reviewed by Bonting,[2] arguments favor

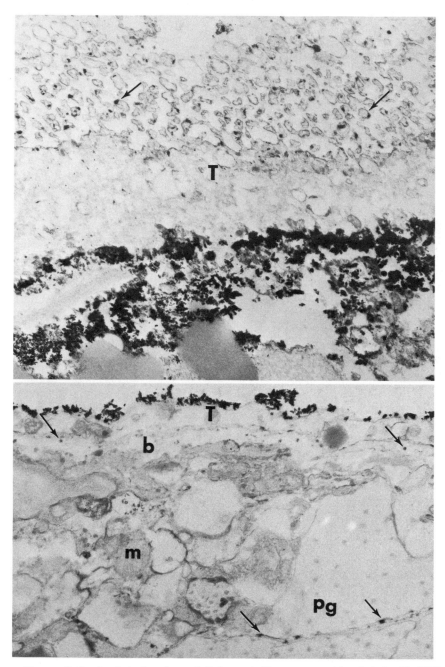

FIGURE 5 (*top*). Apical surface of *S. haematobium* sporocyst incubated with NPP and ouabain. Note that only a few deposits remain restricted to the intracytoplasmic side of the plasma in microvilli (arrows) and in the tegument (T). Compare this the conclusion that Mg-ATPase and Na-K-ATPase are two different enzymes. In addition, from a cytochemical viewpoint, Ernst and Philpott [12] and Leuenberger and Novikoff,[9] among others, have suggested that the extracellular deposition of reaction product found with the Wachstein-Meisel method is most likely due to Mg-ATPase. The present study showed Na-K-ATPase on the intracytoplasmic side of the apical plasma membrane of the sporocyst (FIGURE 2) but not of the cercaria (FIGURE 3). In the work of Krupa and Bogitsh,[7] ATPase activity was found on the outer surface of the cercaria but not of the sporocyst. In light of the above reasons, among others, it is quite possible that the surface ATPase of schistosome intrasporocyst cercariae is actually Mg-ATPase.

The specificity of the Ernst medium to demonstrate Na-K-ATPase has been questioned by Firth,[8] who found both nonspecific alkaline phosphatase and Na-K-ATPase activities in mammalian renal tubules incubated with NPP. In avian salt gland and mammalian cornea tissues incubated in the Ernst medium with GP instead of NPP, no reaction product was found.[6, 9] In contrast, when the present schistosome tissues were incubated with GP, we found few or no deposits in the microvilli and tegument of sporocysts, but dense accumulations were seen in deeper subtegumental regions of the sporocyst body wall (FIGURE 9) and on the outer surface of the tegument of intrasporocyst cercariae (not illustrated). With GP instead of ATP used in the Wachstein-Meisel medium, Krupa and Bogitsh [7] found a fine precipitate on the microvilli, dense deposits in the subtegumental part of the sporocyst body wall, and little or no precipitate on the cercarial tegument. Because both the Ernst and Wachstein-Meisel procedures demonstrate much nonspecific alkaline phosphatase activity in the basal portion of the sporocyst body wall, and little or none on the sporocyst microvilli and tegument, the present results, when considered with the other controls, further strengthen our conviction that K-NPPase activity was demonstrated in the microvilli and tegument of sporocysts incubated with NPP (FIGURES 1, 2 & 4). However, when additional evidence is needed to distinguish suspected alkaline phosphatase and Na-K-ATPase activities that occur at similar sites in tissues incubated with NPP, then, as shown by Firth,[8] it would be desirable to use as a control *l*-tetramisole to specifically inhibit alkaline phosphatase activity. Indeed, it is interesting that in parasites incubated with NPP and ouabain, a nonspecific precipitate was found in the subtegumental portion of the sporocyst body wall (FIGURE 5) and on the outer surface of intrasporocyst cercariae (FIGURE 6). Additional work with *l*-tetramisole would be needed to determine whether these deposits are from hydrolysis of NPP by ouabain-insensitive alkaline phosphatase activity.

In experiments performed before the present work, we inadvertently incubated *S. japonicum* and *S. mansoni* sporocysts with NPP and 200 mM Sr instead of 20 mM Sr, as recommended by Ernst,[6] and found deposits only rarely and on the cytoplasmic side of some sporocyst microvilli. This finding may be

---

image with FIGURES 1 and 2 of the sporocyst incubated without inhibitor. Much nonspecific precipitate is seen in subtegumental regions of the sporocyst body wall in this Figure. ×25,000.

FIGURE 6 (*bottom*). Apical surface of *S. haematobium* cercaria in brood chamber of sporocyst in FIGURE 5 incubated with NPP and ouabain. Many nonspecific deposits are present at the outer surface of the tegument (T). Fewer nonspecific granules (arrows) are seen in the basal lamina (b) and in the intercellular space of plasma membranes of penetration gland cells (Pg). Compare with FIGURE 3. m, Mitochondrion. ×25,000.

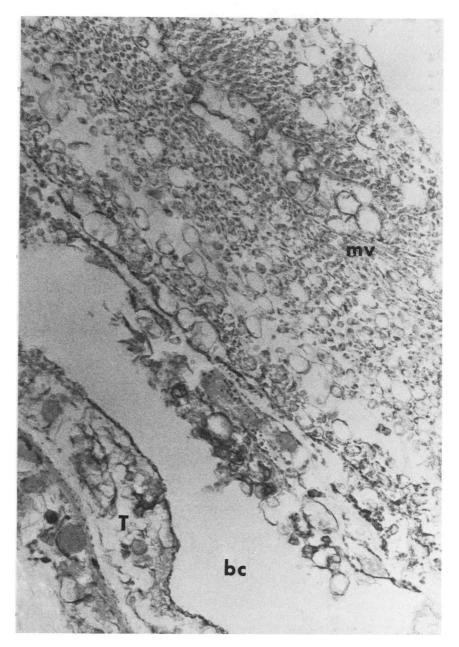

FIGURE 7. Portions of *S. haematobium* sporocyst and intrasporocyst cercaria incubated with NPP but with no K+. K-NPPase activity is greatly reduced or absent from microvilli (mv) and tegument of the sporocyst. T, tegument of cercaria; bc, brood chamber. ×25,000.

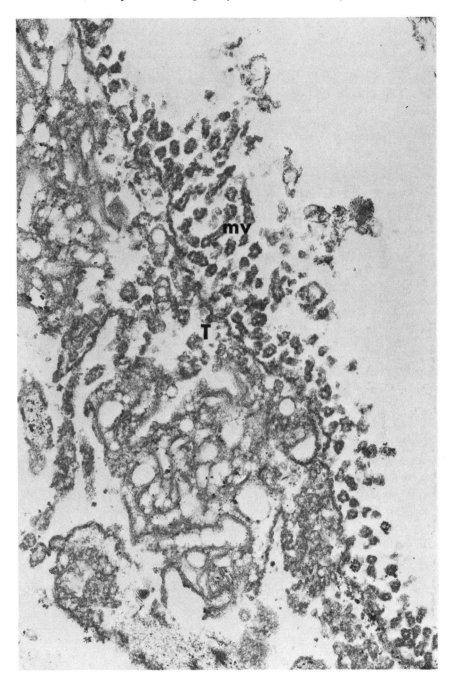

FIGURE 8. Apical portion of *S. haematobium* sporocyst incubated with NPP but with Mg²⁺ deleted. K-NPPase activity is greatly reduced or absent from microvilli (mv) and tegument (T). ×25,000.

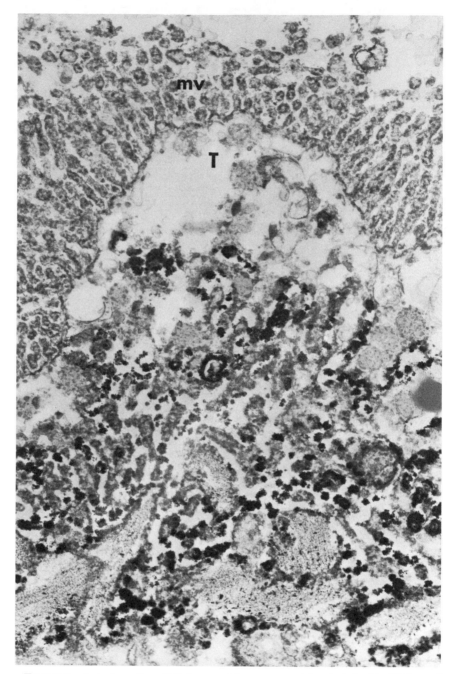

FIGURE 9. Apical portion of *S. haematobium* sporocyst incubated with GP instead of NPP. No deposits are present in microvilli (mv) and tegument (T). Dense non-specific accumulations are seen in more basal, subtegumental regions of the body wall. ×25,000.

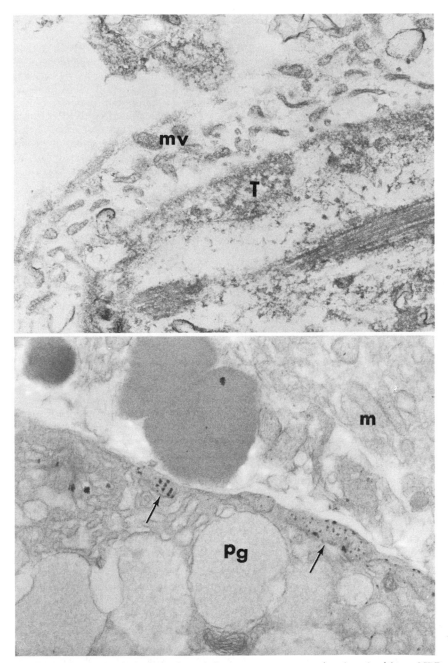

FIGURE 10 (*top*). Apical portion of *S. mansoni* sporocyst incubated with no NPP in the standard incubation medium. No deposits are seen in microvilli (mv) or tegument (T). ×25,000.

FIGURE 11 (*bottom*). Portions of two cells in *S. haematobium* intrasporocyst cercaria incubated with no NPP in standard incubation medium. Nonspecific deposits are detected readily in mitochondria (arrows) of a penetration gland cell (Pg), but few or none are seen in the numerous mitochondria (m) of a neighboring cell. ×25,000.

taken as additional evidence for the specific inhibition of K-NPPase activity, because biochemical evidence [5] showed an increase in the percentage of K-NPPase inhibition with increasing concentrations of Sr when it was used as the heavy metal salt to precipitate phosphate for cytochemistry. A nonenzymatically produced phosphate precipitate was found in our material only in mitochondria of *S. haematobium* cercariae incubated without NPP (FIGURE 11) but not in mitochondria of *S. mansoni* sporocysts and cercariae. Ernst,[6] who observed similar intramitochondrial deposits in all of his incubation groups, considered this finding to be due, in part, to mitochondrial sequestration of lead during postincubatory conversion of SrP to PbP (see his [6] and our MATERIALS AND METHODS).

Various histochemical, biochemical, and morphologic studies have suggested that the sporocyst body wall is specialized for uptake of glucose, amino acids, and other biologically important substances.[20-26] What possible link exists between these previous studies and the present cytochemical demonstration of Na-K-ATPase activity in the surface of schistosome sporocysts? According to recent reviews,[1-3] the concept of active transport systems in cells of higher animals suggests that such cells have a basic economy and simplicity, in that the active pumping of Na+ ions out of a cell may furnish the driving force for the active transport of K+, glucose, amino acids, and other substances into the cell. Thus, high and constant concentrations of intracellular K+ can be maintained, even though external concentrations of Na+ and K+ vary. In addition, glucose and amino acids may be accumulated intracellularly against glucose and amino acid gradients. Uptake of K+ and extrusion of Na+ helps to maintain internal osmotic pressure at the appropriate level.[3] High concentrations of internal K+ are required, among other reasons, for protein synthesis by ribosomes, which need a high concentration of K+ for maximal activity.[3] Thus, it seems reasonable to speculate that, among other functions, the energy from the Na-K-ATPase system in the surface of schistosome sporocysts may prevent osmotic damage to the sporocyst body wall and intrasporocyst cercariae, provide an electrogenic Na+ pump to transport glucose, amino acids, and other nutrients into the sporocyst body wall from where they would pass to developing cercariae, and maintain a concentration of K+ inside the sporocyst for protein synthesis by ribosomes in the production of numerous cercariae.

REFERENCES

1. SKOU, J. C. 1965. Enzymatic basis for active transport of Na+ and K+ across cell membrane. Physiol. Rev. **45:** 596–617.
2. BONTING, S. L. 1970. Sodium-potassium activated adensosinetriphosphatase and cation transport. *In* Membranes and Ion Transport. E. E. Bittar, Ed. Vol. **1:** 257–263. Interscience Publishers. New York, N.Y.
3. LEHNINGER, A. L. 1970. Biochemistry. The Molecular Basis of Cell Structure and Function. Worth Publishers, Inc. New York, N.Y.
4. WACHSTEIN, M. & E. MEISEL. 1957. Histochemistry of hepatic phosphatases at physiologic pH with special reference to the demonstration of bile caniliculi. Amer. J. Clin. Pathol. **27:** 13–23.
5. ERNST, S. A. 1972. Transport adenosine triphosphatase cytochemistry. I. Biochemical characterization of a cytochemical medium for the ultrastructural localization of ouabain-sensitive, potassium-dependent phosphatase activity in the avian salt gland. J. Histochem. Cytochem. **20:** 13–22.
6. ERNST, S. A. 1972. Transport adensosine triphosphatase cytochemistry. II. Cytochemical localization of ouabain-sensitive, potassium-dependent phosphatase

activity in the secretory epithelium of the avian salt gland. J. Histochem. Cytochem. **20**: 23–38.

7. KRUPA, P. L. & B. J. BOGITSH. 1972. Ultrastructural phosphohydrolase activities in *Schistosoma mansoni* sporocysts and cercariae. J. Parasitol. **58**: 495–514.

8. FIRTH, J. A. 1974. Problems of specificity in the use of strontium capture technique for cytochemical localization of ouabain-sensitive, potassium-dependent phosphatase in mammalian renal tubules. J. Histochem. Cytochem. **12**: 1163–1168.

9. LEUENBERGER, P. M. & A. B. NOVIKOFF. 1974. Localization of transport adenosine triphosphatase in rat cornea. J. Cell Biol. **60**: 721–731.

10. PEASE, D. C. 1964. Histological Techniques for Electron Microscopy. Academic Press, Inc. New York, N.Y.

11. SMITH, R. E. & M. FARQUHAR. 1965. Preparation of nonfrozen sections for electron microscope cytochemistry. Sci. Instr. News **10**: 13.

12. ERNST, S. A. & C. W. PHILPOTT. 1970. Preservation of Na-K-activated and Mg-activated triphosphatase activities of avian salt gland and teleost gill with formaldehyde fixative. J. Histochem. Cytochem. **18**: 251–263.

13. ERNST, S. C. 1974. Phosphatases of *Schistosoma mansoni*. Proc. 3rd Int. Cong. Parasitol. Sect. **B4**: 429.

14. ROSENTHAL, A. S., H. L. MOSES, D. L. BEAVER & S. S. SCHUFFMAN. 1966. Lead ion and phosphatase histochemistry. I. Nonenzymatic hydrolysis of nucleoside phosphates by lead ion. J. Histochem. Cytochem. **14**: 698–701.

15. NOVIKOFF, A. B., D. H. HAUSMAN & E. PODBER. 1958. The localization of adenosine triphosphatase in liver: *in situ* staining and cell fractionation studies. J. Histochem. Cytochem. **6**: 61–71.

16. MOSES, H. L. & A. M. ROSENTHAL. 1968. Pitfalls in the use of lead ion for histochemical localization of nucleoside phosphatases. J. Histochem. Cytochem. **16**: 530–539.

17. NOVIKOFF, A. B., E. ESSNER, S. GOLDFISCHER & M. HEUS. 1962. Nucleosidephosphatase activities of cytomembranes. Symp. Int. Soc. Cell Biol. **1**: 149–192.

18. NOVIKOFF, A. B. 1967. Enzyme localizations with Wachstein-Meisel procedures: real or artifact. J. Histochem. Cytochem. **15**: 353, 354.

19. PADYKULA, H. A. & G. F. GAUTHIER. 1963. Cytochemical studies of adenosine triphosphatases in skeletal muscle fibers. J. Cell Biol. **18**: 87–107.

20. CHENG, T. C. & R. SNYDER. 1962. Studies on host-parasite relationships between larval trematodes and their hosts. I. A review. II. The utilization of the host's glycogen by the intramolluscan larvae of *Glypthelmins pennsylvaniensis* Cheng, and associated phenomena. Trans. Amer. Microsc. Soc. **81**: 209–228.

21. CHENG, T. C. & R. SNYDER. 1962. Studies on host-parasite relationships between larval trematodes and their hosts. III. Certain aspects of lipid metabolism in *Helisoma trivolvis* (Say) infected with larvae of *Glypthelmins pennsylvaniensis* Cheng and related phenomena. Trans. Amer. Microsc. Soc. **81**: 327–331.

22. CHENG, T. C. 1963. Biochemical requirements of larval trematodes. Ann. N.Y. Acad. Sci. **113**: 289–321.

23. CHENG, T. C. 1965. Histochemical observations on changes in lipid composition of the American oyster, *Crassostrea virginica* (Gmelin), parasitized by the trematode *Bucephalus* sp. J. Invert. Pathol. **7**: 398–407.

24. NEGUS, M. R. S. 1968. The nutrition of the sporocysts of the trematode *Cercaria doricha* Rothschild, 1935 in the molluscan host *Turitella communis* Risso. Parasitology **58**: 355–386.

25. WATTS, S. D. M. 1970. The amino acid requirements of the redia of *Cryptocotyle lingua* and *Himasthla leptosoma* and of the sporocyst of *Cercaria emasculans* Pelseneer, 1900. Parasitology **61**: 491–497.

26. HOCKLEY, D. J. 1973. Ultrastructure of the tegument of *Schistosoma*. *In* Advances in Parasitology. B. Dawes, Ed. Vol. **11**: 233–305. Academic Press, Inc. New York, N.Y.

27. BOGITSH, B. J. 1975. Personal communication.

BEHAVIORAL AND DEVELOPMENTAL PHYSIOLOGY OF SCHISTOSOME LARVAE AS RELATED TO THEIR MOLLUSCAN HOSTS *

F. J. Etges, O. S. Carter,† and G. Webbe

Department of Biological Sciences
The University of Cincinnati
Cincinnati, Ohio 45221
and The London School of Hygiene and Tropical Medicine
Winches Farm Field Station
St. Albans, Hertshire, England

MIRACIDIA

The life of the schistosome miracidium begins upon its complete embryonation within the egg, some time after being produced by the female parent in the mammalian host. Its first active function in life occurs in the process of hatching; the various environmental factors that condition this process have been described and reviewed recently by Bair and Etges,[1] but the contribution of the miracidium to the process remains poorly understood. The existence of an unidentified hatching factor within schistosome eggs, as suggested by Kusel,[2] remains hypothetical.

The posthatching behavior of schistosome miracidia has been more thoroughly studied; the work of Wright,[3] Chernin and Dunavan,[4] MacInnis,[5] Etges and Decker,[6] among many others,[7-13] serves to show that considerable attention has been given to this phase of the life cycle. Briefly stated, previous studies indicate that hatched miracidia remain infective to their molluscan host for 8–12 hr, swim in a smooth spiral path in a "ranging" phase of host location, and increase their turning rate dramatically when stimulated by chemical agents emitted by snails and other organisms (termed the "excited state"). Excited miracidia thus remain relatively close to the source of chemical stimulation and, upon chance contact with a surface, begin to rotate their bodies vigorously while maintaining contact with the surface by the anterior terebratorium. Secretions of apical glands augment the boring movements and finally permit physical entry of the entire ciliated miracidial body. Should the surface penetrated be a susceptible snail's tegument, the miracidia will metamorphose into a mother sporocyst; otherwise, the miracidia die. Host location, therefore, appears to be the result of characteristic ciliary locomotion of miracidia, conditioned by their orientation to various physical stimuli (light, gravity, contact, and so on), until some chemical substance stimulates them to exhibit excited locomotor behavior; Chernin[8] coined the term "miraxone" to refer to the undefined complex of substances emitted by host snails that produce this effect. Though some earlier

* Supported in part by Research Fellowship F03 AI 51 149–01 (F.J.E.) from the National Institutes of Health.
† Present address: Department of Biology, Vanderbilt University, Nashville, Tenn. 37235.

reports suggested that miracidia were more stimulated by their proper host snail than others,[6] later evidence suggests that stimulation and even penetration can be elicited by a variety of natural and synthetic agents; that is, the stimulus is nonspecific.

Further evidence of the nonspecificity of miracidial responses has recently been noted with freshwater turbellarians. In studies that used the large British turbellarian worm *Dendrocoelum lacteum,* the senior author found that miracidia of both *Schistosoma mansoni* and *S. haematobium* exhibit marked excitement in the presence of these worms or their mucus secretions. Miracidia have been shown to be variously affected by turbellarian species,[7, 11, 12] primarily by immobilizing or even lethal action. Miracidia in contact with mucus from *D. lacteum* behaved differently; they showed typical rapid-turning excitement, followed by active boring motion, which resulted in their penetration of the worms or masses of their mucus. When retrieved from surrounding turbellarian mucus, rinsed in two or three changes of clean water, and transferred to a clean vessel, these miracidia resumed apparently normal swimming movements and remained active for more than 8 hr. Unlike the reaction of *S. mansoni* miracidia described by Chernin and Perlstein[13] after exposure to a nonsusceptible snail

TABLE 1

EFFECT OF EXPOSURE TO MUCUS OF *D. lacteum* * ON INFECTIVITY
OF *S. mansoni* AND *S. haematobium* MIRACIDIA

Number of *B. glabrata* Infected by *S. mansoni* Miracidia (5/snail)		Number of *B. africanus* Infected by *S. haematobium* Miracidia (5/snail)	
Mucus-Treated	Controls	Mucus-Treated	Controls
1/26	17/20	0/32	11/25

* Miracidia exposed for 5–10 min.

(*Helisoma caribaeum*), miracidia exposed to *D. lacteum* did not assume a pyriform shape or round up, nor was their locomotor activity abnormal or slow; their behavior and viability appeared normal.

To test whether some less conspicuous change might have been induced in mucus-exposed miracidia, freshly rinsed specimens were placed in contact with their proper susceptible snail hosts, *Biomphalaria glabrata* and *Bulinus africanus,* respectively. Each snail was exposed to five miracidia of the same age, both in experimental groups and controls, using miracidia but was unexposed to turbellarian mucus. Results of these experiments are summarized in TABLE 1.

These experimental data show that though both species of schistosome miracidia behaved apparently normally and survived as long as untreated specimens, their ability to infect a snail was practically obliterated by exposure to the mucus of *D. lacteum.* It is inferred that not all planarians are nearly so lethal to schistosome miracidia as those previously described. Conversely, *D. lacteum* had a much more pronounced effect on infectivity of miracidia exposed to them than Glaudel and Etges[11] found with miracidia of the avian schistosome, *Gigantobilharzia huronensis,* briefly exposed to four American species of turbellarians.

More recently, one of us (O.S.C.) has made another interesting observation on miracidia of *S. mansoni.* Having demonstrated the presence and distribution of various histochemically active materials in tissues of *B. glabrata,* Falck and Owen's technique for localizing the biogenic amines serotonin and dopamine revealed several areas of yellow-green fluorescence indicative of serotonin. Whereas most activity was observed in expected sites, such as nerve cell bodies and tracts, serotonin was particularly abundant in the tentacle and head-foot epithelia. Numerous fibers were observed to extend to the body surface, between epithelial and mucus gland cells, which suggests that their product (serotonin) may be released into the water that surrounds the snail. To the writers' knowledge, no previous analysis has demonstrated this substance in water in which *B. glabrata* have been kept, that is, "snail-conditioned water" (SCW).

Accordingly, experiments similar to those described by Chernin [8] were conducted to determine what action serotonin might have on *S. mansoni* miracidia. Depression slide wells, 15 mm in diameter, were filled with suspensions of about 50 freshly hatched miracidia. Distribution of miracidia was observed to be random in the chamber, due to uniform fluorescent illumination and lack of any other stimulation. Addition of a moist 1-mm square of filter paper to the chamber produced no change in the distribution of swimming miracidia. When moist filter paper was dipped into crystals of serotonin (5-hydroxytryptamine-creatinine sulfate), several would adhere, and when the filter paper was dropped into the test chamber, it caused an almost instantaneous (15–30 sec) aggregation and excited behavior of miracidia around it. As the serotonin crystals dissolved, dispersal of miracidia occurred; after about 5 min, random distribution had resumed, and miracidia exhibited normal locomotor behavior (see FIGURE 1).

To further test the effect of serotonin on *S. mansoni* miracidia, specimens exposed briefly to serotonin were isolated with their snail host, *B. glabrata,* to determine whether their infectivity had been affected. Fifteen snails were individually exposed to four to six serotonin-treated miracidia; as controls, 15 other snails were similarly exposed to four to six untreated miracidia of the same age, hatched simultaneously with the experimental group. Data from a representative experiment, presented in TABLE 2, show that serotonin reduced miracidial infectivity to a marked degree and suggest that exposed miracidia that do succeed in infecting a snail eventually produce far fewer cercariae.

Present findings on the effects of serotonin on *S. mansoni* miracidia are correlated with previous work. For example, Chiang *et al.*[15] found that serotonin levels are much greater in *B. glabrata* than in several other snail species; accordingly, our observations of the apparent release of serotonin through the epithelia of the tentacles and upper head-foot make feasible the concept that serotonin is a component of Chernin's stimulating substance, miraxone. Chernin's [8] partial characterization of miraxone included a low-molecular-weight (under 500) subtance, and serotonin's molecular weight is 179.1. Further, the very general (nonspecific) occurrence of miraxone in a variety of snail species is paralleled by the general distribution of serotonin in animals. The authors do *not* imply that serotonin is the sole stimulating principle of miraxone; MacInnis' [5] study provides ample evidence of the stimulating action of a variety of amino and other organic acids for schistosome miracidia, and MacInnis *et al.*[16] have further proven that these compounds are found in the secretion-excretion materials released by *B. glabrata,* forming an active component of "snail-conditioned water." Sturrock and Upatham [17] provided evidence of the effects of pH,

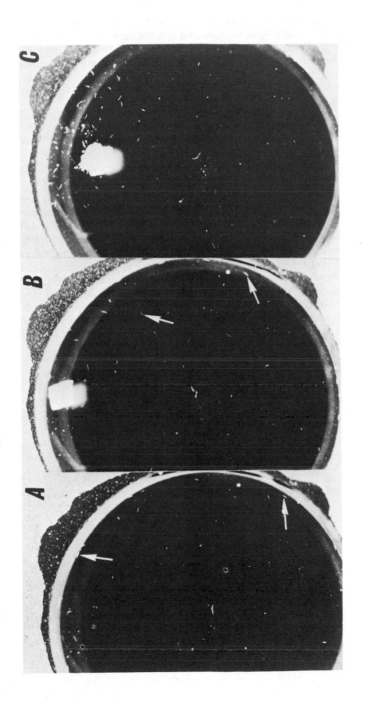

FIGURE 1. A, Random dispersal of *S. mansoni* miracidia in test chamber; B, random dispersal of miracidia in presence of moist filter paper; C, concentration of miracidia around filter paper fragment bearing crystals of serotonin, 30 sec after immersion of test material. Arrows indicate individual miracidia.

salinity, and turbidity on miracidial infectivity in the *S. mansoni-B. glabrata* complex, and Short and Saladin [18] have reported on the apparent stimulatory effect of divalent inorganic cations. Taken together, present evidence suggests that miraxone is a complex of soluble substances emitted by snails and other aquatic animals, which may well include the neurogenic product serotonin. Clearly, the subject of miracidial host-finding-penetration needs further study to resolve the many questions that have been raised.

Snail Fecundity and Growth

One of the more conspicuous impacts of schistosome infections on their snail hosts, prior to killing them, is the dramatic decline in fecundity of the mollusk. Descriptions of this effect in the *S. mansoni-B. glabrata* complex are in general agreement as to the timing of cessation of egg laying, that is, about the fourth to fifth week of infection (see Pan,[19] Wright,[20] Sturrock,[21] Etges and Gresso [22]). The latter authors found that egg laying resumed partially in late stages of infection (notably after 100 days; see Figure 2), whereas the other two reports indicated that infected snails never resumed egg production. That schistosome-infected snails remain potentially fertile is indicated by Pan's [19] description of the relatively undamaged, though atrophied, condition of the ovotestis. Presumably, the difference in these accounts lies in the physiologic condition of the snails involved, and the possibility of strain differences suggests itself. In any event, it is well known that complete "sterilization" does not occur

TABLE 2

Effect of Exposure of *S. mansoni* Miracidia to Serotonin
on Their Infectivity and Development in the Snail, *B. glabrata*

	Numbers of Cercariae Produced by Groups of Snails Exposed to Miracidia Which Were:					
	Serotonin-Treated				Untreated	
Group Snail	A *		Snail	B †		
	Cercariae			Cercariae		
	Day 33	Day 40		Day 33	Day 40	
1	100	86	1	4	—	
2	30	55	2	5	517	
			3	84	1117	
			4	650	1584	
			5	667	1850	
			6	767	2217	
			7	1084	2900	
			8	1400	3300	
			9	1767	3417	
			10	2850	3517	
			11	3083	4500	

* Group A contained 2/12 infected snails on Days 33 and 40 postexposure.
† Group B contained 11/12 infected snails on Day 33 and 10/12 on Day 40 postexposure.

in *Bulinus truncatus* infected with *S. haematobium*,[23] an observation confirmed by Lo [24] in *B. sericinus* and *B. guernei*. Brumpt's [25] original description of infected *B. glabrata* eggs containing living *S. mansoni* cercariae also was confirmed by Etges and Gresso.[22]

Recently, with the adoption of a different strain of *B. glabrata* in our laboratory, the occurrence of cercariae in snail eggs became commonplace; consequently, some attention was given to the phenomenon. The strain (designated W) is an albino, obtained from the Winches Farm Field Station of the London School of Hygiene and Tropical Medicine and presumably of Puerto Rican descent.

Initial experiments were designed to determine the frequency and duration of oviposition in *S. mansoni*-infected *B. glabrata*. Control experiments with uninfected groups of three strains of *B. glabrata* [two Puerto Rican (W and UC) and one Brazilian (LP)], in which all snails were maintained without feeding for 3 weeks, showed a nearly identical pattern of decline and complete cessation of oviposition by the 14th day of starvation (see FIGURE 3); clearly, this pattern differs from inhibition of egg laying induced by schistosome infection (see FIGURE 2). Two groups of 15 W snails were then individually exposed to 10 and 50 miracidia, respectively, and allowed to develop to patency. Beginning with the eighth week, egg clutches were collected and examined daily to establish their fecundity and the occurrence of cercariae in them. Fecundity, as measured by number of eggs and clutches produced daily, differed surprisingly little in infected groups of snails compared with uninfected controls (see FIGURE 4). TABLE 3 further indicates that fecundity remained surprisingly great, with little difference between snails exposed to 10 and 50 miracidia, and the occurrence of cercariae in eggs was almost universal during 3 weeks of observation. These

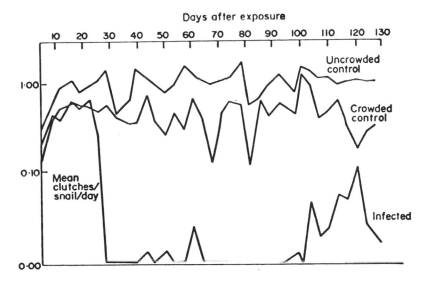

FIGURE 2. Semilog plot of egg clutch production by groups of *B glabrata;* note higher rate of egg laying among uncrowded control snails and extremely poor fecundity in *S. mansoni*-infected snails. (From Etges & Gresso.[22] By permission of *The Journal of Parasitology*.)

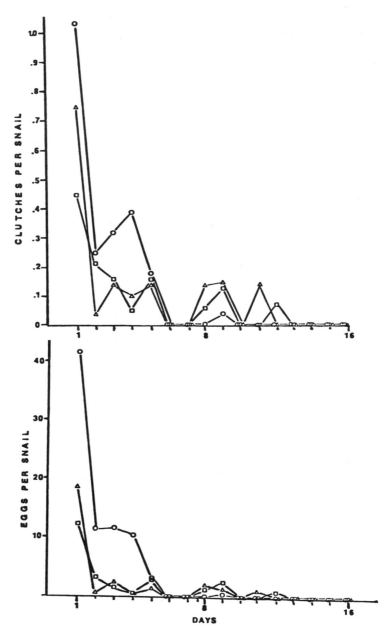

FIGURE 3. Effect of starvation on fecundity of three strains of *B. glabrata*. Upper graph shows dimunution in number of egg clutches produced/snail/day; lower graph shows decline in numbers of eggs produced daily per snail. □, Brazilian strain (LP); △, Puerto Rican strain (UC); ○, Puerto Rican strain (W).

data suggest a marked difference from previous reports of only infrequent appearance of cercaria-containing eggs and profound inhibition of host snail fecundity. Because development and hatching of eggs from infected snails is known to be nearly normal, it is apparent that reproduction of the W strain

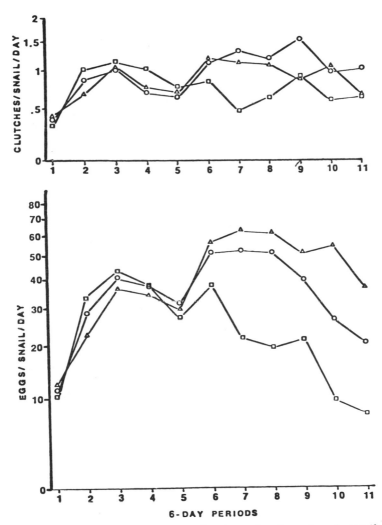

FIGURE 4. Semilog plots of egg clutch number (*upper*) and number of eggs (*lower*) produced/snail/day during the course of infection with *S. mansoni*. △, Uninfected controls; ○, 10 miracidia per snail; □, 50 miracidia per snail.

would hardly be affected by infection with *S. mansoni*. It may be inferred that such a host snail is better adapted to schistosome infection than any strains previously described and that one could not expect such infections to have adverse effects on such host snail populations.

TABLE 3

PRODUCTION OF CLUTCHES THAT CONTAINED *S. mansoni* CERCARIAE IN TWO GROUPS OF INFECTED *B. glabrata* (WINCHES STRAIN): W10 (EXPOSED TO 10 MIRACIDIA PER SNAIL) AND W50 (EXPOSED TO 50 MIRACIDIA PER SNAIL) FOR A 22-DAY PERIOD, BEGINNING DAY 49 POSTMIRACIDIAL EXPOSURE

Groups	Total Clutches Infected/Total Produced (% positive)	
	W10	W50
Days		
49, 50	6/8 (75)	11/11 (100)
51, 52	30/34 (88)	26/26 (100)
53, 54	11/14 (79)	17/17 (100)
55, 56	10/10 (100)	14/14 (100)
57, 58	7/7 (100)	8/8 (100)
59, 60	18/19 (95)	14/14 (100)
61, 62	9/9 (100)	15/16 (94)
63, 64	15/15 (100)	8/8 (100)
65, 66	13/13 (100)	14/14 (100)
67, 68	16/16 (100)	8/8 (100)
69, 70	12/12 (100)	4/4 (100)
Totals	147/157 (93.5)	139/149 (99.3)

To further test the W strain, measurements of growth also were made during infection, with the greatest shell diameter used as an index (a vernier caliper was employed). Previous reports by Pan,[19] Sturrock and Sturrock,[26] and by others have shown a slight increase in growth of *S. mansoni*-infected snails in early stages of infection. The present data, from groups of 15 snails exposed to 10 and 50 miracidia each, showed that there was a marked and consistent increase in shell size during the first 9 weeks of infection (see FIGURE 5) and that the more heavily infected snails were significantly larger than uninfected control snails in the same period. Previous (unpublished) observations in this laboratory, with three other laboratory strains of Puerto Rican *B. glabrata*, never gave this result; consequently, we suggest that the difference lies in the nature of snail strain W and not in our laboratory methods or schistosome strain. Comparison of normal growth and fecundity of W snails with other strains of *B. glabrata* reveals little perceptible difference from the uninfected state. Again, it can be inferred that the W strain is more compatible with *S. mansoni* infection than other strains of *B. glabrata* studied.

SPOROCYSTS

As pointed out by Erasmus,[27] relatively little is known of the physiology of trematode sporocysts generally, and few histochemical studies have been reported until very recently. As exemplified by the work of Pan[19] and Smith and Chernin,[28] the sporocyst tegument has received the most interest. *In vitro* cultivation of *S. mansoni* sporocysts has also received recent attention, beginning with Chernin[29] and more currently by DiConza and Hansen[30] and Hansen.[31, 32] Aside from passing comment on slight motility exhibited by mother sporocysts of *S. mansoni* compared with the more mobile daughter sporocysts, little more is known than Pan's [19] statement that active migration is primarily through loose connective tissues of the snail from the head-foot toward the liver, where the majority of daughter sporocysts mature and produce cercariae. Conversely, Maldonado and Acosta-Matienzo [33] reported that migration of *S. mansoni* sporocysts was *via* passive transport in circulating blood; Lengy's [34] description of sluggish, nonprogressive movement of *S. bovis* sporocysts tended to support the concept of their passive transport. In sites other than the liver and ovotestis, most sporocysts degenerate and die. Olivier and Mao [35] estimated that 200–300 daughter sporocysts may be produced by a single mother sporocyst in a period of 6–7 weeks. Tegumentary sense organs, such as those described in the cercaria and adult stages, and nerve fibers and ganglia, such as those described for the miracidia, cercaria, and adult worms,[36-39] have not been reported in the daughter sporocyst of schistosomes. It is even noted that a modern reference book states that sporocysts lack a nervous system; it is difficult to reconcile such a deficiency with accounts of active locomotor migration of daughter sporocysts from the head-foot through various host tissues, terminating in their localization in the digestive gland and ovotestis. Some degree of coordinated locomotion and perception of environmental stimuli seems essential to such complex behavior. Some recent observations of *S. mansoni* sporocyst migrational behavior in young albino specimens of the W strain of *B. glabrata* may be of interest.

Three groups of ten snails, 10–13 mm in diameter, were exposed individually to 10 *S. mansoni* miracidia. Within 1 week, developing mother sporocysts were observed in the tentacles, head-foot, and mantle collar; the average number

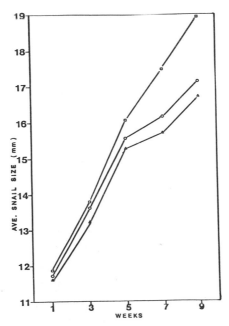

FIGURE 5. Effect of *S. mansoni* infection on growth of *B. glabrata* (strain W). △, Uninfected controls; ○, 10 mircidia per snail; □, 50 miracidia per snail.

of patent mother sporocysts observed was eight per snail. Migration of daughter sporocysts was first noted on the 11th day, but more commonly this movement did not begin until the 13th day of infection. Dissection of five infected snails permitted an estimate of 25–60 daughter sporocysts in 25 isolated mother sporocyst "nests" to be made on the 16th day of infection. Individual daughter sporocysts were easily observed moving actively in the mantle wall of intact albino snails from Days 13–24 of infection, apparently using their anterior tegumentary spines in a manner suggested by Pan.[19] Vigorous, progressive sporocyst movement was also noted in vitro, free of host tissues; they employ strong contractions of the body wall, aided by adhesion of their anterior ends to the glass surface in a progressive, probing kind of euglenoid motion. Observation of apparent adhesion was confirmed by gently flushing isolated sporocysts as they moved on a clean glass surface, showing that some were attached at their anterior end (an ability not likely due to their tegumentary spines). It is inferred that anterior glandular secretions of the sporocysts account for this ability and that such secretions augment the action of body spines in the migratory process and localization in the larger hemal sinuses of the hepatopancreas. As sporocysts moved up the mantle wall, many of them were seen to encounter and enter extensions of the hemocoel; almost immediately, their progress accelerated, until the vessel size was large enough to permit their being swept away in the blood current. Concentrating our observations on the two largest mantle veins (renal and pulmonary), it was possible to watch numerous daughter sporocysts being carried rapidly to the heart; presumably, they soon reached the hepatopancreas or other organs of the body, as determined by which artery they happened to enter after passing the heart. The reader is referred to the descriptions of the venous system of the mantle of Sullivan and Cheng[40] and the arterial system of B. glabrata by Basch[41] for a clear understanding of this route of sporocyst movement.

Based on these findings, it is possible to reconcile the apparently divergent views of Pan[19] and of Maldonado and Acosta-Matienzo[33] as to passive vs active migration of S. mansoni daughter sporocysts. Initially, the sporocysts move through snail tissues by their own locomotor actions from their site of origin in the head-foot toward the mantle; here (or earlier), they may enter small venous vessels and be carried passively for the rest of their journey to the liver or ovotestis, where further growth and development can occur. Not all sporocysts, however, are successful in this process; many of them become trapped and immobile in the mantle wall, growing slightly in length for a few days, but then become granular and opaque, and finally disintegrate after 10 days. Presumably, the same fate awaits most sporocysts that miss the proper arterial route to the liver or ovotestis after passing the heart.

By use of this simple method of direct observation of the migration of sporocysts, it was also possible to make a quantitative estimate of their number as they moved through either the renal or pulmonary veins. This estimate was made in three groups of 10 snails on a daily basis; the number of sporocysts in one of these veins was counted for 5 min per snail. Counts were made at different times of day and night, with no perceptible difference detected in migrational activity in the morning, afternoon, evening, or after midnight; it is inferred that the process is continuous. Data from these experiments are summarized in TABLE 4. Although sporocyst migration was observed in one snail as early as the 11th day of infection, counts were initiated on Day 13 and were continued for 10 days. There appeared to be a peak of migration on the 16th day, after a rapid increase from Days 13 and 14, followed by slowly diminishing numbers. Assuming that the process is reasonably constant, these numbers were used to calculate mean daily migration of sporocysts, which were then totalled for the entire 10-day observation period. Each snail, in which an average of eight mother sporocysts were seen, was found to produce nearly 5000 daughter sporocysts in a 10-day period, based on the assumptions that migration is continuous in each 24-hr period and that equal numbers migrate through the renal and pulmonary veins. This estimate is conservative in that it does not take into account sporocysts that utilize alternative migration routes or those that undoubtedly migrate before and after Days 13–22 of infection. Olivier and Mao [35] estimated that 200–300 daughter sporocysts were produced by each *S. mansoni* mother sporocyst in a period of 6–7 weeks. Though the present study suggests that a considerably greater number of daughter sporocysts mi-

TABLE 4

NUMBERS OF *S. mansoni* SECONDARY SPOROCYSTS MIGRATING VIA
MAJOR MANTLE VEINS * OF *B. glabrata* (W STRAIN) †

Day of Infection	Number of Snails	Sporocysts/ Snail/5 min [range (mean)]	24-Hour Total (calculated)
13	30	0–1 (0.3)	86
14	30	0–3 (0.8)	230
15	30	2–5 (3.0)	864
16	29	2–7 (4.2)	120
17	28	1–4 (1.7)	490
18	28	0–5 (2.1)	605
19	27	1–3 (1.2)	346
20	27	0–6 (1.9)	547
21	25	1–4 (1.2)	346
22	24	0–2 (0.5)	144
		10–day total	4868

* Either the pulmonary or renal vein was observed.
† Three groups of 10 snails, 10–12 mm in diameter, were individually exposed to 10 *S. mansoni* miracidia.

grates than can be accounted for by Olivier and Mao's estimate, or our own count of an average of 40 daughter sporocysts per mother sporocyst nest on the 16th day of infection, two possible explanations are offered. A difference may exist between the schistosome and/or snail strains employed, such that fecundity is greater in one system than in the other. Alternatively, and more likely in the writers' view, some migrating sporocysts that take the "wrong" route in passive transport by the circulatory system may eventually "recycle" one or more times and thus be counted more than once as they pass through the mantle veins. Evidence of such free daughter sporocysts in various organs of the body has been reported,[19] but generally they are assumed to be incapable of further development in organs other than the liver and ovotestis.

In further studies of intramolluscan stages of schistosomes, efforts were made to discern localizations of esterase activity that might suggest the presence

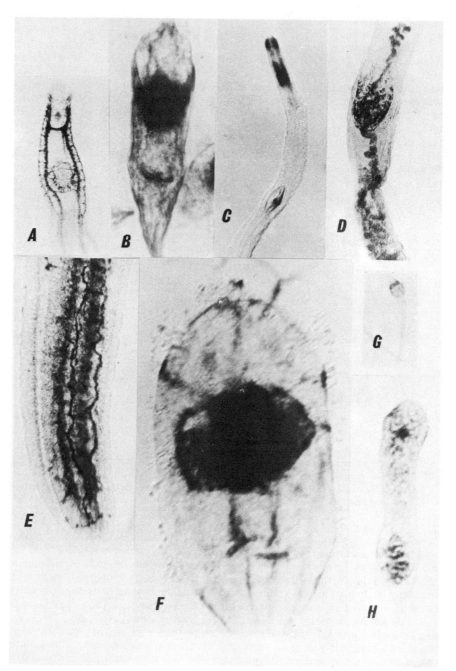

FIGURE 6. A, Adult male *S. haematobium* (BIAc method); B, *S. mansoni* miracidium (BIAc); C, adult female *S. haematobium* with single egg (AcSChI method); D, *S. haematobium* in region of ootype (BIAc); E, *S. haematobium* male posterior

of nervous system structure in them. With a modification of Thompson's [42] bromoindoxyl acetate (BIAc) method for nonspecific esterases and acetylthiocholine iodide (AcSChI) method for acetylcholinesterase, whole specimens of *S. mansoni* (adults, cercariae, miracidia, and secondary sporocysts), *S. haematobium* (adults and miracidia), *S. bovis* (miracidia), and *S. mattheei* (cercariae) were prepared, mounted, and photographed. Fixation, when employed, was by means of Pearson's [43] formalin-sucrose-ammonia solution, but superior results were often obtained with unfixed specimens. Various inhibitors, such as eserine sulfate, sodium fluoride, and isooctamethyl pyrophosphoramide, were used to discriminate between specific and nonspecific esterases, but these compounds revealed that most esterase activity in the miracidia, cercariae, and sporocysts was acetylcholinesterase; only the adults had perceptible amounts of diffuse and localized esterase not blocked by the specific anticholinesterase inhibitor BW 284 C51 dibromide (Wellcome Research Laboratories). FIGURE 6 shows the results of these experiments.

Summarily, it may be seen that the nervous system of adult *S. haematobium* is fundamentally like that of any digenetic trematode: it possesses three pairs of longitudinal nerve trunks (one large ventral pair, one smaller lateral pair, and a minor dorsal pair) interconnected by tranverse commissures; prominent plexi serve the suckers and urinary bladder, and paired cephalic ganglia are located anteriorly. Nonspecific esterase activity is also found in the esophageal glands and testes of males and in the ootype, vitelline cells, uterus, and eggs of female worms; the nervous system in females is less conspicuous than that in males but shows massive ganglia and oral sucker plexus activity. Miracidia of *S. bovis* have large ganglia with fibers that extend laterally and anteriorly to the tegumentary sense organs and the terebratorium; the latter shows acetylcholinesterase activity strongly, as do the two pairs of flame cells. Nonspecific esterase activity of apical gland cells makes the central ganglionic mass appear enlarged. Cercariae of *S. mattheei* exhibit two large anterior ganglia and other more diffuse activity in both the body and base of the tail stem; nonspecific esterases have similar distribution but fail to delineate structural loci well. Young daughter sporocysts of *S. mansoni* dissected from the head-foot of *B. glabrata* possess nonspecific esterase localizations in an unidentified anterior node and in their germ cell mass posteriorly. Specimens taken from the hepatopancreas and ovotestis that had grown only slightly lacked any acetylcholinesterase anteriorly but had multiple sites of nonspecific esterases in their germinal material; the disappearance of the anterior node of esterase-positive material also occurred in migrating sporocysts found trapped in the mantle wall.

Except for observations of loci of esterase activity in actively migrating, young daughter sporocysts of *S. mansoni,* none of these results conflicts with previous descriptions of *S. mansoni;* [36-39] mainly, these data show that species of *Schistosoma* other than *S. mansoni* provide similar results with the esterase methods employed. The finding of a transitory site of esterase activity situated anteriorly in sporocysts, contrary to the report of Kinoti *et al.*[44] in their study of *S. bovis* sporocysts, suggests that nervous elements may be present. Further, critically timed studies are needed to verify or refute the present suggestion that migrational sporocysts may have a nervous center of control for their complex, coordinated, oriented behavior in their brief phase of development.

---

extremity in region of urinary bladder (BIAc); F, *S. bovis* miracidium (BIAc); G, *S. mattheei* cercaria (AcSChI); H, *S. mansoni* daughter sporocyst (BIAc). For descriptive account, please see text.

ACKNOWLEDGMENTS

The senior author extends his thanks to John Preston, Andrew Peterson, and Valerie Gregory for providing some of the living material used in this study and to Robert Etges for photographic assistance.

REFERENCES

1. BAIR, R. D. & F. J. ETGES. 1973. *Schistosoma mansoni:* factors affecting hatching of eggs. Exp. Parasitol. **33:** 155–167.
2. KUSEL, J. R. 1970. Studies on the structure and hatching of the eggs of *Schistosoma mansoni.* Parasitology **60:** 79–88.
3. WRIGHT, C. A. 1958. Host-location by trematode miracidia. Ann. Trop. Med. Parasitol. **53:** 288–292.
4. CHERNIN, E. & C. A. DUNAVAN. 1962. The influence of host-parasite dispersion upon the capacity of *Schistosoma* mansoni miracidia to infect *Australorbis glabratus.* Amer. J. Trop. Med. Hyg. **11:** 455–471.
5. MacINNIS, A. J. 1965. Responses of *Schistosoma mansoni* miracidia to chemical attractants. J. Parasitol. **51:** 731–746.
6. ETGES, F. J. & C. L. DECKER. 1963. Chemosensitivity of the miracidium of *Schistosoma mansoni* to *Australorbis glabratus* and other snails. J. Parasitol. **49:** 114–116.
7. CHERNIN, E. & J. M. PERLSTEIN. 1971. Protection of snails against miracidia of *Schistosoma mansoni* by various aquatic invertebrates. J. Parasitol. **57:** 217–219.
8. CHERNIN, E. 1970. Behavioral responses of miracidia of *Schistosoma mansoni* and other trematodes to substances emitted by snails. J. Parasitol. **56:** 287–296.
9. SHIFF, C. J. & R. L. KRIEL. 1970. A water-soluble product of *Bulinus (Physopsis) globosus* attractive to *Schistosoma haematobium* miracidia. J. Parasitol. **56:** 281–286.
10. UPATHAM, E. S. & R. F. STURROCK. 1973. Field investigations on the effect of other aquatic animals on the infection of *Biomphalaria glabrata* by *Schistosoma mansoni* miracidia. J. Parasitol. **59:** 448–453.
11. GLAUDEL, R. J. & F. J. ETGES. 1973. Toxic effects of freshwater turbellarians on schistosome miracidia. J. Parasitol. **59:** 74–76.
12. MATTES, O. 1932. Uber die Wirkungsweise und die Bedeutung Turbellarien-Hautdrusen. Z. Morphol. Oekol. Tiere **24:** 743–767.
13. CHERNIN, E. & J. M. PERLSTEIN. 1969. Further studies on interference with the host-finding capacity of *Schistosoma mansoni* miracidia. J. Parasitol. **55:** 500–508.
14. FALCK, B. & C. OURMAN. 1965. A detailed methodological description of fluorescence methods for the cellular demonstration of biogenic amines. Acta Univ. Lund. **2**(7).
15. CHIANG, P. K., J. G. BOURGEOIS & E. BUEDING. 1974. 5-Hydroxytryptamine and dopamine in *Biomphalaria glabrata.* J. Parasitol. **60:** 264–271.
16. MacINNIS, A. J., W. M. BETHEL & E. M. CORNFORD. 1974. Identification of chemicals of snail origin that attract *Schistosoma mansoni* miracidia. Nature (London) **248:** 361–363.
17. STURROCK, R. F. & E. S. UPATHAM. 1973. An investigation of the interactions of some factors influencing the infectivity of *Schistosoma mansoni* miracidia to *Biomphalaria glabrata.* Int. J. Parasitol. **3:** 35–41.
18. SHORT, R. B. & K. SALADIN. 1973. Behavior of trematode larval stages to environmental stimuli. J. Parasitol. Progr. Abst. 64.
19. PAN, C.-T. 1965. Studies on the host-parasite relationship between *Schistosoma*

mansoni and the snail *Australorbis glabratus*. Amer. J. Trop. Med. Hyg. **14:** 931–976.

20. WRIGHT, C. A. 1966. The pathogenesis of helminths in the Mollusca. Helminth. Abst. **35:** 207–224.

21. STURROCK, B. M. 1966. The influence of infection with *Schistosoma mansoni* on the growth rate and reproduction of *Biomphalaria pfeifferi*. Ann. Trop. Med. Parasitol. **60:** 187–192.

22. ETGES, F. J. & W. GRESSO. 1965. Effect of *Schistosoma mansoni* infection upon fecundity in *Australorbis glabratus*. J. Parasitol. **51:** 757–760.

23. NAJARIAN, H. H. 1961. Egg-laying capacity of the snail *Bulinus truncatus* in relation to infection with *Schistosoma haematobium*. Texas Rep. Biol. Med. **19:** 327–331.

24. LO, C. T. 1972. Compatibility and host-parasite relationships between species of the genus *Bulinus* (Basommatophora: Planorbidae) and an Egyptian strain of *Schistosoma haematobium* (Trematoda: Digenea). Malacologia **11:** 225–280.

25. BRUMPT, E. 1941. Observations biologiques diverses concernant *Planorbis* (*Australorbis*) *glabratus*, hote intermediare de *Schistosoma mansoni*. Ann. Parasitol. **18:** 9–45.

26. STURROCK, B. M. & R. F. STURROCK. 1970. Laboratory studies of the host-parasite relationship of *Schisotsoma mansoni* and *Biomphalaria glabrata* from St. Lucia, West Indies. Ann. Trop. Med. Parasitol. **64:** 357–363.

27. ERASMUS, D. A. 1972. The Biology of Trematodes. E. Arnold Ltd. Publ. London, England.

28. SMITH, J. H. & E. CHERNIN. 1974. Ultrastructure of young mother and daughter sporocysts of *Schistosoma mansoni*. J. Parasitol. **60:** 85–89.

29. CHERNIN, E. 1964. Maintenance *in vitro* of larval *Schistosoma mansoni* in tissues from the snail, *Australorbis glabratus*. J. Parasitol. **50:** 531–545.

30. DICONZA, J. J. & E. L. HANSEN. 1972. Multiplication of transplanted *Schistosoma mansoni* daughter sporocysts. J. Parasitol. **58:** 181, 182.

31. HANSEN, E. L. 1973. Progeny-daughter sporocysts of *Schistosoma mansoni*. Int. J. Parasitol. **3:** 267, 268.

32. HANSEN, E. L., K. WALEN & E. YARWOOD. 1974. Cell lineage in cultured larval *Schistosoma mansoni*. Amer. Soc. Trop. Med. Hyg. Progr. No. 2.

33. MALDONADO, J. F. & J. ACOSTA-MATIENZO. 1947. The development of *Schistosoma mansoni* in the snail intermediate host, *Australorbis glabratus*. Puerto Rico J. Publ. Health Trop. Med. **22:** 331–373.

34. LENGY, J. 1962. Studies on *Schistosoma bovis* (Sonsino, 1876) in Israel. I. Larval stages from egg to cercaria. Bull. Res. Council Israel Sect. E **10:** 1–36.

35. OLIVIER, L. & C. P. MAO. 1949. The early larval stages of *Schistosoma mansoni* Sambon, 1907 in the snail host, *Australorbis glabratus* (Say, 1818). J. Parasitol. **35:** 267–275.

36. FRIPP, P. J. 1967. Histochemical localization of esterase activity in schistosomes. Exp. Parasitol. **21:** 380–390.

37. BUEDING, E., E. L. SCHILLER & J. G. BOURGEOIS. 1967. Some physioloigcal, biochemical, and morphologic effects of tris (p-aminophenyl) carbonium salts (TAC) on *Schistosoma mansoni*. Amer. J. Trop. Med. Hyg. **16:** 500–515.

38. MORRIS, G. P. & L. T. THREADGOLD. 1967. A presumed sensory structure associated with the tegument of *Schistosoma mansoni*. J. Parasitol. **53:** 537–539.

39. BRUCKNER, D. A. & M. VOGE. 1974. The nervous system of larval *Schistosoma mansoni* as revealed by acetylcholinesterase staining. J. Parasitol **60:** 437–446.

40. SULLIVAN, J. T. & T. C. CHENG. 1974. Structure and function of the mantle cavity of *Biomphalaria glabrata* (Mollusca: Pulmonata). Trans. Amer. Microsc. Soc. **93:** 416–420.

41. BASCH, P. F. 1969. The arterial system of *Biomphalaria glabrata* (Say). Malacologia **7:** 169–181.

42. THOMPSON, S. W. 1966. Selected Histochemical and Histopathological Methods. Charles C Thomas, Publisher. Springfield, Ill.
43. PEARSON, C. K. 1963. A formalin-sucrose-ammonia fixative for cholinesterases. J. Histochem. Cytochem. 11: 665, 666.
44. KINOTI, G. K., R. G. BIRD & M. BARKER. 1971. Electron microscope and histochemical observations on the daughter sporocyst of Schistosoma mattheei and Schistosoma bovis. J. Helminthol. 45: 237–244.

LIGHT AND ELECTRON MICROSCOPY OF THE HOST-PARASITE INTERFACE AND HISTOPATHOLOGY OF *NASSARIUS OBSOLETUS* INFECTED WITH REDIAE OF *HIMASTHLA QUISSETENSIS* *

George P. Hoskin

Department of Biology
Lafayette College
Easton, Pennsylvania 18042

INTRODUCTION

The mudflat snail *Nassarius obsoletus* serves as an intermediate host for several species of digenetic trematodes, including *Austrobilharzia variglandis* (Schistosomatidae), a causative agent of marine dermatitis, and *Himasthla quissetensis* (Echinostomatidae).[1] *H. quissetensis* rediae are potential antagonists of *A. variglandis* sporocysts, because both species are known to occur in double infections of *N. obsoletus*.[2] Direct antagonism that involves a redia and a sporocyst usually results in destruction of the sporocyst.[3]

The role of *H. quissetensis* as a human pathogen is speculative; however, Vogel[4] reported adults of *Himasthla muehlensi* from a patient with gastrointestinal disturbance, and *H. quissetensis* metacercariae or their metabolic byproducts also have been suspected of causing gastrointestinal disturbance in persons eating raw quohogs (*Mercenaria mercenaria*).[5]

There has been a continuing interest in studies on the biochemistry and physiology of *H. quissetensis* rediae;[6-12] however, a detailed description of the body surface of this species has not been reported. Because a thorough understanding of host-parasite relationships between larval trematodes and mollusks is dependent upon elucidation of the structure of the tegument of these larvae, which represents the greatest potential area of host-parasite contact, the following study was undertaken.

MATERIALS AND METHODS

Specimens of *N. obsoletus* were collected from Shore Acres, Rhode Island, during August and September of 1972–74. The shells were cracked with pliers, and the digestive gland-gonad region of each snail was examined. Those that contained rediae of *H. quissetensis* were immediately prepared for microscopy. Certain snails were maintained in the laboratory for 9–12 months, as previously described.[10]

Light Microscopy

Whole infected snails with their shells removed, or daughter rediae isolated from snails, were fixed in cold 10% seawater-formalin, embedded in Tissuemat®,

* Supported in part by a Summer Research Fellowship.

and sectioned at 8 μm. Some of the sections were stained with Harris' hematoxylin and eosin or Mallory's triple connective tissue stain. In addition, the following histochemical tests were performed: the mercuric bromphenol blue method for proteins,[13] the periodic acid-Schiff (PAS)[14] reaction with controls predigested for 40 min in 0.5% malt diastase at 37° C, alcian blue at pH 0.5,[15] 2.6,[16, 17] and 5.7,[18] Sudan black B for bound lipids,[19] and toluidine blue for detection of metachromasia.[20]

Lipoidal material was demonstrated by isolating live rediae, which were immediately submerged in Tissue-Tek® OCT compound (Ames Co.), followed by freezing at −20° C. Subsequently, sections were cut in a cryostat (Lab Tek, Ames Co.), fixed over formalin fumes for 2–3 min, stained with Sudan black B[21] or oil red O,[22] and mounted in glycerin jelly. Control sections were extracted in chloroform-methanol (2:1, v/v) for 5 min before staining.

Transmission Electron Microscopy (TEM)

Freshly isolated daughter rediae or small pieces of snail tissue that contained rediae were fixed for 2–3 hr at 10° C with 2% glutaraldehyde in 30% filtered artificial seawater at pH 7.9. The tissues were rinsed in buffer, postfixed in buffered 5% osmium tetroxide for 2 hr, rinsed in buffer, dehydrated in ethanol or acetone, and embedded in Araldite® or Epon® 812. Sections were cut with glass knives, stained in uranyl acetate and lead citrate, and examined in an electron microscope (Philips 201). Alternatively, tissues were fixed with 2% glutaraldehyde-2% osmium tetroxide, followed by rapid acetone dehydration, and embedded in Epon 812.[23]

Only fully developed daughter rediae that contained cercariae were examined by TEM.

Scanning Electron Microscopy (SEM)

Mature daughter rediae were isolated from *N. obsoletus,* fixed for 2 hr with 2% glutaraldehyde in phosphate buffer at pH 7.9, dehydrated in an acetone-acetylacetone series, and subjected to critical-point freeze drying.[24] The specimens were coated with gold and observed in a scanning electron microscope (ETEC).

RESULTS

Redial Structure

Light Microscopy

Stunkard[25] has provided a general description of the mother and daughter redial stages of *H. quissetensis.* In addition to what he described, each daughter redia possesses both a collar and an oral ring (FIGURE 1). The pharynx is situated between the level of the oral ring and collar (FIGURE 1). This region of the redia is capable of extending and retracting.

Large amounts of lipoidal material are present in the deeper areas of the body wall, although a few droplets also occur in the subsurfacial zone (FIGURES 4 & 5).

Germ balls in intimate association with the redial wall also include considerable lipid (FIGURE 4); however, cercariae in various stages of development contain less lipid than does the heavily stained redial wall (FIGURES 4 & 5).

The outer layer of the redial wall is γ metachromatic when stained with toluidine blue and also stains with alcian blue at pH 0.5, 2.6, and 5.7. However, it is PAS negative. This region is also stained by mercuric bromphenol blue and Sudan black B.

Electron Microscopy

SEM of the surface of the oral ring reveals numerous cilia-like structures, each of which projects from a papilla. A few of these structures also occur on the tegumental surface between the oral ring and collar (FIGURE 2). The surface of the oral ring and pharynx are also covered with microvilli (FIGURE 3). The tegument in this region has undulations and knobs (FIGURE 3). The entire body surface of each redia is carpeted with densely spaced microvilli (FIGURE 6).

TEM has revealed that the body wall between the level of the oral ring and ambulatory buds, which are posteriorly situated, consists of an outer, anucleate cytoplasmic layer that supports the microvilli (FIGURES 8, 13, 14 & 16). These microvilli vary in length but average between 0.5 and 1.0 μm long. A hirsute coat that consists of minute electron-dense granules, each of which measures 100–200 Å in diameter, and filaments is present on the microvilli (FIGURES 16, 23 & 25).

Invaginations are common on the surface of the cytoplasmic syncytium (FIGURES 15 & 16), as are small vesicles just mediad to the external plasma membrane (FIGURE 16, inset). Adhering to the inner surface of the membrane that lines each vesicle are commonly found electron-dense particles that are dimensionally similar to those located on the external surface of the microvilli.

Also embedded within the cytoplasmic syncytium are mitochondria (FIGURES 8, 14 & 17), lipid droplets (FIGURE 13), membrane-bound disks (FIGURES 11 & 16), and granules of varying electron densities.

A basal lamina, which varies between 0.07 and 0.15 μm thick, is situated mediad to the internal plasma membrane of the cytoplasmic syncytium (FIGURES 8, 16 & 17). Complex folds of the basal lamina extend between the bands of circularly oriented muscles (FIGURES 8, 9 & 15). These folds may even completely surround the myofibers (FIGURE 8).

As had been reported in other species of rediae,[26-28] the cytoplasmic syncytium is connected to the cytons, which are mediad to the muscle layers, by cytoplasmic bridges (internuncial processes) (FIGURES 9 & 19).

In addition to the nucleus, each cyton includes α rosettes of glycogen (FIGURE 16), although some β particles are also present. Mitochondria also occur in the cytons; each one measures 0.5–1.5 μm along the longitudinal axis (FIGURES 10, 13 & 15).

Membrane-bound disks, each of which measures 0.15–0.20 μm in greatest diameter, occur in clusters in the cytons (FIGURES 12 & 16) and within internuncial processes. These organelles are identical to those described earlier in the outer cytoplasmic syncytium. Structures of similar size but of varying

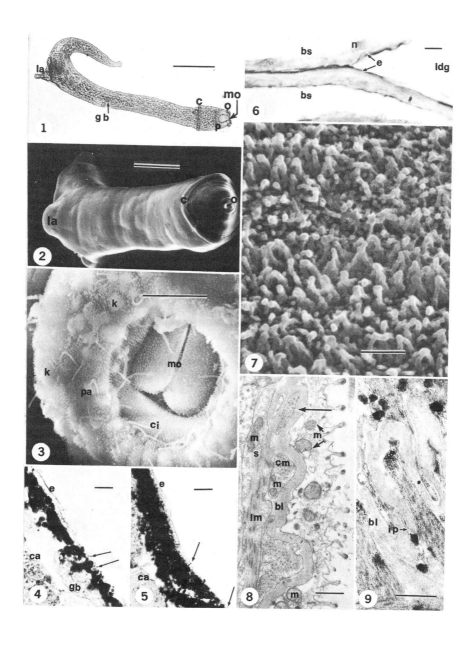

FIGURE 1.† Daughter redia of *H. quissetensis* stained with Harris' hematoxylin. The redia shown is immature; thus, germ balls, but not developed cercariae, are discernible in the brood chamber. Bar = 100 μm.

FIGURE 2. Scanning electron micrograph of mature daughter redia shows oral ring, collar, and ambulatory buds. The region between the oral ring and collar is partially contracted. Bar = 100 μm.

FIGURE 3. Scanning electron micrograph of oral ring of mature daughter redia shows papilliae with cilia and microvilli on the oral ring and pharynx. Bar = 10 μm. (Courtesy of Mrs. Annette G. Pashayan.)

FIGURE 4. Section through a redial wall stained with oil red O shows heavy lipid deposits in wall and developing germ ball but less lipid in developing cercaria. Arrows indicate lipid in outer layer of body wall. Bar = 10 μm.

FIGURE 5. Section through redial wall stained with Sudan black B shows heavy lipid deposits and (arrows) lipid in the outer layer of the body wall. Bar = 10 μm.

FIGURE 6. Section of two rediae in contact shows positive staining of outermost layer of epithelium (e); stained with alcian blue at pH 2.7. Bar = 10 μm.

FIGURE 7. SEM of the body surface of *H. quissetensis* confirms that surface protrusions observed in transmission electron micrographs are microvilli. Bar = 1.0 μm.

FIGURE 8. TEM shows folds in the basal lamina of *H. quissetensis* and mitochondria in the distal cytoplasm and muscles. Bar = 1.0 μm.

FIGURE 9. TEM shows passage of granule along an internuncial process through the basal lamina. Bar = 0.25 μm.

† Figure abbreviations: ag, α glycogen; am, amoebocyte; bg, β glycogen; bl, basal lamina; c, collar; ca, cercaria; ci, cilia; cm, circular muscle; cp, ciliary papilla; dc, distal cytoplasm; e, body surface; eb, electron-dense body; fs, extension of fibroblast; g, Golgi apparatus; gb, germ ball; im, irregular microvillus; ip, internuncial process; k, knob; la, ambulatory bud; lm, longitudinal muscle; lp, lipid; m, mitochondrion; mf, myofibril; mg, membrane-bound granule; mo, mouth; mv, microvillus; n, nucleus; o, oral ring; p, pharynx; pa, papilla; pn, pycnotic nucleus; rb, ribosome; rer, rough endoplasmic reticulum; rf, reticulin-like fiber; s, sarcoplasm; sa, sarcolemma; sl, large lysosome; sm, smooth endoplasmic reticulum; v, vesicle; dm, degenerating mitochondrion.

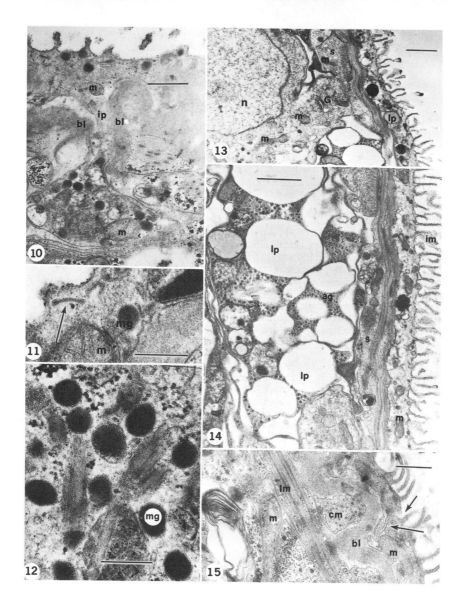

FIGURE 10. TEM of internuncial process through basal lamina shows membrane-bound granules and mitochondria in cyton and distal cytoplasm. Bar=0.5 μm.

FIGURE 11. TEM shows membrane-bound granules in cross section and plane section. Bar=0.25 μm.

FIGURE 12. TEM of membrane-bound granules shows differences in electron opacity. Central granules appear to contain less material than do surrounding granules. Bar=0.25 μm.

FIGURE 13. TEM shows cytoplasmic extension of cyton that contains Golgi apparatus and lipid-like depsit in distal cytoplasm. Bar=1.0 μm.

FIGURE 14. TEM shows large lipid vacuoles adjacent to large deposits of glycogen. Note presence of branched and irregular microvilli and of mitochondria with granules. Bar=1.0 μm.

FIGURE 15. TEM shows pinocytotic channel that terminates near mitochondrion (arrow). Bar=0.5 μm.

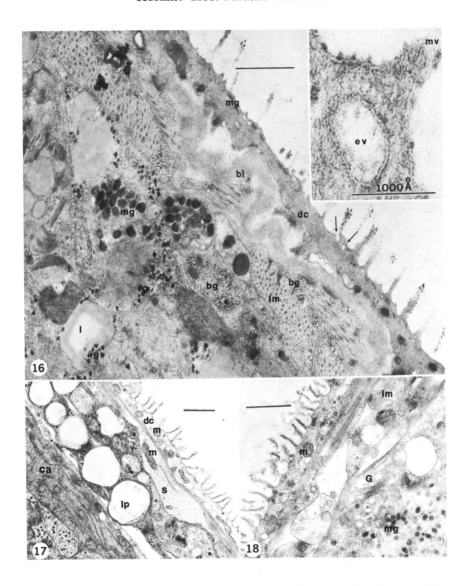

FIGURE 16. TEM of body wall of redia shows deposits of α and β glycogen. Note that only β glycogen is found within the sarcolemma. Pinocytotic vesicle and channel are indicated by arrows. Inset portrays pinocytotic vesicle with granular material adhering to the membrane. Bar = 1.0 μm.

FIGURE 17. TEM of body wall of redia and developing cercaria. Note the presence of large lipid vacuoles in the redial wall and of mitochondria in the distal cytoplasm and muscle of the redia. Bar = 1.0 μm.

FIGURE 18. TEM shows Golgi apparatus in cyton and membrane-bound granules associated with it. Bar = 1.0 μm.

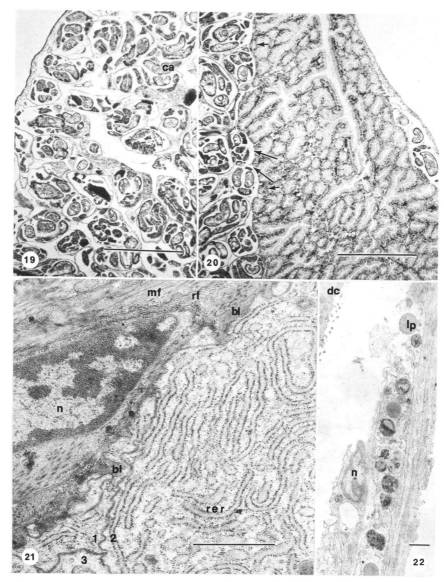

FIGURE 19. Light micrograph of the gonadal region adjacent to the digestive gland shows complete loss of recognizable gonadal tissue; hematoxylin-eosin. Bar=1 mm.

FIGURE 20. Light micrograph of rediae adjacent to the digestive gland. Most rediae occupy the digestive gland-gonadal region. Some rediae also lie between the digestive gland and the tunica propria (*right*). Arrows indicate tissue strands that connect rediae and digestive gland tubules. Shorter arrows indicate compressed tubules with reduced lumina; hematoxylin-eosin. Bar=1 mm.

FIGURE 21. TEM of connective tissue that surrounds basal portions of three digestive gland cells. Cells 1 and 2 are secretory; cell 3 is a digestive cell. Bar=1 μm.

FIGURE 22. TEM of connective tissue shows cells damaged mechanically. Note the normal-appearing fibroblast nucleus and the lipid globules and lysosomes. Bar=1 μm.

electron densities also occur in the cytons. Golgi apparatuses are frequently found associated with the granules in the cytons (FIGURE 18).

Host-Redia Interaction

Light Microscopy

In heavy infections of freshly collected or laboratory maintained snails, the rediae completely replace the gonadal tissue (FIGURE 19). Compression of Leydig cells and digestive gland cells due to the presence of the rediae is apparent, and the lumina of some digestive gland tubules may be nearly occluded as a result of this pressure (FIGURE 20). Strands of tissue may connect rediae with host digestive gland tubules (FIGURE 20).

Many rediae lie adjacent to host tissues. Serial sections of infected snails reveal that many other rediae are completely surrounded by sister rediae and do not make direct contact with host cells.

Electron Microscopy

The normal histology of the digestive gland has been described at the light microscope level.[29] Electron micrographs reveal that each acinar tubule of the digestive gland is ensheathed with a connective tissue layer that includes reticulin-like fibers, nucleated connective tissue cells, and myofibers. A thin basal lamina separates this layer from the basal region of the digestive gland cells (FIGURE 21). Nerve axons and fibroblasts are also present. The digestive gland cells contain mitochondria, Golgi apparatuses, and extensive rough endoplasmic reticulum.

Cells of the connective tissue sheath that are in juxtaposition to rediae may be mechanically disrupted. The contents of these cells spill into the hemolymph sinus (FIGURE 22).

Other forms of cell damage are associated with direct contact between the host tegument and parasite cell membranes. Microvilli adhere to cell membranes of fibroblasts, although cell injury may not be recognizable (FIGURE 23). Contacts between parasite and host cell membranes are also observed where obvious injury to host cells occurs. Specifically, when the connective tissue is damaged, myofibers normally embedded in it are exposed. There is direct contact between the sarcolemma and the parasite's microvilli. Nuclei become pycnotic, and interruptions in the sarcolemma occur (FIGURES 24, 25 & 27). Severe injury to the connective tissue may expose the basal portions of the digestive gland cells. Such injury is accompanied by necrosis of those cells. The plasmalemma is disrupted, the endoplasmic reticulum becomes vacuolated, mitochondria degenerate, nuclei become pycnotic, and lysosomes that contain myelin figures appear (FIGURES 26 & 27). Amoebocytes become associated with sites of necrosis (FIGURE 27). Extensions of an amoebocyte protrude toward the microvilli (FIGURE 27).

DISCUSSION

Redial Structure

The results of histochemical studies of the redial wall indicate that the outermost layer includes sulfated acid mucopolysaccharide. The presence of mucins

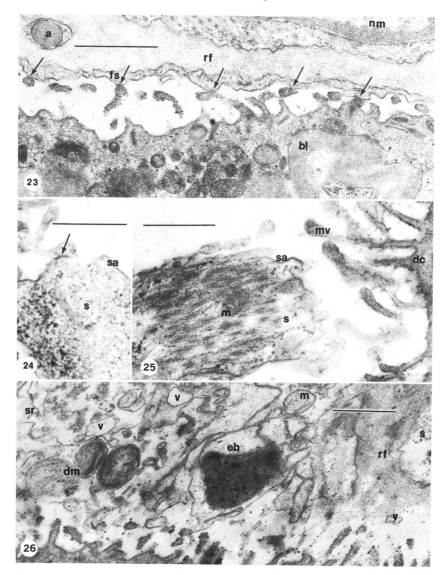

FIGURE 23. TEM shows microvilli in contact with fibroblast cell membrane. Arrows indicate regions of apparent membrane-membrane contact. Lines indicate filaments of microvillar hirsute coat. Bar=1.0 μm.

FIGURE 24. TEM shows apparent contact between host connective tissue sarcolemma and redial microvillus. Bar=0.5 μm.

FIGURE 25. TEM shows exposed connective tissue fiber with disrupted sarcolemma. Note strands that emanate from surface of microvilli. Bar=0.5 μm.

FIGURE 26. TEM shows intermingling of redial microvilli and cytoplasmic extensions of necrotic hepatocyte. Some connective tissue reticular fibers appear at right. Note degenerating mitochondrion, lysosomes that contain myelin figures, vacuolated endoplasmic reticulum, and general lack of definable plasmalemma of hepatocyte. Bar=0.5 μm.

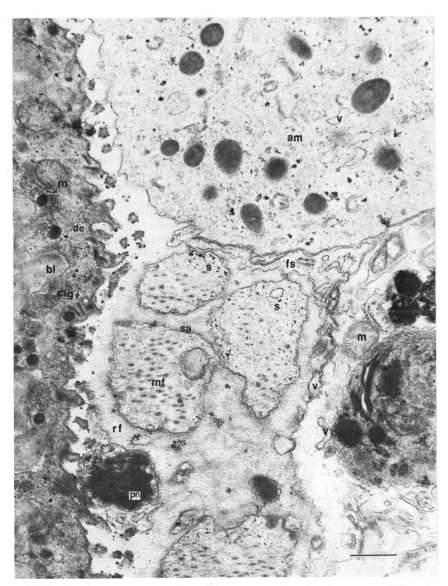

FIGURE 27. TEM shows eroded digestive gland connective tissue, necrotic hepato-cyte, and granular amoebocyte with pseudopodium-like extensions that project toward individual parasite microvilli at (arrows); note the cleft that separates the amoebocyte and digestive gland cell membranes. Bar = 0.5 μm.

is indicated by the γ metachromasia observed after treatment of sections with toluidine blue.[20, 30] This region also is stained a greenish blue color by alcian blue at pH 0.5, which indicates the presence of sulfated polyanions.[15, 31] The reaction of this layer with alcian blue at pH 2.6 indicates the presence of acid mucopolysaccharide.[16, 17] Staining by alcian blue at pH 5.7 indicates the presence of various cationic polyanions;[18, 32] however, this region is PAS negative, which is characteristic of acid mucopolysaccharide.[30] It should be noted that Rahemtulla and Løvtrup[33] have concluded that "over sulfated chondroitin sulfate is the typical acid mucopolysaccharide found in the Platyhelminths."

The positive staining reactions for protein and bound lipid at the redial surface are not contradictory with the conclusion that the surface layer is invested with acid mucopolysaccharide. Electron microscopy has revealed that the surface consists of closely spaced microvilli. The plasmalemma of these microvilli is composed of proteins and lipids; therefore, the microvilli provide a 0.5–1.0-μm thick layer rich in these compounds that take up enough stain to be detectable by light microscopy, although a simple cytomembrane would not do so.

All species of rediae examined exhibit elaboration of the tegument as laminar folds[34] or microvilli.[26–28, 35–40] The functional and phylogenetic significance of these two different structures requires further investigation.

Some conclusions may be reached about the distribution of nutrients stored in the redial wall. Specifically, β glycogen occurs within the muscles, whereas α-glycogen rosettes are prominent throughout the cytoplasm of the cytons. A similar distribution of glycogen is found in *Cryptocotyle lingua* rediae.[34] However, both α and β glycogen are found within the sarcolemma of young rediae of *Neophasis lageniformis*.[27]

Membrane-bound disks abound in cytons of the body wall of *H. quissetensis* rediae. Structures morphologically similar to these disks reported from *Fasciola hepatica* are restricted to cells in the pharyngeal region that apparently secrete them into the lumen of the intestine.[41] Similar structures have been reported from cytons of *N. lageniformis*[27] and *C. lingua*[34] and from the tegument of adult *F. hepatica*[42] and *Leucochloridiomorpha constantiae* metacercariae.[43]

A correlation between the developmental state of the metacercarial tegument of *L. constantiae* and the abundance of inclusions was observed.[43] The significance of the occurrence of such inclusions in the tegument of *H. quissetensis* or other rediae is not clear.

The membrane-bound disks occur in the cytons, within an internuncial process, and within the cytoplasmic syncytium of *H. quissetensis* rediae, which indicates that these cytoplasmic bridges serve to transport material between the perinuclear and the distal cytoplasm.

The morphologic evidence, namely, the presence of microvilli on the tegumental surface, of mitochondria and pinocytotic vesicle-like organelles in the outer cytoplasmic syncytium and of internuncial bridges that connect the syncytium with the cytons, all suggests that the surface of the daughter rediae of *H. quissetensis* functions as a transport epithelium. This function is also suggested by earlier autoradiographic and physiologic studies.[9, 10]

Host-Parasite Interaction

Various histopathologic changes in mollusks infected with larval trematodes have been reported.[44–47] In *N. obsoletus* infected with *Zoogonus rubellus* sporocysts, digestive gland tubules persist, even in the absence of gonadal tissue.[48] The survival of the host is probably prolonged if gonadal rather than digestive gland tissue is destroyed to provide space for the parasites within the confines of the host shell. Relative to this hypothesis, it should be noted that *Lymnaea stagnalis* infected with sporocysts of *Trichobilharzia ocellata* may live even longer than uninfected snails, although egg laying is greatly reduced.[49] Bourns [53] compared the total protein and carbohydrate loss in the form of eggs deposited by uninfected *L. stagnalis* with the total loss of these substances from infected snails as eggs and shed cercariae. He concluded that the nutritional drain is reduced in infected snails. Furthermore, *Littorina saxitalis* and *Littorina littorea* infected with rediae of *C. lingua* show no reduction in nutrient assimilation rates compared with noninfected controls.[50, 51]

In the infected specimens of *N. obsoletus* examined during this study, gonadal tissue was invariably found to be absent, although it was easily recognized in uninfected snails. It is reasonable to conclude that this redial species causes parasitic castration of *N. obsoletus*, although the absence of gonadal tissue in these specimens prevented attempts to describe pathologic changes.

Adherence of host tissues to the tegument of rediae is evident in light and electron micrographs. This contact may be strengthened by the acid mucopolysaccharide present at the redial surface, because this substance serves as a "flexible cement." [52] The acid mucopolysaccharide may also provide a matrix in which enzyme-substrate reactions or reactions involved in transport occur.[54]

Destruction of digestive gland cells by rediae is of four types: mechanical destruction due to pressure, extracorporeal digestion and direct ingestion, lysis caused by parasites' excretions, and autolysis due to starvation.[47]

Mechanical destruction of connective tissue cells is easily recognized. Necrosis of connective tissue cells from other causes also occurs at the interface with the general tegument of *H. quissetensis* rediae.

It can be argued that the presence of rediae at sites of host cellular necrosis is coincidental and that the host cells are undergoing changes associated with normal aging and death. That the observations reported herein are the result of coincidence does not seem likely, however, because the pattern of damage observed involves erosion of the connective tissue sheath that surrounds the digestive gland tubules, followed by pathologic alterations in the digestive gland cells. These alterations include loss of continuity of the host cell membrane. Activities at the host-parasite interface theoretically include excretion-secretion, diffusion, active transport pinocytosis, extracellular digestion, membrane digestion, and molecular mimicry.[55] Information from light and electron micrographs presented in this study provides morphologic evidence that pinocytosis may occur at the redial surface, and necrosis of host cells adjacent to rediae suggests that diffusible parasite-produced molecules affect the host cells. The intimate associations that exist between host and cell membranes raise the intriguing possibility that contact digestion is involved in this relationship.

ACKNOWLEDGMENTS

I am indebted to Mr. Jack Carty for preparing the SEM and light micrographic prints. I also thank Mr. John Sullivan and Mr. Richard Korastinski for technical assistance in preparing the SEM micrographs. Finally, I thank Dr. Thomas C. Cheng and Dr. Bernard Fried for their helpful suggestions on writing portions of this manuscript and Mrs. Joan Clymer and Mrs. Ruth Hekel for typing the drafts and final copy.

REFERENCES

1. MILLER, H. M. & F. E. NORTHUP. 1926. The seasonal infestation of *Nassa obsoleta* (Say) with larval trematodes. Biol. Bull. **50:** 490–508.
2. VERNBERG, W. B., F. J. VERNBERG & F. W. BECKERDITE, JR. 1969. Larval trematodes: double infections in common mud-flat snail. Science **164:** 1287, 1288.
3. LIM, H. K. & D. HEYNEMAN. 1972. Intramolluscan inter-trematode antagonism: a review of factors influencing the host-parasite system and its possible role in biological control. Advan. Parasitol. **10:** 191–268.
4. VOGEL, H. 1933. *Himasthla muehlensi* n. sp., ein neuer menschlicher Trematode der Familie Echinostomatidae. Zentr. Bakteriol. Parasitenk. Abt. I Orig. **127:** 385–391.
5. CHENG, T. C. 1967. Marine molluscs as hosts for symbiosis: with a review of known parasites of commercially important species. Advan. Marine Biol. **5:** 1–424.
6. VERNBERG, W. V. & W. S. HUNTER. 1963. Utilization of certain substrates by larval and adult stages of *Himasthla quissetensis*. Exp. Parasitol. **14:** 311–315.
7. VERNBERG, W. B. 1968. Platyhelminths: respiratory metabolism. Chem. Zool. **III:** 359–393.
8. LUNETTA, J. E. & W. B. VERNBERG. 1971. Fatty acid composition of parasitized and non-parasitized tissue of the mud-flat snail, *Nassarius obsoleta* (Say). Exp. Parasitol. **30:** 244–248.
9. HOSKIN, G. P. & T. C. CHENG. 1974. *Himasthla quissetensis:* uptake and utilization of glucose by rediae as determined by autoradiography and respirometry. Exp. Parasitol. **35**(1): 61–67.
10. HOSKIN, G. P. & T. C. CHENG. 1973. Dehydrogenase activity in the rediae of *Himasthla quissetensis* (Trematoda) as an indicator of substrate utilization. Comp. Biochem. Physiol. **46B:** 361–366.
11. HOSKIN, G. P., T. C. CHENG & I. L. SHAPIRO. 1974. Fatty acid composition of three lipid classes of *Himasthla quissetensis* rediae before and after starvation. Comp. Biochem. Physiol. **47B:** 821–829.
12. HOSKIN, G. P. & T. C. CHENG. 1975. Occurrence of carotenoids in *Himasthla quissetensis* rediae and the host, *Nassarius obsoletus*. J. Parasitol. **61**(2): 381, 382.
13. MAZIA, D., P. A. BREWER & M. ALFERT. 1953. The cytochemical staining and measurement of protein with mercuric bromphenol blue. Biol. Bull. **104:** 57–67.
14. MCMANUS, J. F. A. 1946. Histochemical demonstration of mucin after periodic acid. Nature (London) **158:** 202.
15. CONSTANTINE, V. S. & R. W. MOWRY. 1966. Histochemical demonstration of sialomucin in human exocrine sweat glands. J. Invest. Dermatol. **46:** 536–541.
16. MOWRY, L. W. 1963. The special value of methods that color both acidic and vicinal hydroxyl groups in the histochemical study of mucins. With revised directions for the colloidal iron stain, the use of alcian blue G 8X and their combinations with the periodic acid-Schiff reaction. Ann. N.Y. Acad. Sci. **106:** 402–423.
17. LUNA, L. G. 1968. Manual of Histologic Staining Methods of the Armed Forces Institute of Pathology. 3rd edit. McGraw-Hill Book Company. New York, N.Y.
18. SCOTT, J. E. 1966. Aliphatic ammonium salts in the assay of acid polysaccharides from tissues. Methods Biochem. Anal. **8:** 145–197.
19. BERENBAUM, M. C. 1958. The cytochemistry of bound lipids. Quart. J. Microsc. Sci. **99:** 231–242.
20. KRAMER, H. & G. H. WINDRUM. 1955. The metachromic staining reaction. J. Histochem. Cytochem. **3:** 227–237.
21. CHIFFELLE, T. L. & F. A. PUTT. 1951. Propylene and ethylene glycol as solvents for Sudan IV and Sudan black B. Stain Technol. **26:** 51–56.

22. LILLIE, R. D. 1944. Various oil soluble dyes as fat stains in the supersaturated isopropanol technique. Stain Technol. **19**: 55–58.
23. BUSCHMANN, R. J. 1972. Loss of absorbed lipid during processing of intestine for electron microscopy. *In* Proceedings of the Electron Microscopy Society of America, 13th Annual EMSA Meeting. C. J. Arceneaux, Ed. : 306, 307. Claitors Publishing Division. Baton Rouge, La.
24. RUFFOLO, J. J., JR. 1974. Critical point drying of protozoan cells and other biological specimens for scanning electron microscopy: apparatus and methods of specimen preparation. Trans. Amer. Microsc. Soc. **93**(1): 124–131.
25. STUNKARD, H. W. 1938. The morphology and life cycle of the trematode *Himasthla quissetensis* (Miller and Northup, 1926). Biol. Bull. **75**: 145–164.
26. KRUPA, P. L., G. H. COUSINEAU & A. K. BAL. 1968. Ultrastructural and histochemical observations on the body wall of *Cryptocotyle lingua* rediae (Trematoda). J. Parasitol. **54**: 900–908.
27. KØIE, M. 1971. On the histochemistry and ultrastructure of the redia of *Neophasis lageniformis* (Lebour, 1910) (Trematoda: Acanthocolpidae). Ophelia **9**(1): 113–143.
28. READER, T. A. J. 1972. Ultrastructural and cytochemical observations on the body wall of the redia of *Sphaeridiotrema globulus* (Rudolphi, 1819). Parasitology **65**: 537–546.
29. BROWN, S. 1969. The structure and function of the digestive system of the mudsnail *Nassarius obsoletus* (Say). Malacologia **9**(2): 447–500.
30. PEARSE, A. G. E. 1961. Histochemistry: Theoretical and Applied. Little, Brown and Company. Boston, Mass.
31. LEV, R. & S. SPICER. 1964. Specific staining of sulfate groups with alcian blue at low pH. J. Histochem. Cytochem. **12**: 309.
32. SCOTT, J. E., G. QUINTARELLI & M. C. DELLOVO. 1964. The chemical and histochemical properties of alcian blue staining. Histochemie **4**: 73–85.
33. RAHEMTULLA, F. & S. LØVTRUP. 1974. The comparative biochemistry of invertebrate mucopolysaccharides. I. Methods: platyhelminths. Comp. Biochem. Physiol. **49**(b): 631–637.
34. KRUPA, P. L., A. K. BAL & G. H. COUSINEAU. 1967. Ultrastructure of the redia of *Cryptocotyle lingua*. J. Parasitol. **53**: 725–734.
35. BILS, R. F. & W. E. MARTIN. 1966. Fine structure and development of the trematode tegument. Trans. Amer. Microsc. Soc. **85**: 78–88.
36. GINETSINSKAYA, T. A., A. A. DOBOROVOLSKI & V. F. MASHANSKI. 1965. Ultrastructure of the tissues of trematode larvae. Mater. Nauchn. Konf. Vsesouiz. Obshch. Gelmint. Part **I**: 58–60.
37. GINETSINSKAYA, T. A., A. A. DOBOROVOLSKI, & V. F. MASHANSKI. 1966. Ultrastructure of the wall and method of feeding of rediae and sporocysts (Trematoda). Dokl. Akad. Nauk. SSSR **166**: 1003, 1004.
38. REES, G. 1966. Light and electron microscope studies of the rediae of *Parorchis acanthus* Nicoll. Parasitology **56**: 589–602.
39. REES, G. 1971. The ultrastructure of the epidermis of the rediae and cercaria of *Parorchis acanthus* Nicoll. A study by scanning and transmission electron microscopy. Parasitology **62**: 479–488.
40. DIXON, K. E. 1970. Absorption by developing cercariae of *Cloacitrema narrabeenensis* (Philophthalmidae). J. Parasitol. **56**; *In* 2nd International Congress of Parasitology, Washington, D.C. Proceedings, Part **2**: 416, 417.
41. WILSON, R. A. 1972. Gland cells in the redia of *Fasciola hepatica*. Parasitology **65**: 433–436.
42. THREADGOLD, L. T. 1967. Electron microscope studies of *Fasciola hepatica*. III. Further observations on the tegument and associated structures. Parasitology **57**: 633–637.
43. HARRIS, K. R., T. C. CHENG & A. CALI. 1974. An electron microscope study of the tegument of the metacercaria and adult of *Leucochloridiomorpha constantiae* (Trematoda: Brachylaemidae). Parasitology **68**: 57–67.

44. WRIGHT, C. A. 1966. The pathogenesis of helminths in the Mollusca. Helminth. Abst. **35:** 207–224.
45. MEULEMAN, E. 1972. Host-parasite interrelationships between the freshwater pulmonate *Biomphalaria pfeifferi* and the trematode *Schistosoma mansoni*. Neth. J. Zool. **22**(4): 355–427.
46. READER, T. A. J. 1971. The pathological effects of sporocysts, rediae and metacercariae on the digestive gland of *Bithynia tentaculata* (Mollusca: Gastropoda). Parasitology **63:** 483–489.
47. MALEK, E. A. & T. C. CHENG. 1975. Medical and Economic Malacology. Academic Press, Inc. New York, N.Y.
48. CHENG, T. C., J. T. SULLIVAN & K. R. HARRIS. 1973. Parasitic castration of the marine prosobranch gastropod *Nassarius obsoletus* by sporocysts of *Zoogonus rubellus* (Trematoda): histopathology. J. Invert. Pathol. **21**(2): 183–190.
49. MCCELLAND, G. & T. K. R. BOURNS. 1969. Effects of *Trichobilharzia ocellata* on growth, reproduction, and survival of *Lymnaea stagnalis*. Exp. Parasitol. **24:** 37–146.
50. PLATT, P. 1968. The effect of endoparasitism by *Cryptocotyle lingua* (Creplin) on digestion in the snail, *Littorina littorea*. M.Sc. Thesis. Dalhousie University. Halifax, Nova Scotia, Canada.
51. DAVIS, D. S. & J. FARLEY. 1973. The effect of parasitism by the trematode *Cryptocotyle lingua* (Creplin) on digestive efficiency in the snail host, *Littorina saxitalis* (Olivi). Parasitology **66:** 191–197.
52. LEHNINGER, A. L. 1970. Biochemistry. Worth Publishers, Inc. New York, N.Y.
53. BOURNS, T. K. R. 1974. Carbohydrate and protein in *Lymnaea stagnalis* eggs and *Trichobilharzia ocellata* cercariae. J. Parasitol. **60**(6): 1046, 1047.
54. REVEL, J. P. & S. ITO. 1967. The surface components of cells. *In* The Specificity of Cell Surfaces. Prentice-Hall, Inc. Englewood Cliffs, N.J.
55. SMYTH, J. D. 1973. Some interface phenomena in parasitic protozoa and platyhelminths. Can. J. Zool. **51**(3): 367–377.

IN VITRO CULTIVATION OF CELLS AND A
MICROSPORIDIAN PARASITE OF BIOMPHALARIA
GLABRATA (PULMONATA: BASOMMATOPHORA) *

C. J. Bayne and A. Owczarzak

Department of Zoology
Oregon State University
Corvallis, Oregon 97331

W. E. Noonan

Department of Biology
Whitman College
Walla Walla, Washington 99362

INTRODUCTION

During research directed toward the establishment of a cell line from *Biomphalaria glabrata*, a snail responsible for the transmission of *Schistosoma mansoni*, we have simultaneously propagated a microsporidian that has not been previously described. Whereas the infected snail colony feeds and reproduces like a healthy population, cultures obtained from primary explants exhibit varying degrees of microsporidian infection. In some cases, sectors of the cultures show high incidences of infection. The presence of the intracellular protozoan appears to have little effect on the well-being of the cultures.

The growth of microsporidia in tissue culture was first reported by Trager;[1] more recently, insect pathologists have extended this work in studies of microsporidian life cycles.[2,3] Michelson[4] was the first to report a microsporidian parasite of a basommatophoran snail, though there have been both earlier and subsequent reports of hyperparasitized trematode parasites of such mollusks.[5,7] Michelson[4] was unable to infect *B. glabrata* with *Plistophora hussey*, from physid snails. In 1973, Richards and Sheffield[8] reported the presence of a microsporidian, *Steinhausia*, in vivo in *B. glabrata*, and Basch and Di Conza[9] reported unidentified microsporidia in the cells of embryonic *B. glabrata* cultured *in vitro*. Microsporidian parasites of *B. glabrata* are of potential value in the fight against schistosomiasis, because they may interact competitively with the intramolluscan stages of the trematode. Sohi and Wilson[10] have shown the value of *in vitro* studies on microsporidia in determining tolerance ranges to pharmacologic and physiologic variables.

In this paper, we shall describe the procedures used to establish long-lived cultures of young *Biomphalaria* cells (at the time of writing, several cultures have passed the 1-year mark), several aspects of the biology and ultrastructure of the microsporidian, and the results of efforts with various pharmaceuticals to control the growth of this symbiont.

* Supported by National Institutes of Health, NIAID Contract NIH-NIAID-22-527 and Grant AI-12409-2.

513

Establishment of Snail Cell Cultures

Juvenile snails (maximum diameter of shell, 11 mm) were scrubbed free of surface contaminants in distilled water and were soaked for 1 hr in a mixture of penicillin (100 IU/ml), streptomycin (100 μg/ml), and Fungizone® (2.5 μg/ml) [(PSF) BioQuest] in dechlorinated water. By sterile procedures and working with a dissecting microscope in a sterile hood, the shell was broken over the heart and gonad, and the organs were pulled out and cut free. The organs were further sterilized by passing them through six 10-min washes of PSF in NCTC 109 (Difco) diluted 1:1 with distilled water.

After 60 min in PSF medium, the organs were cut into explants 1 mm³, rinsed in three changes of complete medium composed of reconstituted NCTC medium 109 diluted 1:1 with double distilled water, and placed into Costar T 30 plastic flasks (Microbiological Associates). TC medium 199 (Difco) minus the vertebrate salts and dissolved in Noonan's balanced salt solution (composed of 1500 mg NaCl, 150 mg KCl, 450 mg $MgSO_4$, 350 mg $NaHCO_3$, 530 mg $CaCl_2$, 70 mg $NaHPO_4$, 1 l double distilled water) has also been used successfully. The flasks were prepared by the addition of 2 ml of the complete medium that contained 5% by volume of fetal calf serum (Microbiological Associates) and 1% by volume of PSF. The osmolal concentration of the medium was between 140 and 145 mOsm. After the culture surface of the flasks had been wetted with the medium, the flasks were inverted. The explants were transferred from the last rinse and placed on the wetted surface, where they were allowed to adhere. The flasks were gassed with a mixture of 95% N_2-5% CO_2 until the pH of the medium was 7.0–7.2 and were left inverted overnight at room temperature ($\sim$21° C). The next morning, the flasks were carefully righted, thereby covering the explants with the medium. Emigration of cells will occur at a wide range of temperature (15–27° C). After 3 days, a zone of cellular outgrowth surrounded each explant. Every week, half of the medium was removed and replaced with new medium. "Feeding" the cells at shorter or longer intervals did not improve the condition of the cultures.

Photomicroscopy

Flask cultures were monitored for mitotic activity and cell behavior by time-lapse photocinematography. Cover slip cultures, grown in Leighton tubes, were used for high-resolution light microscopy. For staining, the cultures were fixed in Zenker's and stained with Giemsa according to the method of Price, as outlined by Luna,[11] with McManus' periodic acid-Schiff (PAS) with diastase controls,[12] and by the Feulgen technique.[13] For photomicrography of living cells and their microsporidian parasites, the cover slips were removed from their tubes and inverted over nutrient medium on a 3 × 1 glass slide and examined under phase-contrast oil immersion objectives. Microsporidian polar tubes were extruded under the influence of sodium hydroxide, which was placed on the slide adjacent to the cover slip and allowed to diffuse into the surrounding medium. One culture was subjected to four separate techniques that permitted the localization of neutral fats (oil red O), phase-contrast microscopy, identification of the polar cap by the PAS reaction, and scanning electron microscopy

(SEM) (FIGURES 1–6). This was accomplished by mounting the culture in glycerine jelly for the first three steps and using the critical-point method for the fourth (SEM).

Electron Microscopy

Flasks that contained microsporidia were prepared for transmission electron microscopy (TEM) by removal of the culture medium and fixation by 3% glutaraldehyde in 0.1 M phosphate buffer (pH 7.2) at room temperature for 30 min. After rinsing, the cultures can either be stored in the buffer at refrigerator temperatures or immediately postfixed in 1% osmic acid phosphate buffer (pH 7.2) for 30 min, also at room temperature. Subsequent treatment, performed at room temperature on a 15-min schedule, included a buffer rinse, dehydration in 20, 50, 70, and 95% ethanol plus four changes of absolute ethanol, and infiltration by four changes of complete Araldite® embedding medium,[14] as suggested by Trotter,[15] at 35° C. After the last change of plastic, the upper wall of the flask was perforated [16] to promote the removal of volatiles. Embedding was in the same Araldite mixture at 35° C overnight, followed by an overnight curing at 60° C. Previously marked areas were cut from the final embedment, and the wall of the flask was removed prior to pegging the specimen. Thin sections were mounted on uncoated grids, stained with uranyl acetate and lead citrate, and examined with an electron microscope. Thick sections were stained with Mallory's azure II-methylene blue,[17] air dried, mounted in immersion oil, and examined with the light microscope. A Wratten 22 (orange) filter used during observation and photography gave contrasts identical to those of the electron micrographs.

Drug Therapy

Benomyl® (Du Pont de Nemours) and fumadil B (Abbott Laboratories) have been shown to successfully control microsporidian infections in insect cell cultures.[10] Benomyl was added to our culture medium at 25, 50, or 100 µg/ml. Fumadil B was added at 25 or 50 µg/ml. The drugs were assayed separately by maintaining cultures with the drug for extended periods of time: 8 weeks for Benomyl and 15 weeks for fumadil B. The success or failure of the drug concentration was determined microscopically on living cultures, by observing the presence or absence of the microsporidian.

RESULTS

Both gonadal and heart tissues, when explanted *in vitro,* yield large numbers of cells that actively emigrate onto the culture surface (FIGURE 7). Time-lapse records reveal that some of the cells are actively amoeboid, but for most cells, locomotion is limited to a very gradual gliding movement away from the explants. Whereas surface blebbing reminiscent of mitotic cells in anaphase has been observed in the time-lapse films, actual divisions have not been observed. This failure is due to the very small size of the mitotic figures. Metaphase figures measure 6.2 × 2.7 µm, and anaphase/telophase figures measure

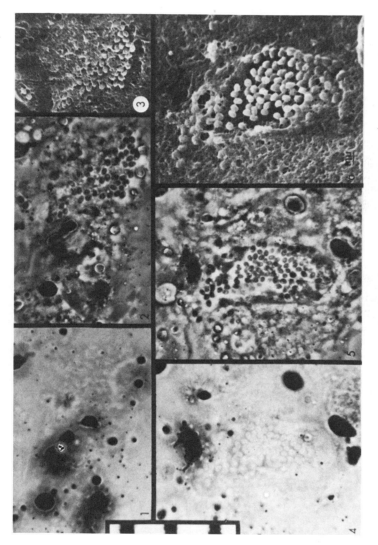

FIGURES 1–6. Pansporoblasts in snail cells viewed by three microscopic methods. FIGURES 1 & 4. Bright-field illumination of oil red O-stained culture shows dark droplets of neutral lipids and faint outlines of spores. FIGURES 2 & 5. The same preparations, observed by phase-contrast microscopy, illustrate relationships of the spores to one another and to host cell contents. FIGURES 3 & 6. Scanning electron micrograph of the same preparations clearly shows the dimensions and topography of the spores. Scale divisions, 10 μm (FIGURES 1–5); bar (FIGURE 6), 1 μm.

2.8 × 1.6 μm. The figures in FIGURE 8 are from Giemsa-stained Leighton tube cultures. The cell populations are not prolifically mitotic, even under challenge of mitogens and mutagens. The following agents and concentrations were used without recognizable success: phytohemagglutinin, 1, 10, 50, 100 μg/ml; concanavalin A, 1, 10, 50, 100, 500 μg/ml; pokeweed mitogen, 1, 5, 10, 25 mg/ml; dibenzanthracene, 1, 10, 50, 100 μg/ml; nitrosoguanidine, 1, 10, 50, 100, 500 μg/ml; cyclic AMP, 1, 10, 100 μg/ml; cyclic GMP, 1, 10, 100 μg/ml; papaverine, <1 mmole.

It has been characteristic that molluscan cells cultured in several laboratories tolerate rather wide ranges of pH, temperature, and osmotic concentrations of the medium. In this laboratory, the cells appear most healthy at pH

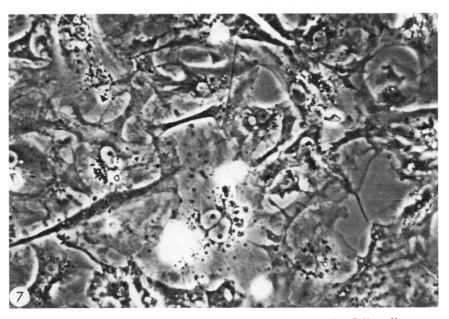

FIGURE 7. Cultured snail gonad cells in the area of outgrowth. Cell outlines, nuclei, and dense nucleoli are clearly visible. Age of culture is 1 week; phase-contrast microscopy.

7.0–7.2, 23 ± 2° C, and 140 ± 10 mOsm, but they survive for several days at pH 6.0–8.0, temperatures of 15–27° C, and osmolal concentrations of 110–180 mOsm.

The microsporidian, when present, tolerates the above extremes in culture on a par with the host cells. However, the simultaneous presence of various stages of spore maturation in single pansporoblasts suggests that physiologic inadequacies may exist under our culture conditions. The spore structure is characteristically microsporidian. Counts reveal that pansporoblasts may contain from 8 to 128 spores (FIGURES 9–13). It is possible that endogenous sporogeny occurs and that pansporoblasts with few spores represent earlier stages of the life cycle. This belief is supported by the presence, in the pansporo-

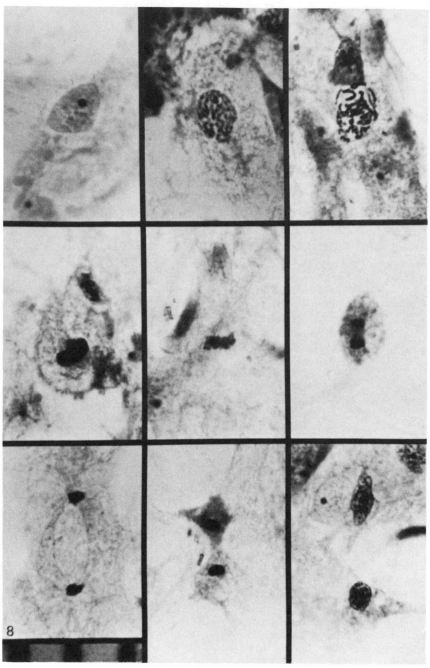

FIGURE 8. Cells in various stages of mitotic division, as seen in the area of outgrowth of cultured snail gonad. From top left to bottom right, one can trace sequential stages of mitosis; photographs are of separate cells. Geimsa stained; scale division, 10 μm.

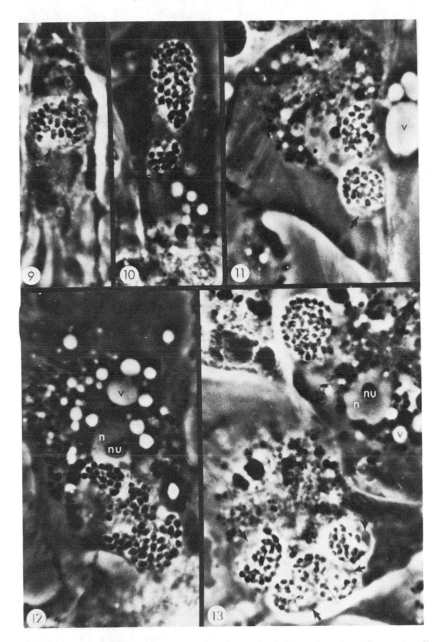

FIGURES 9–13. Microsporidian pansporoblasts in living cultured snail gonad cells. The number of individuals per cell differs, as do their size and the number of spores produced. The sporoblastic areas are indicated by arrows. The magnification scales of FIGURES 1–6 and 8 are applicable to these Figures. Abbreviations (host cell organelles): n, nucleus; nu, nucleolus; v, vacuole.

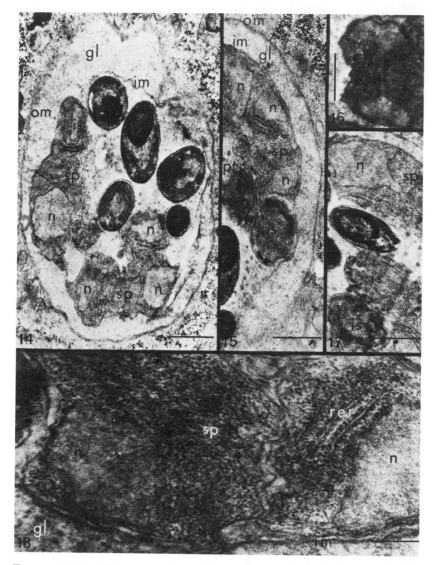

FIGURES 14–18. Ultrastructure of microsporidian pansporoblasts. FIGURES 14 & 15. The peripheral granular layer (gl) that lies between the inner (im) and outer membranes (om) of the pansporoblast is shown, as are the sporoblastic and sporogenous zones. Nuclei (n) lying in a common sporoplasm (sp) plus various developmental stages of spores are illustrated. FIGURE 15 also includes the polar tube (pt) of an immature spore (is). FIGURE 16 illustrates sporogenous nuclear division. A lengthy isthmus connects the two daughter nuclei. FIGURE 17 shows early, middle, and late spore development. The nucleus of the sporogenous tissue bears a protrusion to the right, which may be a segment of the interconnecting isthmus. FIGURE 18 is a high-magnification micrograph of the sporoplasm at the top of FIGURE 15 which gives details of two nuclei, the ribosome-rich sporoplasm, and the rough endoplasmic reticulum (rer) of two very early spores. Bars (FIGURES 14–17), 1 µm; bar in FIGURE 18 equals 1/4 µm.

blasts, of areas of differentiating sporogenous material, immature spores, and fully differentiated spores (FIGURES 9, 10 & 13–18). The species may, however, be mictosporous, as reported for *Stempellia*.[18] It has proven difficult to accumulate knowledge of the vegetative stages; nothing firm is known about the nuclear events in the life cycle.

It would appear from both light and electron micrographs that more than one pansporoblast may be present in a single snail cell (FIGURES 10–13).

The mode of spore release remains obscure; however, it has been possible, with time-lapse cinematography, to follow the fate of released spores. Film sequences suggest that the spores may be forcibly ejected into the surrounding medium, after which they move erratically, as is typical of particles in Brownian movement. One film sequence suggests the fusion or engulfment of a spore by a snail cell (FIGURE 19). Very small motile bodies seen in the movies may represent secondary infective forms of the parasite, but there is no way of differentiating them from snail cell fragments broken from the cells on release of adhesion.

It has been possible to induce polar tube and sporoplasm extrusion by the addition of alkali to the culture medium (FIGURE 20). Measurements indicate a mean tube length of 24 μm $\pm$ 5.5 SD. This figure agrees with calculations made from electron micrograph measurements.

It is not known how the infection is transmitted in the snail colonies.

The structure of the pansporoblast is revealed in FIGURE 14. The sporogenous sector to which reference was made earlier is seen to contain endoplasmic reticulum, ribosomes, and nuclear material. The presence of both early and late stages of spore maturation in single pansporoblasts has not been described previously for any microsporidian, and its visibility in living material shows that it is not an artifact (FIGURES 9, 11 & 13). A second unusual feature of this species is the presence of a granular layer between the inner and outer membrane pairs of the pansporoblast (FIGURES 14 & 15).

Production of spores involves a nuclear division, which in microsporidia occurs without the breakdown of the nuclear membrane. Dumbbell-shaped nuclei and others that possess processes suggestive of the isthmus between sister nuclei occur in the sporogonial plasmodium (FIGURES 16 & 17). Sporoblast limiting membranes appear to be formed *de novo* around the products of division in the manner of endogenous sporogeny (FIGURES 14, 15, 17 & 18). Morphogenesis of spore organelles follows; the exospore is formed last (FIGURES 15 & 17).

The size of the mature spore, as determined from light micrographs of living materials, differs from that obtained from TEM micrographs: $1.87 \pm 0.05 \times 1.17 \pm 0.05$ μm vs $1.50 \pm 0.02 \times 0.86 \pm 0.01$ μm. The shrinkage of 23% is undoubtedly due to the rigors of fixation and embedding for TEM. The outer wall of the spore is composed of an electron-opaque layer, the exospore, a wider electron-transparent layer, and an inner electron-dense layer, the endospore (FIGURES 21–24). The body of the spore consists of the sporoplasm, which is composed of a structureless ground cytoplasm that contains numerous ribosomes, a single nucleus, and the organelles of infection, all of which will be described below. Occasionally, membranes suggestive of the Golgi apparatus appear in close juxtaposition with a segment of the polar tube (FIGURE 23). A similar configuration associated with the developing tubule of nematocysts in coelenterates [19] hints at an analogous mechanism for the origin of this part of the inoculative apparatus.

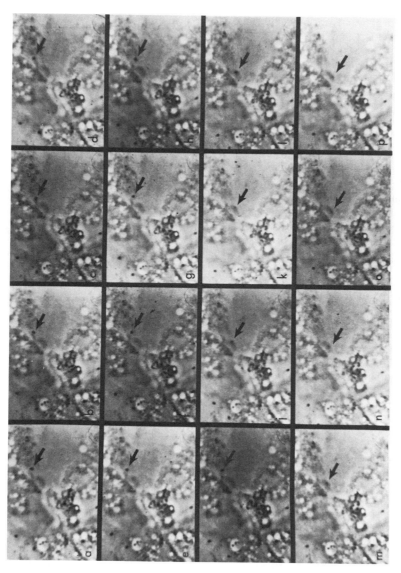

FIGURE 19. Cinematographic sequence of microsporidian spore engulfment by a snail gonad cell. Time-lapse interval of 10 sec between frames. One spore that shows Brownian movement is indicated by arrows. A bleb on the surface of the snail cell is seen to the left of the spore. Contact and engulfment occur in frame j. Although the spore is visible inside the bleb in the following frames, complete viewing of the film reveals that it is stationary and slowly disappears from view inside the cell cytoplasm.

The polaroplast takes the form of an ovoid group of very tightly packed smooth membranes that are markedly electron dense after the preparative procedures we use (FIGURES 21–24). It has a small opening under the polar cap to which the polar tube is attached (FIGURE 21). Another opening appears at one side, through which the polar tube passes from the center of the polaroplast to the more basal regions of the spore (FIGURE 24).

There is a clearly distinguished PAS-positive polar cap, in the form of a bowl, at the apex of the spore (FIGURES 21 & 23). It is as electron dense as the polaroplast but is not contiguous with it. It is clear that the polar tube attaches here (FIGURE 21).

The polar tube can be subdivided into three regions: a short straight length

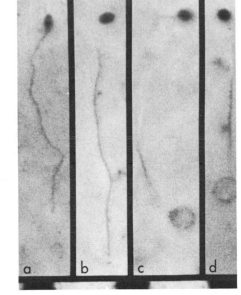

FIGURE 20. Spores after alkali-induced eversion of the polar tube; in c and d, the sporoplasm is seen at the end of the tube. Scale divisions, 10 μm.

proximal to and attached to the polar cap and encompassed by the polaroplast (FIGURE 21) and with a diameter of 0.06 ± 0.004 μm, a lengthy spiral portion of seven to 11 gyres that abut the plasma membrane with diameters of 0.08 ± 0.003 × 0.06 ± 0.004 μm (FIGURES 22 & 23), and a short distal segment, 0.06 ± 0.006 × 0.04 ± 0.006 μm in diameter, adjacent to the posterior vacuole (FIGURE 23).

The posterior vacuole, which is considered to play a role in polar tube extrusion that involves osmotic swelling, rests pressed against the cell membrane at the posterior end of the spore (FIGURES 22 & 23).

The nucleus appears to be devoid of definable structures. It lies beneath the polaroplast enveloped by a very RNA granule-rich but otherwise structureless cytoplasm (FIGURES 21–24).

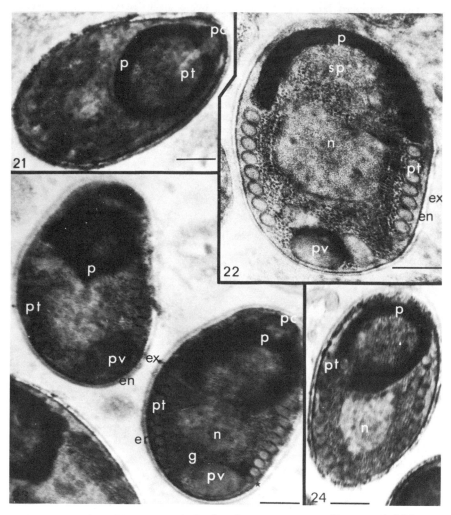

FIGURES 21–24. Ultrastructural details of mature spores. Bars equal 0.25 μm. FIGURE 21 shows the attachment of the polar tube (pt) to the polar cap (pc) via a pore in the polaroplast (p). FIGURE 22 illustrates detail of the internal organization of a spore. The nucleus (n), with slight internal differentiation, lies centrally in a ribosome-rich sporoplasm (sp). Note the alignment of ribosomes at the sides of the spore between the nucleus and cross sections of the polar tube (pt). The polaroplast (p) in this case appears abnormal; it assumes the form of an inverted bowl rather than a perforated spheroid, as in the other Figures. The presence of an electron-opaque cap on the anterior surface of the polar vacuole (pv) is also unusual. The spore wall consists of the endospore (en), an electron-transparent zone, and the exospore (ex). FIGURE 23 directs attention to the smaller-diameter portions of the polar tube (*) adjacent to the posterior vacuole (pv). A cup-shaped pair of membranes (g) suggestive of the Golgi apparatus encompasses part of the polar tube (pt) in the right-hand spore. FIGURE 24 shows the point at which the polar tube (pt) passes posteriorly through the base of the polaroplast (p).

Effect of Drugs

The microsporidian has not been eliminated from our cultures by the use of either Benomyl or fumadil B. This result is not surprising, because the work of Sohi and Wilson [10] demonstrates that the drugs merely inhibit further growth of the sporozoan: in the presence of abundant dividing insect cells, the overall effect is to eliminate the parasite through the practice of serial subculturing. The snail cells in our cultures are not actively mitotic; therefore, the microsporidian, even if arrested, remains evident.

DISCUSSION

Stimulated by the increasing spread of schistosomiasis in tropical regions, considerable effort has recently been applied toward establishing a cell line from one of the snail intermediate hosts of *Schistosoma* sp. Until recently, the work of Chernin [20] remained the only readily repeatable achievement in this area. The work of Benex [21] (reviewed in Reference 22), which utilized explants of *B. glabrata in vitro,* was constructive but was more concerned with organ culture. In 1973, both Basch and Di Conza [9] and Cheng and Arndt [23] reported maintenance of *B. glabrata* cells for periods that exceeded those achieved by Chernin.[20] More recently, Hansen [4] has reported successful establishment of a cell line from embryonic snails, but a cell line from adult cells remains elusive.

The significant accomplishment of our cell culture work is notably our ability to maintain cells derived from juvenile snails in an apparently healthy condition for periods of up to 1 year, which is strikingly longer than any published account. With such prolonged maintenance, we have provided a tool of potential value in the study of schistosome-snail cell interactions and in more basic studies of cell physiology and behavior.

The attractiveness of the concept of biologic control for *B. glabrata* has, of course, led us to consider the possibility of using the microsporidian contaminant to this end. It appears, however, that the snail colony that is the source of our infected tissues is as healthy as noninfected colonies. Thus, without selective genetic experiments, it is not conceivable that snail control may be achieved with this agent.

Mollusks appear to have an astounding capacity to tolerate physiologic insults from parasites or from the extraneous environment that appear excessive to us, without showing adverse effects. Microsporidians may be tolerated as well as schistosomes, but the possibility of lowered fecundity of trematodes in snails that carry microsporidian infections is certainly worthy of investigation.

One of the unusual features of this microsporidian is the concurrent presence of both mature and developing spores in the pansporoblasts. We consider this characteristic to be generic, but it is conceivable that the microsporidian is not entirely compatible with our culture conditions and that all spores are therefore not developing to maturity in a synchronous manner. The organism otherwise most closely resembles members of the genus *Plistophora*.

SUMMARY

Cells from juvenile heart and gonads of *B. glabrata* have been grown *in vitro* for more than 1 year. These cell cultures are not actively mitotic but show other characteristics normal for metazoan cells in culture. They are tolerant of widely variable culture conditions. Challenges with mitogens, mutagens, and altered cyclic nucleotide levels have failed to induce mitosis. A microsporidian parasite grows intracellularly *in vitro*. The ultrastructural details of sporogeny and pansporoblastic maturation are described. Several pansporoblasts can occur in one snail cell; maturation of spores within a pansporoblast is not synchronous, which is a highly unusual feature. Time-lapse cinemicrography reveals engulfment of free spores by snail cells. Polar tube and sporoplasm release are reported photographically. Drug therapy failed to eliminate the protozoan. The potential value of microsporidia in schistosome control programs is evaluated as slight.

ACKNOWLEDGMENTS

The technical assistance of Peggy C. Salvatore is appreciated. Analysis of photographic materials benefited from discussions with Don Morrison, Victor Sprague, Jiri Vavra, C. S. Richards, and Ann Cali. We are grateful to Ann Cali also for FIGURES 14, 15, 17, 18, and 22.

REFERENCES

1. TRAGER, W. 1937. The hatching of spores of *Nosema bombycis* Naegeli and the partial development of the organism in tissue cultures. J. Parasitol. **23:** 226, 227.
2. ISHIHARA, R. 1969. The life cycle of *Nosema bombycis* as revealed in tissue culture of *Bombyx mori*. J. Invert. Pathol. **14:** 316–320.
3. SOHI, S. S. 1972. *In vitro* cultivation of hemocytes of *Malcosoma disstria* Hubner (Lepidoptera: Lasiocampidae). Can. J. Zool. **49:** 1355–1358.
4. MICHELSON, E. H. 1963. *Plistophora husseyi sp. no.*, a microsporidian parasite of aquatic pulmonate snails. J. Insect Pathol. **5:** 28–38.
5. CORT, W. W., K. L. HUSSEY & D. J. AMEEL. 1960. Studies on a microsporidian hyperparasite of strigeoid trematodes. I. Prevalence and effect on the parasitized trematodes. J. Parasitol. **46:** 317–325.
6. CANNING, E. U., L. P. FOON & L. K. JOE. 1974. Microsporidian parasites of trematode larvae from aquatic snails in West Malaysia. J. Protozool. **21:** 19–25.
7. CANNING, E. U. & P. F. BASCH. 1968. *Perezia helminthorum sp. nov.*, a microsporidian hyperparasite of trematode larve from Malaysian snails. Parasitology **58:** 341–347.
8. RICHARDS, C. S. & H. G. SHEFFIELD. 1970. Unique host relations and ultrastructure of a new microsporidian of the genus *Coccospora* infecting *Biomphalaria glabrata*. *In* Proceedings of the IVth International Colloquium on Insect Pathology. : 439–452.
9. BASCH, P. F. & J. J. DI CONZA. 1973. Primary cultures of embryonic cells from the snail *Biomphalaria glabrata*. Amer. J. Trop. Med. Hyg. **22:** 805–813.
10. SOHI, S. S. & G. G. WILSON. 1974. Propagation of *Nosema* and other protozoan pathogens of insects in tissue culture. Presented to Society for Invertebrate Pathology, Tempe, Arizona.
11. LUNA, L. G. 1968. Manual of Histologic Staining Method of the Armed Forces Institute of Pathology. 3rd edit. McGraw-Hill Book Company. New York, N.Y.
12. BARKA, T. & P. J. ANDERSON. 1963. Histochemistry: Theory, Practice, and Bibliography. Harper & Row, Publishers. New York, N.Y.

13. GURR, E. 1960. Methods of Analytical Histology and Histo-Chemistry. The Williams & Wilkins Co. Baltimore, Md.
14. LUFT, J. 1961. Improvements in epoxy resin embedding methods. J. Biophys. Biochem. Cytol. **9:** 409–414.
15. TROTTER, J. 1974. Personal communication.
16. KEEN, L. N., R. REYNOLDS, W. L. WHITTLE & P. F. KRUSE. 1973. Vertical sectioning B. Cells in plastic flasks. *In* Tissue Culture Methods and Application. P. E. Kruse & M. K. Patterson, Jr., Eds. : 448–451. Academic Press, Inc. New York, N.Y.
17. RICHARDSON, K. C., L. JARETT & E. H. FINKE. 1960. Embedding in epoxy resins for ultrathin sectioning in electron microscopy. Stain Technol. **35:** 313–323.
18. KUDO, R. 1924. A biologic and taxonomic study of the microsporidia. Illinois Biol. Mon. **9:** 11–199.
19. DAVIS, L. E. 1973. Ultrastructural changes during dedifferentiation and redifferentiation in the regenerating, isolated gastrodermis. *In* The Biology of Hydra. A. L. Burnett, Ed. : 171–219. Academic Press, Inc. New York and London.
20. CHERNIN, E. 1963. Observations on hearts explanted *in vitro* from the snail *Australorbis glabratus.* J. Parasitol. **49:** 353–364.
21. BENEX, J. 1967. Les possibilités de la culture organo-typique en milieu liquide dans l'étude des problèmes parasitaires. Ann. Parasitol. Hum. Comp. **41:** 351–378.
22. BAYNE, C. J. 1968. Molluscan organ culture. Malacol. Rev. **1:** 125–135.
23. CHENG, T. C. & R. J. ARNDT. 1973. Maintenance of cells of *Biomphalaria glabrata* (Mollusca) *in vitro.* J. Invert. Pathol. **22:** 308–310.
24. HANSEN, E. L. 1974. A cell line from the freshwater snail *Biomphalaria glabrata.* Int. Res. Commun. Systems **2:** 1703.
25. BASCH, P. F. 1971. Transmission of microsporidian infection in the snail *Indoplanorbis exustus* in West Malaysia. S.E. Asian J. Trop. Med. Publ. Health **2:** 380–383.

ENVIRONMENTAL SIGNIFICANCE OF *BACULOVIRUS* INFECTIONS IN ESTUARINE AND MARINE SHRIMP *

John A. Couch,† Max D. Summers,‡ and Lee Courtney †

† *Gulf Breeze Environmental Research Laboratory*
United States Environmental Protection Agency
Sabine Island, Gulf Breeze, Florida 32561
and ‡ *Cell Research Institute*
University of Texas
Austin, Texas 78712

INTRODUCTION

Certain enveloped, rod-shaped DNA viruses have long been known as pathogens of insects under the descriptive term "nuclear polyhedrosis viruses." [1] These viruses have been extensively and intensively studied since Berghold's [2] early reports in 1947. Subsequent to Berghold's classic early studies, many rod-shaped viruses associated with polyhedral inclusion bodies of a crystalline nature have been described from different species of insects that represent several orders of Insecta. At present, The International Committee on Nomenclature of Viruses places the nuclear polyhedrosis viruses of arthropods in subgroup A under the genus or group name *Baculovirus*.[1] Prior to 1973, there were no reports of viruses that resemble baculoviruses in animals other than insects or mites. In 1973 and 1974, the first reports [3, 4] were made of baculovirus-like particles and associated polyhedral inclusion bodies in a noninsect arthropod host. The new host was the pink shrimp, *Penaeus duorarum,* from Florida waters of the northern Gulf of Mexico. These reports indicated for the *Baculovirus* group a host range extension into the arthropod class Crustacea.

In regard to specific characterization and identification of the shrimp virus, it is pertinent to report that not all of Koch's postulates have been satisfied. Koch's postulates, however, were meant to be used to show specificity of a microorganism as an etiologic agent for a disease condition and not specifically to determine phylogenetic affinity or identity of the microorganism. The latter task (identification) includes determination of biologic, morphologic, chemical, and physical characteristics. Much of our effort has gone into these determinations for the shrimp virus. The first of Koch's postulates (that of association or presence of a microorganism with a disease condition) has been satisfied for patent virus infections in shrimp; that is, inclusion bodies and virions are present in all patent infections that exhibit cytopathologic characteristics. The second of Koch's postulates (that of isolation and pure culture of the microorganism) has not been satisfied for the shrimp virus and poses a severe problem because of the lack of continuous cell cultures of crustacean tissues in which to isolate and grow the virus. At present, we are attempting to use established insect cell lines in which to grow the shrimp virus.

The baculoviruses have attracted much attention in recent years largely because some microbiologists and entomologists consider these viruses to be

* Contribution 253, Gulf Breeze Environmental Research Laboratory.

promising biologic control agents for numerous insect pests.[5-7] The insect baculoviruses have shown narrow host specificity,[8] and all experimental attempts so far to infect noninsect species with insect baculoviruses have failed.[9]

The purpose of the present paper is to consider, in light of our present knowledge, the significance of the shrimp virus in regard to the ecology of its crustacean host.

VIRAL EFFECTS

The capability for recognition of patent virus infections with light microscopy has made possible the harvesting of viral material from feral shrimp. Patently infected shrimp are those in which hepatopancreatic cell nuclei show hypertrophy (FIGURE 2) and in which many of these nuclei possess characteristic virus-associated polyhedral inclusion bodies (PIBs) (FIGURE 3). In producing these effects and in its fine structure, the shrimp *Baculovirus* is similar to other well-described baculoviruses.

Aspects of the cytopathologic effects in shrimp have been described in detail elsewhere.[3, 4] Here, however, it is of value to review certain changes induced by the virus that reveal the extent of impact of the virus on shrimp hepatopancreatic cells. Nuclear hypertrophy, chromatin diminution and margination, and nucleolar loss are the obvious signs of infection prior to the appearance of the PIB in the nucleus. These signs are apparent in heavily infected shrimp with both bright-field and phase-contrast microscopy (FIGURES 1–4). As cellular infections progress in lightly to heavily infected shrimp, tetrahedra (PIBs) from 0.5 to 20 μm in width appear in nuclei in numbers relative to infection intensity (FIGURES 3 & 4).

Electron microscopy reveals both the striking fine structural changes that occur in host cells and the structure of the PIBs and associated virions (FIGURES 5–7). The ultimate cytopathologic effect of the virus is destruction of the host cell. Damage is obvious in loss of the cell's structural and functional integrity and growth of the PIB to a size too great for cellular accommodation (FIGURE 5). TABLE 1 gives a list of cytopathologic alterations of infected hepatopancreatic cells visible with light and electron microscopy.

BIOCHEMICAL CHARACTERISTICS

The shrimp virus has an enveloped nucleocapsid that appears similar to those of insect baculoviruses that have been characterized biochemically (FIGURE 7). Although not yet determined, nucleic acid of the virus is probably double-stranded DNA, as is the case with other baculoviruses.[1] Biochemical and serologic investigations are underway to compare the nucleic acid, virus structural proteins, and inclusion body proteins of the shrimp virus to several species of insect baculoviruses.

CELL CULTURE

A preliminary attempt has been made to introduce virus via ultrafiltrates of infected hepatopancreas into tissue culture cells of *Trichoplusia ni, Spodoptera*

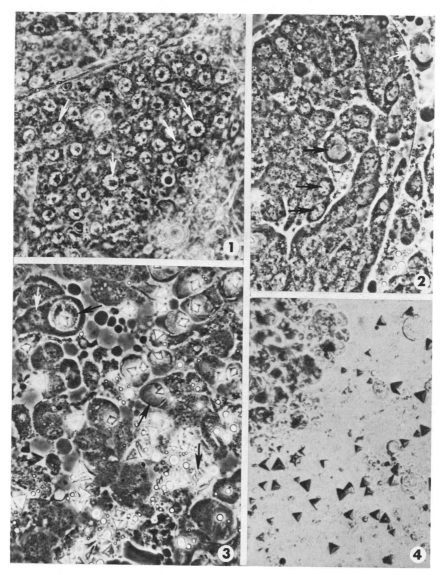

FIGURES 1–4. Light photomicrographs of fresh squash preparation of shrimp hepatopancreas. FIGURE 1 shows uninfected, normal cells nuclei (arrows) of hepatopancreas; note conspicuous nucleoli and chromatin; phase-contrast microscopy (×275). FIGURE 2 illustrates early patent infection (black arrows); note nuclear hypertrophy and loss of chromatin and nucleoli; white arrow points to early PIB formation in a nucleus adjacent to basement membrane of hepatopancreatic acinus; phase-contrast microscopy (×275). FIGURE 3 shows advanced patent infection with many PIBs in hypertrophied nuclei and released from nuclei (black arrows); white arrow points to normal nucleus; phase-contrast microscopy (×275). FIGURE 4 shows PIBs free of cells; bright-field microscopy (×250).

frugiperda, Aedes albopietus, and *Culex solinarius.* Unfortunately, results are uncertain, but cytopathologic effects have been elicited in the *Spodoptera* and in mosquito cells. The question whether the virus or a toxic effect from shrimp protein caused the effect must be answered. No cytopathologic effects have been observed in *T. ni* cells.

LABORATORY ENHANCEMENT OF VIRAL INFECTIONS

Though laboratory transmission of virus from shrimp to shrimp by feeding has been somewhat successful, we are not yet able to depend consistently upon

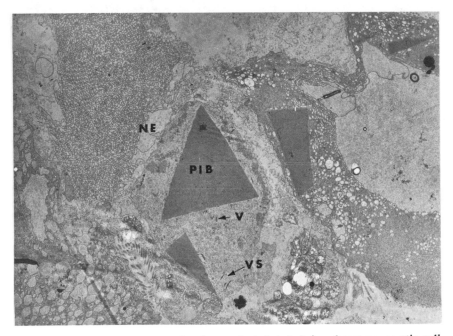

FIGURE 5. Electron micrograph of patently infected shrimp hepatopancreatic cell. PIB, polyhedral inclusion body; NE, nuclear envelope proliferation; VS, virogenic stromata; V, rod shrimp virion in edge of nucleoplasm. ×4000.

feeding of infected tissues to shrimp as a major method to obtain large amounts of virus. On several occasions, we have apparently increased the prevalence of patent infections artificially by holding large samples of shrimp (with initial low prevalence of virus = 0–10%) in small aquaria for up to 40 days. Under crowded, stressful conditions, shrimp with latent infections may develop patent infections, and uninfected shrimp probably become infected by feeding upon carcasses of infected shrimp in these aquaria.

Chemical stress of pink shrimp by laboratory exposures to low levels of organochlorines [11] may increase prevalence of patent infections. This effect

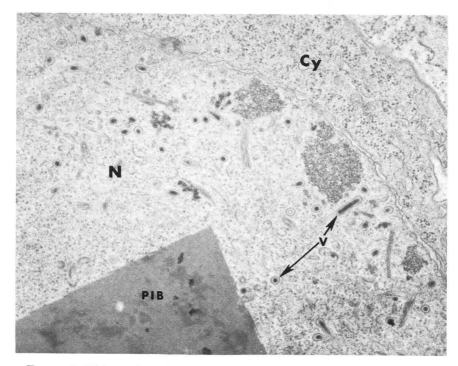

FIGURE 6. Virions, virogenic stages, and PIB in nucleus of patently infected cell. N, nucleoplasm; V, virions in cross and longitudinal sections; Cy, cytoplasm of cell; note many free ribosomes in cytoplasm. ×38,500.

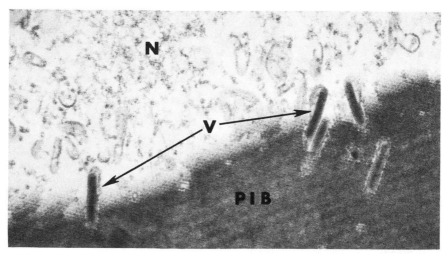

FIGURE 7. Higher magnification of virions at edge of and partially occluded in PIB. ×67,800.

can only really be confirmed, however, in highly controlled *in vivo* and *in vitro* shrimp-virus systems.

DISTRIBUTION AND PREVALENCE OF VIRUS IN NATURE

To date, shrimp have been sampled from waters of the northern Gulf of Mexico and estuaries from Pensacola, Florida eastward to Apalachee Bay near Keaton Beach, Florida. FIGURE 8 shows approximate regions in which virus-infected shrimp have been taken. Only the pink shrimp has shown consistently recoverable natural infections. A single, adult brown shrimp (*Penaeus aztecus*), taken from Escambia Bay, near Pensacola, Florida, was found moderately infected in 1974. White shrimp (*Penaeus setiferus*) and grass shrimp (*Paleo-*

TABLE 1

CYTOPATHOLOGIC EFFECTS OF VIRUS ON SHRIMP HEPATOPANCREATIC CELLS
AS REVEALED BY LIGHT AND ELECTRON MICROSCOPY

Cytopathologic Effect	Light Microscopy	Electron Microscopy
Nuclear hypertrophy	+	+
Chromatin diminution	+	+
Chromatin margination	+	+
Nucleolar loss	+	+
Inclusion body	+	+
Nuclear membrane proliferation (membranous labyrinth)	—	l
Myeloid bodies in cytoplasm	—	+
Increase in free ribosomes	—	+
Reduction in number of mitochondria	—	+
Changes in nucleoplasm		
Fibrillar stroma	—	+
Granular stroma	—	+
Rod-shaped virions in nucleoplasm	—	+

monetes spp.) have not yet been found infected. Other crustacea, such as blue crabs (*Callinectes sapidus*), stone crabs (*Menippe mercenaria*), and mud crabs (*Panopeus* sp. and *Neopanope* sp.), have been found not to harbor the virus.

The prevalences of patently infected pink shrimp in samples taken periodically from various locales along the northern Gulf Coast of Florida since 1970 are given in TABLE 2. Samples taken from Gulf waters near Keaton Beach (Apalachee Bay) have shown the highest prevalence of virus. Our data, to date, indicate no particular seasonal intensification of virus prevalence, although October and January have been productive months for obtaining larger numbers of infected shrimp. Original sample sizes may have influenced this abundance (see TABLE 2).

It is noteworthy that we have not examined specimens from the epicenter of the pink shrimp's geographic distribution in the Gulf of Mexico near the Dry Tortugas and Key West, Florida. These waters maintain the highest known

TABLE 2

NUMBER OF PINK SHRIMP EXAMINED AND PATENT VIRUS INFECTIONS SINCE 1970

Year	Number Examined	Number Patently Infected	Month	Source (all in Florida)
1970	40	12	June	Keaton Beach
	1	1	August	Pensacola
1971	42	0	July	Pensacola
	14	7	August	Keaton Beach
	14	0	September	Keaton Beach
	10	0	October	Keaton Beach
1973	20	0	June	Pensacola
	20	0	August	Pensacola
	42	12	Ocotber	Keaton Beach
	40	6	November	Pensacola
	28	10	November	Port St. Joe
1974	30	0	January	Pensacola
	53	14	January	Keaton Beach
	20	4	February	Keaton Beach
	50	11	March	Keaton Beach
	88	9	May	Keaton Beach
	23	3	August	Keaton Beach
	15	0	September	Keaton Beach
	350	55	October	Keaton Beach
	145	4	October	Port St. Joe
	460	0	November	Pensacola
	298	0	December	Apalachicola
	98	0	December	Pensacola
1975	435	62	January	Keaton Beach
	90	0	January	Pensacola
Totals	2426	210		

pink shrimp densities according to catch per unit of effort of the shrimp fishery.[10] Though pink shrimp sustain a fishery in northern Gulf waters, a study of the virus in more dense populations off southwest Florida should be additionally informative as to the epizootic behavior of the virus in nature. Presence of the virus in southwest Florida pink shrimp is probable because that population merges with the northern Gulf Coast population.

ENVIRONMENTAL SIGNIFICANCE OF SHRIMP VIRUS

Three questions should be considered in regard to discovery of a *Baculovirus* in a marine arthropod. The first is obvious: What is the direct effect of the virus on its natural, feral shrimp host? Thus far, laboratory studies of the shrimp-virus system have not given results that would allow us to predict the effect on pink shrimp populations in nature. There is little doubt that severe cytopathologic effects occur in hepatopancreas of infected individuals. We have some evidence at this time that the virus may cause epizootic mortalities in feral shrimp. Dying shrimp have been found to be heavily infected in laboratory aquaria and large holding tanks. However, other shrimp in the same samples have been found dying with no signs of patent *Baculovirus* infections. Fishery reports [10] indicate that unexplained fluctuations in pink shrimp abundance occur regularly in the northern Gulf of Mexico waters from which virus-infected shrimp have been taken. These fluctuations may be due to any number of causes, but certainly the shrimp virus may be considered as one of the candidates.

The second question is: Are there interactions between stress factors, such as chemical pollutants, and virus infections in shrimp? Further studies must be completed to answer this question. Tests completed to date suggest that the polychlorinated biphenyls may increase prevalence of patent virus infections in test shrimp, whereas other chemicals (methoxychlor) may not.[11] Interactions between natural pathogens and pollutant chemicals may become more apparent in aquatic animals as further studies are completed on chronically polluted estuaries and marine waters. The concept that pollutants act as stressors to lower natural resistance to disease should be explored further with such systems as the shrimp-virus.

The third question is: What are the risks, if any, of not better understanding host specificity in regard to developing viral groups, such as the *Baculovirus* group, for insecticidal uses? Though there appears to be little danger of artificially introducing insect viruses into nontarget species, this question may not have been answered satisfactorily at this time. The discovery of a *Baculovirus* in a marine crustacean suggests that host limitations for this virus group have not been determined absolutely.

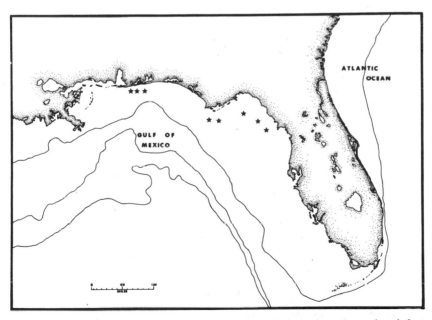

FIGURE 8. Chart that shows areas in northern Gulf of Mexico where virus-infected shrimp have been found; stars indicate approximate sites of collection.

SUMMARY

Pertinent questions must be answered concerning the significance of the discovery of a new *Baculovirus* enzootic in populations of penaeid shrimp in the northern Gulf of Mexico. The virus is rod shaped, both free and occluded in polyhedral inclusion bodies in the nuclei of host hepatopancreatic cells, and is associated with striking cytopathologic effects, but induces no specific gross signs. Samples of pink shrimp taken since 1971 have shown prevalences of from 0 to 50% (shrimp with patent infections/total number of shrimp in sample). The virus has been found in samples of shrimp taken from waters of Apalachee Bay, Port St. Joe, and Pensacola, all in Florida. Attempts to culture the shrimp virus in established insect cell lines are underway; therefore, not all of Koch's postulates have been satisfied for the virus. In the laboratory, virus prevalence in samples of shrimp has been increased by holding the shrimp in large numbers in small aquaria. The major questions that we are attempting to answer about the crustacean *Baculovirus* are:

What direct effect does the virus have on populations of shrimp in nature?

Do pollutant chemicals found in coastal waters enhance the virus effect in shrimp?

What relationship, if any, does the occurrence of a *Baculovirus* in a crustacean have with the development of insect baculoviruses as potential biopesticides?

Other important avenues of investigation have opened. The opportunity has appeared for virologists working with insect baculoviruses to compare these viruses with a *Baculovirus* from a noninsect host.

REFERENCES

1. WILDY, P. 1971. Classification and nomenclature of viruses. First report of the international committee on nomenclature of viruses. Mon. Virol. **5:** 1–81.
2. BERGHOLD, G. H. 1947. Die Isolierung des Polyeder-Virus und die Natur der Polyeder. Z. Naturforsch. **2b:** 122–143.
3. COUCH, J. A. 1974. Free and occluded virus, similar to Baculovirus, in hepatopancreas of pink shrimp. Nature (London) **247:** 229–231.
4. COUCH, J. A. 1974. An enzootic nuclear polyhedrosis virus of pink shrimp: ultrastructure, prevalence, and enhancement. J. Invert. Pathol. **24:** 311–331.
5. JAQUES, R. P. 1970. Application of viruses to soil and foliage for control of the cabbage looper and imported cabbage worm. J. Invert. Pathol. **15:** 328–340.
6. HALL, I. M. 1963. Microbial control. *In* Insect Pathology, An Advanced Treatise. E. A. Steinhaus, Ed. Vol. **2:** 477–517. Academic Press, Inc. New York, N.Y.
7. TANADA, Y. 1956. Microbial control of some lepidopterous pests of crucifers. J. Econ. Entomol. **49:** 320–329.
8. IGNOFFO, C. M. 1968. Specificity of insect viruses. Bull. Entomol. Soc. Amer. **14:** 265–276.
9. LIGHTNER, D. V., R. R. PROCTOR, A. K. SPARKS, J. R. ADAMS & A. M. HEIMPEL. 1973. Testing penaeid shrimp for susceptibility to an insect nuclear polyhedrosis virus. Environ. Entomol. **2:** 611–613.
10. ANONYMOUS. 1969. Gulf of Mexico shrimp atlas. Circular 312. U.S. Department of the Interior, Bureau of Commercial Fish.
11. COUCH, J. A. 1975. Attempts to increase *Baculovirus* prevalences in shrimp by chemical exposure. *In* Progress in Experimental Tumor Research. F. Homburger, Ed. Vol. 19. S. Karger. Geneva, Switzerland.

AFTER DINNER ADDRESS:
INVERTEBRATE PATHOLOGY IN THE INTERNATIONAL
UNION OF BIOLOGICAL SCIENCES

John D. Briggs

Department of Entomology
The Ohio State University
Columbus, Ohio 43210

The International Union of Biological Sciences (IUBS) has the following aims: to promote the study of biological sciences; to initiate, facilitate, and coordinate research and other scientific activities that demand international cooperation; to insure the discussion and dissemination of the results of co-operative research; and to promote the organization of international conferences and to assist in the publication of their reports.

The IUBS comprises several sections and commissions each of which is concerned with a particular discipline in the biological sciences. The sections and commissions are grouped into five divisions: botany, zoology, microbiology, functional and analytical biology, and environmental biology.

In 1973, the Committee on Admissions and Structure of the IUBS in the triennial General Assembly recommended and acted favorably on the establishment of a Commission on Invertebrate Pathology in the Division of Zoology. The recommendation was based on a petition submitted by the Society for Invertebrate Pathology. When the Commission was established in the Division of Zoology, it was suggested that at a later date, the Commission can petition the General Assembly to become an interdivisional commission affiliated also with the Division of Microbiology. Other interdisciplinary commissions are Biohistory, Biological Education, and Biometry. There are several multidisciplinary commissions in the IUBS, namely, the commissions for Culture Collections, Microbial Ecology, and Systematic and Evolutionary Biology. Serving the scientific community as the Commission on Invertebrate Zoology in the Division of Zoology, the Society for Invertebrate Pathology is one of 57 international scientific societies for various biological disciplines that act in the IUBS.

The IUBS is supported by adherent national governments through their academies of sciences or other relevent national organizations. For the United States, the National Research Council and the National Academy of Sciences, through the Division of Biological Sciences, convenes semiannually the United States Committee for the IUBS. In addition to individuals nominated by scientific societies to serve as voting members of the Committee, the Federation of American Societies for Experimental Biology (FASEB) and the American Institute of Biological Sciences (AIBS) each appoint a nonvoting observer to the Committee. Through these individuals in the United States National Committee, contact with the nations' representatives to the IUBS is maintained with the individual biologist. To date, approximately 40 countries are affiliated with the IUBS and support it through their contributions or dues. Additional sources of financial support for the IUBS are grants, and a regular contribution from the United Nations Education Scientific, and Cultural Organization (UNESCO), administered through the International Council of Scientific Unions (ICSU).

The publications of the IUBS are the reports of the General Assemblies, lectures given in the scientific program as a part of the General Assemblies, and the IUBS Newsletter. Information about these publications can be obtained from the permanent offices of the Secretariat in Paris, France.* In addition, a brochure that describes the function and composition of the IUBS is published in several languages.

The Society for Invertebrate Pathology, which serves as the Commission on Invertebrate Pathology in the IUBS, was organized in 1967. The Society's objects are to promote scientific knowledge about the diseases of invertebrate animals and related subjects through scientific meetings, symposia, discussions, reports and publications; to stimulate scientific investigations and their applications; to plan, organize, and administer projects for the advancement of knowledge in invertebrate pathology; to improve professional qualifications; and, especially, to promote international cooperation in achieving these objectives. The publications of the Society are the *Journal of Invertebrate Pathology* and the Society Newsletter. Current membership of the Society is more than 600 persons from approximately 40 nations.

In 1975–76, the plan for action in the Society for Invertebrate Pathology can be specified in five categories: the need for pathology of invertebrates to be included as a core emphasis in educational institutions, the instruction of which should include pathobiology or the biology of diseases; the development of bibliographic services for the infectious and noninfectious diseases of invertebrates; to collaborate with the IUBS Multidisciplinary Commission on Culture Collections for living and preserved collections, and the development of identification services for microorganisms that infect invertebrates; the development and implementation of procedures and methods for disease control or prevention in colonies of invertebrate animals; and to support activities for the biological and physical characterization of microorganisms that affect invertebrates, with an objective to recognize possible hazards of pathogens of invertebrates to nontarget organisms, for example, where pathogens may be employed for regulation of invertebrate populations.

Acting within the framework of the IUBS is a significant responsibility for invertebrate pathology. The IUBS is a nongovernmental organization affiliated with the specialized agencies of the United Nations. For example, serving as a nongovernmental organization to the World Health Organization provides the opportunity for the Commission on Invertebrate Pathology through the IUBS to introduce agenda items for consideration of the World Health Assembly.

In the triennium before the last General Assembly, 1973, the IUBS made loans for the organization of 11 international congresses and received applications for grants to the organizers of more than 20 symposia. It is expected that the loans can be repaid with income from the registration charges paid by the participants. The small grants to assist the organizers of symposia are part of the services provided by the IUBS out of income from the contributions of adhering nations. The Executive Committee of the IUBS, which meets annually, most recently in October 1974 at Paris, approved loans to four international congresses and grants to eight symposia in 1975 and 1976.

The Executive Committee of the IUBS has reaffirmed the role of the IUBS in promoting interdisciplinary communication between divergent branches of

---

* Dr. P. H. Bonnell, M.D., Executive Secretary, International Union of Biological Sciences, 51 Boulevard de Montmorency, Paris 75016, France.

the biological sciences. It is vital that each section and commission within the IUBS give consideration to the interests that they share with other groups of biologists and to seek the possibility of joint meetings at which ideas and information can be freely exchanged. Petitions for support are encouraged for participation in conferences by scientists from developing countries and young scientists who would otherwise not be able to attend. Furthermore, consideration should be given to organize conferences in developing countries.

The IUBS is one union in the International Council of Scientific Unions (ICSU). Support for the IUBS comes in part from the United Nations through UNESCO and the ICSU, and consequently there is concern for the equitable investment of funds for international conferences. One welcome element for the success of international conferences is a resolution passed by the ICSU at a recent General Assembly meeting. This resolution concerns the free circulation of scientists in the world. The resolution draws attention to the following: ". . . an assurance in writing should be obtained from the organizers of conferences who are seeking support from a scientific union, e.g. IUBS, that the country considered for a meeting site will grant the visas to bona fide scientists if proper applications are made;" and ". . . that applications for visas where necessary should be made to the appropriate authorities three months before the date of the meeting, and if these visas are not granted or promised in writing one month before the date of the event, sponsorship by the Union concerned should be withdrawn, and that arrangements for future meetings in any country found unable to comply with these principles should be suspended until more satisfactory circumstances exist."

The results of the General Assemblies, which are held triennually, and annual Executive Committee meetings are seen in the reports of committees presented to these bodies and in the publications of the IUBS. Resolutions introduced by delegates are considered by the Assembly as expressions of needs and concerns in the biological sciences internationally. Resolutions passed by the assemblies of the IUBS should be interpreted as active encouragement for legislative groups and advice to the scientific leadership in the nations associated with the IUBS. Continuity of service by the IUBS to human affairs is exemplified in scientific nomenclature, which is a high-priority activity for the Union. Within the framework of the IUBS, the most important international services are still considered to be nomenclature, for example, for plants, cultivated plants, animals, bacteria, and viruses. The respective international committees on nomenclature receive IUBS support, and necessary bibliographic services for nomenclature are operated under the auspices of the IUBS.

The Commission on Invertebrate Pathology is moving through the existing avenues of the Society of Invertebrate Pathology to support the information systems under development for viruses that affect invertebrates and for the bibliography of spore-forming protozoa Order Microsporida that affect invertebrate and vertebrate animals. One important element that will serve all interests in the pathology of invertebrates is the development of a glossary for invertebrate pathology. The document is to be published with the editorial guidance of a permanent committee appointed by the Editorial Board of the Society for Invertebrate Pathology. The glossary will be developed upon the model provided by *An Abridged Glossary of Terms Used in Invertebrate Pathology*, Second Edition, Pacific Northwest Forest and Range Experiment Station, U.S. Department of Agriculture, Forest Service.

The question "What can go wrong with an invertebrate?" is the focus of attention for biological interests throughout the world. The health of micro-scopic invertebrates in food chains, the well being of invertebrates as sources of proteins for humans, the control of damaging invertebrates with microorga-nisms, and the accurate determination of causes for death of invertebrates are among the international concerns of invertebrate pathologists.

The Commission on Invertebrate Pathology in the IUBS is an additional voice and avenue for action in these matters and others that concern inverte-brates and their pathologies. The Commission may be utilized through the offices of the Society for Invertebrate Pathology or the Secretariat of the IUBS.